# Delivering Health Care in America

## A Systems Approach

### FIFTH EDITION

**Leiyu Shi, DrPH, MBA, MPA**

Professor, Johns Hopkins School of Public Health

Director, Johns Hopkins Primary Care Policy Center for the Underserved

Johns Hopkins University

Baltimore, Maryland

**Douglas A. Singh, PhD, MBA**

Associate Professor, School of Business and Economics

Indiana University South Bend

South Bend, Indiana

JONES & BARTLETT
LEARNING

*World Headquarters*
Jones & Bartlett Learning
5 Wall Street
Burlington, MA 01803
978-443-5000
info@jblearning.com
www.jblearning.com

Jones & Bartlett Learning Canada
6339 Ormindale Way
Mississauga, Ontario L5V 1J2
Canada

Jones & Bartlett Learning International
Barb House, Barb Mews
London W6 7PA
United Kingdom

Jones & Bartlett Learning books and products are available through most bookstores and online booksellers. To contact Jones & Bartlett Learning directly, call 800-832-0034, fax 978-443-8000, or visit our website, www.jblearning.com.

Substantial discounts on bulk quantities of Jones & Bartlett Learning publications are available to corporations, professional associations, and other qualified organizations. For details and specific discount information, contact the special sales department at Jones & Bartlett Learning via the above contact information or send an email to specialsales@jblearning.com.

**Production Credits**
Publisher: Michael Brown
Editorial Assistant: Teresa Reilly
Associate Editor: Maro Gartside
Production Manager: Tracey McCrea
Senior Marketing Manager: Sophie Fleck
Marketing Manager: Grace Richards
Composition: Cenveo Publishing Services
Cover Design: Kate Ternullo
Title Page Image: © Photodisc/Getty Images/Brand X
Cover Image: © Konstantin L/ShutterStock, Inc.
Printing and Binding: Malloy, Inc.
Cover Printing: Malloy, Inc.

**Library of Congress Cataloging-in-Publication Data**
Shi, Leiyu.
  Delivering health care in America : a systems approach / Leiyu Shi, Douglas A. Singh.—5th ed.
    p. ; cm.
  Includes bibliographical references and index.
  ISBN-13: 978-1-4496-2650-1 (pbk.)
  ISBN-10: 1-4496-2650-5 (pbk.)
  1. Medical care—United States. 2. Medical policy—United States. I. Singh, Douglas A., 1946- II. Title.
  [DNLM: 1. Delivery of Health Care—United States. 2. Health Policy—United States. W 84 AA1]
  RA395.A3S485 2012
  362.10973—dc23
                                                                    2011018470

6048
Printed in the United States of America
16 15 14 13 12   10 9 8 7 6 5 4 3

# Contents

**PART V    System Outlook**

# Preface

The Patient Protection and Affordable Care Act (ACA) of 2010 has taken center stage because of its promise to push the American health care system further into the public domain. Signed into law on March 23, 2010 by President Barack Obama, the ACA of 2010 represents the most sweeping commitment of federal and state tax dollars since the creation of the Medicare and Medicaid programs in 1965. Also unique in the history of American health policy making is the manner in which the "Health Care Reform Bill," as it was generally called, was passed by a Democratic majority in Congress without a single Republican vote. Moreover, the American people were not informed of the plan's details. It is quite revealing that one of the chief architects of the bill, Nancy Pelosi, then majority leader in the House of Representatives, stated in a televised speech that the bill had to be passed so the American people could discover what was in it.

Seen as ironic by many, the major provisions of the law are not scheduled to take effect until 2014. In the meantime, the midterm election held in 2010 has changed the political landscape by giving Republicans the majority in the House of Representatives. Another major election, including the one for the presidency, is scheduled for 2012. In the meantime, over one-half of the US states have joined in lawsuits to overturn the ACA of 2010, referred to as ObamaCare by its critics. In December 2010, a federal court in Virginia ruled part of the ACA to be unconstitutional. Just over one month later, in January 2011, the US District Court in Florida declared the entire law to be unconstitutional. Not surprising, about one-half of the American public is also opposed to this law as being too far-reaching and too costly. In the past, incrementalism has been the favored American approach to reform the US health care system. Hence, the ACA of 2010 has opened the proverbial Pandora's box and has aroused public sentiment against a government that is perceived as becoming too large and intrusive. As expected, the Obama Administration has filed legal appeals to have the court decisions rendered in Virginia and Florida overturned by higher courts.

Apart from the legal challenges, the Republicans, who gained control of the House, threatened other measures, such as defunding the ACA's implementation. No doubt, there will be plenty of political fodder to fuel American passions during the 2012 election, which will also have major implications for the future of US health care. Regardless of the ACA's final fate, however, the door for health reform has been opened. Assuming that the ACA becomes unimplementable, forces have been set in motion to make at least some headway toward enabling the uninsured to obtain health insurance.

Conversely, nagging questions remain. Having health insurance (i.e., coverage) and obtaining health care when needed (i.e., access) are two different things. The latter requires an adequate capacity to deliver care when health insurance is extended to millions of additional people. It is uncontested that the United States lacks the capacity to deliver primary care. Retirement of the baby boomers between 2011 and 2030 is another worrisome aspect facing future generations. A true reform of the health care system must address other serious questions: (1) How will a health care system that is lopsided in its focus on medical specialization deal with a mushrooming sector of the population in which the prevention and management of chronic conditions will be of primary importance? (2) How will the nation deal with the impending shortage of qualified workers in just about every area of health care delivery? (3) What can be done to finance long-term care services that over 20% of the US population will start utilizing around 2020 and beyond? (4) Will the nation be able to afford the ongoing development and use of costly new medical technology that may deliver fewer health benefits in relation to its costs? (5) How will a heavily indebted nation deal with the increasing costs of health care?

Other developed nations also face similar dilemmas. Cost control, individual responsibility by following healthy lifestyles and judicious use of health care resources, emphasis on basic health care, and value for the dollar spent should receive much greater emphasis than they have in the past.

Although this book is primarily focused on health care delivery in the United States, the nation is not isolated from global events and the underdeveloped state of health care delivery in poorer countries. The spread of deadly infections does not recognize national borders; natural disasters appear to be taking a toll on human life and health, with greater frequency and severity without warning; and man-made disasters brought on by terrorist activities can happen anywhere and anytime. Dealing with these threats requires international assistance, cooperation, and joint effort. Hence, public health has taken on a new meaning, both in its extent and scope. Without the involvement of public health, any humanitarian efforts remain incomplete.

## New to This Edition

This fifth edition has undergone some major revisions, while maintaining its basic structure and layout that, for almost 15 years, has served quite well in helping readers both at home and overseas understand the complexities of the US health care delivery system. The main thrust of the revisions was to put American health care delivery in the context of current developments in health reform, even though some details will likely change as this major theme continues to evolve. Hence, references to specific provisions of the ACA of 2010 are made in almost all chapters.

As in the past, this edition has been updated throughout with the latest pertinent data, trends, and research findings available at the time the manuscript was prepared. Copious illustrations in the form of examples, facts, figures, tables, and exhibits continue to make the text come alive. Some of the main additions to the text include health care reform in several other countries (Chapter 1); important conceptual frameworks of health determinants and current information on

*Healthy People 2020* (Chapter 2); an overview of the mental asylum in its historical context and the transition to community mental health services (Chapter 3); updates on major issues in health care workforce (Chapter 4); high-deductible health plans; the state of employment-based health insurance; the status of Medicare Hospital Insurance and Supplemental Medical Insurance trust funds; a tabulated summary of the main insurance provisions of the ACA of 2010 (Chapter 6); measurement of and value of primary care; models of patient-centered care; and developments in home health care, community health centers, and alternative medicine (Chapter 7); controversies surrounding physician-owned specialty hospitals; the Magnet Recognition Program® of the American Nurses Credentialing Center (Chapter 8); quality assessment in managed care; accountable care organizations (Chapter 9); updates on racial/ethnic minorities and vulnerable populations (Chapter 11); updates on clinical practice guidelines; CMS's quality initiatives and quality report cards; and state reporting of quality indicators (Chapter 12); and perspectives on the politics of health reform (Chapter 13). To place potential developments in their current context, Chapter 14 has been rewritten almost in its entirety. The chapter begins with a framework that helps understand major forces of change. It discusses the precedents for the ACA of 2010 and evaluates the future of health reform in the context of major constraints. The chapter also explores strategies for implementing emerging models of medical home, community-oriented primary care, and patient-centered care; the skills necessary to prepare the future workforce; challenges in long-term care; innovations

in technology; international issues; and the emerging role of comparative effectiveness research.

Aside from the changes, the book retains the original systems framework to discuss the components of US health care delivery. It also retains the original 14 chapters as major themes following the systems model. Our aim in this textbook is to continue to meet the needs of both graduate and undergraduate students. We have attempted to make each chapter complete without making it overwhelming for beginners. Instructors, of course, will choose the sections they decide are most appropriate for their courses.

As in the past, we invite comments from our readers. Communications can be directed to either or both authors:

Leiyu Shi
Department of Health Policy and
    Management
Bloomburg School of Public Health
Johns Hopkins University
624 North Broadway, Room 409
Baltimore, MD 21205-1996
lshi@jhsph.edu

Douglas A. Singh
School of Business and Economics
Indiana University-South Bend
Wiekamp Hall, Room 2259
1800 Mishawaka Avenue
P.O. Box 7111
South Bend, IN 46634-7111
dsingh@iusb.edu

We appreciate the work of Eunhee Grace Cho and Normalie Barton in providing invaluable assistance in the preparation of selected chapters of this book.

# List of Exhibits

# List of Figures

# List of Tables

# List of Abbreviations/Acronyms

## A

AAA—Area Agencies on Aging

AALL—American Association of Labor Legislation

AAMC—Association of American Medical Colleges

AA/PIs—Asian American and Pacific Islanders

AAs—Asian Americans

ACA—Patient Protection and Affordable Care Act

ACNM—American College of Nurse-Midwives

ACPE—American Council on Pharmaceutical Education

ACS—American College of Surgeons

ADA—American Dental Association

ADA—Americans with Disabilities Act

ADC—adult day care

ADE—adverse drug events

ADL—activities of daily living

ADN—associate's degree nurse

AFC—adult foster care

AFDC—Aid to Families with Dependent Children

AHA—American Hospital Association

AHRQ—Agency for Healthcare Research and Quality

AIDS—acquired immune deficiency syndrome

ALF—assisted living facility

ALOS—average length of stay

AMA—American Medical Association

amfAR—Foundation for AIDS Research

ANA—American Nurses Association

APCs—ambulatory payment classifications

APN—advanced practice nurse

ARRA—American Recovery and Reinvestment Act

ASPR—Assistant Secretary for Preparedness

AZT—zidovudine

## B

BBA—Balanced Budget Act of 1997

BPHC—Bureau of Primary Health Care

BSN—baccalaureate degree nurse

BWC—Biological Weapons Convention

## C

CAH—critical access hospital

CAM—complementary and alternative medicine

CARE Act—Comprehensive AIDS Resources Emergency Act

CAT—computerized axial tomography

CBO—Congressional Budget Office

CCIP—Chronic Care Improvement Program

CCRC—continuing care retirement community

CDC—Centers for Disease Control and Prevention

CEO—chief executive officer

CEPH—Council on Education for Public Health
CF—conversion factor
CHAMPUS—TriCare program
CHAMPVA—Civilian Health and Medical Program of the Department of Veterans Affairs
CHC—community health center
CIA—Central Intelligence Agency
CLASS—Community Living Assistance Services and Support
CMGs—case-mix groups
C/MHCs—Community and Migrant Health Centers
CMS—Centers for Medicare & Medicaid Services
CNA—certified nursing assistant
CNM—certified nurse-midwife
CNSs—clinical nurse specialists
COBRA—Consolidated Omnibus Budget Reconciliation Act of 1985
COGME—Council on Graduate Medical Education
CON—certificate-of-need
COPC—community-oriented primary care
COPD—chronic obstructive pulmonary disease
COTA—certified occupational therapy assistant
COTH—Council of Teaching Hospitals and Health Systems
CPI—consumer price index
CPOE—computerized physician order entry
CPT—current procedural terminology
CQI—continuous quality improvement
CRNA—certified registered nurse anesthetist
CT—computed tomography
CVA—cardiovascular accident

**D**

DC—doctor of chiropractic
DD—developmentally disabled
DDS—Doctor of Dental Surgery

DHHS—Department of Health and Human Services
DHS—Department of Homeland Security
DMD—doctor of dental medicine
DME—durable medical equipment
DoD—Department of Defense
DOs—doctors of osteopathy
DPCs—diagnosis-procedure combinations
DPM—doctor of podiatric medicine
DRA—Deficit Reduction Act of 2005
DRGs—diagnostic-related groups
DSM-IV—Diagnostic and Statistical Manual of Mental Disorders
DTP—diphtheria-tetanus-pertussis

**E**

EBM—evidence-based medicine
EBRI—Employee Benefit Research Institute
ECG—electrocardiogram
ECU—extended care unit
ED—emergency department
EEG—electroencephalogram
EHRs—electronic health records
EIAs—enzyme immunoassays
ELISA—enzyme-linked immunosorbent assay
EMT—emergency medical technician
EMTALA—Emergency Medical Treatment and Labor Act
ENP—elderly nutrition program
EPA—Environmental Protection Agency
EPO—exclusive provider organization
EPSDT—Early Periodic Screening, Diagnosis, and Treatment program
ERISA—Employee Retirement Income Security Act
ESP—Economic Stabilization Program
ESRD—end-stage renal disease
EUA—emergency use authorization

**F**

FBI—Federal Bureau of Investigation
FD&C—Federal Food, Drug, and Cosmetic Act

FDA—Food and Drug Administration
FIW—Federal Interagency Workgroup
FMAP—Federal Medical Assistance
    Percentage
FQHC—Federally Qualified Health Center
FTE—full-time equivalent
FY—fiscal year

**G**

GAO—General Accounting Office
GAT—genome amplification testing
GATS—General Agreement on Trade in
    Services
GDP—gross domestic product
GOAL—National Preparedness Goal
GPs—general practitioners

**H**

HAART—highly active antiretroviral
    therapy
HCBS—home and community based
    services
HCBW—home and community based
    waiver
HCFA—Health Care Financing
    Administration
HCH—Health Care for the Homeless
HCPP—Health Care Prepayment Plan
HDHP—high-deductible health plan
HEDIS—Health Plan Employer Data and
    Information Set
HHCS—Home and Hospice Care Survey
HHRG—home health resource group
HI—hospital insurance
HIAA—Health Insurance Association of
    America
Hib—Haemophilus influenzae B
HIPAA—Health Insurance Portability and
    Accountability Act
HIT—health information technology
HIV—human immunodeficiency virus
HMO—health maintenance organization
HMO Act—Health Maintenance
    Organization Act

HPSAs—Health Professional Shortage
    Areas
HPV—human papillomavirus
HRQL—health-related quality of life
HRSA—Health Resources and Services
    Administration
HSAs—health savings accounts
HSAs—health system agencies
HSEES—hazardous substances emergency
    event surveillance system
HSIs—Health Status Indicators
HTA—health technology assessment
HUD—Department of Housing and Urban
    Development

**I**

IADL—instrumental activities of daily
    living
ICD-9—International Classification of
    Diseases, version 9
ICDs—implantable cardioverter
    defibrillators
ICF—intermediate care facility
ICF/MR—intermediate care facilities for
    mentally retarded
ICSI IVF—intracytoplasmic sperm
    injection in vitro fertilization
IDEA—Individuals with Disabilities
    Education Act
IDS—integrated delivery systems
IDU—injection drug use
IFA—immunofluorescence assay
IHR—International Health Regulations
IHS—Indian Health Service
IMGs—international medical graduates
INS—Immigration and Naturalization
    Service
IOM—Institute of Medicine
IPA—independent practice
    association
IRB—Institutional Review Board
IRF—inpatient rehabilitation facility
IS—information systems
IT—information technology

IUDs—intrauterine devices
IV—intravenous

**J**
JCAHO—Joint Commission on Accreditation of Healthcare Organizations

**L**
LPN—licensed practical nurse
LTC—long-term care
LTCH—long-term care hospital
LVN—licensed vocational nurse

**M**
MAC—mycobacterium avium complex
MA-SNP—Medicare Advantage Special Needs Program
MBA—master of business administration
MCOs—managed care organizations
MDs—doctors of medicine
MDS—minimum data set
MedPAC—Medicare Payment Advisory Commission
MEPS—Medical Expenditure Panel Survey
MFS—Medicare Fee Schedule
MHA—master of health administration
MHPs—multiskilled health practitioners
MHPH—1996 Mental Health Policy Act
MHS—multihospital system
MHSA—master of health services administration
MHSS—Military Health Services System
MIPPA—Medicare Improvements for Patients and Providers Act of 2008
MLP—midlevel provider
MLR—medical loss ratio
MMA—Medicare Prescription Drug, Improvement, and Modernization Act
MMR—measles-mumps-rubella vaccine
MPA—master of public administration/affairs
MPFS—Medicare Physician Fee Schedule

MPH—master of public health
MPPRP—Medicare's Physician Payment Reform Program
MR/DD—mentally retarded, developmentally disabled persons
MRHFP—Medicare Rural Hospital Flexibility Program
MRI—magnetic resonance imaging
MSA—medical savings account
MSA—metropolitan statistical area
MSO—management services organization
MTFs—medical treatment facilities
MUAs—medically underserved areas

**N**
NAB—National Association of Boards of Examiners of Long-Term Care Administrators
NADSA—National Adult Day Services Association
NAPBC—National Action Plan on Breast Cancer
NASA—National Aeronautic and Space Administration
NAT—nucleic acid testing
NCCAM—National Center for Complementary and Alternative Medicine
NCHS—National Center for Health Statistics
NCMS—New Cooperative Medical Scheme
NCQA—National Committee for Quality Assurance
NF—nursing facility
NGC—National Guideline Clearinghouse
NHC—neighborhood health center
NHE—national health expenditures
NHHRC—National Health and Hospitals Reform Commission
NHI—national health insurance
NHS—British National Health Service
NHSC—National Health Service Corps
NHSS—National Health Security Strategy

NIAAA—National Institute of Alcohol Abuse and Alcoholism
NICE—National Institute for Health and Clinical Excellence
NIDA—National Institute on Drug Abuse
NIH—National Institutes of Health
NIMH—National Institute of Mental Health
NIMS—National Incident Management System
NP—nurse practitioner
NPC—nonphysician clinician
NPP—nonphysician practitioner
NRA—Nurse Reinvestment Act of 2002
NRP— National Response Plan

**O**

OAM—Office of Alternative Medicine
OBRA-87—Omnibus Budget Reconciliation Act of 1987
OBRA-89—Omnibus Budget Reconciliation Act of 1989
OBRA-93—Omnibus Budget Reconciliation Act of 1993
OD—doctor of optometry
OI—opportunistic infections
OMB—Office of Management and Budget
OPPS—Outpatient Prospective Payment System
OSHA—Occupational Safety and Health Administration
OT—occupational therapist
OWH—Office on Women's Health

**P**

P4P—pay-for-performance
PA—physician assistant
PACE—Program of All-Inclusive Care for the Elderly
PAHP—Pandemic and All-Hazards Preparedness Act
PASRR—Preadmission Screening and Resident Review

PCCM—primary care case management
PCGs—primary care groups
PCIP—Pre-Existing Condition Insurance Plan
PCM—primary care manager
PCP—pneumocystis carinii
PCP—primary care physician
PCT—primary care trust
PEPFAR—President's Emergency Plan for AIDS Relief
PERS—personal emergency response systems
PET—positron emission tomography
PFFS—private fee-for-service
PharmD—doctor of pharmacy
PhD—doctor of philosophy
PHE—public health emergency
PHI—personal health information
PHO—physician-hospital organization
PhRMA—Pharmaceutical Research and Manufacturers of America
PHS—public health service
PL 107-205—Nurse Reinvestment Act of 2002
PMPM—payment per member per month
PORTS—patient outcomes research teams
POS—point-of-service plan
PPD—per-patient day rate
PPM—physician practice management
PPOs—preferred provider organizations
PPS—prospective payment system
PROs—peer review organizations
PRWORA—Personal Responsibility and Work Opportunity Reconciliation Act
PSO—provider-sponsored organization
PSROs—professional standards review organizations
PsyD—doctor of psychology
PTA—physical therapy assistant
PTCA—percutaneous transluminal coronary angioplasty
PTs—physical therapists

**Q**

QALY—quality-adjusted life year
QDWI—Qualified Disabled and Working
    Individual Program
QI—qualified individual program
QIOs—Quality improvement organizations
QMB—Qualified Medicare Beneficiary
    program

**R**

R&D—research and development
RAI—resident assessment instrument
RBRVS—resource-based relative value
    scales
RFID—radio frequency identification
RICs—rehabilitation impairment categories
RN—registered nurse
RUG-III—Resource Utilization Groups,
    version 3
RUGs—resource utilization groups
RVUs—relative value units
RWJF—Robert Wood Johnson Foundation

**S**

SAMHSA—Substance Abuse and Mental
    Health Services Administration
SARS—severe acute respiratory syndrome
SAV—small area variations
SCHIP—State Children's Health Insurance
    Program
SCN—Sentinel Centers Network
SES—socioeconomic status
SHI—socialized health insurance
S/HMO—social health maintenance
    organization
SIPP—Survey of Income and Program
    Participation
SLMB—specified low-income Medicare
    beneficiary
SMI—supplementary medical insurance

SNF—skilled nursing facility
SNS—Strategic National Stockpile
SPECT—single-photon emission
    computed tomography
SROs—single-room occupancy units
SSI—Supplemental Security Income
STDs—sexually transmitted diseases

**T**

TAH—total artificial heart
TANF—Temporary Assistance for Needy
    Families
TCU—transitional care unit
TEFRA—Tax Equity and Fiscal
    Responsibility Act
TFL—TriCare for Life
TPA—third-party administrator
TQM—total quality management

**U**

UCR—usual, customary, and
    reasonable
UR—utilization review

**V**

VA—Department of Veterans Affairs
VERA—Veterans Equitable Resource
    Allocation
VHA—Veterans Health Administration
VISN—Veterans Integrated Service
    Network
VNA—Visiting Nurses Association
VPS—volume performance standard

**W**

WHO—World Health Organization
WHOCSDH—WHO Commission on
    Social Determinants of Health
WIC—Women, Infants, and Children

# Chapter 1

# A Distinctive System of Health Care Delivery

## Learning Objectives

- To understand the basic nature of the US health care system
- To outline the four key functional components of a health care delivery system
- To discuss the primary characteristics of the US health care system from a free market perspective
- To emphasize why it is important for health care managers to understand the intricacies of the health care delivery system
- To get an overview of the health care systems in other countries
- To introduce the systems model as a framework for studying the health services system in the US

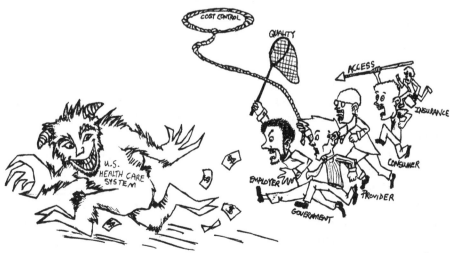

*The US health care delivery system is a behemoth that is almost impossible for any single entity to manage and control.*

## Introduction

The United States has a unique system of health care delivery unlike any other health care system in the world. Most developed countries have national health insurance programs run by the government and financed through general taxes. Almost all citizens in such countries are entitled to receive health care services, depending on the system's capacity to deliver needed services. Such is not yet the case in the United States, where not all Americans are automatically covered by health insurance.

The US health care delivery system is really not a system in its true sense, even though it is called a system when reference is made to its various features, components, and services. Hence, it may be somewhat misleading to talk about the American health care delivery "system" because a true system does not exist (Wolinsky 1988). One main feature of the US health care system is that it is fragmented because different people obtain health care through different means. The delivery system has continued to undergo periodic changes, mainly in response to concerns regarding cost, access, and quality.

Describing health care delivery in the United States can be a daunting task. To facilitate an understanding of the structural and conceptual basis for the delivery of health services, this book is organized according to a systems framework presented at the end of this chapter. Also, the mechanisms of health services delivery in the United States are collectively referred to as a system throughout this book.

The main objective of this chapter is to provide a broad understanding of how health care is delivered in the United States. The overview presented here introduces the reader to several concepts treated more extensively in later chapters.

## An Overview of the Scope and Size of the System

Table 1–1 demonstrates the complexity of health care delivery in the United States. Many organizations and individuals are involved in health care, ranging from educational and research institutions, medical suppliers, insurers, payers, and claims processors to health care providers. Multitudes of providers are involved in the delivery of preventive, primary, subacute, acute, auxiliary, rehabilitative, and continuing care. An increasing number of managed care organizations (MCOs) and integrated networks now provide a continuum of care, covering many of the service components.

The US health care delivery system is massive, with total employment in various health delivery settings over 16 million in 2009. This included over 822,000 professionally active doctors of medicine (MDs), 70,480 osteopathic physicians (DOs), and 2.5 million active nurses (US Census Bureau 2011). The vast number of health care and health services professionals (5.8 million) work in ambulatory health service settings, such as the offices of physicians, dentists, and other health practitioners, medical and diagnostic laboratories, and home health care service locations (US Census Bureau 2011). This is followed by hospitals (4.7 million) and nursing and residential care facilities (3.1 million) (US Census Bureau 2011). The vast array of health care institutions includes 5,815 hospitals, 15,730 nursing homes, and 13,513 substance abuse treatment facilities (US Census Bureau 2011).

Table 1–1  The Complexity of Health Care Delivery

| Education/ Research | Suppliers | Insurers | Providers | Payers | Government |
|---|---|---|---|---|---|
| Medical schools | Pharmaceutical companies | Managed care plans | **Preventive Care** | Blue Cross/ Blue Shield plans | Public insurance financing |
| Dental schools | Multipurpose suppliers | Blue Cross/ Blue Shield plans | Health departments | Commercial insurers | Health regulations |
| Nursing programs | Biotechnology companies | Commercial insurers | **Primary Care** | Employers | Health policy |
| Physician assistant programs | | Self-insured employers | Physician offices | Third-party administrators | Research funding |
| Nurse practitioner programs | | Medicare | Community health centers | State agencies | Public health |
| Physical therapy, occupational therapy, speech therapy programs | | Medicaid | Dentists | | |
| | | VA | Nonphysician providers | | |
| Research organizations | | Tricare | **Subacute Care** | | |
| Private foundations | | | Subacute care facilities | | |
| US Public Health Service (AHRQ, ATSDR, CDC, FDA, HRSA, IHS, NIH, SAMHSA) | | | Ambulatory surgery centers | | |
| | | | **Acute Care** | | |
| | | | Hospitals | | |
| Professional associations | | | **Auxiliary Services** | | |
| Trade associations | | | Pharmacists | | |
| | | | Diagnostic clinics | | |
| | | | X-ray units | | |
| | | | Suppliers of medical equipment | | |
| | | | **Rehabilitative Services** | | |
| | | | Home health agencies | | |
| | | | Rehabilitation centers | | |
| | | | Skilled nursing facilities | | |
| | | | **Continuing Care** | | |
| | | | Nursing homes | | |
| | | | **End-of-Life Care** | | |
| | | | Hospices | | |
| | | | **Integrated** | | |
| | | | Managed care organizations | | |
| | | | Integrated networks | | |

In 2009, 1,131 federally qualified health center grantees, with 123,012 full-time employees, provided preventive and primary care services to approximately 18.8 million people living in medically underserved, rural and urban areas (HRSA 2011). Various types of health care professionals are trained in 159 medical and osteopathic schools, 61 dental schools, over 100 schools of pharmacy, and more than 1,500 nursing programs located throughout the country (US Bureau of Labor Statistics 2011). In 2008, there were 200.9 million Americans with private health insurance coverage, 43 million Medicare beneficiaries, and 42.6 million Medicaid recipients, but 46.3 million people (15.4%) remained without any health insurance (US Census Bureau 2011). Multitudes of government agencies are involved with the financing of health care, medical and health services research, and regulatory oversight of the various aspects of the health care delivery system.

## A Broad Description of the System

US health care does not function as a rational and integrated network of components designed to work together coherently. To the contrary, it is a kaleidoscope of financing, insurance, delivery, and payment mechanisms that remain loosely coordinated. Each of these basic functional components—financing, insurance, delivery, and payment—represents an amalgam of public (government) and private sources. Thus, government-run programs finance and insure health care for select groups of people who meet each program's prescribed criteria for eligibility. To a lesser degree, government programs also deliver certain health care services directly to recipients, such as veterans, military

personnel, and the uninsured who may depend on city and county hospitals or limited services offered by public health clinics. However, the financing, insurance, payment, and delivery functions are largely in private hands.

The market-oriented economy in the United States attracts a variety of private entrepreneurs driven by the pursuit of profits obtained by carrying out the key functions of health care delivery. Employers purchase health insurance for their employees through private sources, and employees receive health care services delivered by the private sector. The government finances public insurance through Medicare, Medicaid, and the Children's Health Insurance Program (CHIP) for a significant portion of the very low-income, elderly, disabled, and pediatric populations. However, insurance arrangements for many publicly insured people are made through private entities, such as HMOs, and health care services are rendered by private physicians and hospitals. The blend of public and private involvement in the delivery of health care has resulted in:

- a multiplicity of financial arrangements that enable individuals to pay for health care services;

- numerous insurance agencies or MCOs that employ varied mechanisms for insuring against risk;

- multiple payers that make their own determinations regarding how much to pay for each type of service;

- a large array of settings where medical services are delivered; and

- numerous consulting firms offering expertise in planning, cost containment, quality, and restructuring of resources.

There is little standardization in a system that is functionally fragmented, and the various system components fit together only loosely. Such a system is not subject to overall planning, direction, and coordination from a central agency, such as the government. Duplication, overlap, inadequacy, inconsistency, and waste exist, leading to complexity and inefficiency, due to the missing dimension of system-wide planning, direction, and coordination. The system does not lend itself to standard budgetary methods of cost control. Each individual and corporate entity within a predominantly private entrepreneurial system seeks to manipulate financial incentives to its own advantage, without regard to its impact on the system as a whole. Hence, cost containment remains an elusive goal. In short, the US health care delivery system is like a behemoth or an economic megalith that is almost impossible for any single entity to manage or control. The US economy is the largest in the world, and, compared to other nations, consumption of health care services in the United States represents a greater proportion of the country's total economic output. Although the system can be credited for delivering some of the best clinical care in the world, it falls short of delivering equitable services to every American.

An acceptable health care delivery system should have two primary objectives: (1) it must enable all citizens to obtain health care services when needed, and (2) the services must be cost effective and meet certain established standards of quality. On one hand, the US health care delivery system falls short of both these ideals. On the other hand, however, certain features of US health care are the envy of the world. The United States leads the world in the latest and the best in medical technology,

training, and research. It offers some of the most sophisticated institutions, products, and processes of health care delivery. These achievements are indeed admirable, but much more remains unaccomplished.

## Basic Components of a Health Services Delivery System

Figure 1–1 illustrates that a health care delivery system incorporates four functional components—financing, insurance, delivery, and payment—necessary for the delivery of health services. The four functional components make up the *quad-function model*. Health care delivery systems differ depending on the arrangement of these components. The four functions generally overlap, but the degree of overlap varies between a private and a government-run system and between a traditional health insurance and managed care-based system. In a government-run system, the functions are more closely integrated and may be indistinguishable. Managed care arrangements also integrate the four functions to varying degrees.

### Financing

Financing is necessary to obtain health insurance or to pay for health care services. For most privately insured Americans, health insurance is employer-based; that is, their employers finance health care as a fringe benefit. A dependent spouse or children may also be covered by the working spouse's or working parent's employer. Most employers purchase health insurance for their employees through an MCO or an insurance company selected by the employer. Small employers may or may not be in a

Figure 1–1  Basic Health Care Delivery Functions.

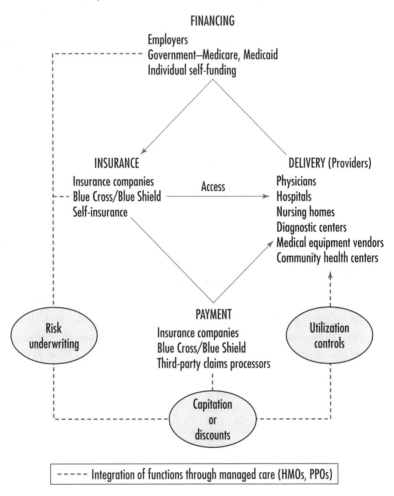

position to afford health insurance coverage for their employees.

## Insurance

Insurance protects the insured against catastrophic risks when needing expensive health care services. The insurance function also determines the package of health services the insured individual is entitled to receive. It specifies how and where health care services may be received. The MCO or insurance company also functions as a claims processor and manages the disbursement of funds to the health care providers.

## Delivery

The term delivery refers to the provision of health care services by various providers. The term *provider* refers to any entity that delivers health care services and can either independently bill for those services or is tax supported. Common examples of providers include physicians, dentists, optometrists, and therapists in private practices, hospitals, and diagnostic and imaging clinics, and suppliers of medical equipment (e.g., wheelchairs, walkers, ostomy supplies, oxygen). With few exceptions, most providers render services to people who have health insurance.

## Payment

The payment function deals with *reimbursement* to providers for services delivered. The insurer determines how much is paid for a certain service. Funds for actual disbursement come from the premiums paid to the MCO or insurance company. The patient is usually required, at the time of service, to pay a small out-of-pocket amount, such as $25 or $30, to see a physician. The remainder is covered by the MCO or insurance company. In government insurance plans, such as Medicare and Medicaid, tax revenues are used to pay providers.

## Uninsured Americans

The United States has a significant number of *uninsured*—those without private or public health insurance coverage. A March 2009 report from Families USA found that 86.7 million, or 1 in 3, Americans under the age of 65 were without health insurance for some period of time between 2008 and 2009 (Families USA 2009).

Since the United States has an employer-based financing system, it is not difficult to see why the unemployed generally have no health insurance. However, even some employed individuals might not have health insurance coverage for two main reasons: (1) In most states, employers are not mandated to offer health insurance to their employees; therefore, some employers, due to economic constraints, do not offer it. Some small businesses simply cannot get group insurance at affordable rates and, therefore, are not able to offer health insurance as a benefit to their employees. (2) In many work settings, participation in health insurance programs is voluntary and does not require employees to join. Some employees choose not to sign up, mainly because they cannot afford the cost of health insurance premiums. Employers rarely pay 100% of the insurance premium; most require their employees to pay a portion of the cost, called *premium cost sharing*. Employees who do not have health insurance offered by their employers or those who are self-employed have to obtain health insurance on their own. Individual rates are typically higher than group rates available to employers, and, in some instances, health insurance is unavailable when adverse health conditions are present.

In the United States, working people earning low wages are the most disenfranchised because most are not eligible for public benefits and cannot afford premium cost sharing. The US government finances health benefits for certain special populations, including government employees, the elderly (people age 65 and over), people with disabilities, some people with very low incomes, and children from low-income families. The program for the elderly and certain disabled individuals is called *Medicare*. The program for the indigent, jointly administered by the federal government and state governments, is named *Medicaid*. The program for children from low-income families, another federal/state partnership, is called the Children's Health Insurance Program (CHIP). For such public programs, the government may function as both financier and insurer, or the insurance function may be carved out to a health maintenance organization (HMO). Private providers, with a few exceptions, render services to these special categories of people, and the government pays for the services, generally, by establishing contractual arrangements with selected intermediaries for the actual disbursement of payments to the providers. Thus, even in government-financed programs, the four functions of financing, insurance, delivery, and payment can be quite distinct.

## Transition from Traditional Insurance to Managed Care

Under traditional insurance, the four basic health delivery functions have been fragmented; that is, the financiers, insurers, providers, and payers have often been different entities, with a few exceptions. During the 1990s, however, health care delivery in the United States underwent a fundamental change involving a tighter integration of the basic functions through managed care.

Previously, fragmentation of the functions meant a lack of control over utilization and payments. The quantity of health care consumed refers to *utilization* of health services. Traditionally, determination of the utilization of health services and the price charged for each service has been left up to the insured individuals and their physicians. Due to rising health care costs, however, current delivery mechanisms have instituted some controls over both utilization and price.

*Managed care* is a system of health care delivery that (1) seeks to achieve efficiencies by integrating the four functions of health care delivery discussed earlier, (2) employs mechanisms to control (manage) utilization of medical services, and (3) determines the price at which the services are purchased and, consequently, how much the providers get paid. The primary financier is still the employer or the government, as the case may be. Instead of purchasing health insurance through a traditional insurance company, the employer contracts with an MCO, such as an HMO or a preferred provider organization (PPO), to offer a selected health plan to its employees. In this case, the MCO functions like an insurance company and promises to provide health care services contracted under the health plan to the enrollees of the plan. The term *enrollee* (member) refers to the individual covered under the plan. The contractual arrangement between the MCO and the enrollee—including the collective array of covered health services that the enrollee is entitled to—is referred to as the *health plan* (or "plan," for short). The health plan uses selected providers from whom the enrollees can choose to receive services.

## Primary Characteristics of the US Health Care System

In any country, certain external influences shape the basic character of the health services delivery system. These forces consist of the political climate of a nation; economic development; technological progress; social and cultural values; physical environment; population characteristics, such as demographic and health trends; and global influences (Figure 1–2). The combined interaction of these environmental forces influences the course of health care delivery.

Figure 1–2 External Forces Affecting Health Care Delivery.

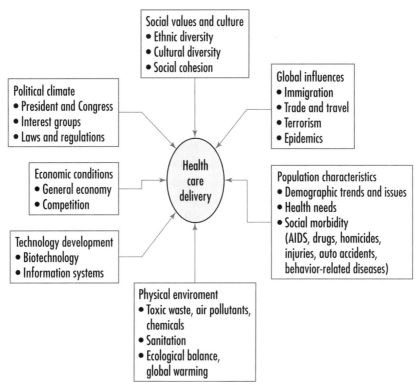

Ten basic characteristics differentiate the US health care delivery system from that of other countries:

1. No central agency governs the system.
2. Access to health care services is selectively based on insurance coverage.
3. Health care is delivered under imperfect market conditions.
4. Third-party insurers act as intermediaries between the financing and delivery functions.
5. The existence of multiple payers makes the system cumbersome.
6. The balance of power among various players prevents any single entity from dominating the system.
7. Legal risks influence practice behavior of physicians.
8. Development of new technology creates an automatic demand for its use.
9. New service settings have evolved along a continuum.
10. Quality is no longer accepted as an unachievable goal in the delivery of health care.

## No Central Agency

The US health care system is not administratively controlled by a department or an agency of the government. Most other developed nations have national health care programs in which every citizen is entitled to receive a defined set of health care services. Availability of "free" services can break a system financially. To control costs, these systems use *global budgets* to determine total health care expenditures on a national scale and to allocate resources within budgetary limits. Availability of services, as well as payments to providers, is subject to such budgetary constraints. The government of these nations also controls the proliferation of health care services, especially costly medical technology. System-wide controls over the allocation of resources determine to what extent government-sponsored health care services are available to citizens. For instance, the availability of specialized services is restricted.

By contrast, the United States has mainly a private system of financing, as well as delivery. Private financing, predominantly through employers, accounts for approximately 54% of total health care expenditures; the government finances the remaining 46% (National Center for Health Statistics 2006). Private delivery of health care means that the majority of hospitals and physician clinics are private businesses, independent of the government. No central agency monitors total expenditures through global budgets or controls the availability and utilization of services. Nevertheless, the federal and state governments in the United States play an important role in health care delivery. They determine public-sector expenditures and reimbursement rates for services provided to Medicaid, CHIP, and Medicare beneficiaries. The government also formulates *standards of participation* through health policy and regulation, meaning providers must comply with the standards established by the government to be certified to provide services to Medicaid, CHIP, and Medicare beneficiaries.

Certification standards are also regarded as minimum standards of quality in most sectors of the health care industry.

## Partial Access

*Access* means the ability of an individual to obtain health care services when needed. In the United States, access is restricted to people who (1) have health insurance through their employers, (2) are covered under a government health care program, (3) can afford to buy insurance with their own private funds, or (4) are able to pay for services privately. Health insurance is the primary means for ensuring access. Although the uninsured can access certain types of services, they often encounter barriers to obtaining needed health care. Federally supported community health centers, for example, provide physician services to anyone regardless of ability to pay. Such centers and other types of free clinics, however, are located only in certain geographic areas. Under US law, hospital emergency departments are required to evaluate a patient's condition and render medically needed services for which the hospital does not receive any direct payments unless the patient is able to pay. Uninsured Americans, therefore, are able to obtain medical care for acute illness. Hence, one can say that the United States does have a form of universal catastrophic health insurance even for the uninsured (Altman and Reinhardt 1996). On the other hand, the uninsured generally have to forego continual basic and routine care, commonly referred to as *primary care*.

Countries with national health care programs provide *universal coverage*; that is, health insurance is available to all citizens. However, access to services when needed may be restricted because no health care system has the capacity to deliver on demand every type of service the citizens may require. Hence, *universal access*—the ability of all citizens to obtain health care when needed—remains mostly a theoretical concept.

Experts generally believe that the inadequate access to basic and routine primary care services particularly by the nation's vulnerable populations (see Chapter 11 for detailed discussion) is one of the main reasons why the United States, in spite of being the most economically advanced country, lags behind other developed nations in measures of population health, such as infant mortality and overall life expectancy. It remains to be seen whether the Patient Protection and Affordable Care Act of 2010 will be able to deliver on the promise of access to health care for all Americans by 2014 (see Chapter 6 for further details).

## Imperfect Market

In the United States, even though the delivery of services is largely in private hands, health care is only partially governed by free market forces. The delivery and consumption of health care in the United States does not quite pass the basic test of a *free market*, as subsequently described. Hence, the system is best described as a quasi-market or an imperfect market. Following are some key features characterizing free markets.

In a free market, multiple patients (buyers) and providers (sellers) act independently, and patients can choose to receive services from any provider. Providers neither collude to fix prices, nor are prices fixed by an external agency. Rather, prices are governed by the free and unencumbered interaction of the forces of supply and demand (Figure 1–3). *Demand*—that is, the quantity of health care purchased—in turn, is driven

by the prices prevailing in the free market. Under free market conditions, the quantity demanded will increase as the price is lowered for a given product or service. Conversely, the quantity demanded will decrease as the price increases.

At casual observation, it may appear that multiple patients and providers do exist. Most patients, however, are now enrolled in either a private health plan or government-sponsored Medicare, Medicaid, or CHIP programs. These plans act as intermediaries for the patients, and the consolidation of patients into health plans has the effect of shifting the power from the patients to the administrators of the plans. The result is that the health plans, not the patients, are the real buyers in the health care services market. Private health plans, in many instances, offer their enrollees a limited choice of providers rather than an open choice.

Theoretically, prices are negotiated between the payers and providers. In practice, however, prices are determined by the payers, such as managed care, Medicare, and Medicaid. Because prices are set by agencies external to the market, they are not governed by the unencumbered forces of supply and demand.

For the health care market to be free, unrestrained competition must occur among providers based on price and quality. Generally speaking, free competition exists among health care providers in the United States. The consolidation of buying power in the hands of private health plans, however, has been forcing providers to form alliances and integrated delivery systems on the supply side. Integrated delivery systems (discussed in Chapter 9) are networks of health services organizations. In certain geographic sectors of the country, a single giant medical system has taken over as the

Figure 1–3  Relationship Between Price, Supply, and Demand Under Free-Market Conditions.

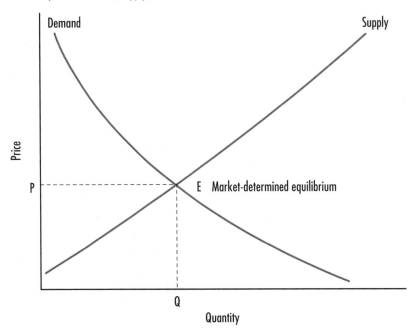

Under free-market conditions, there is an inverse relationship between the quantity of medical services demanded and the price of medical services. That is, quantity demanded goes up when the prices go down and vice versa. On the other hand, there is a direct relationship between price and the quantity supplied by the providers of care. In other words, providers are willing to supply higher quantities at higher prices and vice versa. In a free market, the quantity of medical care that patients are willing to purchase, the quantity of medical care that providers are willing to supply, and the price reach a state of equilibrium. The equilibrium is achieved without the interference of any nonmarket forces. It is important to keep in mind that these conditions exist only under free-market conditions, which are not characterisitic of the health care market.

sole provider of major health care services, restricting competition. As the health care system continues to move in this direction, it appears that only in large metropolitan areas will there be more than one large integrated system competing to get the business of the health plans.

A free market requires that patients have information about the appropriateness of various services. Such information is difficult to obtain because technology-driven medical care has become highly sophisticated. New diagnostic methods, intervention techniques, and more effective drugs fall in the domain of the professional physician. Also, medical interventions are commonly required in a state of urgency. Hence, patients have neither the skills nor the time and resources to obtain accurate information when needed. Channeling all health care needs through a primary care provider is likely to reduce this information gap when the primary care provider acts as the patient's advocate or agent. Conversely, the Internet is becoming a prominent source of medical information, and medical advertising is having an impact on consumer expectations.

In a free market, patients have information on price and quality for each provider. The current system has other drawbacks that obstruct information-seeking efforts. Item-based pricing, instead of package pricing, is one such hurdle. Surgery is a good example to illustrate item-based pricing. Patients can generally obtain the fees the surgeon would charge for a particular operation. But the final bill, after the surgery has been performed, is likely to include charges for supplies, use of the hospital's facilities, and services performed by providers, such as anesthesiologists, nurse anesthetists, and pathologists. These providers, sometimes referred to as *phantom providers*, who function in an adjunct capacity, bill for their services separately. Item billing for such additional services, which sometimes cannot be anticipated, makes it extremely difficult to ascertain the total price before services have actually been received. Package pricing and capitated fees can help overcome these drawbacks, but they have made relatively little headway for pricing medical procedures. *Package pricing* refers to a bundled fee for a package of related services. In the surgery example, this would mean one all-inclusive price for the surgeon's fees, hospital facilities, supplies, diagnostics, pathology, anesthesia, and postsurgical follow-up. With *capitation*, all health care services are included under one set fee per covered individual.

In recent years, quality of health care has received much emphasis. Performance ratings and report cards, however, furnish scant information on the quality of health care providers.

In a free market, patients must directly bear the cost of services received. The purpose of insurance is to protect against the risk of unforeseen catastrophic events. Since the fundamental purpose of insurance is to meet major expenses when unlikely events occur, having insurance for basic and routine health care undermines the principle of insurance. When you buy home insurance to protect your property against the unlikely event of a fire, you do not anticipate the occurrence of a loss. The probability that you will suffer a loss by fire is very small. If a fire does occur and cause major damage, insurance will cover the loss, but the policy does not cover routine wear and tear on the house, such as chipped paint or a leaking faucet. Health insurance, however, generally covers basic and routine services that are predictable. Health insurance coverage for minor services, such as colds and coughs, earaches, and so forth, amounts to prepayment for such services. Health insurance has the effect of insulating patients from the full cost of health care. There is a *moral hazard* that, once enrollees have purchased health insurance, they will use health care services to a greater extent than if they were to bear the full cost of these services.

In a free market for health care, patients make decisions about the purchase of health care services. The main factors that limit the patient's ability to make health care purchase decisions have already been discussed. Even with the best intentions, the circumstances surrounding sickness and injury often prohibit comparative shopping based on price and quality. Further, such information is not easily available. At least two additional factors limit the ability of patients to make decisions. First, decisions about the utilization of health care are often determined by need rather than by price-based demand. *Need* has been defined as the amount of medical care that medical experts believe a person should have to remain or become healthy (Feldstein 1993). Need can also be based on self-evaluation of one's own health status. Second, the delivery of health care can result in demand creation. This follows from self-assessed need, which, coupled with moral hazard, leads to greater utilization, creating an artificial demand because prices are not taken into consideration. Practitioners who have a financial interest in additional treatments also create artificial demand (Hemenway and Fallon 1985), commonly referred to as *provider-induced demand*, or supplier-induced demand. Functioning as patients' agents, physicians exert enormous influence on the demand for health care services (Altman and Wallack 1996). Research studies have pointed to physicians' behavior of creating demand to their own financial benefit (see, for instance, McGuire and Pauly 1991). Demand creation occurs when physicians prescribe medical care beyond what is clinically necessary. This can include practices such as making more frequent follow-up appointments than necessary, prescribing excessive medical tests, or performing unnecessary surgery (Santerre and Neun 1996).

## Third-Party Insurers and Payers

Insurance often functions as the intermediary among those who finance, deliver, and receive health care. Delivery of health care is often viewed as a transaction between the patient and the provider, but insurance and payment functions introduce a *third party* into the transaction (Griffith 1995), the patient being the first party and the provider the second party. Apart from being the payer, the third-party insurer also takes over most other administrative functions associated with the plan. The providers, as well as the enrollees,

must comply with the policies set forth by the insurer in matters related to the delivery of health care and payment for services.

The intermediary role of insurance creates a wall of separation between the financing and delivery functions so that quality of care often remains a secondary concern. In normal economic markets, the consumer is armed with the power to influence demand based on the price and quality of goods and services. Another way to illustrate this concept is to say that, in a free market, consumers vote with their dollars for the best candidate among competing products, based on the price and quality of each product. The insurance intermediary does not have the incentive to be the patient's advocate on either price or quality. At best, employees can air their dissatisfactions with the plan to their employer, who has the power to discontinue the current plan and choose another company. In reality, however, employers may be reluctant to change plans if the current plan offers lower premiums compared to a new plan. National health care programs have even fewer incentives for promoting quality, although they can contain costs by artificially fixing prices.

## Multiple Payers

A national health care system is sometimes also referred to as a *single-payer system*, because there is one primary payer, the government. When delivering services, providers send the bill to an agency of the government that subsequently sends payment to each provider.

By contrast, the United States has a multiplicity of health plans and insurance companies because each employer is free to determine the type of health plan it offers.

Each plan spells out the type of services the enrollee can receive. Some plans make an arbitrary determination of how much will be paid for a certain type of service. For Medicare and Medicaid recipients, the government has its own set of regulations and payment schedules.

Multiple payers often represent a billing and collection nightmare for the providers of services. Multiple payers make the system more cumbersome in several ways:

- It is extremely difficult for providers to keep tabs on the numerous health plans. For example, it is difficult to keep up with which services are covered under each plan and how much each plan will pay for those services.
- Providers must hire a battery of claims processors to bill for services and monitor receipt of payments. Billing practices are not always standardized, and each payer establishes its own format.
- Payments can be denied for not precisely following the requirements set by each payer.
- Denied claims necessitate rebilling.
- When only partial payment is received, some health plans may allow the provider to *balance bill* the patient for the amount the health plan did not pay. Other plans prohibit balance billing. Even when the balance billing option is available to the provider, it triggers a new cycle of billings and collection efforts.
- Providers must sometimes engage in lengthy collection efforts, including writing collection letters, turning delinquent accounts over to collection agencies, and finally writing off as bad debt amounts that cannot be collected.

- Government programs have complex regulations for determining whether payment is made for services actually delivered. Medicare, for example, requires that each provider maintain lengthy documentation on services provided. Medicaid is known for lengthy delays in paying providers.

It is generally believed that the United States spends far more on *administrative costs*—that is the costs associated with billing, collections, bad debts, and maintaining medical records—than the national health care systems in other countries. However, estimates of cost differentials between the US health care system and single-payer systems have been the subject of considerable controversy (Kahn et al. 2005).

## Power Balancing

The US health services system involves multiple players, not just multiple payers. The key players in the system have been physicians, administrators of health service institutions, insurance companies, large employers, and the government. Big business, labor, insurance companies, physicians, and hospitals make up the powerful and politically active special interest groups represented before lawmakers by high-priced lobbyists. Each set of players has its own economic interests to protect. Physicians, for instance, want to maximize their incomes and have minimum interference with the way they practice medicine; institutional administrators seek to maximize reimbursement from private and public insurers. Insurance companies and MCOs are interested in maintaining their share of the health care insurance market; large employers want to minimize the costs they incur providing health insurance as a benefit to their employees. The government tries to maintain or enhance existing benefits for select population groups and simultaneously reduce the cost of providing these benefits. The problem is that self-interests of different players are often at odds. For example, providers seek to maximize government reimbursement for services delivered to Medicare, Medicaid, and CHIP beneficiaries, but the government wants to contain cost increases. Employers dislike rising health insurance premiums. Health plans, under pressure from the employers, may constrain fees for the providers, who resent any cuts in their incomes.

The fragmented self-interests of the various players produce countervailing forces within the system. One positive effect of these opposing forces is that they prevent any single entity from dominating the system. Conversely, each set of players has a large stake in health policy reforms. In an environment that is rife with motivations to protect conflicting self-interests, achieving comprehensive system-wide reforms has been next to impossible, and cost containment has remained a major challenge. Consequently, the approach to health care reform in the United States has been characterized as incremental or piecemeal, and the focus of reform initiatives has been confined to health insurance coverage and payment cuts to providers.

## Legal Risks

America is a litigious society. Motivated by the prospects of enormous jury awards, Americans are quick to drag an alleged offender into a courtroom at the slightest perception of incurred harm. Private health care providers have become increasingly susceptible to litigation. By contrast, in national health care programs, governments are immune to lawsuits. Hence, in the United States, the risk of malpractice lawsuits is a real consideration in the practice of medicine. To protect themselves against the possibility of litigation, it is not uncommon for practitioners to engage in what is referred to as *defensive medicine* by prescribing additional diagnostic tests, scheduling return checkup visits, and maintaining copious documentation. Many of these additional efforts may be unnecessary; hence, they are costly and inefficient.

## High Technology

The United States has been the hotbed of research and innovation in new medical technology. Growth in science and technology often creates demand for new services despite shrinking resources to finance sophisticated care. People generally equate high-tech care to high-quality care. They want "the latest and the best," especially when health insurance will pay for new treatments. Physicians and technicians want to try the latest gadgets. Hospitals compete on the basis of having the most modern equipment and facilities. Once capital investments are made, costs must be recouped through utilization. Legal risks for providers and health plans alike may also play a role in discouraging denial of new technology. Thus, several factors promote the use of costly new technology once it is developed.

## Continuum of Services

Medical care services are classified into three broad categories: curative (e.g., drugs, treatments, and surgeries), restorative (e.g., physical, occupational, and speech therapies), and preventive (e.g., prenatal care, mammograms, and immunizations). Health care service settings are no longer confined to the hospital and the physician's office, where many of the aforementioned services were once delivered. Several new settings, such as home health, subacute care units, and outpatient surgery centers, have emerged in response to the changing configuration of economic incentives. Table 1–2 depicts the continuum of health care services. The health care continuum in the United States remains lopsided, with a heavier emphasis on specialized services than on preventive services, primary care, and management of chronic conditions.

Table 1–2  The Continuum of Health Care Services

| Types of Health Services | Delivery Settings |
| --- | --- |
| Preventive care | Public health programs<br>Community programs<br>Personal lifestyles<br>Primary care settings |
| Primary care | Physician's office or clinic<br>Community health centers<br>Self-care<br>Alternative medicine |
| Specialized care | Specialist provider clinics |
| Chronic care | Primary care settings<br>Specialist provider clinics<br>Home health<br>Long-term care facilities<br>Self-care<br>Alternative medicine |
| Long-term care | Long-term care facilities<br>Home health |
| Subacute care | Special subacute units (hospitals, long-term care facilities)<br>Home health<br>Outpatient surgical centers |
| Acute care | Hospitals |
| Rehabilitative care | Rehabilitation departments (hospitals, long-term care facilities)<br>Home health<br>Outpatient rehabilitation centers |
| End-of-life care | Hospice services provided in a variety of settings |

## Quest for Quality

Even though the definition and measurement of quality in health care are not as clear cut as they are in other industries, the delivery sector of health care has come under increased pressure to develop quality standards and demonstrate compliance with those standards. There are higher expectations for improved health outcomes at the individual and broader community levels. The concept of continual quality improvement has also received much emphasis in managing health care institutions.

## Trends and Directions

Since the final two decades of the 20th century, the US health care delivery system has continued to undergo certain fundamental shifts in emphasis, summarized in Figure 1–4. Later chapters discuss these transformations in greater detail and focus on the factors driving them.

Figure 1–4  Trends and Directions in Health Care Delivery.

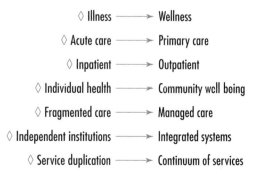

◊ Illness ——→ Wellness
◊ Acute care ——→ Primary care
◊ Inpatient ——→ Outpatient
◊ Individual health ——→ Community well being
◊ Fragmented care ——→ Managed care
◊ Independent institutions ——→ Integrated systems
◊ Service duplication ——→ Continuum of services

Promotion of health at less cost has been the driving force behind these trends. An example of a shift in emphasis is the concept of health itself: The focus is changing from illness to wellness. Such a change requires new methods and settings for wellness promotion, although the treatment of illness continues to be the primary goal of the health services delivery system.

## Significance for Health Care Practitioners and Policymakers

An understanding of the health care delivery system is essential for managers and policy makers. In fact, an understanding of the intricacies within the health services system would be beneficial to all those who come in contact with the system. In their respective training programs, health professionals, such as physicians, nurses, technicians, therapists, dietitians, and pharmacists, as well as others, may understand their own individual roles but remain ignorant of the forces outside their profession that could significantly impact current and future practices. An understanding of the health care delivery system can attune health professionals to their relationship with the rest of the health care environment. It can help them better understand changes and the potential impact of those changes on their own practice. Adaptation and relearning are strategies that can prepare health professionals to cope with an environment that will see ongoing change long into the future.

Policy decisions to address specific problems must also be made within the broader macro context because policies designed to bring about change in one health care sector can have wider repercussions,

both desirable and undesirable, in other sectors of the system. Policy decisions and their implementation are often critical to the future direction of the health care delivery system. However, in a multifaceted system, future issues will be best addressed by a joint undertaking with a balanced representation of the key players in health services delivery: physicians, insurance companies, managed care organizations, employers, institutional representatives, and the government.

## Significance for Health Care Managers

An understanding of the health care system has specific implications for health services managers, who must understand the macro environment in which they make critical decisions in planning and strategic management, regardless of whether they manage a private institution or a public service agency. Such decisions and actions, eventually, affect the efficiency and quality of services delivered. The interactions among the system's key components and the implications of those interactions must be well understood because the operations of health care institutions are strongly influenced, either directly or indirectly, by the financing of health services, reimbursement rates, insurance mechanisms, delivery modes, new statutes and legal opinions, and government regulations.

The environment of health care delivery will continue to remain fluid and dynamic. The viability of delivery settings, and, thus, the success of health care managers, often depends on how the managers react to the system dynamics. Timeliness of action is often a critical factor that can make the difference between failure and success. Following are some more specific reasons why understanding the health care delivery system is indispensable for health care managers.

## Positioning the Organization

Health services administrators need to understand their own organizational position within the macro environment of the system. Senior managers, such as chief executive officers, must constantly gauge the nature and impact of the fundamental shifts illustrated in Figure 1–4. Managers need to consider which changes in the current configuration of financing, insurance, payment, and delivery might affect their organization's long-term stability. Middle and first-line managers also need to understand their role in the current configuration and how that role might change in the future. How should resources be realigned to effectively respond to those changes? For example, these managers need to evaluate whether certain functions in their departments will have to be eliminated, modified, or added. Would the changes involve further training? What processes are likely to change and how? What do the managers need to do to maintain the integrity of their institution's mission, the goodwill of the patients they serve, and the quality of the services? Well thought through and appropriately planned change is likely to cause less turbulence for the providers, as well as the recipients of care.

## Handling Threats and Opportunities

Changes in any of the functions of financing, insurance, payment, and delivery can present new threats or opportunities in the health care market. Health care managers are more effective if they proactively deal with any threats to their institution's profitability and viability. Managers need to find ways to transform certain threats into new opportunities.

## Evaluating Implications

Managers are better able to evaluate the implications of health policy and new reform proposals when they understand the relevant issues and how such issues link to the delivery of health services in the establishments they manage. With the expected expansion of health insurance coverage, more individuals will be brought into the health care system, creating further demand for health services. Planning and staffing for the right mix of health care workforce to meet this anticipated surge in demand is critical.

## Planning

Senior managers are often responsible for strategic planning, regarding which services should be added or discontinued, which resources should be committed to facility expansion, or what should be done with excess capacity. Any long-range planning must take into consideration the current makeup of health services delivery, the evolving trends, and the potential impact of these trends.

## Capturing New Markets

Health care administrators are in a better position to capture new health services markets if they understand emerging trends in the financing, insurance, payment, and delivery functions. New opportunities must be explored before any newly evolving segments of the market get overcrowded. An understanding of the dynamics within the system is essential to forging new marketing strategies to stay ahead of the competition and often to finding a service niche.

## Complying with Regulations

Delivery of health care services is heavily regulated. Health care managers must comply with government regulations, such as standards of participation in government programs, licensing rules, and security and privacy laws regarding patient information, and must operate within the constraints of reimbursement rates. The Medicare and Medicaid programs have, periodically, made drastic changes to their reimbursement methodologies that have triggered the need for operational changes in the way services are organized and delivered. Private agencies, such as the Joint Commission on Accreditation of Healthcare Organizations (JCAHO), also play an indirect regulatory role, mainly in the monitoring of quality of services. Health care managers have no choice but to play by the rules set by the various public and private agencies. Hence, it is paramount that health care managers acquaint themselves with the rules and regulations governing their areas of operation.

## Following the Organizational Mission

Knowledge of the health care system and its development is essential for effective management of health care organizations. By keeping up to date on community needs, technological progress, consumer demand, and economic prospects, managers can be in a better position to fulfill their organizational missions to enhance access, improve service quality, and achieve efficiency in the delivery of services.

## Health Care Systems of Other Countries

Canada and most Western European countries have national health care programs that provide universal coverage. There are three basic models for structuring national health care systems:

1. In a system under *national health insurance* (NHI), such as in Canada, the government finances health care through general taxes, but the actual care is delivered by private providers. In the context of the quad-function model, NHI requires a tighter consolidation of the financing, insurance, and payment functions coordinated by the government. Delivery is characterized by detached private arrangements.

2. In a *national health system* (NHS), such as in Great Britain, in addition to financing a tax-supported NHI program, the government manages the infrastructure for the delivery of medical care. Under such a system, the government operates most of the medical institutions. Most health care providers, such as physicians, are either government employees or are tightly organized in a publicly managed infrastructure. In the context of the quad-function model, NHS requires a tighter consolidation of all four functions.

3. In a *socialized health insurance* (SHI) system, such as in Germany, government-mandated contributions by employers and employees finance health care. Private providers deliver health care. Private not-for-profit insurance companies, called sickness

funds, are responsible for collecting the contributions and paying physicians and hospitals (Santerre and Neun 1996). In a socialized health insurance system, insurance and payment functions are closely integrated, and the financing function is better coordinated with the insurance and payment functions than in the United States. Delivery is characterized by independent private arrangements. The government exercises overall control.

In the remainder of this book, the terms "national health care program" and "national health insurance" are used generically and interchangeably to refer to any type of government-supported universal health insurance program. Table 1–3 presents selected features of the national health care programs in Canada, Germany, and Great Britain compared to the United States. Following is a brief discussion of health care delivery in selected countries from various parts of the world, to illustrate the application of the three models discussed and to provide a sample of the variety of health care systems in the world.

## Australia

In the past, Australia had switched from a universal national health care program to a privately financed system. Since 1984, it has returned to a national program—called Medicare—financed by income taxes and an income-based Medicare levy. The system is built on the philosophy of everyone

Table 1–3 Health Care Systems of Selected Industrialized Countries

|  | United States | Canada | Great Britain | Germany |
|---|---|---|---|---|
| Type | Pluralisitic | National health insurance | National health system | Socialized health insurance |
| Ownership | Private | Public/Private | Public | Private |
| Financing | Voluntary, multipayer system (premiums or general taxes) | Single payer (general taxes) | Single payer (general taxes) | Employer–employee (mandated payroll contributions and general taxes) |
| Reimbursement (hospital) | Varies (DRG, negotiated fee for service, per diem, capitation) | Global budgets | Global budgets | Per diem payments |
| Reimbursement (physicians) | RBRVS, fee for service | Negotiated fee for service | Salaries and capitation payments | Negotiated fee for service |
| Consumer copayment | Small to significant | Negligible | Negligible | Negligible |

*Note:* RBRVS, resource-based relative value scale.

*Source:* Data from R.E. Santerre and S.P. Neun, *Health Economics: Theories, Insights, and Industry Studies*, p. 146, © 1996, Irwin.

contributing to the cost of health care according to his or her capacity to pay. In addition to Medicare, approximately 43% of Australians carry private health insurance (Australian Government 2004) to cover gaps in public coverage, such as dental services and care received in private hospitals (Willcox 2001). Although private health insurance is voluntary, it is strongly encouraged by the Australian government through tax subsidies for purchasers and tax penalties for nonpurchasers (Healy 2002). Public hospital spending is funded by the government, but private hospitals offer better choices. Costs incurred by patients receiving private medical services, whether in or out of the hospital, are reimbursed in whole or in part by Medicare. Private patients are free to choose and/or change their doctors. The medical profession in Australia is composed mainly of private practitioners, who provide care predominantly on a fee-for-service basis (Hall 1999; Podger 1999).

Recent health care reform undertaken by the Australian government has focused mainly on creating a better primary care system with the aim of offsetting the growing prevalence of chronic diseases (Gregory 2010; National Health and Hospitals Reform Commission 2010). Efforts have been launched to improve access and quality. Another objective is to reform the public hospital system by increasing the number of beds and improving productivity.

Information on safety and quality standards, as well as prices, will be accessible to the public and closely monitored to ensure transparency. The reform also created the Australian Commission on Safety and Quality in Health Care, the Independent Hospital Pricing Authority, and the National Performance Authority to help improve system performance. These three divisions have been established for continual improvement, well after the implementation of reform legislation, and to assist Australians in making more informed decisions about health services (Australian Government 2010).

## Canada

Canada implemented its national health insurance system—referred to as Medicare—under the Medical Care Act of 1966. Currently, Medicare is composed of 13 provincial and territorial health insurance plans, sharing basic standards of coverage, as defined by the Canada Health Act (Health Canada 2006). The bulk of financing for Medicare comes from general provincial tax revenues; the federal government provides a fixed amount that is independent of actual expenditures. Taxes are used to pay for nearly 70% of total health care expenditures in Canada. The remaining 30%, which pays for supplementary services, such as drugs, dental care, and vision care, is financed privately (Canadian Institute for Health Information 2005). Many employers offer private insurance for supplemental coverage.

Provincial and territorial departments of health have the responsibility to administer medical insurance plans, determine reimbursement for providers, and deliver certain public health services. Provinces are required by law to provide reasonable access to all medically necessary services and to provide portability of benefits from province to province. Patients are free to select their providers (Akaho et al. 1998). Several provinces have established contracts with providers in the United States for certain specialized services. According to Canada's Fraser Institute, specialist physicians surveyed across 12 specialties and 10 Canadian provinces reported a total waiting time of 18.2 weeks between referral from a general practitioner and delivery of treatment in 2010, an increase from 16.1 weeks in 2009. Patients had to wait the longest to undergo orthopedic surgery (35.6 weeks) (Barua et al. 2010).

Nearly all the Canadian provinces (Ontario being one exception) have resorted to regionalization, by creating administrative districts within each province. The objective of regionalization is to decentralize authority and responsibility to more efficiently address local needs and to promote citizen participation in health care decision making (Church and Barker 1998). The majority of Canadian hospitals are operated as private nonprofit entities run by community boards of trustees, voluntary organizations, or municipalities, and most physicians are in private practice (Health Canada 2006). Most provinces use global budgets and allocate set reimbursement amounts for each hospital. Physicians are paid fee-for-service rates, negotiated between each provincial government and medical association (MacPhee 1996; Naylor 1999).

Over the years, federal financial support to the provinces has been drastically reduced. Under the increasing burden of higher costs, certain provinces, such as Alberta and Ontario, have started small-scale experimentation with privatization. However, in 2003, the Health Council of Canada, composed of representatives of federal, provincial, and territorial governments, as well as health care experts, was established to assess Canada's health care system performance and establish goals for improvement. The Council's 2003 First Ministers' Accord on Health Care Renewal created a 5-year, $16 billion Health Reform Fund targeted at improving primary health care, home care, and catastrophic drug coverage (Health Council of Canada 2005).

Although most Canadians are quite satisfied with their health care system, how to sustain current health care delivery and financing remains a challenge. Spending on health care has increased from approximately 7% of program spending at the provincial level in the 1970s to almost 40% today. It is expected to surpass 50% in every province and territory within the next few years.

## China

Since the economic reforms initiated in the late 1970s, health care in the People's Republic of China has undergone significant changes. In urban China, health insurance has evolved from a predominantly public insurance (either government or public enterprise) system to a multipayer system. Government employees are covered under government insurance as a part of their benefits. Employees for public enterprises are largely covered through public enterprise insurance, but the actual benefits and payments vary according to the financial well-being of the enterprises. Employees of foreign businesses or joint ventures are, typically, well insured through private insurance arrangements. Almost all of these plans contain costs through a variety of means, such as experience-based premiums, deductibles, copayments, and health benefit dollars (i.e., pre-allocated benefit dollars for health care that can be converted into income if not fully used). The unemployed, self-employed, and employees working for small enterprises (public or private) are largely uninsured. They can purchase individual or family plans in the private market or pay for services out of pocket. In rural China, the New Cooperative Medical Scheme (NCMS) (discussed later) has become widespread with funds pooled from national and local government, as well as private citizens. Although the insurance coverage rate is high (reaching over 90%), the actual benefits are still very limited.

Similar to the United States, China has been facing the growing problems of a large uninsured population and health care cost inflation. Although health care funding was increased by 87% in 2006 and 2007, the country has yet to reform its health care system into one that is efficient and effective. Employment-based insurance in China does not cover dependents, nor does it cover migrant workers, leading to high out-of-pocket cost sharing in total health spending. Rural areas in China are the most vulnerable because of a lack of true insurance plans and the accompanying comprehensive coverage. Health care cost inflation is also growing at a rate that is 7% faster than gross domestic product (GDP) growth of 16% per year (Yip and Hsia 2008).

Health care delivery has also undergone significant changes. The former three-tier referral system (primary, second, tertiary) has been largely abolished. Patients can now go to any hospital of their choice as long as they are insured or can pay out of pocket. As a result, large (tertiary) hospitals are typically overutilized, whereas smaller (primary and secondary) hospitals are underutilized. Use of large hospitals contributes to medical cost escalation and medical specialization.

Major changes in health insurance and delivery have made access to medical care more difficult for the poor, uninsured, and underinsured. As a result, wide and growing disparities in access, quality, and outcomes are becoming apparent between rural and urban areas, and between the rich and the poor. Since the severe acute respiratory syndrome (SARS) epidemic in 2003,

the government created an electronic disease reporting system at the district level. In addition, each district in China now has a hospital dedicated to infectious disease. However, flaws still remain, particularly in monitoring infectious disease in the remote localities that comprise some districts (Blumenthal and Hsiao 2005).

To fix some of its problems, the Chinese government has pushed through health reform initiatives in five prominent areas: health insurance, pharmaceuticals, primary care, public health, and public/community hospitals. For example, it created the New Cooperative Medical Scheme to provide rural areas with a government-run voluntary insurance program. It prevents individuals living in these areas from becoming impoverished due to illness or catastrophic health expenses (Yip and Hsia 2008). A similar program was established in urban areas in 2008, called the Urban Resident Basic Medical Insurance scheme. The scheme targets the uninsured children, elderly, and other nonworking urban residents and enrolls them into the program at the household level rather than at the individual level (Wagstaff et al. 2009).

To improve access to primary care, China has reestablished community health centers (CHCs) to provide preventive and primary care services to offset the expensive outpatient services at hospitals. The goal is to reduce hospital utilization in favor of CHCs that can provide prevention, home care, and rehabilitative services (Yip and Hsia 2008; Yip and Mahal 2008). The CHCs have not been very popular among the public because of their perceived lack of quality and reputation. It remains uncertain whether China will restore its previously integrated health care delivery system, aimed at achieving universal access, or continue its current course of medical specialization and privatization.

## Germany

The German health care system is characterized by socialized health insurance (SHI) financed by pooling employer and employee premium contributions through payroll taxes. Nonprofit sickness funds manage the social insurance pool. About 88% of the population has been enrolled in a sickness fund; another 11% either have private health insurance or are government workers with special coverage provisions. Less than 0.2% of Germans are uninsured (Busse 2002). Sickness funds act as purchasing entities by negotiating contracts with hospitals. However, with an aging population, fewer people in the workforce, and stagnant wage growth during recessions, paying for the increasing cost of medical care has been challenging.

During the 1990s, Germany adopted legislation to promote competition among sickness funds (Brown and Amelung 1999). To further control costs, the system employs global budgets for the hospital sector and places annual limits on spending for physician services. Disease management programs are also implemented to standardize care for ailments like diabetes, as well as fixed payments to hospitals that discourage overtreatment.

## Great Britain

Great Britain follows the national health system (NHS) model. Coincidentally, the British health delivery system is also named NHS (National Health Service), which marked 50 years of existence in 1998. The NHS is founded on the principles of primary care and has strong focus on community health services. The system owns its hospitals and employs its hospital-based specialists and other staff on a salaried basis. The primary care physicians, referred to as general practitioners (GPs), are mostly private practitioners.

Delivery of primary care is through primary care trusts (PCTs) in England, local health groups in Wales, health boards in Scotland, and primary care partnerships in Northern Ireland. PCTs have geographically assigned responsibility for community health services, in which each person living in a given geographic area is assigned to a particular PCT. A typical PCT is responsible for approximately 50,000–250,000 patients (Dixon and Robinson 2002). PCTs function independently of the local health authorities and are governed by a consumer-dominated board. A fully developed PCT has its own budget allocations, used for both primary care and hospital-based services. In this respect, PCTs function like MCOs in the United States.

It is also of interest to note that 11.5% of the British population holds private health care insurance (Dixon and Robinson 2002), and approximately 2.2 billion pounds are spent annually in the acute sector of private health care (Doyle and McNeilly 1999). Future "pro-market" reforms in the UK's National Health Service would likely shift decision making to general practitioners, let some hospitals become nonprofit, and give patients more control over their health care.

## Israel

Until 1995, Israel had a system of universal coverage based on the German SHI model, financed through an employer tax and income-based contributions from individuals. When the National Health Insurance (NHI) Law went into effect in 1995, it made insurance coverage mandatory for all Israeli citizens. Adults are required to pay a health tax. General tax revenue supplements the health tax revenue, which the government distributes to the various health plans based on a capitation formula. Each year the government determines how much from the general tax revenue should be contributed toward the NHI. The employer tax for health care was abolished in 1997; as a result, the share of general tax revenue to finance health care rose from 26% in 1995 to 46% in 2000 (Rosen 2003).

Health plans (or sickness funds) offer a predefined basic package of health care services and are prohibited from discriminating against those who have preexisting medical conditions. The capitation formula has built-in incentives for the funds to accept a larger number of elderly and chronically ill members. Rather than relying on a single-payer system, the reform allowed the existence of multiple health plans (today there are four competing, nonprofit sickness funds) to foster competition among funds with the assumption that competition would lead to better quality of care and an increased responsiveness to patient needs. The plans also sell private health insurance to supplement the basic package. The system is believed to provide a high standard of care (Rosen and Merkur 2009; Gross et al. 1998).

Unlike Germany, approximately 85% of the general hospital beds in Israel are owned by the government and the General Sick Fund, the largest of the four sickness funds. Hospitals are reimbursed under the global budget model (Chinitz and Israeli 1997). There was a major effort, in the early 1990s, to shift hospitals from government ownership to independent, nonprofit trusts, but this endeavor failed because of opposition from labor unions. Despite this, government hospitals have been granted more autonomy in the intervening years (Rosen 2003).

## Japan

Since 1961, Japan has been providing universal coverage to its citizens through two main health insurance schemes. The first one is an employer-based system, modeled after Germany's SHI program. The second is a national health insurance program. Generally, large employers (with more than 300 employees) have their own health programs. Nearly 2,000 private, nonprofit health insurance societies manage insurance for large firms. Smaller companies either band together to provide private health insurance or belong to a government-run plan. Day laborers, seamen, agricultural workers, the self-employed, and retirees are all covered under the national health care program. Individual employees pay roughly 8% of their salaries as premiums and receive coverage for about 90% of the cost of medical services, with some limitations. Dependents receive slightly less than 90% coverage. Employers and the national government subsidize the cost of private premiums. Coverage is comprehensive, including dental care and prescription drugs, and patients are free to select their providers (Akaho et al. 1998; Babazono et al. 1998). Providers are paid on a fee-for-service basis with little control over reimbursement (McClellan and Kessler 1999).

Several health policy issues have emerged in Japan, however, in the past few years. First, since 2002, some business leaders and economists urged the Japanese government to lift its ban on mixed public/private payments for medical services, arguing that private payments should be allowed for services not covered by medical insurance (i.e., services involving new technologies or drugs). The Japan Medical Association and Ministry of Health, Labor, and Welfare have argued against these recommendations, stating such a policy would favor the wealthy, create disparities in access to care, and could be a risk to patient safety. Although the ban on mixed payments has not been lifted, Prime Minister Koizumi expanded the existing "exceptional approvals system" for new medical technologies in 2004 to allow private payments for selected technologies not covered by medical insurance (Nomura and Nakayama 2005).

Another recent policy development in Japan is the hospitals' increased use of a new system of reimbursement for inpatient care services, called diagnosis-procedure combinations (DPCs). Using DPCs, hospitals receive daily fees for each condition and treatment, regardless of actual provision of tests and interventions, proportionate to patients' length of stay. It is theorized that the DPC system will incentivize hospitals to provide more efficient, higher quality care to patients (Nomura and Nakayama 2005).

Japan's economic stagnation in the last several years has led to an increased pressure to contain costs (Ikegami and Campbell 2004). In 2005, Japan implemented reform initiatives in long-term care (LTC) delivery to contain costs in a growing sector of health care with rapidly rising costs. The new policy required residents in LTC facilities to pay for room and board. It also established new preventive benefits for seniors with low needs, who are at risk of requiring care in

the future. The preventive benefits were designed to maintain health and independence and to postpone the need for nursing home care. Charging nursing home residents a fee for room and board was a departure from past policies that promoted institutionalization (Tsutsui and Muramatsu 2007).

## Singapore

Prior to 1984, Singapore had a British-style NHS program, in which medical services were provided mainly by the public sector and financed through general taxes. Since then, the nation has designed a system based on market competition and self-reliance. Singapore has achieved universal coverage through a policy that requires mandatory private contributions but little government financing. The program, known as Medisave, mandates every working person, including the self-employed, to deposit a portion of earnings into an individual Medisave account. Employers are required to match employee contributions. These savings can only be withdrawn (1) to pay for hospital services and some selected, expensive physician services or (2) to purchase a government-sponsored insurance plan, called Medishield, for catastrophic (expensive and major) illness. For basic and routine services, people are expected to pay out of pocket. Those who cannot afford to pay receive government assistance (Hsiao 1995). In 2002, the government introduced ElderShield, which defrays out-of-pocket medical expenses for the elderly and severely disabled requiring long-term care (Singapore Ministry of Health 2004). The fee-for-service system of payment is prevalent throughout Singapore (McClellan and Kessler 1999).

## Developing Countries

Developing countries, containing 84% of the world's population, claim only 11% of the world's health spending. Yet, these countries account for 93% of the worldwide burden of disease. The six developing regions of the world are East Asia and the Pacific, Europe (mainly Eastern Europe) and Central Asia, Latin America and the Caribbean, the Middle East and North Africa, South Asia, and Sub-Saharan Africa. Of these, the latter two have the least resources and the greatest health burden. On a per capita basis, industrialized countries have six times as many hospital beds and three times as many physicians as developing countries. People with private financial means can find reasonably good health care in many parts of the developing world. However, the majority of the populations have to depend on limited government services that are often of questionable quality, as evaluated by Western standards. As a general observation, government financing for health services increases in countries with higher per capita incomes (Schieber and Maeda 1999).

---

# The Systems Framework

A *system* consists of a set of interrelated and interdependent, logically coordinated components designed to achieve common goals. Even though the various functional components of the health services delivery structure in the United States are, at best, only loosely coordinated, the main components can be identified using a systems model. The systems framework used here helps one understand that the structure of health care services in the United States is based on some foundations, provides a

logical arrangement of the various components, and demonstrates a progression from inputs to outputs. The main elements of this arrangement are system inputs (resources), system structure, system processes, and system outputs (outcomes). In addition, system outlook (future directions) is a necessary feature of a dynamic system. This systems framework is used as the conceptual base for organizing later chapters in this book (see Figure 1–5).

## System Foundations

The current health care system is not an accident. Historical, cultural, social, and economic factors explain its current structure. These factors also affect forces that shape new trends and developments, as well as those that impede change. Chapters 2 and 3 provide a discussion of the system foundations.

## System Resources

No mechanism for health services delivery can fulfill its primary objective without deploying the necessary human and nonhuman resources. Human resources consist of the various types and categories of workers directly engaged in the delivery of health services to patients. Such personnel— physicians, nurses, dentists, pharmacists, other doctoral trained professionals, and numerous categories of allied health professionals—usually have direct contact with patients. Numerous ancillary workers— billing and collection agents, marketing and public relations personnel, and building maintenance employees—often play an important, but indirect, supportive role in the delivery of health care. Health care managers are needed to manage various

Figure 1–5  The Systems Model and Related Chapters.

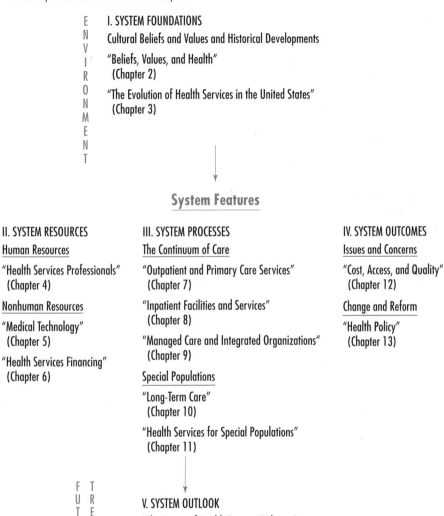

**E N V I R O N M E N T**

**I. SYSTEM FOUNDATIONS**

Cultural Beliefs and Values and Historical Developments

"Beliefs, Values, and Health"
  (Chapter 2)

"The Evolution of Health Services in the United States"
  (Chapter 3)

**System Features**

**II. SYSTEM RESOURCES**

Human Resources

"Health Services Professionals"
  (Chapter 4)

Nonhuman Resources

"Medical Technology"
  (Chapter 5)

"Health Services Financing"
  (Chapter 6)

**III. SYSTEM PROCESSES**

The Continuum of Care

"Outpatient and Primary Care Services"
  (Chapter 7)

"Inpatient Facilities and Services"
  (Chapter 8)

"Managed Care and Integrated Organizations"
  (Chapter 9)

Special Populations

"Long-Term Care"
  (Chapter 10)

"Health Services for Special Populations"
  (Chapter 11)

**IV. SYSTEM OUTCOMES**

Issues and Concerns

"Cost, Access, and Quality"
  (Chapter 12)

Change and Reform

"Health Policy"
  (Chapter 13)

**FUTURE  TRENDS**

**V. SYSTEM OUTLOOK**

"The Future of Health Services Delivery"
  (Chapter 14)

types of health care services. This book primarily discusses the personnel engaged in the direct delivery of health care services (Chapter 4). The nonhuman resources include medical technology (Chapter 5) and health services financing (Chapter 6).

Resources are closely intertwined with access to health care. For instance, in certain rural areas of the United States, access is restricted due to a shortage of health professionals within certain categories. Development and diffusion of technology also determine the caliber of health care to which people may have access. Financing for health insurance and reimbursement to providers affect access indirectly.

## System Processes

System resources influence the development and change in the physical infrastructure—such as hospitals, clinics, and nursing homes—essential for the different processes of health care delivery. Most health care services are delivered in noninstitutional settings, mainly associated with processes referred to as *outpatient care* (Chapter 7). Institutional health services provided in hospitals, nursing homes, and rehabilitation institutions, for example, are predominantly *inpatient services* (Chapter 8). Managed care and integrated systems (Chapter 9) represent a fundamental change in the financing (including payment and insurance) and delivery of health care. Even though managed care represents an integration of the resource and process elements of the systems model, it is discussed as a process for the sake of clarity and continuity of discussions. Special institutional and community-based settings have been developed for long-term care (Chapter 10) and mental health (Chapter 11).

## System Outcomes

System outcomes refer to the critical issues and concerns surrounding what the health services system has been able to accomplish, or not accomplish, in relation to its primary objective, to provide, to an entire nation, cost-effective health services that meet certain established standards of quality. The previous three elements of the systems model play a critical role in fulfilling this objective. Access, cost, and quality are the main outcome criteria to evaluate the success of a health care delivery system (Chapter 12). Issues and concerns regarding these criteria trigger broad initiatives for reforming the system through health policy (Chapter 13).

## System Outlook

A dynamic health care system must be forward looking. In essence, it must project into the future the accomplishment of desired system outcomes in view of anticipated social, economic, political, technological, informational, and ecological forces of change (Chapter 14).

## Summary

The United States has a unique system of health care delivery. The basic features characterizing this system—or rather a patchwork of subsystems—include the absence of a central agency to govern the system; unequal access to health care services, mainly because of a lack of health insurance for all Americans; health care delivery under imperfect market conditions; the existence of multiple payers; third-party insurers functioning as intermediaries between the financing and delivery aspects of health care; a balancing of power among various players; legal risks influencing practice behavior; new and expensive medical technology; a continuum of service settings; and a focus on quality improvement.

No country in the world has a perfect system, and most nations with a national health care program also have a private sector that varies in size. Because of resource limitations, universal access remains a theoretical concept even in countries that offer universal health insurance coverage. The developing countries of the world also face serious challenges due to scarce resources and strong underlying needs for services.

Under free-market conditions, there is an inverse relationship between the quantity of medical services demanded and the price of medical services. Conversely, there is a direct relationship between price and the quantity supplied by the providers of care. In a free market, the quantity of medical care that patients are willing to purchase, the quantity of medical care that providers are willing to supply, and the price reach a state of equilibrium. The equilibrium is achieved without interference of any non-market forces. These conditions exist only under free-market conditions, which are not characteristic of the health care market.

Health care administrators must understand how the health care delivery system works and evolves. Such an understanding improves awareness of the position their organization occupies within the macro environment of the system. This awareness also facilitates strategic planning and compliance with health regulations, enabling them to deal proactively with both opportunities and threats, and enabling them to effectively manage health care organizations. The systems *framework* provides an organized approach to an understanding of the various components of the US health care delivery system.

## Test Your Understanding

### Terminology

| | | |
|---|---|---|
| *access* | *Medicaid* | *provider-induced demand* |
| *administrative costs* | *Medicare* | *quad-function model* |
| *balance bill* | *moral hazard* | *reimbursement* |
| *capitation* | *national health insurance* | *single-payer system* |
| *defensive medicine* | *national health system* | *socialized health insurance* |
| *demand* | *need* | *standards of participation* |
| *enrollee* | *outpatient care* | *system* |
| *free market* | *package pricing* | *third party* |
| *global budget* | *phantom providers* | *uninsured* |
| *health plan* | *premium cost sharing* | *universal access* |
| *inpatient services* | *primary care* | *universal coverage* |
| *managed care* | *provider* | *utilization* |

## Review Questions

1. Why does cost containment remain an elusive goal in US health services delivery?

2. What are the two main objectives of a health care delivery system?

3. Name the four basic functional components of the US health care delivery system. What role does each play in the delivery of health care?

4. What is the primary reason for employers to purchase insurance plans to provide health benefits to their employees?

5. Why is it that, despite public and private health insurance programs, some US citizens are without health care coverage?

6. What is managed care?

7. Why is the US health care market referred to as "imperfect"?

8. Discuss the intermediary role of insurance in the delivery of health care.

9. Who are the major players in the US health services system? What are the positive and negative effects of the often-conflicting self-interests of these players?

10. What main roles does the government play in the US health services system?

11. Why is it important for health care managers and policy makers to understand the intricacies of the health care delivery system?

12. What kind of a cooperative approach do the authors recommend for charting the future course of the health care delivery system?

13. What is the difference between national health insurance (NHI) and a national health system (NHS)?

14. What is socialized health insurance (SHI)?

## REFERENCES

Akaho, E. et al. 1998. A proposed optimal health care system based on a comparative study conducted between Canada and Japan. *Canadian Journal of Public Health* 89, no. 5: 301–307.

Altman, S.H., and U.E. Reinhardt. 1996. Introduction: Where does health care reform go from here? An uncharted odyssey. In: *Strategic choices for a changing health care system*. S.H. Altman and U.E. Reinhardt, eds. Chicago: Health Administration Press. p. xxi–xxxii.

Altman, S.H., and S.S. Wallack. 1996. Health care spending: Can the United States control it? In: *Strategic choices for a changing health care system*. S.H. Altman and U.E. Reinhardt, eds. Chicago: Health Administration Press. p. 1–32.

Australian Government, Department of Health and Ageing. May 2004. *Australia: Selected health care delivery and financing statistics*. Available at: http://www.health.gov/au. Accessed December 15, 2010.

Australian Government, Department of Health and Ageing. 2010. *A national health and hospitals network for Australia's future: Delivering the reforms*. Commonwealth of Australia.

Babazono, A. et al. 1998. The effect of a redistribution system for health care for the elderly on the financial performance of health insurance societies in Japan. *International Journal of Technology Assessment in Health* Care 14, no. 3: 458–466.

Barua, B. et al. 2010. *Waiting your turn: Wait times for health care in Canada 2010 report*. Vancouver, Canada: The Fraser Institute.

Blue Cross Blue Shield Association. 2007. Available at: http://www.bcbs.com/coverage/find/plan. Accessed December 15, 2010.

Blumenthal D., and W. Hsiao. 2005. Privatization and its discontents—The evolving Chinese health care system. *New England Journal of Medicine* 353, no. 11: 1165–1170.

Brown, L.D., and V.E. Amelung. 1999. "Manacled competition": Market reforms in German health care. *Health Affairs* 18, no. 3: 76–91.

Busse, R. 2002. Germany. In: *Health care systems in eight countries: Trends and challenges*. A. Dixon and E. Mossialos, eds. London: The European Observatory on Health Care Systems, London School of Economics & Political Science. p. 47–60.

Canadian Institute for Health Information. 2005. *National health expenditure trends, 1975–2005*. Ottawa, ON: The Institute. p. iii, 7.

Chinitz, D., and A. Israeli. 1997. Health reform and rationing in Israel. *Health Affairs* 16, no. 5: 205–210.

Church, J., and P. Barker. 1998. Regionalization of health services in Canada: A critical perspective. *International Journal of Health Services* 28, no. 3: 467–486.

Dixon, A., and R. Robinson. 2002. The United Kingdom. In: *Health care systems in eight countries: Trends and challenges*. A. Dixon and E. Mossialos, eds. London: The European Observatory on Health Care Systems, London School of Economics & Political Science. p. 103–114.

Doyle, Y.G., and R.H. McNeilly. 1999. The diffusion of new medical technologies in the private sector of the U.K. health care system. *International Journal of Technology Assessment in Health Care* 15, no. 4: 619–628.

Families USA (2009). Americans at risk. Available at: http://www.familiesusa.org/resources /publications/reports/americans-at-risk-findings.html. Accessed January 2011.

Feldstein, P.J. 1993. *Health care economics*. 4th ed. New York: Delmar Publishing.

Gregory, G. 2010. A brief history of "Health reform" in Australia, 2007–2009. *Australian Journal of Rural Health* 18: 49–55.

Griffith, J.R. 1995. *The well-managed health care organization*. Ann Arbor, MI: AUPHA Press/ Health Administration Press.

Gross R. et al. 1998. Evaluating the Israeli health care reform: Strategy, challenges, and lessons. *Health Policy* 45: 99–117.

Hall, J. 1999. Incremental change in the Australian health care system. *Health Affairs* 18, no. 3: 95–110.

Health Canada. 2006. Available at: http://www.hc-sc.gc.ca/hcs-sss/medi-assur/index_e.htmlwhich. Accessed September 2006.

Health Council of Canada. 2005. *Annual report 2005*. Available at: http://www.healthcouncilcanada .ca/en/index.php?option=com_content&task=view&id=51&Itemid=50. Accessed September 2006.

Health Resources and Services Administration (HRSA) 2011. Health center snapshot 2009. Available at: http://www.hrsa.gov/data-statistics/health-center-data/index.html. Accessed January 2011.

Healy, J. 2002. Australia. In: *Health care systems in eight countries: Trends and challenges*. A. Dixon and E. Mossialos, eds. London: The European Observatory on Health Care Systems, London School of Economics & Political Science. p. 3–16.

Hemenway, D., and D. Fallon. 1985. Testing for physician-induced demand with hypothetical cases. *Medical Care* 23, no. 4: 344–349.

Hsiao, W.C. 1995. Medical savings accounts: Lessons from Singapore. *Health Affairs* 14, no. 2: 260–266.

Ikegami N., and J.C. Campbell. 2004. Japan's health care system: Containing costs and attempting reform. *Health Affair* 23: 26–36.

Kahn, J.G. et al. 2005. The cost of health insurance administration in California: Estimates for insurers, physicians, and hospitals. *Health Affairs* 24, no. 6: 1629–1639.

MacPhee, S. 1996. Reform the watchword as OECD countries struggle to contain health care costs. *Canadian Medical Association Journal* 154, no. 5: 699–701.

McClellan, M., and D. Kessler. 1999. A global analysis of technological change in health care: The case of heart attacks. *Health Affairs* 18, no. 3: 250–257.

McGuire, T.G., and M.V. Pauly. 1991. Physician response to fee changes with multiple payers. *Journal of Health Economics* 10, no. 4: 385–410.

National Association of Community Health Centers (NACHC). 2006. *A sketch of community health centers: Chart book, 2006.* Washington, DC: NACHC.

National Center for Health Statistics. 2006. *Health, United States, 2006: With chartbook on trends in the health of Americans.* Hyattsville, MD: Department of Health and Human Services.

National Health and Hospitals Reform Commission. 2010. *A Healthier Future for All Australians— Final Report June 2009.* Commonwealth of Australia. http://www.yourhealth.gov.au/internet/yourhealth/publishing.nsf/Content/nhhrc-report-toc. Accessed April 22, 2011.

Naylor, C.D. 1999. Health care in Canada: Incrementalism under fiscal duress. *Health Affairs* 18, no. 3: 9–26.

Nomura, H., and T. Nakayama. 2005. The Japanese healthcare system. *BMJ* 331: 648–649.

Podger, A. 1999. Reforming the Australian health care system: A government perspective. *Health Affairs* 18, no. 3: 111–113.

Rosen, B. 2003. Israel: Health system review. In: *Health care systems in transition.* S. Tomson and E. Mossialos, eds. Copenhagen: European Observatory on Health Care Systems.

Rosen, B., and S. Merkur. 2009. Israel: Health system review. *Health Systems in Transition* 11: 1–226.

Santerre, R.E., and S.P. Neun. 1996. *Health economics: Theories, insights, and industry studies.* Chicago: Irwin.

Schieber, G., and A. Maeda. 1999. Health care financing and delivery in developing countries. *Health Affairs* 18, no. 3: 193–205.

Singapore Ministry of Health. 2004. *Medisave, Medishield and other subsidy schemes: Overview.* Available at: www.moh.gov.sg/corp/financing/overview.do. Accessed September 2006.

Tsutsui T., and N. Muramatsu. 2007. Japan's universal long-term care system reform of 2005: Containing costs and realizing a vision. *Journal of the American Geriatrics Society* 55: 1458–1463.

US Bureau of Labor Statistics. 2011. *Occupational outlook handbook, 2010–2011.* Available at: http://www.bls.gov/oco/home.htm. Accessed January 2011.

US Census Bureau. 2011. The 2011 Statistical Abstract. Available at: http://www.census.gov/compendia/statab/cats/health_nutrition/health_care_resources.html. Accessed January 2011.

Wagstaff, A. et al. (2009). China's health system and its reform: A review of recent studies. *Health Economics* 18: S7–S23.

Willcox, S. 2001. Promoting private health insurance in Australia. *Health Affairs* 20, no. 3: 152–161.

Wolinsky, F.D. 1988. *The sociology of health: Principles, practitioners, and issues*. 2nd ed. Belmont, CA: Wadsworth Publishing Company.

Yip, W., and W.C. Hsia. (2008). The Chinese health system at a crossroads. *Health Affairs* 27: 460–468.

Yip, W., and A. Mahal. (2008). The health care systems of China and India: Performance and future challenges. *Health Affairs* 27: 921–932.

# PART I

---

# System Foundations

# Chapter 2

# Beliefs, Values, and Health

## Learning Objectives

- To understand the concepts of health and disease
- To examine the determinants of health
- To explore the American beliefs and values related to the delivery of health care
- To appreciate the implications of the meaning of health, its determinants, and beliefs and values for medical care delivery
- To develop a position on the equitable distribution of health care services
- To explore the efforts undertaken to integrate individual and community health
- To understand the basic measures of health status and health services utilization

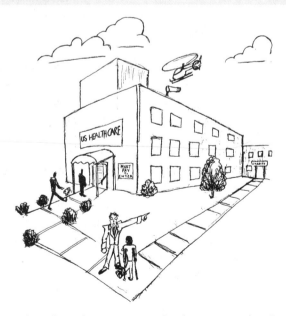

*"This is the market justice system. Social justice is over there."*

# Introduction

From an economic perspective, curative medicine appears to produce decreasing returns in health improvement while increasing health care expenditures (Saward and Sorensen 1980). There has also been a growing recognition of the benefits to society from the promotion of health and prevention of disease, disability, and premature death. However, progress in this direction has been slow because of the prevailing social values and beliefs that still focus on curing diseases rather than promoting health. The common definitions of health, as well as measures for evaluating health status, reflect similar inclinations. This chapter proposes a holistic approach to health, although such an ideal would be quite difficult to fully achieve. For example, it is not easy for a system to enact a change in personal lifestyles and behaviors among the population. Regardless, the health care delivery system must allocate resources and take other measures to bring about a change in course. The 10-year Healthy People initiatives, undertaken by the US Department of Health and Human Services (DHHS) since 1980, illustrate steps taken in this direction, even though these initiatives have been typically strong in rhetoric but weak in actionable strategies or the necessary funding.

Beliefs and values ingrained in the American culture have been influential in laying the foundations of a system that has remained predominantly private, as opposed to a tax-financed national health care program. Discussion on this theme begins in this chapter and continues in Chapter 3, where failures of past proposals to create a nationalized health care system are discussed in the context of cultural beliefs and values. Social norms also help explain how American society views illness and the expectations it has of those who are sick.

This chapter further explores the issue of equity in the distribution of health services, using the contrasting theories of market justice and social justice. The conflict between the principles of market and social justice is reflected throughout US health care delivery. For the most part, strong market justice values prevail, although some components of health care delivery in the United States reflect social justice values. This chapter concludes with an overview of measures commonly used to understand the health status of a population.

# Significance for Managers and Policymakers

Materials covered in this chapter have several implications for health services managers and policymakers: (1) The health status of a population has tremendous bearing on the utilization of health services, assuming the services are readily available. Planning of health services must be governed by demographic and health trends and initiatives toward reducing disease and disability. (2) The basic meaning of health, determinants of health, and health risk appraisal should be used to design appropriate educational, preventive, and therapeutic initiatives. (3) There is a growing emphasis on evaluating the effectiveness of health care organizations based on the contributions they make to community and population health. The concepts discussed in this chapter can guide administrators in implementing programs of most value to their communities. (4) The exercise of justice and equity in making health care available to all Americans remains a lingering concern. This monumental problem requires a joint undertaking from providers, administrators, policymakers, and other key stakeholders. (5) Quantified measures of health status and utilization can be used by managers and policymakers to evaluate the adequacy and effectiveness of existing programs, plan new strategies, measure progress, and discontinue ineffective services.

# Basic Concepts of Health

## Health

In the United States, the concepts of health and health care have largely been governed by the medical model, more specifically referred to as the biomedical model. The *medical model* defines health as the absence of illness or disease. This definition implies that optimum health exists when a person is free of symptoms and does not require medical treatment. However, it is not a definition of health in the true sense but rather a definition of what ill health is not (Wolinsky 1988). This prevailing view of health emphasizes clinical diagnose and medical interventions to treat disease or symptoms of disease, while prevention of disease and health promotion are relegated to a secondary status. Therefore, when the term "health care delivery" is used, in reality it refers to medical care delivery.

Medical sociologists have gone a step further in defining health as the state of optimum capacity of an individual to perform his or her expected social roles and tasks, such as work, school, and doing household chores (Parsons 1972). A person who is unable (as opposed to unwilling) to perform his or her social roles in society is considered sick. However, this concept also tends to view health negatively, because many people continue to engage in their social obligations despite suffering from pain, cough, colds, and other types of temporary disabilities, including mental distress. In other words, a person's engagement in social roles does not necessarily signify that the individual is in optimal health.

An emphasis on both physical and mental dimensions of health is found in the definition of health proposed by the Society for Academic Emergency Medicine, according to which health is "a state of physical and mental well-being that facilitates the achievement of individual and societal goals" (Ethics Committee, Society for Academic Emergency Medicine 1992). This view of health recognizes the importance of achieving harmony between the physiological and emotional dimensions.

The World Health Organization's (WHO) definition of health is most often cited as the ideal for health care delivery systems. WHO defines health as "a state of complete physical, mental and social well-being and not merely the absence of disease or infirmity" (WHO 1948). Since it includes the physical, mental, and social dimensions, WHO's model can be referred to as the biopsychosocial model of health. WHO's definition specifically identifies social well-being as a third dimension of health. In doing so, it emphasizes the importance of positive social relationships. Having a social support network is positively associated with life stresses, self-esteem, and social relations. The social aspects of health also extend beyond the individual level to include responsibility for the health of entire communities and populations. WHO's definition recognizes that optimal health is more than a mere absence of disease or infirmity.

WHO has also defined a health care system as all the activities whose primary purpose is to promote, restore, or maintain health (McKee 2001). As this chapter points out, health care should include much more than medical care. Thus, *health care* can be defined as a variety of services believed to improve a person's health and well-being.

In recent years, there has been a growing interest in *holistic health,* which emphasizes the well-being of every aspect of what makes a person whole and complete. Thus, *holistic medicine* seeks to treat the individual as a whole person (Ward 1995). For example, diagnosis and treatment should take into account the mental, emotional, spiritual, nutritional, environmental, and other factors surrounding the origin of disease (Cohen 2003).

Holistic health incorporates the spiritual dimension as a fourth element—in addition to the physical, mental, and social aspects—as necessary for optimal health (Figure 2–1). A growing volume of medical literature points to the healing effects of a person's religion and spirituality on morbidity and mortality (Levin 1994). Numerous studies point to an inverse association between religious involvement and all-cause mortality (McCullough et al. 2000). Religious and spiritual beliefs and practices have shown a positive impact on a person's physical, mental, and social well-being. These beliefs and practices may affect the incidences, experiences, and outcomes of several common medical problems (Maugans 1996). For instance, people with high levels of general religious involvement are likely to suffer less from depressive symptoms and disorders (McCullough and Larson 1999). Spiritual well-being has also been recognized as an important internal resource for helping people cope with illness. For instance, a study conducted at the University of Michigan found that 93% of the women undergoing cancer treatment indicated that their religious lives helped them sustain their hope (Roberts et al. 1997). Studies have found that a large percentage of patients want their physicians to consider their spiritual needs, and almost half expressed a desire for the physicians to pray with them if they could (see Post et al. 2000). However, many physicians feel that spiritual matters fall outside their expertise or that they would be intruding into patients' private lives. Also, ethical issues and religious coercion are valid concerns, and referral to a chaplain or pastoral leader is often a more appropriate alternative (Post et al. 2000).

The spiritual dimension is frequently tied to one's religious beliefs, values, morals, and practices. Broadly, it is described as meaning, purpose, and fulfillment in life; hope and will to live; faith; and a person's relationship with God (Marwick 1995; Ross 1995; Swanson 1995). A clinically tested scale to measure spiritual well-being included categories such as belief in a power greater than oneself, purpose in life, faith, trust in providence, prayer, meditation, group

Figure 2–1 The Four Dimensions of Holistic Health.

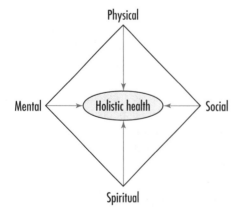

worship, ability to forgive, and gratitude for life (Hatch et al. 1998).

Some of the nation's leading medical schools now offer courses that explore spiritual issues in health care, as well as how to address such issues in patient care delivery (American Physical Therapy Association 1997). Spiritual assessment instruments have been developed to assist physicians and other clinicians in spiritual history taking (Maugans 1996; Puchalski and Romer 2000). The Committee on Religion and Psychiatry of the American Psychological Association has issued a position statement to emphasize the importance of maintaining respect for a patient's religious/spiritual beliefs. For the first time, "religious or spiritual problem" has been included as a diagnostic category in DSM-IV.[1] The holistic approach to health also alludes to the need for incorporating alternative therapies (discussed in Chapter 7) into the predominant medical model.

Tamm (1993) observes that different groups in society—including physicians, nurses, and patients—look at health and disease from partly different vantage points, those that are holistic and those that emphasize illness and disease. Such tensions can have significant implications for the delivery of health services, especially in a pluralistic society such as the United States. Although the medical model plays a key role in the delivery of health care, integration of the concepts of holistic health can optimize well-being and promote early recovery from sickness.

## Quality of Life

The term *quality of life* is used in a denotative sense to capture the essence of overall satisfaction with life during and following a person's encounter with the health care delivery system. Thus, the term is employed in two ways. First, it is an indicator of how satisfied a person is with the experiences while receiving health care. Specific life domains, such as comfort factors, respect, privacy, security, degree of independence, decision-making autonomy, and attention to personal preferences are significant to most people. These factors are now regarded as rights that patients can demand during any type of health care encounter. Second, quality of life can refer to a person's overall satisfaction with life and with self-perceptions of health, particularly after some medical intervention. The implication is that desirable processes during medical treatment and successful outcomes would, subsequently, have a positive effect on an individual's ability to function, carry out social roles and obligations, and have a sense of fulfillment and self-worth.

## Risk Factors and Disease

The occurrence of disease involves more than just a single factor. For example, the mere presence of tubercle bacillus does not mean the infected person will develop tuberculosis. Other factors, such as poverty, overcrowding, and malnutrition, may be essential for development of the disease (Friedman 1980). Hence, tracing *risk factors*—attributes that increase the likelihood of developing a particular disease or negative health condition in the future—requires a broad approach. One useful explanation of disease occurrence (for communicable diseases, in particular) is provided by the tripartite model, sometimes

[1]*Diagnostic and Statistical Manual of Mental Disorders* is the most widely recognized system of classifying mental disorders.

Figure 2–2  The Epidemiology Triangle.

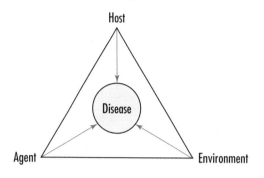

referred to as the Epidemiology[2] Triangle (Figure 2–2). Of the three entities in this model, the *host* is the organism—generally, a human—that becomes sick. Factors associated with the host include genetic make-up, level of immunity, fitness, and personal habits and behaviors. However, for the host to become sick, an *agent* must be present, although presence of an agent does not en-sure that disease will occur. In the previous example, tubercle bacillus is the agent for tuberculosis. Other examples are chemical agents, radiation, tobacco smoke, dietary indiscretions, and nutritional deficiencies. The third entity, *environment*, is external to the host and includes the physical, so-cial, cultural, and economic aspects of the environment. Examples include sanitation, air pollution, cultural beliefs, social equity, social norms, and economic status. The en-vironmental factors play a moderating role that can either enhance or reduce suscepti-bility to disease. Because the three entities often interact to produce disease, disease prevention efforts should focus on a broad approach to mitigate or eliminate risk fac-tors associated with all three entities.

---

[2]Epidemiology is the study of the nature, cause, control, and determinants of the frequency and distribution of disease, dis-ability, and death in human populations (Timmreck 1994, 2).

## Behavioral Risk Factors

Certain individual behaviors and personal lifestyle choices represent important risk factors for illness and disease. For example, smoking has been identified as the leading cause of preventable disease and death in the United States, because it significantly increases the risk of heart disease, stroke, lung cancer, and chronic lung disease (DHHS 2004). Substance abuse, inadequate physical exercise, a high-fat diet, irrespon-sible use of motor vehicles, and unsafe sex are additional examples of behavioral risk factors. (Table 2–1 presents the percentage of the US population with selected behav-ioral risks.)

## Acute, Subacute, and Chronic Conditions

Disease can be classified as acute, subacute, or chronic. An *acute condition* is relatively severe, episodic (of short duration), and of-ten treatable and subject to recovery. Treat-ments are generally provided in a hospital. Examples of acute conditions are a sudden interruption of kidney function or a myo-cardial infarction (heart attack). A *subacute condition* is a less severe phase of an acute illness. It can be a postacute condition, re-quiring treatment after discharge from a hospital. Examples include ventilator and head trauma care. A *chronic condition* is one that persists over time, is not severe, but is generally irreversible. A chronic con-dition may be kept under control through appropriate medical treatment, but if left untreated, the condition may lead to severe and life-threatening health problems. Exam-ples of chronic conditions are hypertension, asthma, arthritis, heart disease, and diabe-tes. Contributors to chronic disease include ethnic, cultural, and behavioral factors and

Table 2–1  Percentage of US Population with Behavioral Risks

| Behavioral Risks | Percentage of Population | Year |
|---|---|---|
| Alcohol (12 years and over) | 51.1 | 2007 |
| Marijuana (12 years and over) | 5.8 | 2007 |
| Cocaine use (12th graders) | 1.9 | 2008 |
| Cocaine use (10th graders) | 1.2 | 2008 |
| Cocaine use (8th graders) | 0.8 | 2008 |
| Cigarette smoking (18 years and over) | 19.7 | 2007 |
| Hypertension (20 years and over) | 31.3 | 2003–06 |
| Overweight (20–74 years) | 66.9 | 2003–06 |
| Serum cholesterol (20 years and over) | 15.6 | 2005–06 |

*Note:* Data are based on household interviews of a sample of the civilian noninstitutionalized population 12 years of age and over in the coterminous United States.

*Source:* Data from National Center for Health Statistics. *Health, United States, 2009.* Hyattsville, MD: Department of Health and Human Services, 2010, pp. 276, 281, 283, 292, 293, 301.

the social and physical environment, discussed later in this chapter.

In the United States, chronic diseases have become the leading cause of death and disability. According to the Centers for Disease Control and Prevention (CDC), almost 50% of Americans have at least one chronic illness, and 7 out of every 10 deaths are attributable to chronic disease (CDC 2010a). Among both the younger and older age groups (ages 18 and up), hypertension was ranked the most common chronic condition, followed by cholesterol disorders. Among children up to age 17, respiratory diseases and asthma were the most common chronic conditions (Agency for Healthcare Research and Quality 2006). The incidence of childhood chronic diseases has almost quadrupled over the past four decades, mostly due to a threefold increase in childhood obesity (PFCD 2009).

It is estimated that 75% of total health expenditures in the United States are attributable to the treatment of chronic conditions (PFCD 2009). In 2007, total health care costs associated with the treatment of chronic diseases were approximately $1.7 trillion. In addition, health disparities continue to be a serious threat to the health and well-being of some population groups. For example, African American, Hispanic, American Indian, and Alaskan Native adults are twice as likely as white adults to have diabetes (CDC 2010a).

There are three main reasons behind the rise of chronic conditions in the US population: (1) New diagnostic methods, medical procedures, and pharmaceuticals have significantly improved the treatment of acute illnesses, survival rates, and longevity, but these achievements have come at the consequence of a larger number of people living with chronic conditions. The prevalence of chronic disease is expected to continue to rise with an aging population and longer life expectancy. (2) Screening and diagnosis have expanded in scope, frequency, and accuracy (Robert Wood Johnson Foundation 2010). (3) Lifestyle choices, such as high-salt and high-fat diets and sedentary lifestyles, are risk factors that contribute to the development of chronic conditions. To address these issues, the DHHS launched a comprehensive initiative with the aid of $650 million allocated under the American Recovery and Reinvestment Act of 2009. The goal of this initiative—Communities Putting Prevention to Work—is to "reduce risk factors, prevent/delay chronic disease, promote wellness in children and adults, and provide positive, sustainable health change in communities" (DHHS 2010a).

## Health Promotion and Disease Prevention

A program of health promotion and disease prevention is built on three main principles: (1) An understanding of risk factors associated with host, agent, and/or environment. Risk factors and their health consequences are evaluated through a process called *health risk appraisal.* Only when the risk factors and their health consequences are known can interventions be developed to help individuals adopt healthier lifestyles. (2) Interventions for counteracting the key risk factors include two main approaches: (a) behavior modification geared toward the goal of adopting healthier lifestyles and (b) therapeutic interventions. Both are discussed in the next paragraph. (3) Adequate public health and social services, as discussed later in this chapter, include all health-related services designed

to minimize risk factors and their negative effects in order to prevent disease, control disease outbreaks, and contain the spread of infectious agents. The goal of public health is to maximize the health of a population.

Various avenues can be used for motivating individuals to alter behaviors that may contribute to disease, disability, or death. Behavior can be modified through educational programs and incentives directed at specific high-risk populations. In the case of cigarette smoking, for example, health promotion aims at building people's knowledge, attitudes, and skills to avoid or quit smoking. It also involves reducing advertisements and other environmental enticements that promote nicotine addiction. Financial incentives, such as a higher cigarette tax, are used to discourage purchase of cigarettes.

Therapeutic interventions fall into three areas of preventive effort: primary prevention, secondary prevention, and tertiary prevention. *Primary prevention* refers to activities undertaken to reduce the probability that a disease will develop in the future (Kane 1988). Its objective is to restrain the development of a disease or negative health condition before it occurs. Therapeutic intervention would include community health efforts to assist patients in smoking cessation and exercise programs to prevent conditions such as lung cancer and heart disease. Teen driver education can prevent disability and death from auto accidents. Safety training and practices can reduce serious workplace injuries. Prenatal care is known to lower infant mortality rates. Immunization has had a greater impact on prevention against childhood diseases and mortality reduction than any other public health intervention besides clean water (Plotkin and Plotkin 1999). Hand washing, refrigeration of foods, garbage collection, sewage treatment, and protection of the water sup-ply are also examples of primary prevention (Timmreck 1994). There have been numer-ous incidents where emphasis on food safety and proper cooking could have prevented out-breaks of potentially deadly episodes, such as those caused by E. coli.

*Secondary prevention* refers to early detection and treatment of disease. Health screenings and periodic health examina-tions are just two examples. The main ob-jective of secondary prevention is to block the progression of a disease or an injury from developing into an impairment or dis-ability (Timmreck 1994). Screening tests, such as hypertension screening, Pap smears, and mammograms, have been instrumental in prescribing early treatment.

*Tertiary prevention* refers to interven-tions that could prevent complications from chronic conditions and prevent further ill-ness, injury, or disability. For example, reg-ular turning of bed-bound patients prevents pressure sores; rehabilitation therapies can prevent permanent disability; and infection control practices in hospitals and nursing homes are designed to prevent *iatrogenic illnesses*, that is, illnesses or injuries caused by the process of health care.

As shown in Table 2–2, prevention, early detection, and treatment efforts helped reduce cancer mortality quite significantly between 1991 and 2007. This decrease was the first sustained decline since record keep-ing was instituted in the 1930s. The decline in breast cancer has been credited to early detection and treatment advances. The drop in cervical cancer has been attributed to the widespread use of Pap screening. Later data, however, show that the declines in cancer death rates are moderating, most likely due to other factors, such as aging.

Table 2–2  Annual Percent Decline in US Cancer Mortality 1991–2007

| Type of Cancer | 1991–95 | 1994–2003 | 1998–2007 |
|---|---|---|---|
| All cancers | 3.0 | 1.1 | 1.4 |
| Breast cancer | 6.3 | 2.5 | 2.2 |
| Cervical cancer | 9.7 | 3.6 | 2.6 |
| Ovarian cancer | 4.8 | 0.5 | 0.8 |
| Prostate cancer | 6.3 | 3.5 | 3.1 |

*Source:* Data from National Center for Health Statistics of the Centers for Disease Control and Prevention, National Cancer Institute, SEER Cancer Statistics Review, 1975–2007.

## Promotion of Developmental Health

*Development* refers to growth in skill and capacity to function normally (Hancock and Mandle 1994). Early childhood develop-ment influences a person's health in later years. The foundations laid in the early years often determine the individual's fu-ture adjustments to life (Berger 1988) and shape individual behaviors. Children who fail to acquire certain skills in childhood of-ten have real difficulties as adults (Wynder and Orlandi 1984). The importance of early childhood development has important im-plications for health services delivery in two main areas: (1) Expectant mothers need adequate prenatal care. The health promo-tion needs of the expectant mother and the fetus are so closely intertwined that the two must be considered one unit (Hancock and Mandle 1994). (2) Adequate child care is needed, especially during the first few years of growth. Immunization, nutrition, family and social interaction, and health care are key developmental elements until a child reaches adulthood. Preventable developmental disabilities impose an undue burden on the health care delivery system.

# Public Health

Public health remains poorly understood by its prime beneficiaries, the public. For some people, public health evokes images of a massive social enterprise or welfare system. To others, the term means health care services for everyone. Still another image of public health is that of a body of knowledge and techniques that can be applied to health-related problems (Turnock 1997). However, none of these ideas adequately reflects what public health is.

The Institute of Medicine (IOM) proposed that the mission of public health is to fulfill "society's interest in assuring conditions in which people can be healthy" (IOM 1988). *Public health* deals with broad societal concerns about ensuring conditions that promote optimum health for the society as a whole. It involves the application of scientific knowledge to counteract disease outbreaks and protect the general population.

Three main distinctions can be seen between the practices of medicine and public health: (1) Medicine focuses on the individual patient—diagnosing symptoms, treating and preventing disease, relieving pain and suffering, and maintaining or restoring normal function. Public health, conversely, focuses on populations (Lasker 1997). (2) The emphases in modern medicine are on the biological causes of disease and developing treatments and therapies. Public health focuses on identifying the environmental, social, and behavioral risk factors that cause disease and on developing and implementing population-wide interventions to minimize those risk factors (Peters et al. 2001). (3) Medicine focuses on the treatment of disease and recovery of health, whereas public health deals with various efforts to prevent disease and promote health.

To promote and protect society's interest in health and well-being, public health activities can range from providing education on nutrition to passing laws that enhance automobile safety. For example, public health includes dissemination to the public and to health professionals of timely and appropriate information about important health issues, particularly when communicable diseases pose potential threats to large segments of a population.

Compared to the delivery of medical services, public health involves a broader range of professionals. The medical sector encompasses physicians, nurses, dentists, therapists, social workers, psychologists, nutritionists, health educators, pharmacists, laboratory technicians, health services administrators, and so forth. In addition to these professionals, public health also involves professionals such as sanitarians, epidemiologists, statisticians, industrial hygienists, environmental health specialists, food and drug inspectors, toxicologists, and economists (Lasker 1997).

## Health Protection and Environmental Health

Health protection is one of the main public health functions. In the 1850s, John Snow successfully traced the risk of cholera outbreaks in London to the Broad Street water pump (Rosen 1993). Since then, *environmental health* has specifically dealt with preventing the spread of disease through water, air, and food (Schneider 2000). Environmental health science, along with other public health measures, was instrumental in reducing the risk of infectious diseases during the 1900s. For example, in 1900, pneumonia, tuberculosis, and diarrhea, along with enteritis, were the top three killers in the United States (CDC 1999); that is no longer the case today (see Table 2–3). With the rapid industrialization during the 20th century, environmental health faced new challenges, due to serious health hazards from chemicals, industrial waste, infectious waste, radiation, asbestos, and other toxic substances.

## Health Protection During Global Pandemics

In 2003, to prevent the introduction, transmission, and spread of severe acute respiratory syndrome (SARS)—a contagious disease that is accompanied by fever and symptoms of pneumonia or other respiratory illness—the White House designated SARS a communicable disease for the apprehension, detention, or conditional release of individuals with the disease.

The global threat of avian influenza has also solicited a public health and government response. The CDC launched a website dedicated to educating the public about avian influenza, how it is spread, and past and current outbreaks. The website contains specific information for health professionals, travelers, the poultry industry, state departments of health, and people with possible exposures to avian influenza (CDC 2007).

After a novel H1N1 influenza virus emerged from Mexico in early April 2009, the first H1N1 influenza patient in the United States was confirmed by CDC on April 15, 2009 (DHHS 2009). Although US

**Table 2–3** Leading Causes of Death, 2006

| Cause of Death | Deaths | Percentage |
| --- | --- | --- |
| All causes | 2,426,264 | 100.0 |
| Diseases of the heart | 631,636 | 26.0 |
| Malignant neoplasms | 559,888 | 23.1 |
| Cerebrovascular diseases | 137,119 | 5.7 |
| Chronic lower respiratory diseases | 124,583 | 5.1 |
| Unintentional injuries | 121,599 | 5.0 |
| Diabetes mellitus | 72,449 | 3.0 |
| Alzheimer's disease | 56,326 | 2.3 |
| Influenza and pneumonia | 72,432 | 3.0 |
| Nephritis, nephrotic syndrome, and nephrosis | 45,344 | 1.9 |
| Septicemia | 34,234 | 1.4 |

*Source:* Data from National Center for Health Statistics. *Health, United States, 2009.* Hyattsville, MD: Department of Health and Human Services, 2010, p. 198.

health officials anticipated and prepared for an influenza pandemic, the H1N1 virus had strained the response capabilities of the public health system. The virus affected every US state, and Americans were left unprotected in the outbreak, due to unavailability of antiviral medications. On April 26, 2009, DHHS declared a nationwide Public Health Emergency (PHE), which enabled the Food and Drug Administration (FDA) to issue Emergency Use Authorizations (EUAs) for certain antiviral medications, such as Tamiflu, Relenza, and Peramivir IV, in vitro diagnostic devices, and respiratory protection products (DHHS 2009). As of July 24, 2009, CDC reported 43,771 confirmed and probable cases, with 5,011 hospitalizations and 302 deaths (DHHS 2009).

# Bioterrorism and Disaster Preparedness

Since the horrific events of what is now commonly referred to as 9/11 (September 11, 2001), America has opened a new chapter in health protection. As the nation was still recovering from the shock of the attacks on New York's World Trade Center, attempts to disseminate anthrax through the US Postal Service were discovered. In June 2002, former President Bush signed into law the Public Health Security and Bioterrorism Response Act of 2002. The term *bioterrorism* encompasses the use of chemical, biological, and nuclear agents to cause harm to relatively large civilian populations. Dealing with such a threat requires large-scale preparations, which include appropriate tools and training for workers in medical care, public health, emergency care, and civil defense agencies at the federal, state, and local levels. It requires national initiatives to develop countermeasures, such as new vaccines, a

robust public health infrastructure, and coordination among numerous agencies. It requires an infrastructure to handle large numbers of casualties and isolation facilities for contagious patients. Hospitals, public health agencies, and civil defense must be linked together through information systems. Containment of infectious agents, such as smallpox, would require quick detection, treatment, isolation, and organized efforts to protect the unaffected population. Rapid cleanup, evacuation of the affected population, and transfer of victims to medical care facilities require detailed plans and logistics.

The Homeland Security Act of 2002, signed into law in November 2002 by the Bush Administration, created the Department of Homeland Security (DHS) and called for a major restructuring of the nation's resources with the primary mission of helping prevent, protect against, and respond to any acts of terrorism in the United States. It also provided better tools to contain attacks on the food and water supplies; protect the nation's vital infrastructures, such as nuclear facilities; and track biological materials anywhere in the United States.

Over the past several years, the United States has witnessed unprecedented efforts to prepare for and respond to natural and man-made disasters. Following the creation of DHS in 2002 and the establishment of the National Incident Management System (NIMS) and the National Response Framework (NRF) in 2008, the nation confronted major natural disasters, such as hurricanes Katrina, Rita, and Wilma in 2005. In December 2006, President Bush signed the Pandemic and All-Hazards Preparedness Act (PAHPA) "to improve the nation's public health and medical preparedness and response capabilities for emergencies, whether deliberate, accidental, or natural" (DHHS

2010b). The Act authorized a new Assistant Secretary for Preparedness and Response (ASPR) within DHHS and called for the establishment of a quadrennial National Health Security Strategy (NHSS), with specific planning provisions that included National Preparedness Goal implementation and the Strategic National Stockpile (SNS).

In 2007, in response to a call from Homeland Security Presidential Directive 21 to enhance the nation's ability to detect and respond to health-related threats, CDC and DHHS developed the National Biosurveillance Strategy for Human Health. Six priority areas were established: electronic health information exchange, electronic laboratory information exchange, unstructured data, integrated biosurveillance information, global disease detection and collaboration, and biosurveillance workforce. A progress report shows that most states and localities have strong biological laboratory capabilities and capacities, with nearly 90% of laboratories in the Laboratory Response Network reachable around the clock (CDC 2010b).

Notable progress has also been made in the detection of hazardous substances. The Hazardous Substances Emergency Event Surveillance system (HSEES), which was established in 1998 to reduce injury and death among first responders, employees, and the general public, tracked 8,150 hazardous substance incidents, 2,290 injuries, and 67 fatalities sustained from hazardous substance incidents. In addition, 606 incidents led to the evacuation of 48,464 people in 14 states in 2008 (CDC 2010b).

## Determinants of Health

*Health determinants* are major factors that, over time, affect the health and well-being of individuals. Individual health eventually determines, at an aggregate level, the health of communities and even larger populations. An understanding of health determinants is necessary for any positive interventions necessary to improve health and longevity at both the individual and population levels.

### Blum's Model of Health Determinants

In 1974, Blum (1981) proposed an "Environment of Health" model, later called the "Force Field and Well-Being Paradigms of Health" (Figure 2–3). Blum proposed four major inputs that contributed to health and well-being. These main influences (called "force fields") are environment, lifestyle, heredity, and medical care, all of which must be considered simultaneously when addressing the health status of an individual or a population. In other words, there is no single pathway to better health, because health determinants interact in complex ways. Consequently, improvement in health requires a multipronged approach.

The four wedges in Figure 2–3 represent the four major force fields. The size of each wedge signifies its relative importance. Thus, the most important force field, according to this model, is environment, followed by lifestyles and heredity. Medical care has the least impact on health and well-being.

### Environment

Environmental factors encompass the physical, socioeconomic, sociopolitical, and sociocultural dimensions. Among physical environmental factors are air pollution, food and water contaminants, radiation, toxic chemicals, wastes, disease vectors, safety hazards, and habitat alterations.

Figure 2–3 The Force Field and Well-Being Paradigms of Health.

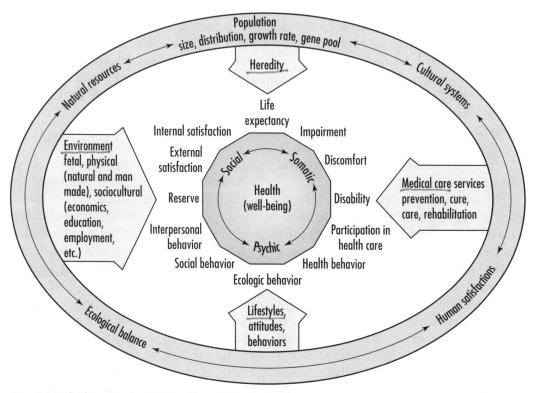

The relationship of socioeconomic status (SES) to health and well-being may be explained by the general likelihood that people who have better education also have higher incomes. They live in better homes and locations where they are less exposed to environmental risks. They have better access to health care and are more likely to avoid risky behaviors, such as smoking and drug abuse. The greater the economic gap between the rich and the poor in a given geographic area, the worse the health status of the population in that area is likely to be. It has been suggested that wide income gaps produce less social cohesion, greater psychosocial stress, and, consequently, poorer

health (Wilkinson 1997). For example, social cohesion—characterized by a hospitable social environment in which people trust each other and participate in communal activities—is linked to lower overall mortality and better self-rated health (Kawachi et al. 1997, 1999). Researchers have postulated that a political and policy context that creates income inequality is a precursor to health inequalities (Dye 1991). However, even countries with national health insurance programs, such as Britain, Australia, Denmark, and Sweden, experience persistent and widening disparities in health according to socioeconomic status (Pincus et al. 1998). The joint relationship of income inequality and availability of primary care has also been found to be significantly associated with individuals' self-rated health status (Shi et al. 2002).

The relationship between education and health status has been well established. Less educated Americans die younger, compared to their better educated counterparts. Unemployment may affect social health because of reduced social functioning; mental health because of increased levels of stress; and physical health due to various stress-related illnesses. Pincus and colleagues (1998) proposed that poor health in sociologically disadvantaged populations results more from unfavorable social conditions and ineffective self-management than from limitations in access to medical care.

The environment can also have a significant influence on developmental health. It has been shown, for example, that children who are isolated and do not socialize much with their peers tend to be overrepresented in groups of delinquents and adults with mental health problems (Wynder and Orlandi 1984). Research points out that the experiences that children have and the way adults interact with them in early years have a major impact on children's mental and emotional development. Neuroscientists have found that good nurturing and stimulation in the first 3 years of life—a prime time for brain development—activate neural pathways in the brain that might otherwise atrophy and may even permanently increase the number of brain cells. Hence, the importance of quality of child care provided in the first 3 years of life is monumental (Shellenbarger 1997).

## ②Lifestyle

Lifestyle, or behavioral risk factors, were previously discussed. This section provides

some illustrations of how lifestyle factors are related to health. Studies have shown that diet and foods, for example, play a major role in most of the significant health problems of today. Heart disease, diabetes, stroke, and cancer are but some of the diseases with direct links to dietary choices. Throughout the world, incidence and mortality rates for many forms of cancer are rising. Yet research has clearly indicated that a significant portion of cancer is preventable. The role of diet and nutrition in cancer prevention has been one of the most exciting and promising research areas over the past few years. Researchers estimated that 40 to 60% of all cancers, and as many as 35% of cancer deaths, are linked to diet (American Institute for Cancer Research 1996). Current research also shows that a diet rich in fruits, vegetables, and low-fat dairy foods, and with reduced saturated and total fat, can substantially lower blood pressure (see, for example, the DASH Eating Plan recommended by DHHS; available at http://www.nhlbi.nih.gov/health/public/heart/hbp/dash/new_dash.pdf as of April 2011). Thus, a nutritional approach can be effective in both preventing and treating hypertension and other diseases. The role of exercise and physical activity as a potentially useful, effective, and acceptable method for reducing the risk of colon cancer is also significant (Macfarlane and Lowenfels 1994). Research findings have also confirmed the association between recreational and/or occupational physical activity and a reduced risk of colon cancer (White et al. 1996).

## ③ Heredity

Genetic factors predispose individuals to certain diseases. For example, cancer occurs when the body's healthy genes lose their ability to suppress malignant growth or when other genetic processes stop working properly, although this does not mean that cancer is entirely a disease of the genes (Davis and Webster 2002).

A person can do little about the genetic makeup he or she has inherited. However, lifestyles and behaviors that a person may currently engage in can have significant influences on future progeny. Advances in gene therapy hold the promise of treating a variety of inherited or acquired diseases.

## Medical Care

Even though the other three factors are more important in the determination of health, well-being, and susceptibility to premature death, medical care is, nevertheless, a key determinant of health. Both individual and population health are closely related to having access to adequate preventive and curative health care services. Despite the fact that medical care, compared to the other three factors, has the least impact on health and well-being, Americans' attitudes toward health improvement focus on more medical research, development of new medical technology, and spending more on high-tech medical care. Yet, significant declines in mortality rates were achieved well before the modernization of Western medicine and the escalation in medical care expenditures.

The availability of primary care may be one alternative pathway through which income inequality influences population-level health outcomes. Shi and colleagues (1999, 2001) examined the joint relationships among income inequality, availability of primary care, and certain health indicators. The results suggest that access to primary care physicians, in addition to income inequality, significantly correlates with reduced mortality, increased life expectancy, and improved birth outcome. In the United States, individuals living in states with a higher primary care physician-to-population ratio are more likely to report good health than those living in states with a lower ratio (Shi et al. 2002).

## Contemporary Models of Health Determinants

Although Blum's model lays the foundation for understanding the determinants of health and wellness, more recent models have built upon this foundation. For example, the model proposed by Dahlgren and Whitehead (2006) states that age, sex, and genetic makeup are fixed factors, but other factors in the surrounding layers can be modified to positively influence population health. Individual lifestyle factors have the potential to promote or damage health, and social interactions can sustain people's health; but living and working conditions; food supplies; access to essential goods and services; and the overall economic, cultural, and environmental conditions have wider influences on individual and population health.

Ansari and colleagues (2003) proposed a public health model of the social determinants of health in which the determinants are categorized into four major groups: social determinants, health care system attributes, disease inducing behaviors, and health outcomes (Ansari et al. 2003).

The WHO Commission on Social Determinants of Health (WHOCSDH) (2007) concluded that "the social conditions in which people are born, live, and work are the single most important determinant of one's health status." The WHO model provides a conceptual framework for understanding the socioeconomic and political contexts; structural determinants; intermediary determinants (including material circumstances,

Figure 2–4  WHO Commission on Social Determinants of Health Conceptual Framework.

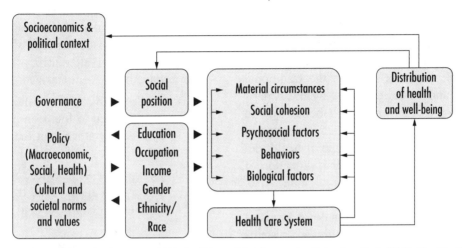

*Source:* Centers for Disease Control and Prevention. 2010. *Establishing a Holistic Framework to Reduce Inequities in HIV, Viral Hepatitis, STDs, and Tuberculosis in the United States.*

social-environmental circumstances, behavioral and biological factors, social cohesion, and the health care system); and the impact on health equity and well-being measured as health outcomes.

In the United States, government agencies, such as CDC and DHHS, have recognized the need to address health inequities. CDC's National Center for HIV/AIDS, Viral Hepatitis, STD, and TB Prevention adopted the WHO framework on social determinants of health to use as a guide for its activities (see Figure 2–4). The Patient Protection and Affordable Care Act of 2010 and Healthy People 2020 also focus on health determinants that may create new opportunities to apply a comprehensive approach to address health disparities.

### Overarching Factors and Implications for Health Care Delivery

The force fields illustrated in Blum's model (Figure 2–3) are affected by broad national and international factors, such as a nation's population characteristics, natural resources, ecological balance, human satisfactions, and cultural systems. Among these factors, type of health care delivery system can also be included. In the United States, the preponderance of health care expenditures is devoted to the treatment of medical conditions rather than to the prevention and control of factors that produce those medical conditions in the first place. This misdirection can be traced to the conflicts that often result from the beliefs and values ingrained in the American culture.

## Cultural Beliefs and Values

A value system orients the members of a society toward defining what is desirable for that society. It has been observed that even a society as complex and highly differentiated as in the United States can be said to have a relatively well-integrated system of institutionalized common values at the societal level (Parsons 1972). Although such a view may still prevail, American society now has several different subcultures that have grown in size due to a steady influx of immigrants from different parts of the world.

The current system of health services delivery traces its roots to the traditional beliefs and values espoused by the American people. The value and belief system governs the training and general orientation of health care providers, type of health delivery settings, financing and allocation of resources, and access to health care. Also, beliefs and values have historically led Americans to oppose any major reforms of the health care system. Health care systems in other countries also reflect deeply rooted beliefs and values. For example, Canadians prefer increased spending on health and social programs to receiving a tax cut from the government. Conversely, Americans are skeptical of any heavy-handed government involvement in the health care system.

Some of the main beliefs and values predominant in the American culture are outlined as follows:

1. A strong belief in the advancement of science and the application of scientific methods to medicine were instrumental in creating the medical model that primarily governs health care delivery in the United States. In turn, the medical model has fueled the tremendous growth in medical science and technological innovation. As a result, the United States has been leading the world in medical breakthroughs. These developments have had numerous implications for health services delivery:

    a. They increase the demand for the latest treatments and raise patients' expectations for finding cures.

    b. Medical professionals have been preoccupied, almost exclusively, with clinical interventions, whereas the holistic aspects of health and use of alternative therapies have been deemphasized.

    c. Health care professionals have been trained to focus on physical symptoms rather than the underlying causes of disease.

    d. Few attempts have been made to integrate diagnosis and treatment with health education and disease prevention.

    e. The concern with diseases has funneled most research efforts away from the pursuit of health into development of sophisticated medical technology. Commitment of resources to the preservation and enhancement of health and well-being has lagged far behind.

    f. Medical specialists, using the latest technology, are held in higher esteem and earn higher incomes than general practitioners and health educators.

    g. The desirability of health care delivery institutions, such as hospitals, is often evaluated by their acquisition of advanced technology.

    h. Whereas biomedicine has taken central stage, diagnosis and treatment of mental health have been relegated to a lesser status.

    i. The biomedical model has isolated the social and spiritual elements of health.

2. America has been a champion of capitalism. Due to a strong belief in capitalism, health care has largely

been viewed as an economic good (or service), not as a public resource.

3. A culture of capitalism promotes entrepreneurial spirit and self-determination. Hence, individual capabilities to obtain health services have largely determined the production and consumption of health care—which services will be produced, where and in what quantity, and who will have access to those services. Some key implications are:

   a. Financing of health care largely through private health insurance has made access to health care a social privilege.

   b. A clear distinction exists between the types of services for poor and affluent communities and between those in rural and urban locations.

   c. The culture of individualism emphasizes individual health rather than population health. Medical practice, therefore, has been directed at keeping the individual healthy rather than keeping the entire community healthy.

4. A concern for the most underprivileged classes in society—the poor, the elderly, the disabled, and children—led to the creation of the public programs Medicare, Medicaid, and CHIP.

5. Principles of free enterprise and a general distrust of big government have kept the delivery of health care largely in private hands. Hence, a separation also exists between public health functions and the private practice of medicine.

# Equitable Distribution of Health Care

Scarcity of economic resources is a central economic concept. From this perspective, health care can be viewed as an economic good. Two fundamental questions arise with regard to how scarce health care resources ought to be used: (1) How much health care should be produced? (2) How should health care be distributed? The first question concerns the appropriate combination in which health services ought to be produced in relation to all other goods and services in the overall economy. If more health care is produced, a society may have to do less with some other goods, such as food, clothing, and transportation. The second question affects individuals at a more personal level. It deals with who can receive which type of medical service, and how access to services will be restricted.

The production, distribution, and subsequent consumption of health care must be perceived as equitable. No society has found a perfectly equitable method to distribute limited economic resources. In fact, any method of resource distribution leaves some inequalities. Societies, therefore, try to allocate resources according to some guiding principles acceptable to each society. Such principles are ingrained in a society's value and belief system. It is recognized that not everyone can receive everything medical science has to offer. The fundamental question that deals with distributive justice or equity is who should receive the medical goods and services that society produces (Santerre and Neun 1996). By extension, this basic question about equity includes not only who should receive medical care but also which type of services and in what quantity.

A just and fair allocation of health care poses conceptual and practical difficulties; hence, a theory of justice needs to resolve the problem of health care allocation (Jonsen 1986). The principle of justice derives from ethical theories, especially those advanced by John Rawls, who defined justice as fairness (Darr 1991). Even though various ethical principles can be used to guide decisions pertaining to just and fair allocation of health care in individual circumstances, the broad concern about equitable access to health services is addressed by the theories referred to as market justice and social justice. These two contrasting theories govern the production and distribution of health care services.

## Market Justice

The principle of *market justice* ascribes the fair distribution of health care to the market forces in a free economy. Medical care and its benefits are distributed based on people's willingness and ability to pay (Santerre and Neun 1996). In other words, people are entitled to purchase a share of the available goods and services that they value. They are to purchase these valued goods and services by means of wealth acquired through their own legitimate efforts. This is how most goods and services are distributed in a free market. The free market implies that giving people something they have not earned would be morally and economically wrong.

Chapter 1 discussed several characteristics that describe a free market. Those market characteristics are a precondition to the distribution of health care services according to market justice principles. It should be added that health care in the United States is not delivered in a free market; rather it is delivered in a quasi-market (see Chapter 1). Hence, market justice principles are only

partially applicable to the US health care delivery system. Distribution of health care according to market justice is based on the following key assumptions:

- Health care is like any other economic good or service, the distribution and consumption of which are determined by free market forces of supply and demand.

- Individuals are responsible for their own achievements. From the rewards of their achievements, people are free to obtain various economic goods and services, including health care. When individuals pursue their own best interests, the interests of society as a whole are best served (Ferguson and Maurice 1970).

- People make rational choices in their decisions to purchase health care products and services. People demand health care because it can rectify a health problem and restore health, can reduce pain and discomfort and make people feel better, and can reduce anxiety about their health and well-being. Therefore, people are willing to purchase health care services. Grossman (1972) proposed that health is also an investment commodity. People consider the purchase of health services as an investment. For example, the investment has a monetary payoff when it reduces the number of sick days, making extra time available for productive activities, such as earning a living. Or it can have a utility payoff—a payoff in terms of satisfaction—when it makes life more enjoyable and fulfilling.

- People, in consultation with their physicians, know what is best for them. This assumption implies that people place a certain degree of trust in their physicians and that the physician–patient relationship is ongoing.

- The marketplace works best with minimum interference from the government. In other words, the market, rather than the government, can allocate health care resources in the most efficient and equitable manner.

The classical ethical theory known as *deontology* may be applied to market justice. Deontology asserts that it is an individual's duty (from the Greek word "deon") to do what is right. The results are not important. Deontology emphasizes individual responsibilities, as in a physician–patient relationship. A physician is duty bound to do whatever is necessary to restore a patient's health. The patient is responsible for compensating the physician for his or her services. The destitute and poor may be served by charity, but deontology largely tends to ignore the importance of societal good. It does not address what responsibilities people have toward the society.

Market justice may also be associated with the libertarian view that equity is achieved when resources are distributed according to merits. That is, health care should be distributed according to minimum standards and financed according to willingness to pay. According to this view, equality in health status need not be a central priority (Starfield 1998).

Under market justice, the production of health care is determined by how much the consumers are willing and able to purchase at the prevailing market prices. It follows that, in a free market system, individuals without sufficient income face a financial barrier to obtaining health care (Santerre and Neun 1996). Thus, prices and ability to pay ration the quantity and type of health

care services people consume. The uninsured and those who lack sufficient income to pay privately face barriers to obtaining health care. Such limitations to obtaining health care are referred to as "rationing by ability to pay" (Feldstein 1994), *demand-side rationing*, or price rationing.

The key characteristics and their implications under the system of market justice are summarized in Table 2–4. Market justice emphasizes individual, rather than collective, responsibility for health. It proposes private, rather than government, solutions to social problems of health.

## Social Justice

The idea of social justice is at odds with the principles of capitalism and market justice. The term "social justice" was invented in the 19th century by the critics of capitalism to describe the "good society" (Kristol 1978). According to the principle of *social justice*, the equitable distribution of health care is a societal responsibility, which is best achieved by letting a central agency, generally the government, take over the production and distribution of health care. Social justice regards health care as a social good—as opposed to an economic good—that should be collectively financed and available to all citizens regardless of the individual recipient's ability to pay for that care. Canadians and Europeans, for example, long ago reached a broad social consensus that health care is a social good (Reinhardt 1994). Public health also has a social justice orientation (Turnock 1997). Under the social justice system, inability to obtain medical services because of a lack of financial resources is considered inequitable. A just distribution of health care must be based on need, not simply on one's ability to purchase in the marketplace

Table 2–4  Comparison of Market Justice and Social Justice

| Market Justice | Social Justice |
|---|---|
| **Characteristics** | |
| • Views health care as an economic good | • Views health care as a social resource |
| • Assumes free-market conditions for health services delivery | • Requires active government involvement in health services delivery |
| • Assumes that markets are more efficient in allocating health resources equitably | • Assumes that the government is more efficient in allocating health resources equitably |
| • Production and distribution of health care determined by market-based demand | • Medical resource allocation determined by central planning |
| • Medical care distribution based on people's ability to pay | • Ability to pay inconsequential for receiving medical care |
| • Access to medical care viewed as an economic reward of personal effort and achievement | • Equal access to medical services viewed as a basic right |
| **Implications** | |
| • Individual responsibility for health | • Collective responsibility for health |
| • Benefits based on individual purchasing power | • Everyone is entitled to a basic package of benefits |
| • Limited obligation to the collective good | • Strong obligation to the collective good |
| • Emphasis on individual well-being | • Community well-being supersedes that of the individual |
| • Private solutions to social problems | • Public solutions to social problems |
| • Rationing based on ability to pay | • Planned rationing of health care |

(demand). Need for health care is determined either by the patient or by a health professional. The principle of social justice is also based on certain assumptions:

• Health care is different from most other goods and services. Health-seeking behavior is governed primarily by need rather than by ability to pay.

• Responsibility for health is shared. Individuals are not held completely responsible for their condition because factors outside their control may have brought on the condition. Society is held responsible because individuals cannot control certain environmental factors, such as economic inequalities, unemployment, unsanitary conditions, or air pollution.

• Society has an obligation to the collective good. The well-being of the community is superior to that of the individual. An unhealthy individual is a burden on society. A person carrying a deadly infection, for example, is a threat to society. Society, therefore, is obligated to cure the problem by providing health care to the individual because, by doing so, the whole society would benefit.

• The government rather than the market can better decide through rational planning how much health care to produce and how to distribute it among all citizens.

Social justice is consistent with the theory of *utilitarianism*, a teleological principle (from the Greek, "telos," meaning end). Utilitarianism emphasizes happiness and welfare for the masses; it ignores the individual. Society's goal is to achieve the greatest good for the greatest number of people. In this case, the greatest good for the greatest number of people is thought to be achieved when the well-being of the whole community supersedes the well-being of individuals. By implication, the government is thought to distribute health care resources more equitably than the market.

Social justice finds its ethical roots in the egalitarian view that equity is achieved when resources are distributed according to needs. That is, more resources are made available to populations that need more services because of their greater social or health disadvantage (Starfield 1998).

Under social justice, how much health care to produce is determined by the government; however, no country can afford to provide unlimited amounts of health care to all its citizens (Feldstein 1994). The government then also finds ways to limit the availability of certain health care services by deciding, for instance, how technology will be dispersed and who will be allowed access to certain types of high-tech services, even though basic services may be available to all. To distribute limited health care resources, the government engages in *supply-side rationing*, which is also referred to as *planned rationing*, or nonprice rationing. The government makes deliberate attempts, often referred to as "health planning," to limit the supply of health care services, particularly those beyond the basic level of care. It is because of the necessity to ration health care that citizens of a country can be given universal coverage but not universal access (see Chapter 1). Even when a covered individual has a medical need, depending on the nature of health services required, he or she may have to wait until services become available. The main characteristics and implications of social justice are summarized in Table 2–4.

## Justice in the US Health Delivery System

In a quasi- or imperfect market, which characterizes health care delivery in the United States, elements of both market and social justice exist, but the principles of market justice are dominant. In some areas, the principles of market and social justice complement each other. In other areas, the two are in conflict.

### Health Insurance

In a society with strong market justice values, individuals paying for their own care would predominantly finance the medical care system, and a multitude of private health insurance plans would prevail. In a society with strong social justice principles, the government would finance the medical care system through general tax revenues (Long 1994).

In the United States, the principles of market justice and social justice complement each other with private, employer-based health insurance for mainly middle-income Americans (market justice); publicly financed Medicaid, Medicare, and CHIP coverage for certain disadvantaged groups; and workers' compensation for those injured at work (social justice). The Patient Protection and Affordable Care Act is also based on the principles of social justice. The main objectives of this law are threefold: (1) to expand health coverage; (2) to ensure access to quality, affordable health care; and (3) to contain the growth in health care costs through transformations within the health care system (Kaiser Family Foundation 2010).

## Organization of Health Care Delivery

In a market justice-dominant society, the number and type of physicians produced by the educational system are determined by the desires of would-be physicians and their assessment of chances for future success. Physicians themselves decide where they will be located to practice, without necessarily taking into account the needs of the population (Long 1994). Physicians are compensated mostly on a fee-for-service basis, the fees being established by the physicians themselves. Similarly, hospital location and operations are influenced by financial viability without regard to duplication or shortages of services and technology. In a society with strong social justice values, the number, type, and location of physicians and hospitals; reimbursement to providers; and distribution of medical technology are determined by the government, supposedly based on the health needs of the populations.

In the United States, private and government health insurance programs enable the covered populations to access health care services delivered by private practitioners and private institutions (market justice). Tax-supported county and city hospitals, public health clinics, and community health centers can be accessed by the uninsured in areas where such services are available (social justice). Publicly run institutions, generally, operate in large inner cities and certain rural areas. Conflict between the two principles of justice arises in small cities and towns and large rural sections where such services are not available. Medicare and Medicaid make their own determinations on how much is paid for services. These characteristics do not fully harmonize with market justice principles.

## Limitations of Market Justice

The principles of market justice work well in the allocation of economic goods when their unequal distribution does not affect the larger society. For example, based on individual success, people live in different sizes and styles of homes, drive different types of automobiles, and spend their money on a variety of things, but the allocation of certain resources has wider repercussions for society. In these areas, market justice has severe limitations:

1. Market justice principles fail to rectify critical human concerns. Pervasive social problems, such as crime, illiteracy, and homelessness, can significantly weaken the fabric of a society. Indeed, the United States has recognized such issues and instituted programs based on social justice to combat the problems through added police protection, publicly supported education, and subsidized housing for the poor and elderly. Health care is an important social issue because it not only affects human productivity and achievement but also provides basic human dignity.

2. Market justice does not always protect a society. Individual health issues can have negative consequences for society because ill health is not always confined to the individual. The acquired immune deficiency syndrome (AIDS) epidemic is an example in which society can be put at serious risk. Initial spread of the SARS epidemic in Beijing was largely due to patients with SARS symptoms being turned away by hospitals because they were not able to pay in advance for the cost of the treatment. Similar to clean air and water, health care is a social concern that, in the long run, protects against the burden of preventable disease and disability, a burden that is ultimately borne by society.

3. Market justice does not work well in health care delivery. A growing national economy and prosperity in the past did not materially reduce the number of uninsured Americans. On the other hand, the number of uninsured increases during economic downturns. For example, during the 2007–2009 recession, 5 million Americans lost employment-based health insurance (Holahan 2011).

# Integration of Individual and Community Health

It has been recognized that typical emphasis on the treatment of acute illness in hospitals, biomedical research, and high technology has not significantly improved the population's health. Consequently, it has been proposed that the medical model should be replaced with a disease-prevention, health-promotion, primary care-based model (Shortell et al. 1995). More precise, this is a call for integration of the two models rather than a total abandonment of the medical model in favor of another. Society will always need the benefits of modern science and technology for the treatment of disease. Disease prevention, health promotion, and primary care can prevent certain health problems, delay the onset of disease, and prevent disability and premature death. An integrated approach will improve the overall health of the population, enhance people's quality of life, and conserve health care resources.

The real challenge for the health care delivery system is to incorporate the medical and wellness models within the holistic context of health. The Ottawa Charter for Health Promotion, for instance, mentions caring, holism, and ecology as essential issues in developing strategies for health promotion (de Leeuw 1989). "Holism" and "ecology" refer to the complex relationships that exist among the individual; the health care delivery system; and the physical, social, cultural, and economic environmental factors. In addition, as the increasing body of research points out, the spiritual dimension must be incorporated into the integrated model.

Another equally important challenge for the health care delivery system is to focus on both individual and population health outcomes. The nature of health is complex, and the interrelationships among the physical, mental, social, and spiritual dimensions are not well understood. How to translate this multidimensional framework of health into specific actions that are efficiently configured to achieve better individual and community health is the greatest challenge any health care system could possibly face.

Figure 2–5  Integrated Model for Holistic Health.

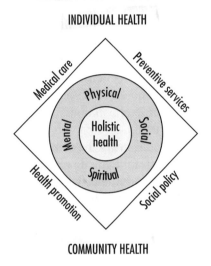

INDIVIDUAL HEALTH

COMMUNITY HEALTH

For an integrated approach to become reality, resource limitations make it necessary to deploy the best US ingenuity toward health-spending reduction, elimination of wasteful care, promotion of individual responsibility and accountability for one's health, and improved access to services. In a broad sense, these services include medical care, preventive services, health promotion, and social policy to improve education, lifestyle, employment, and housing (Figure 2–5). The Ottawa Charter has proposed achieving health objectives through social public policy and community action. An integrated approach also necessitates creation of a new model for training health care professionals by forming partnerships with the community (Henry 1993). The subsequent paragraphs describe examples of community partnership reflected in community health assessment and Healthy People initiatives.

## Community Health Assessment

*Community health assessment* is a method used to conduct broad assessments of populations at a local or state level. For integrating individual and community health, the assessment is best conducted by collaboration among public health agencies, hospitals, and other health care providers. Community hospitals, in particular, are increasingly held accountable for the health status of the communities in which they are located. To fulfill this mission, hospitals must first conduct a health assessment of their communities. Such assessments provide broad perspectives of the populations' health and point to specific needs that health care providers can address. These assessments can help pinpoint interventions that should be given priority to improve the populations' health status or address critical issues pertaining to certain groups within the populations.

## Healthy People Initiatives

Since 1980, the United States has undertaken 10-year plans outlining certain key national health objectives to be accomplished during each of the 10-year periods. These initiatives have been founded on the integration of medical care with preventive services, health promotion, and education; integration of personal and community health care; and increased access to integrated services. Accordingly, the objectives are developed by a consortium of national and state organizations under the leadership of the US Surgeon General. The first of these programs, with objectives for 1990, provided national goals for reducing premature deaths and for preserving the independence of older adults.

*Healthy People 2000: National Health Promotion and Disease Prevention Objectives*, released in 1990, identified health improvement goals and objectives to be reached by the year 2000. As part of this process, standardized Health Status Indicators (HSIs) were developed to facilitate the comparison of health status measures at national, state, and local levels over time. According to the final review, the major accomplishments of Healthy People 2000 included surpassing the targets for reducing deaths from coronary heart disease and cancer; meeting the targets for incidence rates for AIDS and syphilis, mammography exams, violent deaths, and tobacco-related deaths; nearly meeting the targets for infant mortality and number of children with elevated levels of lead in blood; and making progress reducing health disparities among special populations.

*Healthy People 2010: Healthy People in Healthy Communities*, launched in January 2000, continued in the earlier traditions as an instrument to improve the health of the American people in the first decade of the 21st century. It focused on two broad goals: (1) to increase quality and years of healthy life and (2) to eliminate health disparities. It went a step beyond the previous initiatives, by emphasizing the role of community partners—businesses; local governments; and civic, professional, and religious organizations—as effective agents for improving health in their local communities (DHHS 1998). A final report on Healthy People 2010 is to be released in 2011.

Healthy People 2020 was launched in 2010 under the direction of the Secretary of Health and Human Services' Advisory Committee on National Health Promotion and Disease Prevention Objectives for 2020 and the Federal Interagency Workgroup (FIW). The Vision Statement for Healthy People 2020 is "A society in which all people live long, healthy lives." Its mission

statement is "Healthy People 2020 strives to: (1) Identify nationwide health improvement priorities; (2) Increase public awareness and understanding of the determinants of health, disease, and disability and the opportunities for progress; (3) Provide measurable objectives and goals that can be used at the national, state, and local levels; (4) Engage multiple sectors to take actions that are driven by the best available evidence and knowledge; (5) Identify critical research and data collection needs." Its four overarching goals are to:

1. Attain high-quality, longer lives free of preventable disease, disability, injury, and premature death.

2. Achieve health equity, eliminate disparities, and improve the health of all groups.

3. Create social and physical environments that promote good health for all.

4. Promote quality of life, healthy development, and healthy behaviors across all life stages.

The overarching goals are in line with the tradition of earlier Healthy People initiatives but place particular emphasis on the determinants of health. Figure 2–6 illustrates the Action Model to Achieve Healthy People 2020 Overarching Goals.

This model illustrates that interventions (i.e., policies, programs, information) influence the determinants of health at four levels: (1) individual; (2) social, family, and community; (3) living and working conditions; and (4) broad social, economic, cultural, health, and environmental conditions, leading to improvement in outcomes. Results are to be demonstrated through

Figure 2–6  Action Model to Achieve US Healthy People 2020 Overarching Goals.

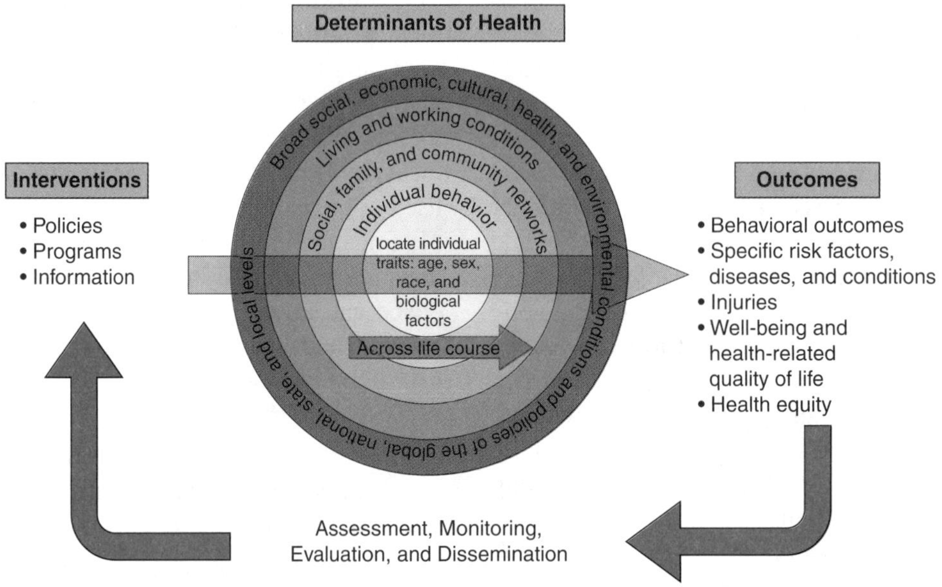

**Determinants of Health**

Broad social, economic, cultural, health, and environmental conditions

Living and working conditions

Social, family, and community networks

Individual behavior

locate individual traits: age, sex, race, and biological factors

Across life course

Promotion and policies of the global, national, state, and local levels

**Interventions**
- Policies
- Programs
- Information

**Outcomes**
- Behavioral outcomes
- Specific risk factors, diseases, and conditions
- Injuries
- Well-being and health-related quality of life
- Health equity

Assessment, Monitoring, Evaluation, and Dissemination

*Source:* Department of Health and Human Services.

assessment, monitoring, and evaluation, and the dissemination of findings would provide feedback for the intervention stage.

Healthy People 2020 is differentiated from previous Healthy People initiatives by including multiple new topic areas to its objective list, such as adolescent health, genomics, global health, health communication and health information technology, and social determinants of health. Healthy People 2020 has 42 topic areas, with 13 new areas (underlined in Table 2–5).

Healthy People 2020 also establishes four foundational health measures to monitor progress toward achieving its goals. The foundational health measures include general health status, health-related quality of life and well-being, determinants of health, and disparities. Measures of general health status include life expectancy, healthy life expectancy, years of potential life lost, physically and mentally unhealthy days, self-assessed health status, limitation of activity, and chronic disease prevalence. Measures of health-related quality of life and well-being include physical, mental, and social health-related quality of life; well-being/satisfaction; and participation in common activities. Healthy People 2020 defines determinants of health as "a range of personal, social, economic, and environmental factors that influence health status. Determinants of health include such things as biology, genetics, individual behavior, access to health services, and the environment in which people are born, live, learn, play, work, and age." Measures of disparities and inequity include differences in health status based on race/ethnicity, gender, physical and mental ability, and geography (DHHS 2010c).

**Table 2–5** List of Healthy People 2020 Topic Areas

1. Access to Health Services
2. Adolescent Health
3. Arthritis, Osteoporosis, and Chronic Back Conditions
4. Blood Disorders and Blood Safety
5. Cancer
6. Chronic Kidney Disease
7. Dementias, Including Alzheimer's Disease
8. Diabetes
9. Disability and Health
10. Early and Middle Childhood
11. Educational and Community-Based Programs
12. Environmental Health
13. Family Planning
14. Food Safety
15. Genomics
16. Global Health
17. Health Communication and Health Information Technology
18. Healthcare-Associated Infections
19. Health-Related Quality of Life and Well-Being
20. Hearing and Other Sensory or Communication Disorders
21. Heart Disease and Stroke
22. HIV
23. Immunization and Infectious Diseases
24. Injury and Violence Prevention
25. Lesbian, Gay, Bisexual, and Transgender Health
26. Maternal, Infant, and Child Health
27. Medical Product Safety
28. Mental Health and Mental Disorders
29. Nutrition and Weight Status
30. Occupational Safety and Health
31. Older Adults
32. Oral Health
33. Physical Activity
34. Preparedness
35. Public Health Infrastructure
36. Respiratory Diseases
37. Sexually Transmitted Diseases
38. Sleep Health
39. Social Determinants of Health
40. Substance Abuse
41. Tobacco Use
42. Vision

# Measures of Health Status

Certain quantitative measures commonly apply to health, health status, and the utilization of health care. It is one thing to conceptually define health but quite a different thing to measure health status or the health state of a population. The conceptual approaches for defining health and its distribution help form a vision for the future, but objective measures are needed to evaluate the success of various programs, as well as to direct future planning activities. Practical approaches for measuring health are, however, quite limited, and mental health is more difficult to quantify and measure than physical health. An objective evaluation of social and spiritual health is even more obscure. Approaches presented for quantifying the latter are mere illustrations.

The concept of population, as it applies to population health, has been borrowed from the disciplines of statistics and epidemiology. The term "population" is not restricted to describing the total population. Although commonly used in that way, the term may also apply to a defined subpopulation, for example, age groups, marital categories, income levels, occupation categories, racial/ethnic groups, a group of people having a common disease, people in a certain risk category, or people in a certain community or geographic region of a country. The main advantage of studying subpopulations is tracing the existence of health problems to a defined group in the total population. Doing so avoids concealing serious problems in a minority group within the favorable statistics of the majority. By pinpointing health problems in certain well-defined groups, targeted interventions and new policy initiatives can be deployed in the most effective manner.

## Measures of Physical Health

Physical health status is often interpreted through *morbidity* (disease and disability) and *mortality* (death) rates. In addition, self-perceived health status is a commonly used indicator of health and well-being. Respondents are asked to rate their health as excellent, very good, good, fair, or poor. Self-perceived health status is highly correlated with many objective measures of health status. It is also a good predictor of patient-initiated physician visits, including general medical and mental health visits.

### Longevity

*Life expectancy*—a prediction of how long a person will live—is widely used as a basic measure of health status. The two common measures are life expectancy at birth

Table 2–6  US Life Expectancy at Birth—1999 and Future Projections

| Year | Total | Male | Female |
|------|-------|------|--------|
| 1999 | 76.7 | 73.9 | 79.4 |
| White | 77.3 | 74.6 | 79.9 |
| Black | 71.4 | 67.8 | 74.7 |
| 2003 | 77.5 | 74.8 | 80.1 |
| White | 78.0 | 75.3 | 80.5 |
| Black | 72.7 | 69.0 | 76.1 |
| 2010 | 77.9 | 74.1 | 80.6 |

*Sources:* Data from National Center for Health Statistics, *Health, United States, 1996–1997 and Injury Chartbook.* Hyattsville, MD: 1997, p. 108; *Health, United States, 2002,* p. 116; and *Health, United States, 2006,* p. 176.

(Table 2–6)—or how long a newborn can expect to live—and life expectancy at age 65—expected remaining years of life for someone at age 65. These measures are actuarially determined and published by government agencies such as the National Center for Health Statistics. The US Census Bureau projected that life expectancy in the United States will increase from 76.0 years in 1993 to 82.6 years in 2050 (http://www.census.gov/population/www/pop-profile/natproj.html, accessed December 29, 2010).

### Morbidity

The measurement of morbidity or disease, such as cancer or heart disease, is expressed as a ratio or proportion of those who have the problem and the *population at risk*. The population at risk includes all the people in the same community or population group who could acquire a disease or condition

(Smith 1979). Incidence and prevalence are two widely used indicators for the number of *cases*, that is, people who end up acquiring a negative health condition. *Incidence* counts the number of new cases occurring in the population at risk within a certain period of time, such as a month or a year (Smith 1979; see Formula 2–1). Incidence describes the extent to which, in a given population, people who do not have a disease develop the disease during the specified time period (Timmreck 1994). Incidence is particularly useful in estimating the magnitude of conditions of relatively short duration. Decreased levels of incidence point to success of health promotion and disease prevention efforts, because they prevent new cases (Ibrahim 1985). High levels of incidence may suggest an impending *epidemic*, that is, a large number of people who get a specific disease from a common source. The second measure of morbidity, *prevalence*, determines the total number of cases at a specific point in time, in a defined population (see Formula 2–2). Prevalence is useful in quantifying the magnitude of illnesses of a relatively long duration. Decreased prevalence indicates success of treatment programs by shortening the duration of illness (Ibrahim 1985). Both incidence and prevalence rates can apply to disease, disability, or death.

Formula 2–1

Incidence = Number of new cases during a specified period/Population at risk

Formula 2–2

Prevalence = Total number of cases at a specific point in time/Specified population

The calculation of rates often requires dividing a small number by a large number representing a defined population. The result is a fraction. To make the fractions meaningful and interpretable, they are multiplied by 100 (to get a percentage), 1,000 (to get a rate per 1,000 people), 10,000 (to get a rate per 10,000 people), or a higher multiple of 10.

## Disability

Disease and injury can lead to temporary or permanent, as well as partial or total, disability. Although the idea of morbidity includes disabilities, as well as disease, there are specific measures of disability. Some common measures are the number of days of bed confinement, days missed from work or school, and days of restricted activity. All measures are in reference to a specific time period, such as a year.

One of the most widely used measures of physical disability among the elderly is the *activities of daily living* (ADL) scale. The ADL scale is appropriate for evaluating disability in both community-dwelling and institutionalized adults. The classic ADL scale, developed by Katz and Akpom (1979), includes six basic activities to determine whether an individual needs assistance. The six basic activities are eating, bathing, dressing, using the toilet, maintaining continence, and transferring from bed to chair (Katz and Akpom 1979). To evaluate disability in community-dwelling adults, a modified Katz scale is commonly used. It consists of seven items (Ostir et al. 1999). Five of these items—feeding, bathing, dressing, using the toilet, and transferring from bed to chair—have been retained from the original Katz scale. The additional two items are grooming and walking a distance of 8 feet. Thus, it includes items measuring self-care and mobility. The ADLs identify personal care functions with which a disabled person may need assistance. Depending on the extent of disability, personal care needs can be met through adaptive devices; care rendered by another individual, such as a family member; or care in a nursing facility.

Another commonly used measure of physical function is the *instrumental activities of daily living* (IADL) scale. This scale measures activities that are necessary for living independently in the community, such as using the telephone, driving a car or traveling alone on a bus or in a taxi, shopping, preparing meals, doing light housework, taking medicine, handling money, doing heavy housework, walking up and down stairs, and walking a half-mile without help. These 10 items categorize activities a person is (a) able or (b) unable to do. IADLs, typically, require higher cognitive functioning than ADLs and, as such, are not purely physical tests of functional disability. IADLs are not, generally, used in institutional settings, because institutionalized persons are not required to perform many IADL tasks (Ostir et al. 1999). The IADL scale measures the level of functioning in activities that are important for self-sufficiency.

## Mortality

Death rates are computed in different forms as indicators of population health. *Crude rates* refer to the total population; they are not specific to any age group or disease category (Formula 2–3).

### Formula 2–3

Crude death rate = Total deaths (usually in 1 year)/ Total population

Specific rates are useful because death rates vary greatly by race, sex, age, and type of disease or condition. Specific rates allow health care professionals to target programs at the appropriate population subgroups (Dever 1984). Examples of specific rates are age-specific mortality rate (Formula 2–4) and cause-specific mortality rate (Formula 2–5). The age-specific mortality rate provides a measure of the risk (or probability) of dying when a person is in a certain age group. The cause-specific mortality rate provides a measure of the risk (or probability) of dying from a specific cause. Table 2–3 provides the 10 leading causes of death in the United States.

### Formula 2–4

Age-specific mortality rate = Number of deaths within a certain age group/Total number of persons in that age group

### Formula 2–5

Cause-specific mortality rate = Number of deaths from a specific disease/Total population

Infant mortality rate (actually a ratio; Formula 2–6) is another important indicator. It reflects the health status of the mother and the child through pregnancy and the birth process. It also reflects the level of prenatal and postnatal nutritional care (Timmreck 1994).

### Formula 2–6

Infant mortality rate = Number of deaths from birth to 1 year of age (in 1 year)/Number of live births during the same year

## Demographic Change

In addition to measures of disease and mortality, changes in the composition of a population over time are important to planning of health services. Population change involves three components: births, deaths, and migration (Dever 1984). For example, the migration of the elderly to the southern states requires planning of adequate retirement and long-term care services in those states. Longevity is also an important factor that determines demographic change. For example, lower death rates, lower birth rates, and greater longevity, together, indicate an aging population. The subsequent section presents measures of births and migration, whereas measures of death were previously discussed.

## Births

Natality and fertility are two measures associated with births. *Natality*, or birth rate, is useful in assessing the influence of births on demographic change and measured by the crude birth rate (Formula 2–7).

### Formula 2–7

Crude birth rate = Number of live births (usually in 1 year)/Total population

*Fertility* refers to the capacity of a population to reproduce (see Formula 2–8 for fertility rate). Fertility is a more precise measure than natality, because fertility relates actual births to the sector of the population capable of giving birth.

### Formula 2–8

Fertility rate = Number of live births (usually in 1 year)/Number of females aged 15–44

## Migration

*Migration* refers to the geographic movement of populations between defined geographic units and involves a permanent change of residence. The net migration rate (Formula 2–9) defines the change in the population as a result of *immigration* (in migration) and *emigration* (out migration) (Dever 1984, 249). The rate is calculated for a specified period, such as 1 year, 2 years, 5 years, and so on.

### Formula 2–9

Net migration rate = (Number of immigrants – Number of emigrants)/Total population (during a specific period of time)

## Measures of Mental Health

Measurement of mental health is less objective than measurement of mortality and morbidity, because mental health often encompasses feelings that cannot be observed. Physical functioning, by contrast, reflected in behaviors and performances, can be more readily observed. Hence, measurement of mental health more appropriately refers to assessment rather than measurement. Mental health can be assessed by the presence of certain symptoms, including both psychophysiologic and psychological symptoms. Examples of psychophysiologic symptoms are low energy, headache, and upset stomach. Examples of psychological symptoms are nervousness, depression, and anxiety.

Self-assessment of one's own psychological state may also be used for mental health assessment. Self-assessment can be obtained through self-reports of frequency and intensity of psychological distress, anxiety, depression, and psychological well-being.

## Measures of Social Health

Measures of social health extend beyond the individual to encompass the extent of social contacts across various facets of life, such as family life, work life, and community life.

Breslow (1972) attempted to measure social health along four dimensions: (1) employability, based on educational achievement, occupational status, and job experience; (2) marital satisfaction; (3) sociability, determined by the number of close friends and relatives; and (4) community involvement, which encompassed attendance at religious services, political activity, and organizational membership.

Social health status is sometimes evaluated in terms of social contacts and social resources. *Social contacts* are evaluated in terms of the number of social contacts or social activities a person engages in within a specified period. Examples are visits with friends and relatives, as well as attendance at social events, such as conferences, picnics, or other outings. *Social resources* refer to social contacts that can be relied on for support, such as relatives, friends, neighbors, and members of a religious congregation. Social contacts can be observed, and they represent the more objective of the two categories; however, one criticism of social contact measures is their focus on events and activities themselves, with little consideration of how the events are personally experienced. Unlike social contacts, social resources cannot be directly observed and are best measured by asking the individuals direct questions. Evaluative questions include whether these individuals can rely on their social contacts to provide tangible support and needed companionship and whether they feel cared for, loved, and wanted.

## Measures of Spiritual Health

Within a person's individual, social, and cultural context, spiritual well-being can have a large variety of connotations. Such variations make it extremely difficult to propose standardized approaches for measuring the spiritual dimension. Attempts to measure this dimension are illustrated in the General Social Survey, which includes people's self-perceptions about happiness; religious experiences; and their degree of involvement in activities, such as prayer and attending religious services. The spiritual well-being scale developed by Vella-Brodrick and Allen (1995) evaluates items, such as reaching out for spiritual intervention; engaging in meditation, yoga, or prayer; duration of meditation or prayer for inner peace; frequency of meditation or prayer; reading about religion; and discussions or readings about ethical and moral issues.

## Measures of Health Services Utilization

*Utilization* refers to the consumption of health care services and the extent to which health care services are used. Measures of utilization can be used to determine which individuals in a population group receive certain types of medical services, which do not receive services, and why. A health care provider, such as a hospital, can find out the extent to which its services are used. Measures of utilization can help managers decide whether certain services should be added or eliminated, and health planners can determine whether programs have been effective in reaching their targeted populations. Measures of utilization, therefore, play a critical role in the planning of health care delivery capacity, for example, how many hospital beds are required to meet the acute care needs of a given population (Pasley et al. 1995). Measures of utilization are too numerous to be covered here, but some selected common measures are provided (Formulas 2–10 to 2–16).

## Crude Measures of Utilization

### Formula 2–10

Access to primary care services = Number of persons in a given population who visited a primary care provider in a given year/Size of the population

(This measure is generally expressed as a percentage, i.e., the fraction is multiplied by 100.)

### Formula 2–11

Utilization of primary care services = Number of primary care visits by people in a given population in a given year/Size of the population

(This measure is generally expressed as number of visits per person per year.)

## Specific Measures of Utilization

### Formula 2–12

Utilization of targeted services = Number of people (visits) using special services targeted at a specific population group/Size of the targeted population group

(The fraction obtained is multiplied by 100, 1000, or a higher multiple of 10 to facilitate interpretation of the result.)

### Formula 2–13

Utilization of specific inpatient services = Number of inpatient days/Size of the population

(The fraction obtained is multiplied by 100, 1000, or a higher multiple of 10 to facilitate interpretation of the result.)

## Measures of Institution-Specific Utilization

### Formula 2–14

Average daily census = Total number of inpatient days in a given time period/Number of days in the same time period

### Formula 2–15

Occupancy rate = Total number of inpatient days in a given time period/Total number of available beds during the same time period

or

Average daily census/Total number of beds in the facility

(This measure is expressed as a percentage, i.e., the fraction is multiplied by 100.)

### Formula 2–16

Average length of stay = Total number of inpatient days during a given time period/Total number of patients served during the same time period

## Summary

The delivery of health care is primarily driven by the medical model, which emphasizes illness rather than wellness. Holistic concepts of health, along with the integration of medical care with preventive and health promotional efforts, need to be adopted to significantly improve the health of Americans. Such an approach would also require individual responsibility for one's own health-oriented behaviors, as well as community partnerships to improve both personal and community health. An understanding of the determinants of health, health education, community health assessment, and national initiatives, such as Healthy People, are essential to accomplishing these goals. Healthy People 2020, launched in 2010, continues its goals of improving health and eliminating disparities. Public health has gained increased importance because of a growing recognition of its role in health protection,

*+ demand-side rationing = -economic theory that advocates use of gov. spending + growth in money supply to stimulate demand for goods + services to expand econ. activity*

environmental health, and preparedness for natural disasters and bioterrorism.

The broad concern about equitable access to health services is addressed by two contrasting theories of market justice and social justice. Countries offering universal coverage have adopted the theory of social justice under which the government determines the distribution of health care services. However, because no country can afford to provide unlimited amounts of health care to all citizens, supply-side rationing becomes inevitable. In the United States, the principles of market justice are dominant, but social justice is also apparent in publicly financed programs, mainly Medicare, Medicaid, and CHIP. Under market justice,

not all citizens have health insurance coverage, a phenomenon called demand-side rationing. Many of the peculiarities of the US health care system trace back to the beliefs and values underlying the American culture.

Commonly used measures of health status and health care utilization provide quantitative means for evaluating health status and measuring progress. Most measures available today apply to the physical dimension of health. Assessment of mental health is less objective than measuring mortality, morbidity, and disability that apply to physical health. Scales to assess social health and spiritual health have also been developed.

---

## Terminology

**Test Your Understanding**

| | | |
|---|---|---|
| *activities of daily living* | *health care* | *natality* |
| *acute condition* | *health determinants* | *planned rationing* |
| *agent* | *health risk appraisal* | *population at risk* |
| *bioterrorism* | *holistic health* | *prevalence* |
| *cases* | *holistic medicine* | *primary prevention* |
| *chronic condition* | *host* | *public health* |
| *community health* | *iatrogenic illnesses* | *quality of life* |
| *assessment* | *immigration* | *risk factor* |
| *crude rates* | *incidence* | *secondary prevention* |
| *demand-side rationing* | *instrumental activities of* | *social contacts* |
| *deontology* | *daily living* | *social justice* |
| *development* | *life expectancy* | *social resources* |
| *emigration* | *market justice* | *subacute condition* |
| *environment* | *medical model* | *supply-side rationing* |
| *environmental health* | *migration* | *tertiary prevention* |
| *epidemic* | *morbidity* | *utilitarianism* |
| *fertility* | *mortality* | *utilization* |

# Review Questions

1. What is the role of health risk appraisal in health promotion and disease prevention?

2. Health promotion and disease prevention may require both behavioral modification and therapeutic intervention. Discuss.

3. Discuss the definitions of health presented in this chapter, in terms of their implications for the health care delivery system.

4. What implications does early childhood development have for health care delivery?

5. What are the main objectives of public health?

6. Discuss the significance of an individual's quality of life from the health care delivery perspective.

7. What "preparedness" related measures have been taken to cope with potential natural and man-made disasters since the tragic events of 9/11? Assess their effectiveness.

8. The Blum model points to four key determinants of health. Discuss their implications for health care delivery.

9. What has been the main cause of the dichotomy in the way physical and mental health issues have traditionally been addressed by the health care delivery system?

10. Discuss the main cultural beliefs and values in American society that have influenced health care delivery and how they have shaped the health care delivery system.

11. Briefly describe the concepts of market justice and social justice. In what way do the two principles complement each other and in what way are they in conflict in the US system of health care delivery?

12. Describe how health care is rationed in the market justice and social justice systems.

13. To what extent do you think the objectives set forth in Healthy People initiatives can achieve the vision of an integrated approach to health care delivery in the United States?

14. What are the major differences of *Healthy People 2020* from the previous Healthy People initiatives?

15. How can health care administrators and policymakers use the various measures of health status and service utilization? Please illustrate your answer.

16. Using the data given below:
    a. Compute crude birth rates for 2005 and 2010.
    b. Compute crude death rates for 2005 and 2010.
    c. Compute cancer mortality rates for 2005 and 2010.
    d. Answer the following questions:
        (i) Did the infant death rates improve between 2005 and 2010?

(ii) What conclusions can you draw about the demographic change in this population?

(iii) Have efforts to prevent death from heart disease been successful in this population?

| Population | 2005 | 2010 |
|---|---|---|
| Total | 248,710 | 262,755 |
| Male | 121,239 | 128,314 |
| Female | 127,471 | 134,441 |
| Whites | 208,704 | 218,086 |
| Blacks | 30,483 | 33,141 |
| Number of live births | 4,250 | 3,840 |
| Number of infant deaths (birth to 1 year) | 39 | 35 |
| Number of total deaths | 1,294 | 1,324 |
| Deaths from heart disease | 378 | 363 |
| Deaths from cancer | 336 | 342 |

## REFERENCES

Agency for Healthcare Research and Quality. 2006. The Medical Expenditure Panel Survey. Available at: http://www.ahrq.gov/. Accessed December 2008.

American Institute for Cancer Research. 1996. *Food, nutrition and the prevention of cancer: A global perspective.* Washington, DC. Available at: http://www.aicr.org/site/PageServer. Accessed December 2000.

American Physical Therapy Association. 1997. Religion called valuable health tool. *PT Bulletin*, 10 October, p. 7.

Ansari, Z. et al. 2003. A public health model of the social determinants of health. *Sozial und Präventivmedizin/Social and Preventive Medicine* 48, no. 4: 242–251.

Berger, K.S. 1988. *The developing person through the lifespan.* 2nd ed. New York: Worth Publishers.

Blum, H.L. 1981. *Planning for health.* 2nd ed. New York: Human Sciences Press.

Breslow, L. 1972. A quantitative approach to the World Health Organization definition of health: Physical, mental and social well-being. *International Journal of Epidemiology* 1, no. 4: 347–355.

Centers for Disease Control and Prevention (CDC). 1999. *Morbidity and mortality weekly report* 48, no. 29.

Centers for Disease Control and Prevention (CDC). 2007. Avian influenza (bird flu). Available at: http://www.cdc.gov/flu/avian/. Accessed January 2007.

Centers for Disease Control and Prevention (CDC). 2010a. Establishing a holistic framework to reduce inequities in HIV, Viral Hepatitis, STDs, and Tuberculosis in the United States. Available at: www.cdc.gov/socialdeterminants. Accessed November 2010.

Centers for Disease Control and Prevention (CDC). 2010b. Office of Public Health Preparedness and Response. Public health preparedness: Strengthening the Nation's emergency response state by state. Available at: http://www.bt.cdc.gov/publications/2010phprep. Accessed November 2010.

Cohen, M.H. 2003. *Future medicine*. Ann Arbor: University of Michigan Press.

Dahlgren, G., and M. Whitehead. 2006. European strategies for tackling social inequities in health: Concepts and principles for tackling social inequities in health: Levelling up (part 2). Denmark: World Health Organization: Studies on Social and Economic Determinants of Population Health no. 3. Available at: http://www.euro.who.int/__data/assets/pdf_file/0018/103824 /E89384.pdf. Accessed December 2010.

Darr, K. 1991. *Ethics in health services management*. Baltimore, MD: Health Professions Press.

Davis, D.L., and P.S. Webster. 2002. The social context of science: Cancer and the Environment. *The Annals of the American Academy of Political and Social Science* 584, November 13–34.

de Leeuw, E. 1989. Concepts in health promotion: The notion of relativism. *Social Science and Medicine* 29, no. 11: 1281–1288.

Department of Health and Human Services (DHHS). 1998. *Healthy People 2010 objectives: Draft for public comment*. Washington, DC: US Government Printing Office.

Department of Health and Human Services (DHHS). 2004. *The Health consequences of smoking: A report of the Surgeon General*. Available at: http://www.surgeongeneral.gov/library /smokingconsequences/. Accessed December 2010.

Department of Health and Human Services (DHHS). 2009. *Testimony on 2009-H1N1* influenza: *HHS* preparedness and response *efforts*. Available at: http://www.hhs.gov/asl/testify/2009/07 /t20090729b.html. Accessed November 2010.

Department of Health and Human Services (DHHS). 2010a. *Summary of the prevention and wellness initiative*. Available at: http://www.hhs.gov/recovery/programs/cdc/chronicdisease.html. Accessed November 2010.

Department of Health and Human Services (DHHS). 2010b. *Office of the Assistant Secretary for Preparedness and Response. 2010. Pandemic and All Hazards Preparedness Act*. Available at: http://www.phe.gov/Preparedness/legal/pahpa/Pages/default.aspx. Accessed November 2010.

Department of Health and Human Services (DHHS). 2010c. Healthy People 2020. Available at: http://healthypeople.gov/2020. Accessed December 2010.

Dever, G.E. 1984. *Epidemiology in health service management*. Gaithersburg, MD: Aspen Publishers, Inc.

Dye, T.R. 1991. *Politics in states and communities*. 7th ed. Englewood Cliffs, NJ: Prentice-Hall.

Ethics Committee, Society for Academic Emergency Medicine. 1992. An ethical foundation for health care: An emergency medicine perspective. *Annals of Emergency Medicine* 21, no. 11: 1381–1387.

Feldstein, P.J. 1994. *Health policy issues: An economic perspective on health reform*. Ann Arbor, MI: AUPHA/HAP.

Ferguson, C.E., and S.C. Maurice. 1970. *Economic analysis*. Homewood, IL: Richard D. Irwin.

Friedman, G.D. 1980. *Primer of epidemiology*. New York: McGraw-Hill.

Grossman, M. 1972. On the concept of health capital and the demand for health. *Journal of Political Economy* 80, no. 2: 223–255.

Hancock, L.A., and C.L. Mandle. 1994. Overview of growth and development framework. In: *Health promotion through the lifespan*. C.L. Edelman and C.L. Mandle, eds. St. Louis, MO: Mosby–Year Book.

Hatch, R.L. et al. 1998. The spiritual involvement and beliefs scale: Development and testing of a new instrument. *Journal of Family Practice* 46: 476–486.

Henry, R.C. 1993. Community partnership model for health professions education. *Journal of the American Podiatric Medical Association* 83, no. 6: 328–331.

Holahan, J. 2011. The 2007-09 recession and health insurance coverage. *Health Affairs* 30, no. 1: 145–152.

Ibrahim, M.A. 1985. *Epidemiology and health policy*. Gaithersburg, MD: Aspen Publishers, Inc.

Institute of Medicine, National Academy of Sciences (IOM). 1988. *The future of public health*. Washington, DC: National Academy Press.

Jonsen, A.R. 1986. Bentham in a box: Technology assessment and health care allocation. *Law, Medicine, and Health Care* 14, no. 3–4: 172–174.

Kaiser Family Foundation. 2010. *Summary of New Health Reform Law*. Available at: http://www.kff.org/healthreform/upload/8061.pdf. Accessed November 2010.

Kane, R.L. 1988. Empiric approaches to prevention in the elderly: Are we promoting too much? In: *Health promotion and disease prevention in the elderly*. R. Chernoff and D.A. Lipschitz, eds. New York: Raven Press. p. 127–141.

Katz, S., and C.A. Akpom. 1979. A measure of primary sociobiological functions. In: *Sociomedical health indicators*. J. Elinson and A.E. Siegman, eds. Farmingdale, NY: Baywood Publishing Co. p. 127–141.

Kawachi, I. et al. 1997. Social capital, income inequality, and mortality. *American Journal of Public Health* 87: 1491–1498.

Kawachi, I. et al. 1999. Social capital and self-rated health: A contextual analysis. *American Journal of Public Health* 89: 1187–1193.

Kristol, I. 1978. A capitalist conception of justice. In: *Ethics, free enterprise, and public policy: Original essays on moral issues in business*. R.T. De George and J.A. Pichler, eds. New York: Oxford University Press. p. 57–69.

Lasker, R.D. 1997. *Medicine and public health: The power of collaboration*. New York: The New York Academy of Medicine.

Levin, J.S. 1994. Religion and health: Is there an association, is it valid, and is it causal? *Social Science and Medicine* 38, no. 11: 1475–1482.

Long, M.J. 1994. *The medical care system: A conceptual model*. Ann Arbor, MI: Health Administration Press.

Macfarlane, G.J., and A.B. Lowenfels. 1994. Physical activity and colon cancer. *European Journal of Cancer Prevention* 3, no. 5: 393–398.

Marwick, C. 1995. Should physicians prescribe prayer for health? Spiritual aspects of well-being considered. *Journal of the American Medical Association* 273, no. 20: 1561–1562.

Maugans, T.A. 1996. The SPIRITual history. *Archives of Family Medicine* 5, no. 1:11–16.

McCullough, M.E., and D.B. Larson. 1999. Religion and depression: A review of the literature. *Twin Research* 2: 126–136.

McCullough, M.E. et al. 2000. Religious involvement and mortality: A meta-analytic review. *Health Psychology* 19, no. 3: 211–222.

McKee, M. 2001. Measuring the efficiency of health systems. *British Medical Journal* 323, no. 7308: 295–296.

Ostir, G.V. et al. 1999. Disability in older adults 1: Prevalence, causes, and consequences. *Behavioral Medicine* 24, no. 4: 147–156.

Parsons, T. 1972. Definitions of health and illness in the light of American values and social structure. In: *Patients, physicians and illness: A sourcebook in behavioral science and health*. 2nd ed. E.G. Jaco, ed. New York: Free Press.

Partnership to Fight Chronic Disease (PFCD). 2009. *Almanac of Chronic Disease.*

Pasley, B.H. et al. 1995. Excess acute care bed capacity and its causes: The experience of New York State. *Health Services Research* 30, no. 1: 115–131.

Peters, K.E. et al. 2001. *Cooperative actions for health programs: Lessons learned in medicine and public health collaboration.* Chicago: American Medical Association. Available at: http://fightchronicdisease.wardhealth.com/resources/almanac-chronic-disease-0. Accessed April 25, 2011.

Pincus, T. et al. 1998. Social conditions and self-management are more powerful determinants of health than access to care. *Annals of Internal Medicine* 129, no. 5: 406–411.

Plotkin, S.L., and S.A. Plotkin. 1999. A short history of vaccination. In: *Vaccines*, 3rd ed. S.A. Plotkin and W.A. Orenstein, eds. Philadelphia, PA: W.B. Saunders.

Post, S.G. et al. 2000. Physicians and patient spirituality: Professional boundaries, competency, and ethics. *Annals of Internal Medicine* 132, no. 7: 578–583.

Puchalski, C., and A.L. Romer. 2000. Taking a spiritual history allows clinicians to understand patients more fully. *Journal of Palliative Medicine* 3, no. 1: 129–137.

Reinhardt, U.E. 1994. Providing access to health care and controlling costs: The universal dilemma. In: *The nation's health*, 4th ed. P.R. Lee and C.L. Estes, eds. Boston: Jones & Bartlett Publishers. p. 263–278.

Robert Wood Johnson Foundation. 2010. *Chronic care: Making the case for ongoing care.* Available at: http://www.rwjf.org/pr/product.jsp?id=50968. Accessed April 25, 2011.

Roberts, J.A. et al. 1997. Factors influencing the views of patients with gynecologic cancer about end-of-life decisions. *American Journal of Obstetrics and Gynecology* 176: 166–172.

Rosen, G. 1993. *A history of public health*. Baltimore, MD: Johns Hopkins University Press.

Ross, L. 1995. The spiritual dimension: Its importance to patients' health, well-being and quality of life and its implications for nursing practice. *International Journal of Nursing Studies* 32, no. 5: 457–468.

Santerre, R.E., and S.P. Neun. 1996. *Health economics: Theories, insights, and industry studies.* Chicago: Irwin.

Saward, E., and A. Sorensen. 1980. The current emphasis on preventive medicine. In: *Issues in health services*. S.J. Williams, ed. New York: John Wiley & Sons. p. 17–29.

Schneider, M.J. 2000. *Introduction to public health*. Gaithersburg, MD: Aspen Publishers, Inc.

Shellenbarger, S. 1997. Good, early care has a huge impact on kids, studies say. *The Wall Street Journal*, 9 April, B1.

Shi, L., and B. Starfield. 2001. Primary care physician supply, income inequality, and racial mortality in US metropolitan areas. *American Journal of Public Health* 91, no. 8: 1246–1250.

Shi, L. et al. 1999. Income inequality, primary care, and health indicators. *Journal of Family Practice* 48, no. 4: 275–284.

Shi, L. et al. 2002. Primary care, self-rated health, and reduction in social disparities in health. *Health Services Research* 37, no. 3: 529–550.

Shortell, S.M. et al. 1995. Reinventing the American hospital. *The Milbank Quarterly* 73, no. 2: 131–160.

Smith, B.C. 1979. *Community health: An epidemiological approach.* New York: Macmillan Publishing Co. p. 197–213.

Starfield, B. 1998. *Primary care and health services.* Oxford: Oxford University Press.

Swanson, C.S. 1995. A spirit-focused conceptual model of nursing for the advanced practice nurse. *Issues in Comprehensive Pediatric Nursing* 18, no. 4: 267–275.

Tamm, M.E. 1993. Models of health and disease. *British Journal of Medical Psychology* 66, no. 3: 213–228.

Timmreck, T.C. 1994. *An introduction to epidemiology.* Boston: Jones & Bartlett Publishers.

Turnock, B.J. 1997. *Public health: What it is and how it works.* Gaithersburg, MD: Aspen Publishers, Inc.

Vella-Brodrick, D.A., and F.C. Allen. 1995. Development and psychometric validation of the mental, physical, and spiritual well-being scale. *Psychological Reports* 77, no. 2: 659–674.

Ward, B. 1995. Holistic medicine. *Australian Family Physician* 24, no. 5: 761–762, 765.

White, E. et al. 1996. Physical activity in relation to colon cancer in middle-aged men and women. *American Journal of Epidemiology* 144, no. 1: 42–50.

Wilkinson, R.G. 1997. Comment: Income, inequality, and social cohesion. *American Journal of Public Health* 87: 1504–1506.

Wolinsky, F. 1988. *The sociology of health: Principles, practitioners, and issues.* 2nd ed. Belmont, CA: Wadsworth Publishing.

WHO Commission on Social Determinants of Health. 2007. V. CSDH framework for Action. In: *A Conceptual Framework for Action on the Social Determinants of Health.* Geneva, Switzerland: World Health Organization, 15–49, 71–75. Available at: http://www.who.int/social_determinants/resources/csdh_framework_action_05_07.pdf. Accessed November 4, 2009.

World Health Organization (WHO). 1948. *Preamble to the constitution.* Geneva, Switzerland: Author.

Wynder, E.L., and M.A. Orlandi. 1984. *The American Health Foundation guide to lifespan health: A family program for physical and emotional well-being.* New York: Dodd, Mead & Company.

# Chapter 3

# The Evolution of Health Services in the United States

## Learning Objectives

- To discover historical developments that have shaped the nature of the US health care delivery system
- To evaluate why the system has been resistant to national health insurance reforms
- To explore developments associated with the corporatization of health care
- To speculate on whether the era of socialized medicine has dawned in the United States

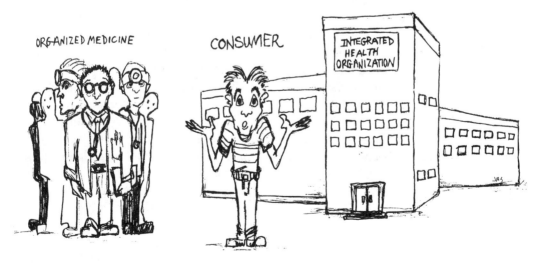

*"Where's the market?"*

# Introduction

The health care delivery system of the United States evolved quite differently from the systems in Europe. American values and the social, political, and economic antecedents on which the US system is based have led to the formation of a unique system of health care delivery, as described in Chapter 1. This chapter discusses how these forces have been instrumental in shaping the current structure of medical services and how they are likely to shape its future. The evolutionary changes discussed here illustrate the American beliefs and values (discussed in Chapter 2) in action, within the context of broad social, political, and economic changes. Because social, political, and economic contexts are not static, their shifting influences lend a certain dynamism to the health care delivery system. Conversely, beliefs and values remain relatively stable over time. Consequently, in the American health care delivery experience, initiatives toward a national health care program have failed to make significant inroads. However, social, political, and economic forces have led to certain compromises, as seen in the creation of Medicare, Medicaid, and other public programs to extend health insurance to certain defined groups of people. Could major social or economic shifts eventually usher in a national health care system? It is anyone's guess. Given the right set of conditions, a national health care system could become a reality in the United States, as recently seen with the passage of the Patient Protection and Affordable Care Act (ACA) of 2010, which promises to reduce the number of uninsured by 32 million (Henry J. Kaiser Family Foundation 2011). Cultural beliefs and values are strong forces against attempts to initiate fundamental changes in the financing and delivery of health care. Therefore, enactment of major health system reforms requires consensus among Americans on basic values and ethics (Kardos and Allen 1993). Ironically, American beliefs and values were not allowed a chance to play out in the political maneuvering that led to the passage of the ACA of 2010 (see Chapter 13).

The growth of medical science and technology (discussed in Chapter 5) has also played a key role in shaping the US health care delivery system. Stevens (1971) points out that the technological revolution has been primarily responsible for bringing medicine into the public domain. Advancement of technology has influenced other factors, as well, such as medical education, growth of institutions, and urban development. Hence, American medicine did not emerge as a professional entity until the beginning of the 20th century, with the progress in biomedical science. Since then, the US health care delivery system has been a growth enterprise. Debates over issues such as methods of financing health care, quality improvement, and the appropriate role of government have also been rooted in the presumed importance of gaining access to ever-rising levels of scientific medicine (Somers and Somers 1977).

This chapter traces the evolution of health care delivery through three major historical phases, each demarcating a major change in the structure of the delivery system. The first phase is the preindustrial era from the middle of the 18th century to the latter part of the 19th century. The second phase is the postindustrial era beginning in the late 19th century. The third, most recent and current phase, is marked by the growth of managed care, organizational integration, the information revolution, and globalization, called the corporate era.

The practice of medicine is central to the delivery of health care; therefore, a major portion of this chapter is devoted to tracing the transformations in medical practice from a weak and insecure trade to an independent, highly respected, and lucrative profession. Delivery of medical services through managed care and the corporatization of physician practices, however, have made a significant impact on practice styles and have compromised the autonomy that physicians have historically enjoyed. The medical profession has also consolidated into larger organizational units, away from the solo practice of medicine that had once prevailed.

## Medical Services in Preindustrial America

From Colonial times to the beginning of the 20th century, American medicine lagged behind the advances in medical science, experimental research, and medical education that were taking place in Britain, France, and Germany. While London, Paris, and Berlin were flourishing as major research centers, Americans had a tendency to neglect research in basic sciences and to place more emphasis on applied science (Shryock 1966). In addition, American attitudes about medical treatment placed strong emphasis on natural history and conservative common sense (Stevens 1971). Consequently, the practice of medicine in the United States had a strong domestic, rather than professional, character. Medical services, when deemed appropriate by the consumer, were purchased out of one's private funds, because there was no health insurance. The health care market was characterized by competition among providers, and the consumer decided who the provider would be.

Thus, the consumer was sovereign in the health care market and health care was delivered under free market conditions.

Five main factors explain why the medical profession remained largely an insignificant trade in preindustrial America:

1. Medical practice was in disarray.
2. Medical procedures were primitive.
3. An institutional core was missing.
4. Demand was unstable.
5. Medical education was substandard.

## Medical Practice in Disarray

The early practice of medicine could be regarded more as a trade than a profession. It did not require the rigorous course of study, clinical practice, residency training, board exams, or licensing, without which it is impossible to practice today. At the close of the Civil War (1861–1865), "anyone who had the inclination to set himself up as a physician could do so, the exigencies of the market alone determining who would prove successful in the field and who would not" (Hamowy 1979). The clergy, for example, often combined medical services and religious duties. The generally well-educated clergyman or government official was more learned in medicine than physicians were at the time (Shryock 1966). Tradesmen, such as tailors, barbers, commodity merchants, and those engaged in numerous other trades, also practiced the healing arts by selling herbal prescriptions, nostrums, elixirs, and cathartics. Midwives, homeopaths, and naturalists could also practice medicine without restriction. The red-and-white striped poles (symbolizing blood and bandages) seen outside barbershops are reminders that barbers also functioned as surgeons at one time, using the same blade to cut hair, shave beards, and bleed the sick.

This era of medical pluralism has been referred to as a "war zone" by Kaptchuk and Eisenberg (2001) because it was marked by bitter antagonism among the various practicing sects. Later, in 1847, the American Medical Association (AMA) was founded with the main purpose of erecting a barrier between orthodox practitioners and the "irregulars" (Rothstein 1972).

In the absence of minimum standards of medical training, entry into private practice was relatively easy for both trained and untrained practitioners, creating intense competition. Medicine as a profession was weak and unorganized. Hence, physicians did not enjoy the prestige, influence, and incomes that they later earned. Many physicians found it necessary to engage in a second occupation because income from medical practice alone was inadequate to support a family. It is estimated that most physicians' incomes in the mid-19th century placed them at the lower end of the middle class (Starr 1982). It is estimated that in 1830 there were 6,800 physicians serving primarily the upper classes (Gabe et al. 1994). It was not until 1870 that medical education was reformed and licensing laws were passed in the United States.

## Primitive Medical Procedures

Up until the mid-1800s, medical care was based more on primitive medical traditions than science. In the absence of diagnostic tools, a theory of "intake and outgo" served as an explanation for all diseases (Rosenberg 1979). It was believed that diseases needed to be expelled from the body. Hence, bleeding, use of emetics (to induce vomiting) and diuretics (to increase urination), and purging with

enemas and purgatives (to clean the bowels) were popular forms of clinical therapy.

When George Washington became ill with an inflamed throat in 1799, he too was bled by physicians. One of the attending physicians argued, unsuccessfully, in favor of making an incision to open the trachea, which today would be considered a more enlightened procedure. The bleeding most likely weakened Washington's resistance, and historians have debated whether it played a role in his death (Clark 1998).

Surgeries were limited because anesthesia had not yet been developed and antiseptic techniques were not known. Stethoscopes and X-rays had not been discovered, clinical thermometers were not in use, and microscopes were not available for medical diagnosis. Physicians relied mainly on their five senses and experience to diagnose and treat medical problems. Hence, in most cases, physicians did not possess any technical expertise greater than that of the mothers and grandparents at home or experienced neighbors in the community.

## Missing Institutional Core

In the United States, no widespread development of hospitals occurred before the 1880s. A few isolated hospitals were either built or developed in rented private houses in large cities, such as Philadelphia, New York, Boston, Cincinnati, New Orleans, and St. Louis. By contrast, general hospital expansion began much before the 1800s in France and Britain (Stevens 1971). In Europe, medical professionals were closely associated with hospitals. New advances in medical science were being pioneered, which European hospitals readily adopted. The medical profession came to be supremely regarded because of its close association with an establishment that was scientifically advanced. In contrast, American hospitals played only a small part in medical practice because most hospitals served a social welfare function by taking care of the poor, those without families, or those who were away from home on travel.

## The Almshouse and the Pesthouse

In the United States, the *almshouse* was the precursor of hospitals, but it was not a hospital in the true sense. Almshouses, also called poorhouses because they served primarily the poor, existed in almost all cities of moderate size and were run by the local governments. These institutions served, primarily, general welfare functions by providing food and shelter to the destitute. Therefore, the main function of the almshouse was custodial. Caring for the sick was incidental because some of the residents would inevitably become ill and would be cared for in an adjoining infirmary. Almshouses were unspecialized institutions that admitted poor and needy persons of all kinds: the elderly, the orphaned, the insane, the ill, and the disabled. Hence, the early hospital-type institutions emerged mainly to take care of indigent people whose families could not care for them.

Another type of institution, the *pesthouse,* was operated by local governments to quarantine people who had contracted a contagious disease, such as cholera, smallpox, typhoid, or yellow fever. Located primarily in seaports, the primary function of a pesthouse was to isolate people with contagious diseases so disease would not spread among the inhabitants of a city. These institutions were the predecessors of contagious-disease and tuberculosis hospitals.

## The Dispensary

Dispensaries were established to provide free care to those who could not afford to pay. Urban workers and their families often depended on such charity (Rosen 1983). Dispensaries operated independently of hospitals, hence, medical practice in the United States was not legitimized because it lacked organizational affiliation.

Starting with Philadelphia in 1786, dispensaries gradually spread to other cities. They were private institutions, financed by bequests and voluntary subscriptions. Their main function was to provide basic medical care and to dispense drugs to ambulatory patients (Raffel 1980). Generally, young physicians and medical students desiring clinical experience staffed these dispensaries, as well as hospital wards, on a part-time basis for little or no income (Martensen 1996), which served a dual purpose. It provided needed services to the poor and enabled both physicians and medical students to gain experience diagnosing and treating a variety of cases. Later, as the practice of specialized medicine, as well as teaching and research, was transferred to hospital settings, many dispensaries were gradually absorbed into hospitals as outpatient departments. Indeed, outpatient or ambulatory care departments became an important locale for specialty consultation services within large hospitals (Raffel 1980).

## The Mental Asylum

Mental health care was seen, primarily, as the responsibility of state and local governments. At this time, little was known about what caused mental illness or how to treat it. Although almshouses were used to accommodate some mental health patients, asylums were built by states for patients with untreatable, chronic mental illness. The first such asylum was built around 1770 in Williamsburg, Virginia. When the Pennsylvania Hospital opened in Philadelphia in 1752, its basement was used as a mental asylum. Attendants in these asylums employed physical and psychological techniques in an effort to return patients to some level of rational thinking. Techniques such as bleeding, forced vomiting, and hot and ice-cold baths were also used. Between 1894 and World War I, the State Care Acts were passed, centralizing financial responsibility for mentally ill patients in every state government. Local governments took advantage of this opportunity to send all those with a mental illness, including dependent, older citizens, to the state asylums. The quality of care in public asylums deteriorated rapidly, as overcrowding and underfunding ran rampant (US Surgeon General 1999).

## The Dreaded Hospital

Not until the 1850s were hospitals similar to those in Europe developed in the United States. These early hospitals had deplorable conditions due to a lack of resources. Poor sanitation and inadequate ventilation were hallmarks of these hospitals. Unhygienic practices prevailed because nurses were unskilled and untrained. These early hospitals had an undesirable image of being houses of death. The mortality rate among hospital patients, both in Europe and America, stood around 74% in the 1870s (Falk 1999). People went into hospitals because of dire consequences, not by personal choice. It is not hard to imagine why members of the middle and upper classes, in particular, shunned such establishments.

## Unstable Demand

Professional services suffered from low demand in the mainly rural, preindustrial society, and much of the medical care was provided by people who were not physicians. The most competent physicians were located in more populated communities (Bordley and Harvey 1976). In the small communities of rural America, a spirit of strong self-reliance prevailed. Families and communities were accustomed to treating the sick, often using folk remedies passed from one generation to the next. It was also common to consult books and published pamphlets on home remedies (Rosen 1983).

The market for physicians' services was also limited by economic conditions. Many families could not afford to pay for medical services. Two factors contributed to the high cost associated with obtaining professional medical care: (1) The indirect costs of transportation and the "opportunity cost" of travel (i.e., forgone value of time that could have been used for something more productive) could easily outweigh the direct costs of physicians' fees. (2) The costs of travel often doubled because two people, the physician and an emissary, had to make the trip back and forth. For a farmer, a trip of 10 miles into town could mean an entire day's work lost. Physicians passed much of their day traveling along backcountry roads. Farmers had to cover travel costs and the opportunity cost of time spent traveling. Mileage charges amounted to four or five times the basic fee for a visit if a physician had to travel 5 to 10 miles. Hence, most families obtained only occasional intervention from physicians, generally for nonroutine and severe conditions (Starr 1982).

Personal health services had to be purchased without the help of government or private insurance. Private practice and *fee for service*—the practice of billing separately for each individual type of service performed—was firmly embedded in American medical care. Similar to physicians, dentists were private entrepreneurs who made their living by private fee-for-service dental practice, but their services were not in great demand because there was little public concern about dental health (Anderson 1990).

## Substandard Medical Education

From about 1800 to 1850, medical training was largely received through individual apprenticeship with a practicing physician, referred to as a preceptor, rather than through university education. Many of the preceptors were themselves poorly trained, especially in basic medical sciences (Rothstein 1972). By 1800, only four small medical schools were operating in the United States: College of Philadelphia (which was established in 1756 and later became the University of Pennsylvania), King's College (which was established in 1768 and later became Columbia University), Harvard University (opened in 1783), and Dartmouth College (started in 1797).

American physicians later initiated the establishment of medical schools in large numbers. This was partly to enhance professional status and prestige and partly to enhance income. Medical schools were inexpensive to operate and often quite profitable. All that was required was a faculty of four or more physicians, a classroom, a back room to conduct dissections, and legal authority to confer degrees. Operating expenses were met totally out of student fees that were paid directly to the physicians (Rothstein 1972). Physicians would affiliate with a local college for the conferral of degrees and use of classroom facilities. Large numbers of men entered medical practice as education in medicine became readily available and unrestricted entry into the profession was still possible (Hamowy 1979). Gradually, as physicians from medical schools began to outnumber those from the apprenticeship system, the Doctor of Medicine (MD) degree became the standard of competence. The number of medical schools tripled between 1800 and 1820 and tripled again between 1820 and 1850, numbering 42 in 1850 (Rothstein 1972). Academic preparation gradually replaced apprenticeship training.

At this point, medical education in the United States was seriously deficient in science-based training, unlike European medical schools. Medical schools in the United States did not have laboratories, and clinical observation and practice were not part of the curriculum. In contrast, European medical schools, particularly those in Germany, were emphasizing laboratory-based medical research. At the University of Berlin, for example, professors were expected to conduct research, as well as teach, and were paid by the state. In American medical schools, students were taught by local practitioners, who were ill-equipped in education and training. Unlike Europe, where medical education was financed and regulated by the government, proprietary medical schools in the United States set their own standards (Numbers and Warner 1985). A year of medical school in the United States, generally, lasted only 4 months and required only 2 years for graduation. In addition, American medical students customarily repeated the same courses they had taken during their first year again during their second year (Numbers and Warner 1985; Rosner 2001). The physicians' desire to keep their schools profitable also contributed to low standards and a lack of rigor. It was feared that higher standards in medical education would drive enrollments down, which could lead the schools into bankruptcy (Starr 1982).

# Medical Services in Postindustrial America

In the postindustrial period, American physicians, unlike other physicians in the world, were highly successful in retaining private practice of medicine and resisting national health care. Physicians also became an organized medical profession and delivered scientifically and technically advanced services to insured patients. Notably, much of this transformation occurred in the aftermath of the Civil War. Social and scientific changes in the period following the war were accompanied by a transition from a rural, agricultural economy to a system of industrial capitalism. Mass production techniques used in the war were applied to peacetime industries. Railroads linked the east and west coasts, and small towns became cities (Stevens 1971).

The American system for delivering health care took its current shape during this period. Private practice of medicine became firmly entrenched as physicians grew into a cohesive profession and gained power and prestige. The well-defined role of employers in providing workers' compensation for work-related injuries and illnesses, together with other economic considerations, was instrumental in the growth of private health insurance. Rising costs of health care, however, prompted Congress to create the publicly financed programs, such as Medicare and Medicaid, for the most vulnerable members of the population. Cost considerations also motivated the formation of prototypes for modern managed care organizations (MCOs).

## Growth of Professional Sovereignty

The 1920s may well mark the consolidation of physicians' professional power. During and after World War I, physicians' incomes grew sharply, and their prominence as a profession finally emerged. This prestige and power, however, did not materialize overnight. Through the years, several factors interacted in the gradual transformation of medicine from a weak, insecure, and isolated trade into a profession of power and authority. Seven key factors contributed to this transformation:

1. urbanization,
2. science and technology,
3. institutionalization,
4. dependency,
5. cohesiveness and organization,
6. licensing, and
7. educational reform.

## Urbanization

Urbanization created increased reliance on the specialized skills of paid professionals. First, it distanced people from their families and neighborhoods where family-based care was traditionally given. Women began working outside the home and could no longer care for sick members of the family. Second, physicians became less expensive to consult as telephones, automobiles, and paved roads reduced the opportunity cost of time and travel and medical care became more affordable. Urban development attracted more and more Americans to the growing towns and cities. In 1840, only 11% of the US population lived in urban areas; by 1900, the proportion of the US population living in urban areas grew to 40% (Stevens 1971). The trend away from home visits to office practice also began to develop around this time (Rosen 1983). Physicians moved to cities and towns in large numbers to be closer to their growing markets. Better geographic proximity of patients enabled physicians to see more patients in a given amount of time. Whereas physicians in 1850 only saw an average of 5 to 7 patients a day, by the early 1940s, the average patient load of general practitioners had risen to 18 to 22 patients a day (Starr 1982).

## Science and Technology

Exhibit 3–1 summarizes some of the groundbreaking scientific discoveries in medicine. Advances in bacteriology, antiseptic surgery, anesthesia, immunology, and diagnostic techniques, along with an expanding repertoire of new drugs, gave medicine an aura of legitimacy and complexity, and the therapeutic effectiveness of scientific medicine became widely recognized.

When advanced technical knowledge becomes essential to practice a profession and the benefits of professional services are widely recognized, a greater acceptance and a legitimate need for the services of that

**Exhibit 3-1** Groundbreaking Medical Discoveries

- The discovery of anesthesia was instrumental in advancing the practice of surgery. Nitrous oxide (laughing gas) was first employed as an anesthetic around 1846 for tooth extraction by Horace Wells, a dentist. Ether anesthesia for surgery was first successfully used in 1846 at the Massachusetts General Hospital. Before anesthesia was discovered, strong doses of alcohol were used to dull the sensations. A surgeon who could do procedures, such as limb amputations, in the shortest length of time was held in high regard.

- Around 1847, Ignaz Semmelweis, a Hungarian physician practicing in a hospital in Vienna, implemented the policy of handwashing. Thus, an aseptic technique was born. Semmelweis was concerned about the high death rate from puerperal fever among women after childbirth. Even though the germ theory of disease was unknown at this time, Semmelweis surmised that there might be a connection between puerperal fever and the common practice by medical students of not washing their hands before delivering babies and right after doing dissections. Semmelweis's hunch was right.

- Louis Pasteur is generally credited with pioneering the germ theory of disease and microbiology around 1860. Pasteur demonstrated sterilization techniques, such as boiling to kill microorganisms and withholding exposure to air to prevent contamination.

- Joesph Lister is often referred to as the father of antiseptic surgery. Around 1865, Lister used carbolic acid to wash wound, and popularized the chemical inhibition of infection (antisepsis) during surgery.

- Advances in diagnostics and imaging can be traced to the discovery of X-rays in 1895 by Wilhelm Roentgen, a German professor of physics. Radiology became the first machine-based medical specialty. Some of the first training schools in X-ray therapy and radiography in the United States attracted photographers and electricians to become Doctors in Roentgenology (from the inventor's name).

- Alexander Fleming discovered the antibacterial properties of penicillin in 1929.

profession are simultaneously created. *Cultural authority* refers to the general acceptance of and reliance on the judgment of the members of a profession (Starr 1982) because of their superior knowledge and expertise. Cultural authority legitimizes a profession in the eyes of common people. Advances in medical science and technology bestowed this legitimacy on the medical profession because medical practice could no longer remain within the domain of lay competence.

Scientific and technological change also required improved therapeutic competence of physicians in the diagnosis and treatment of disease. Developing these skills was no longer possible without specialized training. Science-based medicine created an increased demand for advanced services that were no longer available through family and neighbors.

Physicians' cultural authority was further bolstered when medical decisions became necessary in various aspects of health care delivery. For example, physicians decide whether a person should be admitted to a hospital or nursing home and for how long, whether surgical or nonsurgical treatments should be used, and which medications should be prescribed. Physicians' decisions have a profound impact on other providers and nonproviders alike. The judgment and opinions of physicians even affect aspects of a person's life outside the delivery of health care. For example, physicians often evaluate the fitness of persons for jobs during pre-employment physicals many employers demand. Physicians assess the disability of the ill and the injured in workers' compensation cases. Granting of medical leave for sickness and release back to work require authorizations from physicians. Payment of medical claims requires physicians' evaluations. Other health care professionals, such as nurses, therapists, and dietitians, are expected to follow physicians' orders for treatment. Thus, during disease and disability, and sometimes even in good health, people's lives have become increasingly governed by decisions made by physicians.

## Institutionalization

The evolution of medical technology and the professionalization of medical and nursing staff enabled advanced treatments that necessitated the pooling of resources in a common arena of care (Burns 2004). Rapid urbanization was another factor that necessitated the institutionalization of medical care. As had already occurred in Europe, in the United States, hospitals became the core around which the delivery of medical services was organized. Thus, development of hospitals as the center for the practice of scientific medicine and the professionalization of medical practice became closely intertwined. Indeed, physicians and hospitals developed a symbiotic relationship.

For economic reasons, as hospitals expanded, their survival became increasingly dependent on physicians to keep the beds filled because the physicians decided where to hospitalize their patients. Therefore, hospitals had to make every effort to keep the physicians satisfied, which enhanced physicians' professional dominance, even though they were not employees of the hospitals. This gave physicians enormous influence over hospital policy. Also, for the first time, hospitals began conforming to both physician practice patterns and public expectations about medicine as a modern scientific enterprise. The expansion of surgery, in particular, had profound implications for hospitals, physicians, and the public. As hospitals added specialized facilities and staff, their regular use became indispensable to physicians and surgeons, who earlier had been able to manage their practices with little reference to hospitals (Martensen 1996). Affiliation with establishments symbolizing the scientific cutting edge of medicine lent power and prestige to the medical profession.

Hospitals in the United States did not expand and become more directly related to medical care until the late 1890s. However, as late as the 1930s, hospitals incurred frequent deaths due to infections that could not be prevented or cured. Nevertheless, hospital use was on the rise due to the great influx of immigrants into large American cities (Falk 1999). From only a few score in 1875, the number of general hospitals in the United States expanded to 4,000 by 1900 (Anderson 1990) and to 5,000 by 1913 (Wright 1997).

## Dependency

Patients depend on the medical profession's judgment and assistance. First, dependency is created because society expects a sick person to seek medical help and try to get well. The patient is then expected to comply with medical instructions. Second, dependency is created by the profession's cultural authority because its medical judgments must be relied on to (1) legitimize a person's sickness; (2) exempt the individual from social role obligations, such as work or school, and (3) provide competent medical care so the person can get well and resume his or her social role obligations. Third, in conjunction with the physician's cultural authority, the need for hospital services for critical illness and surgery also creates dependency when patients are transferred from their homes to a hospital or surgery center.

Once physicians' cultural authority became legitimized, the sphere of their influence expanded into nearly all aspects of health care delivery. For example, laws were passed that prohibited individuals from obtaining certain classes of drugs without a physician's prescription. Health insurance paid for treatments only when they were rendered or prescribed by physicians. Thus, beneficiaries of health insurance became dependent on physicians to obtain covered services. More recent, the referral role (gatekeeping) of primary care physicians in managed care plans has increased patients' dependency on primary care physicians for referral to specialized services.

## Cohesiveness and Organization

Toward the end of the 1800s, social and economic changes brought about greater cohesiveness among medical professionals. With the growth of hospitals and specialization, physicians needed support from each other for patient referrals and for access to facilities to admit their patients. Standardization of education also advanced a common core of knowledge among physicians. They no longer remained members of isolated and competing medical sects. Greater cohesiveness, in turn, advanced their professional authority (Starr 1982).

For a long time, physicians' ability to remain free of control from hospitals and insurance companies remained a prominent feature of American medicine. Hospitals and insurance companies could have hired physicians on salary to provide medical services, but individual physicians who took up practice in a corporate setting were castigated by the medical profession and pressured to abandon such practices. In some states, courts ruled that corporations could not employ licensed physicians without engaging in the unlicensed practice of medicine, a legal doctrine that became known as the "corporate practice doctrine" (Farmer and Douglas 2001). Independence from corporate control enhanced private entrepreneurship and put American physicians in an enviable strategic position in relation to hospitals and insurance companies. Later, a formally organized medical profession was in a much better position to resist control from outside entities.

The AMA was formed in 1847, but it had little strength during its first half-century of existence. Its membership was small, with no permanent organization and scant resources. The AMA did not attain real strength until it was organized into county and state medical societies and until state societies were incorporated, delegating greater control at the local level. As part of the organizational reform, the AMA also began, in 1904, to concentrate attention on medical education (Bordley and Harvey 1976). Since then, it has been the chief proponent for the practitioners of conventional medicine in the United States. Although the AMA often stressed the importance of raising the quality of care for patients and protecting the uninformed consumer from "quacks" and "charlatans," its principal goal—like that of other professional associations—was to advance the professionalization, prestige, and financial well-being of its members. The AMA vigorously pursued its objectives by promoting the establishment of state medical licensing laws and the legal requirement that, to be licensed to practice, a physician must be a graduate of an AMA-approved medical school. The concerted activities of physicians through the AMA are collectively referred to as *organized medicine,* to distinguish them from the uncoordinated actions of individual physicians competing in the marketplace (Goodman and Musgrave 1992).

## Licensing

Under the Medical Practice Acts established in the 1870s, medical licensure in the United States became a function of the states (Stevens 1971). By 1896, 26 states had enacted medical licensure laws (Anderson 1990). Licensing of physicians and upgrading of medical school standards developed hand in hand. At first, licensing required only a medical school diploma. Later, candidates could be rejected if the school they had attended was judged inadequate. Finally, all candidates were required to present an acceptable diploma and pass an independent state examination (Starr 1982). Through both licensure and upgrading of medical school standards, physicians obtained a clear monopoly on the practice of medicine (Anderson 1990). The early licensing laws served to protect physicians from the competitive pressures posed by potential new entrants into the medical profession. Physicians led the campaign to restrict the practice of medicine. As biomedicine gained political and economic ground, the biomedical community expelled providers such as homeopaths, naturopaths, and chiropractors from medical societies; prohibited professional association with them; and encouraged prosecution of such providers for unlicensed medical practice (Rothstein 1972). In 1888, in a landmark Supreme Court decision, *Dent v. West Virginia,* Justice Stephen J. Field wrote that no one had the right to practice "without having the necessary qualifications of learning and skill" (Haber 1974). In the late 1880s and 1890s, many states revised laws to require all candidates for licensure, including those holding medical degrees, to pass an examination (Kaufman 1980).

## Educational Reform

Advanced medical training was made necessary by scientific progress. Reform of medical education started around 1870, with the affiliation of medical schools with universities. In 1871, Harvard Medical School, under the leadership of a new university president, Charles Eliot, completely revolutionized the system of medical education. The academic year was extended from 4 to 9 months, and the length of medical education was increased from 2 to 3 years. Following the European model, laboratory instruction and clinical subjects, such as chemistry, physiology, anatomy, and pathology, were added to the curriculum.

Johns Hopkins University took the lead in further reforming medical education when it opened its medical school in 1893, under the leadership of William H. Welch, who trained in Germany. Medical education, for the first time, became a graduate training course, requiring a college degree, not a high school diploma, as an entrance requirement. Johns Hopkins had well-equipped laboratories, a full-time faculty for the basic science courses, and its own teaching hospital (Rothstein 1972). Standards at Johns Hopkins became the model of medical education in other leading institutions around the country. The raising of standards made it difficult for proprietary schools to survive, and, in time, proprietary schools were closed.

The Association of American Medical Colleges (AAMC) was founded in 1876 by 22 medical schools (Coggeshall 1965).

Later, the AAMC set minimum standards for medical education, including a 4-year curriculum, but it was unable to enforce its recommendations. In 1904, the AMA created the Council on Medical Education, which inspected the existing medical schools and found that less than half provided acceptable levels of training. The AMA did not publish its findings but obtained the help of the Carnegie Foundation for the Advancement of Teaching to provide a rating of medical schools (Goodman and Musgrave 1992). The Foundation appointed Abraham Flexner to investigate medical schools located in both the United States and Canada. The Flexner Report, published in 1910, had a profound effect on medical education reform. The report was widely accepted by both the profession and the public. Schools that did not meet the proposed standards were forced to close. State laws were established, requiring graduation from a medical school accredited by the AMA as the basis for a license to practice medicine (Haglund and Dowling 1993).

Once advanced graduate education became an integral part of medical training, it further legitimized the profession's authority and galvanized its sovereignty. Stevens (1971) noted that American medicine moved toward professional maturity between 1890 and 1914, mainly as a direct result of educational reform.

## Specialization in Medicine

Specialization has been a key hallmark of American medicine. As a comparison, in 1931, 17% of all physicians in the United States were specialists, whereas today, the proportion of specialists to generalists is approximately 58:42 (Bureau of Labor

Statistics 2011), and many generalists also have a subspecialty focus. The growth of allied health care professionals has also diversified, both in medical specialization— such as laboratory and radiological technologists, nurse anesthetists, and physical therapists—as well as in new or expanded specialist fields—such as occupational therapists, psychologists, dietitians, and medical social workers (Stevens 1971).

Lack of a rational coordination of medical care in the United States has been one consequence of the preoccupation with specialization. The characteristics of the medical profession in various countries often shape and define the key attributes of their health care delivery systems. The role of the primary care physician (PCP), the relationship between generalists and specialists, the ratio of practicing generalists to specialists, the structure and nature of medical staff appointments in hospitals, and the approach to group practice of medicine have all been molded by the evolving structure and ethos of the medical profession. In Britain, for example, the medical profession has divided itself into general practitioners (GPs) practicing in the community and consultants holding specialist positions in hospitals. This kind of stratification did not develop in American medicine. PCPs in America were not assigned the role that GPs had in Britain, where patients could consult a specialist only by referral from a GP. Unlike Britain, where GPs hold a key intermediary position in relation to the rest of the health care delivery system, the United States has lacked such a gatekeeping role. Only since the early 1990s, under health maintenance organizations (HMOs), has the *gatekeeping* model requiring initial contact with a generalist and the generalist's referral to a specialist gained prominence. The

distinctive shaping of medical practice in the United States explains why the structure of medicine did not develop around a nucleus of primary care.

## From the Asylum to Community Mental Health

At the turn of the 20th century, the scientific study and treatment of mental illnesses, called neuropathology, had just begun. Later, in 1946, federal funding was made available under the National Mental Health Act for psychiatric education and research. This Act led to the creation, in 1949, of the National Institute of Mental Health (NIMH). Early treatment of mental disorders was championed, and the concept of community mental health was born. By this time, new drugs for treating psychosis and depression had become available. Reformers of the mental health system argued that long-term institutional care had been neglectful, ineffective, and even harmful (US Surgeon General 1999). Passage of the Community Mental Health Centers Act of 1963 lent support to the joint policies of "community care" and "deinstitutionalization." From 1970 to 2000, state-run psychiatric hospital beds dropped from 207 to 21 beds per 100,000 persons (Manderscheid et al. 2004). The deinstitutionalization movement further intensified after the 1999 US Supreme Court decision in *Olmstead v. L.C.* that directed US states to provide community-based services to people with mental illness.

## The Development of Public Health

Historically, public health practices in the United States have concentrated on sanitary regulation, the study of epidemics, and vital statistics. The growth of urban centers for the purpose of commerce and industry, unsanitary living conditions in densely populated areas, inadequate methods of sewage and garbage disposal, limited access to clean water, and long work hours in unsafe and exploitative industries led to periodic epidemics of cholera, smallpox, typhoid, tuberculosis, yellow fever, and other diseases. Such outbreaks led to arduous efforts to protect the public interest. For example, in 1793, the national capital had to be moved out of Philadelphia due to a devastating outbreak of yellow fever. This epidemic prompted the city to develop its first board of health that same year. In 1850, Lemuel Shattuck outlined the blueprint for the development of a public health system in Massachusetts. Shattuck also called for the establishment of state and local health departments. A threatening outbreak of cholera in 1873 mobilized the New York City Health Department to alleviate the worst sanitary conditions within the city. Previously, cholera epidemics in 1832 and 1848–1849 had swept through American cities and towns within a few weeks, killing thousands (Duffy 1971). Until about 1900, infectious diseases posed the greatest health threat to society. The development of public health played a major role in curtailing the spread of infection among populations. Simultaneously, widespread public health measures and better medical care reduced mortality and increased life expectancy.

By 1900, most states had health departments that were responsible for a variety of public health efforts, such as sanitary inspections, communicable disease control, operation of state laboratories, vital statistics, health education, and regulation of food and water (Turnock 1997; Williams 1995). Public health functions were later extended to fill gaps in the medical care system. Such

functions, however, were limited mainly to child immunizations, care of mothers and infants, health screening in public schools, and family planning. Federal grants were also made available to state and local governments for programs in substance abuse, mental health, and community prevention services (Turnock 1997).

Public health has remained separate from the private practice of medicine because of the skepticism of private physicians that the government could take control of the private practice of medicine. Physicians realized that the boards of health could be used to control the supply of physicians and to regulate the practice of medicine (Rothstein 1972). Fear of government intervention, loss of autonomy, and erosion of personal incomes created a wall of separation between public health and private medical practice. Under this dichotomous relationship, medicine has concentrated on the physical health of the individual, whereas public health has focused on the health of whole populations and communities. The extent of collaboration between the two has been largely confined to the requirement by public health departments that private practitioners report cases of contagious diseases, such as sexually transmitted diseases, human immunodeficiency virus (HIV) infection, and acquired immune deficiency syndrome (AIDS), and any outbreaks of cases such as West Nile virus and other types of infections.

## Health Services for Veterans

Shortly after World War I, the government started to provide hospital services to veterans with service-related disabilities and for nonservice-related disabilities if the veteran declared an inability to pay for private care.

At first, the federal government contracted for services with voluntary hospitals, but, over time, the Department of Veterans Affairs (formerly called Veterans Administration) built its own hospitals, outpatient clinics, and nursing homes. (Additional details are provided in Chapter 6.)

## Birth of Workers' Compensation

The first broad-coverage health insurance in the United States emerged in the form of workers' compensation programs initiated in 1914 (Whitted 1993). Workers' compensation was originally concerned with cash payments to workers for wages lost due to job-related injuries and disease. Compensation for medical expenses and death benefits to the survivors were added later (discussed in Chapter 6). Between 1910 and 1915, workers' compensation laws made rapid progress in the United States (Stevens 1971). Looking at the trend, some reformers believed that, since Americans had been persuaded to adopt compulsory insurance against industrial accidents, they could also be persuaded to adopt compulsory insurance against sickness. Workers' compensation served as a trial balloon for the idea of government-sponsored, universal health insurance in the United States. However, the growth of private health insurance, along with other key factors discussed later, has prevented any proposals for a national health care program from taking hold.

## Rise of Private Health Insurance

Private health insurance was commonly referred to as *voluntary health insurance*, in contrast to proposals for a government-sponsored compulsory health insurance system. The initial role of private health insurance was income protection during sickness and temporary disability. Some private insurance coverage limited to bodily injuries was also available since approximately 1850. By 1900, health insurance policies became available, but their primary purpose was to protect against loss of income during sickness (Whitted 1993). Later, coverage was added for surgical fees, but emphasis remained on replacing lost income due to sickness or injury. Thus, the coverage was, in reality, disability insurance rather than health insurance (Mayer and Mayer 1984).

As detailed in subsequent sections, technological, social, and economic factors created a general need for health insurance. However, certain economic conditions that prompted private initiatives, self-interests of a well-organized medical profession, and the momentum of a successful health insurance enterprise, gave private health insurance a firm footing in the United States. Coverage for hospital and physician services began separately and was later combined under the auspices of Blue Cross and Blue Shield. Later, economic conditions during the World War II period laid the foundations for health insurance to become an employment-based benefit.

## Technological, Social, and Economic Factors

The health insurance movement of the early 20th century was the product of three converging developments: the technological, the social, and the economic. From a technological perspective, medicine offered new and better treatments. Because of its well-established healing values, medical care had become individually and socially desirable, which created a growing demand for medical services. From an economic perspective, people could predict neither their future needs for medical care nor the costs, both of which had been gradually increasing. In short, scientific and technological advances made health care more desirable but less affordable. These developments pointed to the need for some kind of insurance that could spread the financial risks over a large number of people.

## Early Blanket Insurance Policies

In 1911, insurance companies began to offer blanket policies for large industrial populations, usually covering life insurance, accidents and sickness, and nursing services. A few industrial and railroad companies set up their own medical plans, covering specified medical benefits, as did several unions and fraternal orders; however, the total amount of voluntary health insurance was minute (Stevens 1971). Between 1916 and 1918, 16 state legislatures, including New York and California, attempted to enact legislation compelling employers to provide health insurance, but these efforts were unsuccessful (Davis 1996).

## Economic Necessity and the Baylor Plan

The Great Depression, which started at the end of 1929, forced hospitals to turn from philanthropic donations to patient fees for support. Patients now faced not only loss of income from illness but also increased debt from medical care costs when they became sick. People needed protection from the economic consequences of sickness and hospitalization. Hospitals also needed protection from economic instability (Mayer and Mayer 1984). During the Depression, occupancy rates in hospitals fell, income from endowments and contributions dropped sharply,

and the charity load almost quadrupled (Richardson 1945).

In 1929, the blueprint for modern health insurance was established when J.F. Kimball began a hospital insurance plan for public school teachers at the Baylor University Hospital in Dallas, Texas. Kimball was able to enroll more than 1,200 teachers, who paid 50 cents a month for a maximum of 21 days of hospital care. Within a few years, it became the model for Blue Cross plans around the country (Raffel 1980). At first, other independent hospitals copied Baylor and started offering single-hospital plans. It was not long before communitywide plans, offered jointly by more than one hospital, became more popular because they provided consumers a choice of hospitals. The hospitals agreed to provide services in exchange for a fixed monthly payment by the plans. Hence, in essence, these were prepaid plans for hospital services. A *prepaid plan* is a contractual arrangement under which a provider must provide all needed services to a group of members (or enrollees) in exchange for a fixed monthly fee paid in advance.

## Successful Private Enterprise—The Blue Cross Plans

A hospital plan in Minnesota was the first to use the name Blue Cross in 1933 (Davis 1996). The American Hospital Association (AHA) lent support to the hospital plans and became the coordinating agency to unite these plans into the Blue Cross network (Koch 1993; Raffel 1980). The Blue Cross plans were nonprofit—that is, they had no shareholders who would receive profit distributions—and covered only hospital charges, as not to infringe on the domain of private physicians (Starr 1982).

Later, control of the plans was transferred to a completely independent body, the Blue Cross Commission, which later became the Blue Cross Association (Raffel 1980). In 1946, Blue Cross plans in 43 states served 20 million members. Between 1940 and 1950 alone, the proportion of the population covered by hospital insurance increased from 9 to 57% (Anderson 1990).

## Self Interests of Physicians—Birth of Blue Shield

Voluntary health insurance had received the AMA's endorsement, but the AMA had also made it clear that private health insurance plans should include only hospital care. It is, therefore, not surprising that the first Blue Shield plan designed to pay for physicians' bills was started by the California Medical Association, which established the California Physicians Service in 1939 (Raffel 1980). By endorsing hospital insurance and by actively developing medical service plans, the medical profession committed itself to private health insurance as the means to spread the financial risk of sickness and to ensure that its own interests would not be threatened.

From the medical profession's point of view, voluntary health insurance, in conjunction with private fee-for-service practice by physicians, was regarded as a desirable feature of the evolving health system (Stevens 1971). Throughout the Blue Shield movement, physicians dominated the boards of directors not only because they underwrote the plans but also because the plans were, in a very real sense, their response to the challenge of national health insurance. In addition, the plans met the AMA's stipulation of keeping medical matters in the hands of physicians (Raffel and Raffel 1994).

## Combined Hospital and Physician Coverage

Even though Blue Cross and Blue Shield developed independently and were financially and organizationally distinct, they often worked together to provide hospital and physician coverage (Law 1974). In 1974, the New York Superintendent of Insurance approved a merger of the Blue Cross and Blue Shield plans of Greater New York (Somers and Somers 1977). Since then, similar mergers have occurred in most states, and in nearly every state Blue Cross and Blue Shield plans are joint corporations or have close working relationships (Davis 1996).

The for-profit insurance companies were initially skeptical of the Blue Cross plans and adopted a wait-and-see attitude. Their apprehension was justified because no actuarial information was available to predict losses. But within a few years, lured by the success of the Blue Cross plans, commercial insurance companies also started offering health insurance.

## Employment-Based Health Insurance

Three main factors explain how health insurance in the United States became employment based: (1) To control high inflation in the economy during the World War II period, Congress imposed wage freezes. In response, many employers started offering health insurance to their workers in lieu of wage increases. (2) In 1948, the Supreme Court ruled that employee benefits, including health insurance, were a legitimate part of the union–management bargaining process. Health insurance then became a permanent part of employee benefits in the postwar era (Health Insurance Association of America 1991). (3) According to a 1954 revision to the Internal Revenue Code, employer contributions for the purchase of employee health insurance became exempt from taxable income for the employee. In other words, employees could get noncash income without having to pay taxes on this income.

Employment-based health insurance expanded rapidly. The economy was strong during the postwar years of the 1950s, and employers started offering more extensive benefits. This led to the birth of "major medical" expense coverage to protect against prolonged or catastrophic illness or injury (Mayer and Mayer 1984). Thus, private health insurance became the primary vehicle for the delivery of health care services in the United States.

## Failure of National Health Care Initiatives: A Historical Overview

Starting with Germany in 1883, compulsory sickness insurance had spread throughout Europe by 1912. Health insurance in European countries was viewed as a natural outgrowth of insurance against industrial accidents. Hence, it was considered logical that Americans would also be willing to espouse a national health care program to protect themselves from the high cost of sickness and accidents occurring outside employment.

The American Association of Labor Legislation (AALL) was founded in 1906. Although the AALL took no official position on labor unions, its membership did include prominent labor leaders (Starr 1982). Its relatively small membership, however, was mainly academic, including some leading economists and social scientists, whose all-important agenda was to bring about social reform through government action. The

AALL was primarily responsible for leading the successful drive for workers' compensation. It then spearheaded the drive for a government-sponsored health insurance system for the general population (Anderson 1990) and supported the Progressive movement headed by former President Theodore Roosevelt, who was again running for the presidency in 1912 on a platform of social reform. Roosevelt, who might have been a national political sponsor for compulsory health insurance, was defeated by Woodrow Wilson, but the Progressive movement for national health insurance did not die.

The AALL continued its efforts toward a model for national health insurance by appealing to both social and economic concerns. The reformers argued that national health insurance would relieve poverty because sickness usually brought wage loss and high medical costs to individual families. Reformers also argued that national health insurance would contribute to economic efficiency by reducing illness, lengthening life, and diminishing the causes of industrial discontent (Starr 1982). Leadership of the AMA, at the time, showed outward support for a national plan, and the AALL and the AMA formed a united front to secure legislation. A standard health insurance bill was introduced in 15 states in 1917 (Stevens 1971).

As long as compulsory health insurance was only under study and discussion, potential opponents paid no heed to it; but, once bills were introduced into state legislatures, opponents expressed vehement disapproval. Eventually, support for the AMA's social change proved only superficial.

Historically, repeated attempts to pass national health insurance legislation in the United States have failed for several reasons, which can be classified under four broad categories: political inexpediency, institutional dissimilarities, ideological differences, and tax aversion.

## Political Inexpediency

Before embarking on their national health programs, countries in Western Europe, notably Germany and England, were experiencing labor unrest that threatened political stability. Social insurance was seen as a means to obtain workers' loyalty and ward off political instability. Political conditions in the United States were quite different. There was no threat to political stability. Unlike countries in Europe, the American government was highly decentralized and engaged in little direct regulation of the economy or social welfare. Although Congress had set up a system of compulsory hospital insurance for merchant seamen as far back as 1798, it was an exceptional measure.* Matters related to health and welfare were typically left to state and local governments, and as a general rule, these levels of government left as much as possible to private and voluntary action.

The entry of America into World War I, in 1917, provided a final political blow to the health insurance movement as anti-German feelings were aroused. The US government denounced German social insurance, and opponents of health insurance called it a Prussian menace, inconsistent with American values (Starr 1982).

After attempts to pass compulsory health insurance laws failed at the state levels in California and New York, by 1920, the AALL itself lost interest in an obviously lost cause. Also in 1920, the AMA's House of Delegates approved a resolution condemning compulsory health insurance that would be regulated by the government (Numbers 1985). This AMA resolution opposing national health insurance solidified the profession against government interference with the practice of medicine.

## Institutional Dissimilarities

The preexisting institutions in Europe and America were dissimilar. Germany and England had mutual benefit funds to provide sickness benefits. These benefits reflected an awareness of the value of insuring against the cost of sickness among a sector of the working population. Voluntary sickness funds were less developed in the United States than in Europe, reflecting less interest in health insurance and less familiarity with it. More important, American hospitals were mainly private, whereas in Europe they were largely government operated (Starr 1982).

Dominance of private institutions of health care delivery is not consistent with national financing and payment mechanisms. For instance, compulsory health insurance proposals of the AALL were regarded by individual members of the medical profession as a threat to their private practice because such proposals would shift the primary source of income of medical professionals from individual patients to the government (Anderson 1990). Any efforts that would potentially erode the fee-for-service payment system and let private practice of medicine be controlled by a powerful third party—particularly the government—were opposed.

---

*Important seaports, such as Boston, were often confronted with many sick and injured seamen, who were away from their homes and families. Congress enacted a law requiring that 20 cents a month be withheld from the wages of each seaman on American ships to support merchant marine hospitals (Raffel and Raffel 1994).

Other institutional forces were also opposed to government-sponsored universal coverage. The insurance industry feared losing the income it derived from disability insurance, some insurance against medical services, and funeral benefits[*] (Anderson 1990). The pharmaceutical industry feared the government as a monopoly buyer, and retail pharmacists feared that hospitals would establish their own pharmacies under a government-run national health care program (Anderson 1990). Employers also saw the proposals as contrary to their interests. Spokespersons for American business rejected the argument that national health insurance would add to productivity and efficiency. It may seem ironic, but the labor unions—the American Federation of Labor in particular—also denounced compulsory health insurance at the time. Union leaders were afraid they would transfer over to the government their own legitimate role of providing social benefits, thus weakening the unions' influence in the workplace. Organized labor was the largest and most powerful interest group at that time, and its lack of support is considered instrumental in the defeat of national health insurance (Anderson 1990).

## Ideological Differences

The American value system is based largely on the principles of market justice (as discussed in Chapter 2). Individualism and self-determination, distrust of government, and reliance on the private sector to address social concerns are typical American ideologies that have stood as a bulwark against

anything perceived as an onslaught on individual liberties. The cultural and ideological values represent the sentiments of the American middle class, whose support is necessary for any broad-based reform. Without such support, a national health care program was unable to withstand the attacks of its well-organized opponents (Anderson 1990). Conversely, during times of national distress, such as the Great Depression, pure necessity may have legitimized the advancement of social programs, such as the New Deal programs of the Franklin Roosevelt era (for example, Social Security legislation providing old-age pensions and unemployment compensation).

In the early 1940s, during Roosevelt's presidency, several bills on national health insurance were introduced in Congress, but all the proposed bills died. Perhaps the most notable bill was the Wagner-Murray-Dingell bill, drafted in 1943 and named after the bill's congressional sponsors. However, this time, World War II diverted the nation's attention to other issues, and without the president's active support the bill died quietly (Numbers 1985).

In 1946, Harry Truman became the first president to make an appeal for a national health care program (Anderson 1990). Unlike the Progressives, who had proposed a plan for the working class, Truman proposed a single health insurance plan that would include all classes of society. At the president's behest, the Wagner-Murray-Dingell bill was redrafted and reintroduced. The AMA was vehement in opposing the plan. Other health care interest groups, such as the AHA, also opposed it. By this time, private health insurance had expanded. Initial public reaction to the Wagner-Murray-Dingell bill was positive; however, when a government-controlled medical plan was

[*] Patients admitted to a hospital were required to pay a burial deposit so the hospital would not have to incur a burial expense if they died (Raffel and Raffel 1994). Therefore, many people bought funeral policies from insurance companies.

compared to private insurance, polls showed that only 12% of the public favored extending Social Security to include health insurance (Numbers 1985).

During this era of the Cold War,[*] any attempts to introduce national health insurance were met with the stigmatizing label of *socialized medicine*, a label that has since become synonymous with any large-scale government-sponsored expansion of health insurance or intrusion in the private practice of medicine. The Republicans took control of Congress in 1946, and any interest in enacting national health insurance was put to rest. However, to the surprise of many, Truman was reelected in 1948, promising national health insurance if the Democrats would be returned to power (Starr 1982). Fearing the inevitable, the AMA levied a $25 fee on each of its members toward a war chest of $3.5 million (Anderson 1990). It hired the public relations firm of Whitaker and Baxter and spent $1.5 million, in 1949 alone, to launch one of the most expensive lobbying efforts in American history. The campaign directly linked national health insurance with Communism until the idea of socialized medicine was firmly implanted in the public's minds. Republicans proposed a few compromises in which neither the Democrats nor the AMA was interested. By 1952, the election of a Republican president, Dwight Eisenhower, effectively ended any further debate over national health insurance. Failure of government-sponsored universal health care coverage is often presented as a classic case of the tremendous influence of interest groups in American politics, especially in major health policy outcomes.

---

[*]Rivalry and hostility after World War II between the United States and the then Soviet Union.

## Tax Aversion

An aversion to increased taxes to pay for social programs is another reason middle-class Americans, who are already insured, have opposed national initiatives to expand health insurance coverage. According to polls, Americans have been found to support the idea that the government ought to help people who are in financial need to pay for their medical care. However, most Americans have not favored an increase in their own taxes to pay for such care. This is perhaps why health reform failed in 1993.

While seeking the presidency in 1992, Governor Bill Clinton made health system reform a major campaign issue. Not since Harry Truman's initiatives in the 1940s had such a bold attempt been made by a presidential candidate. As long as the electorate had remained reasonably satisfied with health care—with the exception of uninsured Americans, who have not been politically strong—elected officials had feared the political clout of big interest groups and had refrained from raising tough reform issues. In the Pennsylvania US Senate election in November 1991, however, the victory of Democrat Harris Wofford over Republican Richard Thornburgh sent a clear signal that the time for a national health care program might be ripe. Wofford's call for national health insurance was widely supported by middle-class Pennsylvanians. Election results in other states were not quite as decisive on the health reform issue, but various public polls seemed to confirm that, after the economy (America was in a brief recession at the time), health care was the second most pressing concern on the minds of the American people. One national survey, conducted by Louis Harris and Associates, reported some disturbing findings about health care delivery. Substantial numbers of insured and relatively affluent people said they had not received the services they needed. The poll also suggested that the public was looking to the federal government, not the states or private sector, to contain rising health care costs (Smith et al. 1992). In other opinion polls, Americans expressed concerns that they might not be adequately insured in the future (Skocpol 1995). Against this backdrop, both Bill Clinton and the running incumbent, President George (Herbert Walker) Bush, advanced health care reform proposals.

After taking office, President Clinton made health system reform one of his top priorities. Policy experts and public opinion leaders have since debated over what went wrong. Some of the fundamental causes for the failure of the Clinton plan were no doubt historical in nature, as discussed previously in this chapter. One seasoned political observer, James J. Mongan, however, remarked that reform debates in Congress have never been about the expansion of health care services but rather have been about the financing of the proposed services:

> Thus, the most important cause of health care reform's demise was that avoiding tax increases and their thinly veiled cousin, employer mandates, took priority over expanding coverage. . . . There undoubtedly would have been pitched legislative battles over other issues—how to pay doctors and hospitals, the role of health insurers, the structure of (regional health) alliances—but these debates never happened in detail. The first and only battle . . . was how to pay for reform. . . . What explains this unwillingness to pay for expanded coverage, on the part of citizens and government alike? Any answer must take into account the economic, social, and political context of the past two decades. . . . The social context is that people tend to take for granted the

progress achieved through social insurance programs such as Medicare and Social Security, and they perceive little progress or achievement from welfare expenditures targeted on low-income people. Politically, politicians from the courthouse to the White House have played to an anti-tax sentiment and have convinced Americans and American businesses that they are staggering under an oppressive burden of taxation that saps most productive effort. Although there is little evidence from other countries to support this belief, it is widely held. This climate fosters a self-centeredness—a focus more on the individual's needs than on the community's needs. Some liberals might use a harsher, more grating word— selfishness—to describe this state of mind. But many conservatives would use the phrase *rugged individualism* to describe the same phenomenon. . . . Somewhere in here is where health reform died. . . . Until we as a nation make the right diagnosis and begin an honest dialogue about our national values, about the balance between self-interest and community interests, we will not see our nation join almost all others in guaranteeing health coverage to all of its citizens (Mongan 1995, 99–101).

When American polls indicated that a fundamental reform was needed, the people did not have in mind more government regulation or any significant redistribution of income through increased taxes. Most important, they did not wish to have a negative effect on their own access to care or the quality of care they were receiving (Altman and Reinhardt 1996).

## Creation of Medicaid and Medicare

Before 1965, private health insurance was the only widely available source of payment for health care, and it was available primarily to middle-class working people and their families. The elderly, the unemployed, and the poor had to rely on their own resources, on limited public programs, or on charity from hospitals and individual physicians. Often, when charity care was provided, private payers were charged more to make up the difference, a practice referred to as *cost-shifting* or *cross-subsidization*. In 1965, Congress passed the amendments to the Social Security Act and created the Medicare and Medicaid programs. Thus, for the first time in US history, the government assumed direct responsibility to pay for some of the health care on behalf of two vulnerable population groups—the elderly and the poor (Potter and Longest 1994).

Through the debates over how to protect the public from rising costs of health care and the opposition to national health insurance, one thing had become clear: Government intervention was not desired insofar as it pertained to how most Americans received health care, with one exception. Less opposition would be encountered if reform initiatives were proposed for the underprivileged classes. In principle, the poor were considered a special class who could be served through a government-sponsored program. The elderly—those 65 years of age and over—were another group who started to receive increased attention in the 1950s. On their own, most of the poor and the elderly could not afford the increasing costs of health care. Also, because the health status of these population groups was significantly worse than that of the general population, they required a higher level of health care services. The elderly, particularly, had higher incidence and prevalence of disease compared to younger groups. It was also estimated that less than one-half of the elderly population were covered by private health insurance. By this

time, the growing elderly middle class was also becoming a politically active force.

Government assistance for the poor and the elderly was sought once it became clear that the market alone would not ensure access for these vulnerable population groups. A bill introduced in Congress by Aime Forand, in 1957, provided momentum for including necessary hospital and nursing home care as an extension of Social Security benefits (Stevens 1971). The AMA, however, undertook a massive campaign to portray a government insurance plan as a threat to the physician–patient relationship. The bill was stalled, but public hearings around the country, which were packed by the elderly, produced an intense grassroots support to push the issue onto the national agenda (Starr 1982). A compromised reform, the Medical Assistance Act (Public Law 86–778), also known as the Kerr-Mills Act, went into effect in 1960. Under the Act, federal grants were given to the states to extend health services provided by the state welfare programs to those low-income elderly who previously did not qualify (Anderson 1990). Since the program was based on a *means test* that confined eligibility to people below a predetermined income level, it was opposed by liberal congressional representatives as a source of humiliation to the elderly (Starr 1982). Within 3 years, the program was declared ineffective because many states did not even implement it (Stevens 1971). In 1964, health insurance for the aged and the poor became top priorities of President Johnson's Great Society programs.

During the debate over Medicare, the AMA developed its own "Eldercare" proposal, which called for a federal–state program to subsidize private insurance policies for hospital and physician services. Representative John W. Byrnes introduced yet another proposal, dubbed "Bettercare." It proposed a federal program based on partial premium contributions by the elderly, with the remainder subsidized by the government. Other proposals included tax credits and tax deductions for health insurance premiums.

In the end, a three-layered program emerged. The first two layers constituted Part A and Part B of *Medicare*, or *Title XVIII* of the Social Security Amendment of 1965 to provide publicly financed health insurance to the elderly. Based on Forand's initial bill, the administration's proposal to finance hospital insurance providing hospital care and partial nursing home coverage for the elderly through Social Security became *Part A* of Medicare. The Byrnes proposal to cover physicians' bills through government-subsidized insurance became *Part B* of Medicare. An extension of the Kerr-Mills program of federal matching funds to the states, based on each state's financial needs, became *Medicaid*, or *Title XIX* of the Social Security Amendment of 1965. The Medicaid program was for the indigent, based on means tests established by each state, but it was expanded to include all age groups, not just the poor elderly (Stevens 1971).

Although adopted together, Medicare and Medicaid reflected sharply different traditions. Medicare was upheld by broad grassroots support and, being attached to Social Security, had no class distinction. Medicaid, however, was burdened by the stigma of public welfare. Medicare had uniform national standards for eligibility and benefits; Medicaid varied from state to state in terms of eligibility and benefits. Medicare allowed physicians to *balance bill*, that is, charge the patient the amount above the program's set fees and recoup the difference. Medicaid prohibited balance billing and, consequently, had limited participation from physicians (Starr 1982). Medicaid, in essence, has created a two-tier system of medical care delivery because some physicians refuse to accept Medicaid patients due to low fees set by the government.

Not long after Medicare and Medicaid were in operation, national spending for health services began to rise, as did public outlays of funds in relation to private spending for health services (Anderson 1990). For example, national health expenditures (NHE), which had increased by 50% from 1955 to 1960, and again from 1960 to 1965, jumped by 78% from 1965 to 1970, and by 71% from 1970 to 1975. Similarly, public expenditures for health care, which were stable at 25% of NHE for 1955, 1960, and 1965, increased to 36.5% of NHE in 1970, and to 42.1% of NHE in 1975 (based on data from Bureau of the Census 1976).

## Regulatory Role of Public Health Agencies

With the expansion of publicly financed Medicare and Medicaid programs, the regulatory powers of government have increasingly encroached upon the private sector. This is because the government provides financing for the two programs, but services are delivered by the private sector. After the federal government developed the standards for participation in the Medicare program, states developed regulations in conjunction with the Medicaid program. The regulations often overlapped, and the federal government delegated authority to the states to carry out the monitoring of regulatory compliance. As a result, the regulatory powers assigned to state public health agencies increased dramatically. Thus, most institutions of health care delivery are subject to annual scrutiny by public health agencies under the authority delegated to them by the federal and state governments.

## Prototypes of Managed Care

Even though the early practice of medicine in the United States was mainly characterized by private solo practice, three subsequent developments in medical care delivery are noteworthy: contract practice, group practice, and prepaid group practice. All three required some sort of organizational integration, which was a departure from solo practice. These innovative arrangements can also be regarded as early precursors of managed care and integrated organizations (discussed in Chapter 9).

### Contract Practice

In 1882, Northern Pacific Railroad Beneficial Association was one of the first employers to provide medical care expense coverage (Davis 1996). Between 1850 and 1900, other railroad, mining, and lumber enterprises developed extensive employee medical programs. Such companies conducted operations in isolated areas where physicians were unavailable. Inducements, such as a guaranteed salary, were commonly offered to attract physicians. Another common arrangement was to contract with independent physicians and hospitals at a flat fee per worker per month, referred to as *capitation*. The AMA recognized the necessity of contract practice in remote areas, but elsewhere contract practice was regarded as a form of exploitation because it was assumed that physicians would bid against each other and drive down the price. Offering services at reduced rates was regarded by the AMA as an unethical invasion of private practice. When group health insurance

became common in the 1940s through collective bargaining, the medical profession was freed from the threat of direct control by large corporations. Health insurance also enabled workers to go to physicians and hospitals of their choice (Starr 1982).

Corporate practice of medicine—that is, provision of medical care by for-profit corporations—was generally prohibited by law. It was labeled as commercialism in medicine. In 1917, however, Oregon passed the Hospital Association Act, which permitted for-profit corporations to provide medical services. Whereas health insurance companies, functioning as insurers and payers, acted as intermediaries between patients and physicians, the hospital associations in Oregon contracted directly with physicians and exercised some control over them. Utilization was managed by requiring second opinions for major surgery and by reviewing length of hospital stays. The corporations also restricted medical fees, refusing to pay prices deemed excessive. In short, they acted as a countervailing power in the medical market to limit physicians' professional autonomy. Even though physicians resented controls, they continued to do business with the hospital associations due to guaranteed payments (Starr 1982).

Early contract practice arrangements and the Oregon hospital associations can be viewed as prototypes of managed care. Since the 1980s and 1990s, MCOs have successfully replaced the traditional fee-for-service payment arrangements by capitation and discounted fees. Mechanisms to control excessive utilization are another key feature of managed care.

### Group Practice

Group medicine represented another form of corporate organization for medical care.

Group practice changed the relationship among physicians by bringing them together with business managers and technical assistants in a more elaborate division of labor (Starr 1982). The Mayo Clinic, started in Rochester, Minnesota, in 1887, is regarded as a prototype of the consolidation of specialists into group practice. The concept of a multispecialty group presented a threat to the continuation of general practice. It also presented competition to specialists who remained in solo practice. Hence, the development of group practice met with widespread professional resistance (Stevens 1971). Although specialist group practice did not become a movement, sharing of expenses and incomes, along with other economic advantages, has caused group practices to continue to grow.

## Prepaid Group Plans

In time, the efficiencies of group practice led to the formation of prepaid group plans, in which an enrolled population received comprehensive services for a capitated fee. The HIP Health Plan of New York, started in 1947, stands as one of the most successful programs, providing comprehensive medical services through organized medical groups of family physicians and specialists (Raffel 1980). Similarly, Kaiser-Permanente, started in 1942, has grown on the West Coast. Other examples are the Group Health Cooperative of Puget Sound in Seattle, operating since 1947, which is a consumer-owned cooperative prepaid group practice (Williams 1993), and the Labor Health Institute in St. Louis, started in 1945, which is a union-sponsored group practice scheme (Stevens 1971).

The idea of prepaid group practice had limitations. It required the sponsorship of large organizations. HIP, for example, was created by New York's Mayor Fiorello La Guardia for city employees. Industrialist Henry Kaiser initially set up his prepaid plan to provide comprehensive health care services to his own employees, but the health plan was later extended to other employers.

In 1971, President Nixon singled out prepaid group practice organizations as the model for a rational reorganization in the delivery of health services. They became the prototype of HMOs (Somers and Somers 1977). During the Nixon Administration, the use of HMOs in the private sector was encouraged by federal legislation, the Health Maintenance Organization Act (HMO Act) of 1973. The HMO Act required employers to offer an HMO alternative to conventional health insurance (Goodman and Musgrave 1992). MCOs still attempt to combine the efficiencies of contract and group arrangements with the objective of delivering comprehensive health care services at predetermined costs.

# Medical Care in the Corporate Era

The latter part of the 20th century and start of the 21st century have been marked by the growth and consolidation of large business corporations and tremendous advances in global communications, transportation, and trade. These developments are starting to change the way health care is delivered in the United States and, indeed, around the world. The rise of multinational corporations, the information revolution, and globalization have been interdependent phenomena. The World Trade Organization's General Agreement on Trade in Services (GATS), which came into effect in 1995, aims to gradually remove all barriers to international trade in services. In health care services, GATS may regulate health insurance, hospital services, telemedicine, and acquisition of medical treatment abroad. GATS negotiations, however, have met controversy, as various countries fear that it may shape their domestic health care systems (Belsky et al. 2004), although most analysts predict that GATS is likely to produce future market liberalization (Mutchnick et al. 2005).

## Corporatization of Health Care Delivery

Corporatization here refers to the ways in which health care delivery in the United States has become the domain of large organizations. These corporations may operate either on a for-profit or nonprofit basis, yet they are driven, for the most part, by the common goal of maximizing their revenues. At least one benefit of this corporatization has been the ability of these organizations to deliver sophisticated modern health care in comfortable and pleasant surroundings. But, one main expectation of delivering the same quality of health care at lesser cost remains largely unrealized.

On the supply side, until the mid-1980s, physicians and hospitals clearly dominated the medical marketplace. Since then, managed care has emerged as a dominant force by becoming the primary vehicle for insuring and delivering health care to the majority of Americans. The rise of managed care consolidated immense purchasing power on the demand side. To counteract this imbalance, providers began to consolidate, and larger, integrated health care organizations began forming (see Chapter 9). A second, influential factor behind health care integration was reimbursement cuts for inpatient acute care hospital services in the mid-1980s. To make up for lost revenues in the inpatient sector, hospitals developed various types of outpatient services, such as primary care, outpatient surgery, and home health care, and expanded into other differentiated health care services, such as long-term care and specialized rehabilitation. Together, managed care and integrated delivery organizations have, in reality, corporatized the delivery of health care in the United States.

In a health care landscape that has been increasingly dominated by corporations, individual physicians have struggled to preserve their autonomy. As a matter of survival, many physicians consolidated into large clinics, formed strategic partnerships with hospitals, or started their own specialty hospitals. A growing number of physicians have become employees of large medical corporations. Proliferation of these new models of health care delivery has made it increasingly difficult for states to maintain outright bans on the employment of physicians (Farmer and Douglas 2001).

Both managed care and corporate delivery of medicine have made the health care system extremely complex from the consumer's standpoint. Managed care was supposed to be a market-based reform, but it has stripped the primary consumer, the patient, of practically all marketplace power. Dominance by any entity, whether organized medicine or integrated health organizations, subverts the sovereignty of the health care consumer. In this so-called market-driven integration, the consumer continues to wonder, "Where's the market?"

## Information Revolution

The delivery of health care is being transformed in unprecedented and irreversible ways by telecommunication. The use of telemedicine and telehealth is on the rise (see Chapter 5). These technologies integrate telecommunication systems into the practice of protecting and promoting health, which may or may not incorporate actual physician–patient interactions.

Telemedicine dates back to the 1920s, when shore-based medical specialists were radio linked to address medical emergencies at sea (Winters 1921). Telemedicine came to the forefront in the 1990s, with the technological advances in the distant transmission of image data and the recognition that there was inequitable access to medical care in rural America. Federal dollars were poured into rural telemedicine projects.

Telehealth consultations can occur in real time. Videoconferencing is now replacing telephone consultation as the preferred vehicle for behavioral telehealth or telepsychiatry. *E-health* has also become an unstoppable force that is driven by consumer demand for health care information and services offered over the Internet by professionals and non-professionals alike (Maheu et al. 2001). The Internet has created a new revolution that is increasingly characterized by patient empowerment. Access to expert information is no longer strictly confined to the physician's domain, which in some ways has led to a dilution of the dependent role of the patient.

## Globalization

*Globalization* refers to various forms of cross-border economic activities. It is driven by global exchange of information, production of goods and services more economically in developing countries, and increased interdependence of mature and emerging world economies. It confers many advantages but also has its downsides.

From the standpoint of cross-border trade in health services, Mutchnick and colleagues (2005) identified four different modes of economic interrelationships: (1) Use of advanced telecommunication infrastructures in telemedicine transfers information cross-border for instant answers and services. For example, teleradiology (the electronic transmission of radiological images over a distance) now enables physicians in the United States to transmit radiological images to Australia, where they are interpreted and reported back the next day (McDonnell 2006). Innovative telemedicine consulting services in pathology and radiology are being delivered to other parts of the world by cutting-edge US medical institutions, such as Johns Hopkins. (2) Consumers travel abroad to receive medical care. Specialty hospitals, such as the Apollo chain in India and Bumrungrad International Hospital in Thailand, offer state-of-the-art medical facilities to foreigners at a fraction of the cost for the same procedures done in the United States or Europe. Physicians and hospitals outside the United States have clear competitive advantages: reasonable malpractice costs, minimum regulation, and lower costs of labor. As a result of these efficiencies, Indian specialty hospitals can do quality liver transplants for one-tenth of the cost in US hospitals (Mutchnick et al. 2005). Some health insurance companies have also started to explore cheaper options for their covered members to receive certain costly services overseas. Conversely, dignitaries and other wealthy foreigners come to multispecialty centers in the United States, such as the Mayo Clinic, to receive highly specialized services. (3) Foreign direct investment in health services enterprises benefits foreign citizens. For example, Chindex International, a US corporation, provides medical equipment, supplies, and clinical care in China. Chindex opened the Beijing

United Family Hospital and Clinics in 1997 (Mutchnick et al. 2005). (4) Health professionals move to other countries that present high demand for their services and better economic opportunities than their native countries. For example, nurses from other countries are moving to the United States to relieve the existing personnel shortage. Migration of physicians from developing countries helps alleviate at least some of the shortage in underserved locations in the developed world.

To the above list, we can add two more: (1) Corporations based in the United States have increasingly expanded their operations overseas. As a result, an increasing number of Americans are now working overseas as expatriates. Health insurance companies based in the United States are, in turn, having to develop benefit plans for these expatriates. According to a survey of 87 insurance companies, health care is also becoming one of the most sought after employee benefits worldwide, even in countries that have national health insurance programs. Also, the cost of medical care overseas is rising at a faster rate than the rate of inflation in the general economy (Cavanaugh 2008). Hence, the cost-effective delivery of health care is becoming a major challenge worldwide. (2) Medical care delivery by US providers is in demand overseas. American providers, such as Johns Hopkins, Cleveland Clinic, Mayo Clinic, Duke University, and several others, are now delivering medical services in various developing countries.

Globalization has also produced some negative effects. The developing world pays a price when emigration leaves these countries with shortages of trained professionals. The burden of disease in these countries is often greater than it is in the developed world, and emigration only exacerbates the ability of these countries to provide adequate health care to their own populations (Norcini and Mazmanian 2005). Tobacco use is on the decline in many developed countries, yet economic development in emerging markets provides new targets for multinational tobacco companies. In addition, as developing countries become more prosperous, they acquire Western tastes and lifestyles. In some instances, negative health consequences follow. For example, increased use of motorized vehicles results in a lack of physical exercise, which, along with changes in diet, greatly increases the prevalence of chronic diseases, such as heart disease and diabetes, in the developing world. Conversely, better information about health promotion and disease prevention, as well as access to gyms and swimming pools, in developing countries is making a positive impact on the health and well-being of their middle-class citizens. Globalization has also posed some new threats. For instance, the threat of infectious diseases has increased, as diseases appearing in one country can spread rapidly to other countries. HIV/AIDS, hepatitis B, and hepatitis C infections have spread worldwide. New viral infections, such as avian flu and SARS, have at times threatened to create worldwide pandemics.

## Has the Era of Socialized Medicine Arrived?

Perhaps it has arrived, but only time can tell. Despite the obstacles to national health insurance, discussed previously in this chapter, on March 21, 2010, the House Democrats in Congress successfully passed, by a 219 to 212 vote, the Patient Protection and

Affordable Care Act, which was signed into law 2 days later by President Obama. Not a single Republican voted in favor of the legislation.

Among many campaign promises to bring change to America, Barack Obama stated his goal of drastically reducing the number of Americans who had no health insurance coverage. Details of any "plan" to accomplish this, however, were left unstated. President Obama was sworn into office in January 2009. A Democratic president also had Democrat majority in both houses of Congress for the first time since 1993, the year in which President Clinton had proposed a massive overhaul of the US health care system. Unlike the defeat of Clinton's reform proposals, which were criticized by some congressional leaders in his own party, Obama was able to maneuver the passage of his health care agenda by uniting his party behind a common cause. Support for the bill required backroom deals with waffling members of the Democratic Party and with interest groups representing the hospital and pharmaceutical industries. Surprisingly, the AMA sheepishly pledged its support for the legislation, which was a complete reversal of its historic stance toward national health insurance. According to one commentator, the AMA has tried to protect itself. The AMA is no longer the powerful organization it once was; it now represents only 17% of the physicians in the United States. It is plausible that the AMA has tried to protect its monopoly over the medical coding system that health care providers must use to get paid, which generates an annual income of over $70 million for the organization (Scherz 2010). The American public was also kept in the dark about the details buried in the 2,700 pages filled by the final legislation.

Over one-half of the states and some private parties filed lawsuits challenging the constitutionality of the new law. In December 2010, a federal judge in Virginia ruled that at least certain provisions of the law were unconstitutional because they force individuals to purchase health insurance. In January 2011, a federal judge in Florida ruled in a lawsuit, joined by 26 states, that the entire law was unconstitutional. Many legal scholars think the matter will be finally settled by the Supreme Court.

Polls showed that nearly two-thirds of Americans opposed the legislation as too ambitious and too costly (Page 2010). A more current Gallup poll showed that 46% of Americans were in favor of repealing the law; 40% opposed repealing it (Jones 2011).

In the 2010 midterm elections, Republicans gained control of the House, whereas the Democrats held their majority in the Senate. The balance of power shifted. The Republicans, taking advantage of their majority in the House, voted to repeal the health care law, but the Senate rejected this measure by a vote of 51 to 47 in favor of not repealing the law. Miller (2010) describes the stalemate in health reform as a "cease-fire in a political hundred years' war." The cease-fire may not last for too long.

## Summary

Figure 3–1 provides a snapshot of the historical developments in US health care delivery. The evolution of health care services has been strongly influenced by the advancement of scientific research and technological development. Early scientific discoveries were pioneered in Europe, but they were not readily adopted in the United States.

Figure 3–1  Evolution of the US Health Care Delivery System.

Development of science and technology

| Mid-18th to late 19th century | Late 19th to late 20th century | Late 20th to 21st century |
|---|---|---|
| • Open entry into medical practice<br>• Intense competition<br>• Weak and unorganized profession<br>• Apprenticeship training<br>• Undeveloped hospitals<br>• Private payment for services<br>• Low demand for services<br>• Private medical schools providing only general education | • Scientific basis of medicine<br>• Urbanization<br>• Emergence of the modern hospital<br>• Emergence of organized medicine<br>• Emergence of scientific medical training<br>• Licensing<br>• Development of public health<br>• Specialization in medicine<br>• Emergence of workers' compensation<br>• Emergence of private insurance<br>• Failure of national health insurance<br>• Medicaid and Medicare<br>• Prototypes of managed care | • **Corporatization**<br>  Managed care<br>  Health care integration<br>  Diluted physician autonomy<br>  Complexity for the patient<br>• **Information revolution**<br>  Telemedicine<br>  E-health<br>  Patient empowerment<br>• **Globalization**<br>  Global telemedicine<br>  Medical travel<br>  Foreign investment in health care<br>  Migration of professionals<br>  Exportation of lifestyles<br>  Challenge of new diseases<br>  Bioterrorism |
| Consumer sovereignty | Professional dominance | Corporate dominance |

Beliefs and values/Social, economic, and political  constraints

Therefore, medicine had a largely domestic, rather than professional, character in preindustrial America. The absence of standards of practice and licensing requirements allowed the trained and untrained alike to deliver medical care. Hospitals were more akin to places of refuge than centers of medical practice. The demand for professional services was relatively low because services had to be purchased privately, without the help of government or health insurance. Medical education was seriously deficient in providing technical training based on scientific knowledge. The medical profession faced intense competition; it was weak, unorganized, and insecure.

Scientific and technological advances led to the development of sophisticated institutions, where better-trained physicians could practice medicine. The transformation of America from a mainly rural, sparsely populated country to one with growing centers of urban population created increased reliance on the specialized skills that only trained professionals could offer. Simultaneously, medical professionals banded together into a politically strong organization, the AMA. The AMA succeeded in controlling the practice of medicine, mainly through its influence on medical education, licensing of physicians, and political lobbying.

In Europe, national health insurance has been an outgrowth of generous social programs. In the United States, by contrast, the predominance of private institutions, ideologies founded on the principles of market justice, and an aversion to tax increases have been instrumental in maintaining a health care delivery system that is mainly privately financed and operated. The AMA and other interest groups have also wielded enormous influence in opposing efforts to initiate comprehensive reforms based on national health insurance. Access to health services in the United States is achieved, primarily, through private health insurance; however, two major social programs, Medicaid and Medicare, were expediently enacted to provide affordable health services to vulnerable populations.

The corporate era in health care dawned in the latter part of the 20th century. The rise of multinational corporations, the information revolution, and globalization have marked this current era. Managed care represents corporatization of health care delivery on the demand side. On the supply side, providers have been integrated into various types of consolidated arrangements. The information revolution is characterized by the growth of telemedicine and E-health. Globalization has made the mature and the emerging world economies more interdependent, which has both advantages and disadvantages.

In 2010, thanks to control of Congress and the presidency by the Democratic Party, a sweeping health care reform legislation was passed. However, amid legal challenges, loss of control of the House of Representatives by the Democratic Party, and public opposition, the fate of this new law remains uncertain.

## Test Your Understanding

### Terminology

| | | |
|---|---|---|
| *almshouse* | *gatekeeping* | *pesthouse* |
| *balance bill* | *globalization* | *prepaid plan* |
| *capitation* | *means test* | *socialized medicine* |
| *cost-shifting* | *Medicaid* | *Title XVIII* |
| *cross-subsidization* | *Medicare* | *Title XIX* |
| *cultural authority* | *organized medicine* | *voluntary health insurance* |
| *E-health* | *Part A* | |
| *fee for service* | *Part B* | |

## Review Questions

1. Why did the professionalization of medicine start later in the United States than in some Western European nations?

2. Why did medicine have a domestic, rather than professional, character in the preindustrial era? How did urbanization change that?

3. Which factors explain why the demand for the services of a professional physician was inadequate in the preindustrial era? How did scientific medicine and technology change that?

4. How did the emergence of general hospitals strengthen the professional sovereignty of physicians?

5. Discuss the relationship of dependency within the context of the medical profession's cultural and legitimized authority. What role did medical education reform play in galvanizing professional authority?

6. How did the organized medical profession manage to remain free of control by business firms, insurance companies, and hospitals until the latter part of the 20th century?

7. In general, discuss how technological, social, and economic factors created the need for health insurance.

8. Which conditions during the World War II period lent support to private health insurance in the United States?

9. Discuss, with particular reference to the roles of (a) organized medicine, (b) the middle class, and (c) American beliefs and values, why reform efforts to bring in national health insurance have historically been unsuccessful in the United States.

10. Which particular factors that earlier may have been somewhat weak in bringing about national health insurance later led to the passage of Medicare and Medicaid?

11. On what basis were the elderly and the poor regarded as vulnerable groups for whom special government-sponsored programs needed to be created?

12. Discuss the government's role in the delivery and financing of health care, with specific reference to the dichotomy between public health and private medicine.

13. Explain how contract practice and prepaid group practice were the prototypes of today's managed care plans.

14. Discuss the main ways in which current delivery of health care has become corporatized.

15. How has the information revolution affected the practice of medicine?

16. In the context of globalization in health services, what main economic activities are discussed in this chapter?

---

## REFERENCES

Altman, S.H., and U.E. Reinhardt, eds. 1996. *Strategic choices for a changing health care system.* Chicago: Health Administration Press.

Anderson, O.W. 1990. *Health services as a growth enterprise in the United States since 1875.* Ann Arbor, MI: Health Administration Press.

Belsky, L. et al. 2004. The general agreement on trade in services: Implications for health policymakers. *Health Affairs* 23, no. 3: 137–145.

Bordley, J., and A.M. Harvey. 1976. *Two centuries of American medicine 1776–1976.* Philadelphia, PA: W.B. Saunders Company.

Bureau of the Census. 1976. *Statistical abstract of the United States, 1976.* Washington, DC: US Department of Commerce.

Bureau of Labor Statistics. 2011. *Occupational outlook handbook, 2010-11.* Available at: http://www.bls.gov/oco/home.htm. Accessed January 2011.

Burns, J. 2004. Are nonprofit hospitals really charitable? Taking the question to the state and local level. *Journal of Corporate Law* 29, no. 3: 665–683.

Cavanaugh, B.B. 2008. Building the worldwide health network. *Best's Review* 108, no. 12: 32–37.

Clark, C. 1998. A bloody evolution: Human error in medicine is as old as the practice itself. *The Washington Post,* 20 October, Z10.

Coggeshall, L.T. 1965. *Planning for medical progress through education.* Evanston, IL: Association of American Medical Colleges.

Davis, P. 1996. The fate of Blue Shield and the new blues. *South Dakota Journal of Medicine* 49, no. 9: 323–330.

Duffy, J. 1971. Social impact of disease in the late 19th century. *Bulletin of the New York Academy of Medicine* 47: 797–811.

Falk, G. 1999. *Hippocrates assailed: The American health delivery system.* Lanham, MD: University Press of America, Inc.

Farmer, G.O., and J.H. Douglas. 2001. Physician "unionization"—A primer and prescription. *Florida Bar Journal* 75, no. 7: 37–42.

Gabe, J. et al. 1994. *Challenging medicine.* New York: Routledge.

Goodman, J.C., and G.L. Musgrave. 1992. *Patient power: Solving America's health care crisis.* Washington, DC: CATO Institute.

Haber, S. 1974. The professions and higher education in America: A historical view. In: *Higher education and labor markets.* M.S. Gordon, ed. New York: McGraw-Hill Book Co.

Haglund, C.L., and W.L. Dowling. 1993. The hospital. In: *Introduction to health services.* 4th ed. S.J. Williams and P.R. Torrens, eds. New York: Delmar Publishers. pp. 135–176.

Hamowy, R. 1979. The early development of medical licensing laws in the United States, 1875–1900. *Journal of Libertarian Studies* 3, no. 1: 73–119.

Health Insurance Association of America. 1991. *Source book of health insurance data.* Washington, DC: Health Insurance Association of America.

Henry J. Kaiser Family Foundation. 2011. *Summary of coverage provisions in the Patient Protection and Affordable Care Act.* Available at: http://kff.org/healthreform/upload/8023-R.pdf. Accessed April 2011.

Jones, J.M. 2011. In U.S., 46% favor, 40% oppose repealing healthcare law. Available at: http://www.gallup.com/poll/145496/Favor-Oppose-Repealing-Healthcare-Law.aspx. Accessed April 2011.

Kaptchuk, T.J., and D.M. Eisenberg. 2001. Varieties of healing 1: Medical pluralism in the United States. *Annals of Internal Medicine* 135, no. 3: 189–195.

Kardos, B.C., and A.T. Allen. 1993. Healthy neighbors: Exploring the health care systems of the United States and Canada. *Journal of Post Anesthesia Nursing* 8, no. 1: 48–51.

Kaufman, M. 1980. American medical education. In: *The education of American physicians: Historical essays.* R.L. Numbers, ed. Los Angeles: University of California Press.

Koch, A.L. 1993. Financing health services. In: *Introduction to health services.* 4th ed. S.J. Williams and P.R. Torrens, eds. New York: Delmar Publishers. pp. 299–331.

Law, S.A. 1974. *Blue Cross: What went wrong?* New Haven, CT: Yale University Press.

Maheu, M.M. et al. 2001. *E-health, telehealth, and telemedicine: A guide to start-up and success.* San Francisco: Jossey-Bass.

Manderscheid, R.W. et al. 2004. Highlights of organized mental health services in 2000 and major national and state trends. In: *Mental health, United States, 2002.* R.W. Manderscheid and M.J. Henderson, eds. Washington, DC: US Government Printing Office.

Martensen, R.L. 1996. Hospital hotels and the care of the "worthy rich." *Journal of the American Medical Association* 275, no. 4: 325.

Mayer, T.R., and G.G. Mayer. 1984. *The health insurance alternative: A complete guide to health maintenance organizations.* New York: Putnam Publishing Group.

McDonnell, J. 2006. Is the medical world flattening? *Ophthalmology Times* 31, no. 19: 4.

Miller, T.P. 2010. Health reform: Only a cease-fire in a political hundred years' war. *Health Affairs* 29, no. 6: 1101–1105.

Mongan, J.J. 1995. Anatomy and physiology of health reform's failure. *Health Affairs* 14, no. 1: 99–101.

Mutchnick, I.S. et al. 2005. Trading health services across borders: GATS, markets, and caveats. *Health Affairs* – Web Exclusive 24, suppl. 1: W5-42–W5-51.

Norcini, J.J., and P.E. Mazmanian. 2005. Physician migration, education, and health care. *Journal of Continuing Education in the Health Professions* 25, no. 1: 4–7.

Numbers, R.L. 1985. The third party: Health insurance in America. In: *Sickness and health in America: Readings in the history of medicine and public health.* J.W. Leavitt and R.L. Numbers, eds. Madison, WI: The University of Wisconsin Press.

Numbers, R.L., and J.H. Warner. 1985. The maturation of American medical science. In: *Sickness and health in America: Readings in the history of medicine and public health.* J.W. Leavitt and R.L. Numbers, eds. Madison, WI: The University of Wisconsin Press.

Page, S. 2010. Health care law too costly, most say (USA Today). Available at: http://www .usatoday.com/news/washington/2010-03-29-health-poll_N.htm. Accessed January 2011.

Potter, M.A., and B.B. Longest. 1994. The divergence of federal and state policies on the charitable tax exemption of nonprofit hospitals. *Journal of Health Politics, Policy and Law* 19, no. 2: 393–419.

Raffel, M.W. 1980. *The U.S. health system: Origins and functions.* New York: John Wiley & Sons.

Raffel, M.W., and N.K. Raffel. 1994. *The U.S. health system: Origins and functions.* 4th ed. Albany, NY: Delmar Publishers.

Richardson, J.T. 1945. *The origin and development of group hospitalization in the United States, 1890–1940.* University of Missouri Studies XX, no. 3.

Rosen, G. 1983. *The structure of American medical practice 1875–1941.* Philadelphia, PA: University of Pennsylvania Press.

Rosenberg, C.E. 1979. The therapeutic revolution: Medicine, meaning, and social change in nineteenth-century America. In: *The therapeutic revolution.* M.J. Vogel, ed. Philadelphia, PA: The University of Pennsylvania Press.

Rosner, L. 2001. The Philadelphia medical marketplace. In: *Major problems in the history of American medicine and public health.* J.H. Warner and J.A. Tighe, eds. Boston: Houghton Mifflin Company.

Rothstein, W.G. 1972. *American physicians in the nineteenth century: From sect to science.* Baltimore, MD: Johns Hopkins University Press.

Scherz, H. 2010. Why the AMA wants to muzzle your doctor (*The Wall Street Journal*). Available at: http://online.wsj.com/article/SB10001424052748703961104575226323909364054.html. Accessed April 2011.

Shryock, R.H. 1966. *Medicine in America: Historical essays.* Baltimore, MD: The Johns Hopkins Press.

Skocpol, T. 1995. The rise and resounding demise of the Clinton plan. *Health Affairs* 14, no. 1: 66–85.

Smith, M.D. et al. 1992. Taking the public's pulse on health system reform. *Health Affairs* 11, no. 2: 125–133.

Somers, A.R., and H.M. Somers. 1977. *Health and health care: Policies in perspective.* Germantown, MD: Aspen Systems.

Starr, P. 1982. *The social transformation of American medicine.* Cambridge, MA: Basic Books.

Stevens, R. 1971. *American medicine and the public interest.* New Haven, CT: Yale University Press.

Turnock, B.J. 1997. *Public health: What it is and how it works.* Gaithersburg, MD: Aspen Publishers, Inc. pp. 3–38.

US Surgeon General. 1999. *Mental health: A report of the Surgeon General. Overview of mental health services.* Available at: http://www.surgeongeneral.gov/library/mentalhealth/chapter2/sec2.html. Accessed February 2011.

Whitted, G. 1993. Private health insurance and employee benefits. In: *Introduction to health services.* 4th ed. S.J. Williams and P.R. Torrens, eds. New York: Delmar Publishers. pp. 332–360.

Williams, S.J. 1993. Ambulatory health care services. In: *Introduction to health services.* 4th ed. S.J. Williams and P.R. Torrens, eds. New York: Delmar Publishers.

Williams, S.J. 1995. *Essentials of health services.* Albany, NY: Delmar Publishers. pp. 108–134.

Winters, S.R. 1921. Diagnosis by wireless. *Scientific American* 124: 465.

Wright, J.W. 1997. *The New York Times almanac.* New York: Penguin Putnam, Inc.

# PART II

---

# System Resources

# Chapter 4

---

# Health Services Professionals

## Learning Objectives

- To recognize the various types of health services professionals and their training, practice requirements, and practice settings
- To differentiate between primary care and specialty care and identify the causes for an imbalance between primary care and specialty care in the United States
- To learn about the extent of maldistribution in the physician labor force and to comprehend the reasons for such maldistribution
- To identify various remedies to help overcome the problems of physician imbalance and maldistribution
- To understand the role of nonphysician providers in health care delivery
- To appreciate allied health professionals and their role in health care delivery
- To discuss the functions and qualifications of health services administrators

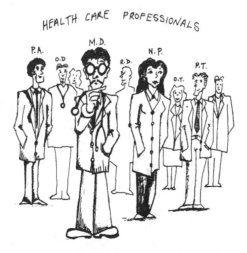

*"Hmm, they're all beginning to look like me."*

# Introduction

The US health care industry is the largest and most powerful employer in the nation. It constitutes more than 3% of the total labor force in the United States. In terms of total economic output, in 2009, the health care sector in the United States contributed 17.6% to the gross domestic product (Martin et al. 2010). The US Bureau of Labor Statistics (2005) projects 7 of the 10 fastest growing occupations for 2004–2014 are health related. Although jobs in many areas of the US economy shrank since the beginning of an economic recession in December 2007, the health care sector grew, adding 613,000 jobs. The growth has been most pronounced in the hospital industry. As the elderly population continues to grow, the demand for health care services will also increase. Hence, several health care and related occupations are projected to grow substantially. The Bureau of Labor Statistics projects the "healthcare practitioners and technical occupations" to grow by 21.4% and the "healthcare support occupations" by 28.8% during 2008–2018, whereas the entire US workforce is projected to grow by 10.1% during this period (US Bureau of Labor Statistics 2009).

Health services professionals include physicians, nurses, dentists, pharmacists, optometrists, psychologists, podiatrists, chiropractors, nonphysician practitioners (NPPs), health services administrators, and a variety of allied health professionals. The latter category incorporates therapists, laboratory and radiology technicians, social workers, and health educators. Health professionals are among the most well-educated and diverse of all labor groups. Almost all of these practitioner groups are now represented by their respective professional associations, which are listed in Appendix 4–A at the end of this chapter.

Health services professionals work in a variety of health care settings that include hospitals, managed care organizations (MCOs), nursing care facilities, mental health institutions, insurance firms, pharmaceutical companies, outpatient facilities, community health centers, migrant health centers, mental health centers, school clinics, physicians' offices, laboratories, voluntary health agencies, professional health associations, colleges of medicine and allied health professions, and research institutions. Most health professionals are employed by hospitals (41.3%), followed by nursing and personal care facilities (11.8%) and physicians' offices and clinics (10.3%) (Table 4–1).

Growth of health care services is closely linked to the demand for health services professionals. The expansion of the number and types of health services professionals closely follows population trends, advances in research and technology, disease and illness trends, and changes in health care financing and delivery of services. Population growth and the aging of the population enhance the demand for health services. Advances in scientific research contribute to new methods of preventing, diagnosing, and treating illness. New and complex medical techniques and machines are constantly introduced, and health services professionals must continually learn how to use these innovations. Specialization in medicine has contributed to the proliferation of different types of medical technicians. The changing patterns of disease, from acute to chronic, have led to a greater need for professionals who are formally prepared to address behavioral risk factors, their consequences, and their prevention. The widespread availability of insurance, from both the public and

Table 4–1  Persons Employed in Health Service Sites (145,362 employed civilians in 2008)

| Site | 2000 | | 2008 | |
| --- | --- | --- | --- | --- |
| | Number of Persons (in thousands) | Percentage Distribution | Number of Persons (in thousands) | Percentage Distribution |
| All employed civilians | 136,891 | 100.0 | 145,362 | 100.0 |
| All health service sites | 12,211 | 100.0 | 15,108 | 100.0 |
| Offices and clinics of physicians | 1,387 | 11.4 | 1,562 | 10.3 |
| Offices and clinics of dentists | 672 | 5.5 | 774 | 5.1 |
| Offices and clinics of chiropractors | 120 | 1.0 | 139 | 0.9 |
| Offices and clinics of optometrists | 95 | 0.8 | 110 | 0.7 |
| Offices and clinics of other health practitioners | 143 | 1.2 | 195 | 1.3 |
| Outpatient care centers | 772 | 6.3 | 1,107 | 7.3 |
| Home health care services | 548 | 4.5 | 881 | 5.8 |
| Other health care services | 1,027 | 8.4 | 1,647 | 10.9 |
| Hospitals | 5,202 | 42.6 | 6,241 | 41.3 |
| Nursing care facilities | 1,593 | 13.0 | 1,779 | 11.8 |
| Residential care facilities, without nursing | 652 | 5.3 | 673 | 4.5 |

*Source:* Data from *Health, United States, 2009*, p. 374.

the private sectors, has contributed to the increase in medical care utilization, which has created a greater demand for health services professionals. Changes in reimbursement, from retrospective to prospective payment methods (see Chapter 6), and increased enrollment in managed care have contributed to a slowdown in cost escalation, a shift from inpatient to outpatient care, and an emphasis on the role of primary care providers.

This chapter provides an overview of the large array of health services professionals employed in a vast assortment of health delivery settings. It briefly discusses the training and practice requirements for the various health professionals, their major roles, the practice settings in which they are employed, and some critical issues concerning their professions. Emphasis is placed on physicians because they play a leading role in the delivery of health care. There has been increased recognition of the role NPPs play in the delivery of primary care services. Notably, some basic medical functions that were traditionally performed by physicians alone are now performed by other trained professionals.

The US health care delivery system is characterized by an imbalance between primary and specialty care services, which has contributed to an imbalance in the ratio of generalists to specialists. There is also a geographic maldistribution of practitioners. This chapter discusses the main causes for these disparities and explores possible solutions. Although a detailed discussion of primary care is provided in Chapter 7, this chapter highlights some of the main differences between primary and specialty care.

## Physicians

In the delivery of health services, physicians play a central role by evaluating a patient's health condition, diagnosing abnormalities, and prescribing treatment. Some physicians are engaged in medical education and research to find new and better ways to control and cure health problems. Many are involved in the prevention of illness.

All states require physicians to be licensed to practice. The licensure requirements include graduation from an accredited medical school that awards a Doctor of Medicine (MD) or Doctor of Osteopathic Medicine (DO) degree, successful completion of a licensing examination governed by either the National Board of Medical Examiners or the National Board of Osteopathic Medical Examiners, and completion of a supervised internship/residency program (Stanfield et al. 2009). The term *residency* refers to graduate medical education in a specialty that takes the form of paid on-the-job training, usually in a hospital. Before entering a residency, which may last 2 to 6 years, most DOs serve a 12-month rotating internship after graduation.

The number of active physicians, both MDs and DOs, has steadily increased from 14.1 physicians per 10,000 population in 1950 to 30.4 per 10,000 population in 2005 (Table 4–2). Of the 159 medical schools in the United States, 133 teach allopathic medicine and award a Doctor of Medicine (MD) degree; 29 teach osteopathic medicine and award the Doctor of Osteopathic Medicine (DO) degree (US Bureau of Labor Statistics 2011).

## Similarities and Differences Between MDs and DOs

Both MDs and DOs use accepted methods of treatment, including drugs and surgery. The two differ mainly in their philosophies and approaches to medical treatment. *Osteopathic medicine,* practiced by DOs, emphasizes the musculoskeletal system of the body, such as correction of joints or tissues. In their treatment plans, DOs stress preventive medicine, such as diet and environment as factors that might influence natural resistance. They take a holistic approach to patient care. MDs are trained in *allopathic medicine,* which views medical treatment as active intervention to produce a counteracting reaction in an attempt to neutralize the effects of disease. MDs, particularly generalists, may also use preventive medicine, along with allopathic treatments. About 5% of all active physicians are osteopaths (American Association of Colleges of Osteopathic Medicine 2007). About 42% of MDs and more than one-half of DOs work in primary care (US Bureau of Labor Statistics 2011).

## Generalists and Specialists

Most DOs are generalists and most MDs are specialists. In the United States, physicians

Table 4–2  Active US Physicians, According to Type of Physician and Number per 10,000 Population

| Year | All Active Physicians | Doctors of Medicine | Doctors of Osteopathy | Active Physicians per 10,000 Population |
|---|---|---|---|---|
| 1950 | 219,900 | 209,000 | 10,900 | 14.1 |
| 1960 | 259,500 | 247,300 | 12,200 | 14.0 |
| 1970 | 326,500 | 314,200 | 12,300 | 15.6 |
| 1980 | 427,122 | 409,992 | 17,130 | 19.0 |
| 1990 | 567,610 | 539,616 | 27,994 | 22.4 |
| 1995 | 672,859 | 637,192 | 35,667 | 25.0 |
| 2000 | 772,296 | 727,573 | 44,723 | 27.0 |
| 2001 | 793,263 | 751,689 | 41,574 | 27.4 |
| 2005* | 902,053 | 844,604 | 57,449 | 30.4 |

*Sources:* Data from *Health, United States, 1995,* p. 220; *Health, United States, 2002,* p. 274; and *Health, United States, 2006,* p. 358.
*Source:* American Medical Association. *Physician Characteristics and Distribution in the US,* 2007 Edition.

trained in family medicine/general practice, general internal medicine, and general pediatrics are considered primary care physicians (PCPs) or *generalists* (Rich et al. 1994). In general, PCPs provide preventive services (e.g., health examinations, immunizations, mammograms, Papanicolaou smears) and treat frequently occurring and less severe problems. Problems that occur less frequently or that require complex diagnostic or therapeutic approaches may be referred to specialists.

Physicians in nonprimary care specialties are referred to as *specialists.* Specialists must seek certification in an area of medical specialization, which commonly requires additional years of advanced residency training, followed by several years of practice in the specialty. A specialty board examination is often required as the final step in becoming a board certified specialist. The common medical specialties, along with brief descriptions, are listed in Exhibit 4–1. Medical specialties may be divided into six major functional groups: (1) the subspecialties of internal medicine; (2) a broad group of medical specialties; (3) obstetrics and gynecology; (4) surgery of all types; (5) hospital-based radiology, anesthesiology, and pathology; and (6) psychiatry (Cooper 1994). The distribution of physicians by specialty appears in Table 4–3. PCPs often coordinate referrals with members of these specialty groups based on an initial evaluation of the patient's medical needs.

## Work Settings and Practice Patterns

Physicians practice in a variety of settings and arrangements. Some work in hospitals

Exhibit 4–1   Definitions of Medical Specialties and Subspecialties

| | |
|---|---|
| Allergists | Treat conditions and illnesses caused by allergies or related to the immune system |
| Anesthesiologists | Use drugs and gases to render patients unconscious during surgery |
| Cardiologists | Treat heart diseases |
| Dermatologists | Treat infections, growths, and injuries related to the skin |
| Emergency Medicine | Work specifically in emergency departments, treating acute illnesses and emergency situations, for example, trauma |
| Family Physicians | Are prepared to handle most types of illnesses and involve the care of the patient as a whole |
| General Practitioners | Similar to family physicians — examine patients or order tests and have X-rays done to diagnose illness and treat the patient |
| Geriatricians | Specialize in problems and diseases that accompany aging |
| Gynecologists | Specialize in the care of the reproductive system of women |
| Internists | Treat diseases related to the internal organs of the body, for example, conditions of the lungs, blood, kidneys, and heart |
| Neurologists | Treat disorders of the central nervous system and order tests necessary to detect diseases |
| Obstetricians | Work with women throughout their pregnancy, deliver infants, and care for the mother after the delivery |
| Oncologists | Specialize in the diagnosis and treatment of cancers and tumors |
| Ophthalmologists | Treat diseases and injuries of the eye |
| Otolaryngologists | Specialize in the treatment of conditions or diseases of the ear, nose, and throat |
| Pathologists | Study the characteristics, causes, and progression of diseases |
| Pediatricians | Provide care for children from birth to adolescence |
| Preventive Medicine | Includes occupational medicine, public health, and general preventive treatments |
| Psychiatrists | Help patients recover from mental illness and regain their mental health |
| Radiologists | Perform diagnosis and treatment by the use of X-rays and radioactive materials |
| Surgeons | Operate on patients to treat disease, repair injury, correct deformities, and improve the health of patients |
| General Surgeons | Perform many different types of surgery, usually of relatively low degree of difficulty |
| Neurologic Surgeons | Specialize in surgery of the brain, spinal cord, and nervous system |
| Orthopaedic Surgeons | Specialize in the repair of bones and joints |
| Plastic Surgeons | Repair malformed or injured parts of the body |
| Thoracic Surgeons | Perform surgery in the chest cavity, for example, lung and heart surgery |
| Urologists | Specialize in conditions of the urinary tract in both sexes and of the sexual/reproductive system in males |

*Source:* Adapted from Stanfield, P.S. 1995. *Introduction to the Health Professions,* 2nd ed. Boston, MA: Jones and Bartlett Publishers. Available at www.jbpub.com. Reprinted with permission.

Table 4–3  US Physicians, According to Activity and Place of Medical Education, 2004

| Activity and Place of Medical Education | Numbers | Percentage | Distribution |
|---|---|---|---|
| Doctors of medicine (professionally active)* | 776,554 | 100.0 | |
| Place of medical education: | | | |
| US medical graduates | 580,336 | 74.7 | |
| International medical graduates | 196,218 | 25.3 | |
| Activity | | | |
| *Patient care* | 732,234 | 100.0 | |
| *Office-based practice* | 562,897 | 76.9 | 100.0 |
| General and family practice | 75,952 | | 13.5 |
| Cardiovascular diseases | 17,504 | | 3.1 |
| Dermatology | 9,036 | | 1.6 |
| Gastroenterology | 10,042 | | 1.8 |
| Internal medicine | 108,552 | | 19.3 |
| Pediatrics | 52,095 | | 9.3 |
| Pulmonary diseases | 7,490 | | 1.3 |
| General surgery | 25,434 | | 4.5 |
| Obstetrics and gynecology | 34,405 | | 6.1 |
| Ophthalmology | 15,852 | | 2.8 |
| Orthopaedic surgery | 19,299 | | 3.4 |
| Otolaryngology | 8,177 | | 1.5 |
| Plastic surgery | 6,100 | | 1.1 |
| Urological surgery | 8,796 | | 1.6 |
| Anesthesiology | 31,617 | | 5.6 |
| Diagnostic radiology | 17,327 | | 3.1 |
| Emergency medicine | 20,036 | | 3.6 |
| Neurology | 10,476 | | 1.9 |
| Pathology, anatomical/clinical | 11,191 | | 2.0 |
| Psychiatry | 27,492 | | 4.9 |
| Radiology | 6,913 | | 1.2 |
| Other specialty | 39,111 | | 6.9 |
| *Hospital-based practice* | 169,337 | 23.1 | 100.0 |
| Residents and interns | 98,688 | | 56.5 |
| Full-time hospital staff | 70,649 | | 41.7 |

*Excludes inactive, not classified, and address unknown.
*Source:* Data from *Health, United States, 2009*, p. 376.

as medical residents or staff physicians. Others work in the public sector, such as federal government agencies, public health clinics, community and migrant health centers, schools, and prisons. Most physicians, however, are office-based practitioners, and most physician contacts occur in physician offices. An increasing number of physicians are partners or salaried employees under contractual arrangements, working in various outpatient settings, such as group practices, freestanding ambulatory care clinics, diagnostic imaging centers, and MCOs.

Figure 4–1 shows that, in 2007, physicians in general/family practice accounted for the greatest proportion of ambulatory care visits, followed by those in internal medicine and pediatrics.

Other medical practice characteristics appear in Table 4–4. For example, physicians in obstetrics and gynecology spent the most hours in patient care per week, even exceeding those in surgery. Surgeons, however, had the highest average annual net income. Operating expenses and malpractice insurance premiums were the highest in obstetrics/gynecology.

## Differences Between Primary and Specialty Care

*Primary care* may be distinguished from *specialty care*, according to the time, focus, and scope of the services provided to patients. The five main areas of distinction are as follows:

1.  In linear time sequence, primary care is first-contact care and is regarded as the portal to the health care system (Kahn et al. 1994). Specialty care, when needed, generally follows primary care.

2.  In a managed care environment in which health services functions are integrated, PCPs serve as gatekeepers, an important role in controlling cost, utilization, and the rational allocation of resources. In the gatekeeping model, specialty care requires referral from a primary care physician.

Figure 4–1  Ambulatory Care Visits to Physicians According to Physician Specialty, 2007.

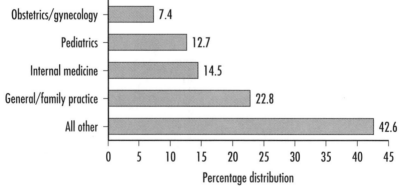

| Specialty | Percentage distribution |
|---|---|
| Obstetrics/gynecology | 7.4 |
| Pediatrics | 12.7 |
| Internal medicine | 14.5 |
| General/family practice | 22.8 |
| All other | 42.6 |

*Source:* Data from *Health, United States, 2002*, pp. 343–344.

Table 4–4  Medical Practice Characteristics by Selected Specialty, 1999

| Characteristics | All Physicians | General/ Family Practice | Internal Medicine | Surgery | Pediatrics | Obstetrics/ Gynecology |
|---|---|---|---|---|---|---|
| Mean patient visits | | | | | | |
| per week (1999) | 106.7 | 122.9 | 103.0 | 95.8 | 120.5 | 101.8 |
| per week (2003–04) | 73.8 | 84.9 | | 66.9 | | |
| Mean hours in patient | | | | | | |
| care per week | 51.6 | 50.6 | 54.2 | 53.3 | 49.5 | 59.0 |
| Mean net income | | | | | | |
| ($1,000) 1998 | 194.4 | 142.5 | 182.1 | 268.2 | 139.6 | 214.4 |
| Mean liability premium | | | | | | |
| ($1,000) 1998 | 16.8 | 10.9 | 16.5 | 22.8 | 9.0 | 35.8 |

*Sources:* Data from *Statistical Abstracts of the United States: 2002*, p. 108.
CDC. Characteristics of Office-Based Physicians and Their Practices: United States, 2003–04. *Vital Health Statistics.* Series 13, No. 164, Jan. 2007.

3. Primary care is longitudinal. In other words, primary care providers follow through the course of treatment and coordinate various activities, including initial diagnosis, treatment, referral, consultation, monitoring, and follow-up. Primary care providers serve as patient advisors and advocates (Williams 1994). Their coordinating role is especially important in the provision of continuing care for chronic conditions. Specialty care is episodic and, thus, more focused and intense.

4. Primary care focuses on the person as a whole, whereas specialty care centers on particular diseases or organ systems of the body. Primary care is holistic in nature and provides an integrating function. Patients often have multiple problems, a condition referred to as *comorbidity*. In such cases, attention from a specialist focusing on one problem may make another problem worse. Primary care, in essence, seeks to balance the multiple requirements a patient's condition might call for and refers patients to appropriate specialty care when needed. Specialty care, by contrast, tends to be limited to illness episodes, the organ system, or the disease process involved. Consequently, specialists, such as oncologists and cardiologists, deal only with specific diseases and body organs (Hibbard and Nutting 1991). Specialty care is also associated with secondary and tertiary levels of services (see *secondary care* and *tertiary care* in the Glossary).

5. The difference in scope is reflected in how primary and specialty care providers are trained. Primary care students spend a significant amount of time in ambulatory care settings, familiarizing themselves with a variety of patient conditions and problems. Students in medical subspecialties spend significant time in inpatient hospitals, where they are exposed to state-of-the-art medical technology.

## The Expanding Role of Hospitalists

Since the mid-1990s, an increasing amount of inpatient medical care in the United States has been delivered by *hospitalists*, physicians who specialize in the care of hospitalized patients (Schneller 2006). Hospitalists do not usually have a relationship with the patient prior to hospitalization. Essentially, the patient's primary care provider entrusts the oversight of the patient's care to a hospitalist upon admission, and the patient returns to the regular physician after discharge (Freed 2004). Approximately 12,000 hospitalists practice in the United States, and the field is estimated to soon grow to 30,000, exceeding the number of cardiologists (Sehgal and Wachter 2006).

The growth of hospitalists is influenced by the desire of hospital executives, HMOs, and medical groups to reduce inpatient costs and increase efficiency, without compromising quality or patient satisfaction. Published research shows that using hospitalists does, in fact, achieve these goals (Wachter 2004). Research findings have also put to rest initial concerns from PCPs, who were accustomed to the traditional method of rounding on their hospitalized patients. PCPs had voiced concerns about discontinuity of care and patients' acceptance of the new practice

(Wachter 2004). Recently, the debate over hospitalists has largely shifted from quality and efficiency to optimizing hospitalists' skills and expanding their roles (Sehgal and Wachter 2006). Hospitalists are not yet certified as a distinct subspecialty of medicine. However, hospitalists convene for large annual meetings and have their own textbook, journal (the *Journal of Hospital Medicine*), and specialty society (Sehgal and Wachter 2006). Their role in the American medical system is expected to continue to increase in importance.

## Issues in Medical Practice, Training, and Supply

### Medical Practice

Research has shown that the way physicians practice medicine and prescribe treatments for similar conditions varies significantly because clinical decisions made by physicians are not always based on strong evidence founded on clinical research (Field and Lohr 1992). Physicians have at their disposal an increasing number of therapeutic options because of the exponential growth in medical science and technology. Conversely, increasing health care costs continue to threaten the viability of the health care delivery system. The responsibilities placed on physicians to perform difficult balancing acts between the availability of the most advanced treatment plans, uncertainties about their potential benefits, and whether the higher costs of treatment are justified have created a confusing environment. Hence, support has been growing for the development and refinement of standardized clinical guidelines to streamline clinical decision making and improve quality of care (discussed in Chapter 12). However, there have been some criticisms about the applicability, flexibility, and objectivity of some guidelines. Although the number of conditions for which guidelines are available is steadily increasing, guidelines for combinations of conditions are not often available. Furthermore, many of the recommendations incorporated in the most well-accepted clinical guidelines permit much flexibility to practicing physicians, making it difficult to determine whether the care physicians decide to give complies with recommendations in the guidelines (Garber 2005). To address this issue, the Medicare Improvements for Patients and Providers Act of 2008 (MIPPA) (Sec. 304(b)) required the secretary of DHHS to conduct a study with the Institute of Medicine (IOM) to ensure that "objective, scientifically valid, and consistent" approaches are employed by organizations that develop clinical practice guidelines (Redhead and Williams 2010).

## Medical Training

The principal source of funding for graduate medical education is the Medicare program, which provides explicit payments to teaching hospitals for each resident in training. The government, however, does not mandate how these physicians should be trained. By contrast, in Great Britain, the government finances all residency slots and controls the number of positions by specialty. In Canada, the number of positions funded by the provincial ministries of health is determined in negotiations among the medical schools, provincial governments, and physician associations.

Emphasis on hospital-based training in the United States has produced too many specialists. In the meanwhile, the health care delivery system is evolving toward primary care orientation. The result is that many physicians in the workforce today are ill-prepared to practice in the wellness-oriented, ambulatory-based environment (American Physical Therapy Association 1998).

## Aggregate Physician Oversupply

Aided by tax-financed subsidies, the United States has experienced a sharp increase in its physician labor force. Between 1950 and 1990, the supply of physicians increased by 173% (Health Resources and Services Administration 1996), and it has steadily increased since then (Figure 4–2). In 1950, there were 142 physicians per 100,000 population. By 2008, this number had increased to 270 per 100,000 population (US Census Bureau 2010). This number far surpasses the estimated 145 to 185 physicians per 100,000 population that the United States actually needs, according to the Council on Graduate Medical Education (COGME). The number of active physicians under age 75 is expected to grow from approximately 817,500 in 2005 to 951,700 by 2020 (HRSA/BHP 2006). The growth, however, has been mainly for specialists. The COGME has warned that there could be a physician deficit of 85,000 by 2020 and has recommended increases in medical school and residency output. On the other hand, contributions of other clinicians and changes in how medical care is delivered in the future would likely offset physician deficits (Phillips et al. 2005).

## Maldistribution

A surplus of physicians leads to unnecessary increases in health care expenditures. A shortage, however, adversely affects the delivery

Figure 4–2  Supply of US Physicians, Including International Medical Graduates (IMGs), per 100,000 Population, 1985–2007.

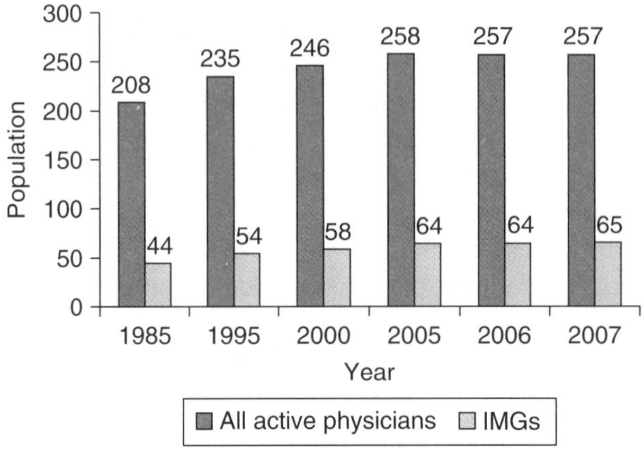

Source: Health, United States, 2009, p. 376. Statistical Abstracts of the United States, 2004, 2008, 2009.

of health services. However, there are maldistributions in terms of both geography and specialty. *Maldistribution* refers to either a surplus or a shortage of the type of physicians needed to maintain the health status of a given population at an optimum level.

## Geographic Maldistribution

One of the ironies of excess physician supply is that localities outside metropolitan areas (that is, counties with <50,000 residents) continue to have a shortage of physicians. Non-metropolitan areas have 59 PCPs/100,000 population compared to 94 PCPs/100,000 population in metropolitan areas (General Accounting Office 2003). Rural areas, particularly, lack an adequate supply of physicians, including primary care physicians, although residents in rural areas have greater medical need, being sicker, older, and poorer than those in non-rural areas. Whereas 20% of the US population lives in rural areas, only 9% of physicians practice there (AHRQ 2005).

Physicians are more likely to concentrate in metropolitan and suburban areas than in rural and inner city areas because the former offer greater prospects for high income; professional interaction; access to modern facilities and technology; continuing education and professional growth; higher standards of living; and such social amenities as cultural diversity, recreational activities, and quality of education for children. Also, rural areas lack the economic capacity to support additional physicians. Problems contributing to the difficulties in recruiting physicians in rural areas include long working hours, requirements to frequently be on call, smaller financial rewards, and a greater degree of professional isolation, such as limited access to high technology, which is more commonly available in urban medical centers (Kohler 1994).

Several federal programs have demonstrated success in increasing the supply of primary care services in rural areas. Some of these programs are discussed in Chapter 11. They include the National Health Service

Corps, which makes scholarship support conditional on a commitment to future service in an underserved area; the Migrant and Community Health Center Programs, designated to provide primary care services to the poor and underserved using federal grants; and the support of primary care training programs and Area Health Education Centers.

Other policy options include regulation of health care professions, reimbursement policies, targeted programs for underserved areas, and health professional schools (Cohen 1993; Kindig and Yan 1993; Weiner 1993; Wennberg et al. 1993). Regulations governing the health professions specify the types of tasks different practitioners are permitted to perform. Of particular significance is the expansion of the scope of practice for advanced nurses, such as nurse practitioners (NPs), physician assistants (PAs), and pharmacists. Such a scope can include the right to prescribe drugs.

Reimbursement policies affect practice-related choices of current and future physicians. Typically, financial rewards in rural settings are lower, compared to more affluent urban areas. Hence, positive incentives are needed to attract professionals to rural locations. Differential rewards to providers who choose to practice in less desirable areas or care for socially disadvantaged populations can be attractive to some physicians. Reimbursement is also crucial to nonphysician health professionals, such as NPs and PAs. A powerful incentive for attracting and retaining nurses with advanced training would be reimbursement rates that are comparable to those paid to physicians for the same procedures.

Research indicates that physicians' personal characteristics play a significant role in their practice location decision (Crandall et al. 1990; Eisenberg 1985; Samuels and Shi 1993). Physicians are more likely to be attracted to rural practice if they have a rural background or exposure to rural practice settings in their clinical training. To ensure a sufficient supply of rural physicians, a comprehensive approach is recommended. Such an approach would facilitate admission to medical schools for students from rural communities, foster premedical training in rural settings, create and use rural preceptorships or externships and rural residency training programs to expose medical students to the practice of medicine among disadvantaged populations.

Targeted programs for underserved areas include setting up task forces or commissions, offices of rural health, and increased funding for training and incentive programs to encourage health professionals to choose primary care and practice in rural and underserved areas. Schools that train health professionals can incorporate the concerns of practicing in underserved areas into medical curricula. Specific training can be directed at practice management, cost-effective care, preventive care, and the coordination of community resources and services. Continued efforts are needed for medical schools to find ways to recruit underserved minority groups, such as African Americans and Hispanics (see Table 4–5 for the racial distribution of medical school enrollment). Although various steps can be taken to address the issue, unfortunately, distributional shortages of physicians are likely to persist in many rural and selected inner city areas.

## Specialty Maldistribution

Besides geographic maldistribution of physicians, a considerable imbalance exists between primary and specialty care in the

Table 4–5  Percentage of Total Enrollment of Students for Selected Health Occupations, 2006–2007

| Race | Allopathic | Osteopathic | Dentistry | Pharmacy | Nursing Baccalaureate |
|---|---|---|---|---|---|
| All races | 100.0 | 100.0 | 100.0 | 100.0 | 100.0 |
| White, non-Hispanic | 62.9 | 71.1 | 61.3 | 60.2 | 75.2 |
| Black, non-Hispanic | 7.3 | 4.1 | 5.8 | 6.7 | 12.4 |
| Hispanic | 7.6 | 3.8 | 5.9 | 3.9 | 5.4 |
| American Indian | 0.9 | 0.6 | 0.6 | 0.5 | 0.7 |
| Asian | 21.2 | 16.8 | 22.4 | 21.2 | 6.3 |

*Source:* Data from *Health, United States, 2009*, p. 381.

United States. Approximately 42% of physicians work in primary care; the remaining 58% are specialists (US Bureau of Labor Statistics 2011). In other industrialized countries, only 25 to 50% of physicians are specialists (Schroeder 1992).

Figure 4–3 illustrates trends in the supply of PCPs. From 1979 to 1999, the supply of family practitioners per 100,000 people in the United States increased only 18%, whereas the supply of medical specialists increased by 118% (Goodman 2004). The

Figure 4–3  Trend of US Primary Care Generalists of Medicine.

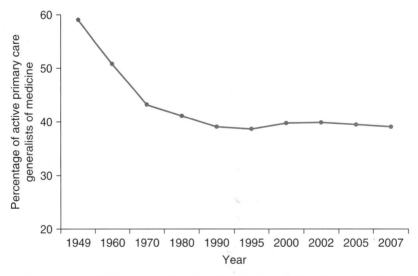

*Source:* Data from National Center for Health Statistics, Hyattsville, MD: *Health, United States, 2008*, p. 397; *Health, United States, 2009*, p. 377.

number of positions filled in family practice residency programs showed an increase during the first few years of the 1990s, but there has been a slow decline since 1998 (Pugno et al. 2001). A decreasing number of physicians have been entering primary care. Also, about one in six general internists leave their practice by midcareer either due to dissatisfaction or by moving into a subspecialty of internal medicine (Bylsma et al. 2010). An increasing number of international medical graduates (IMGs) practicing in the United States have helped alleviate the shortage of PCPs.

Specialty maldistribution has become ingrained in the US health care delivery system for three main reasons: (1) medical technology, (2) reimbursement methods and remuneration, and (3) specialty-oriented medical education. Conversely, the need for PCPs is determined mainly by the demographics of the general population.

The major driving force behind the increasing number of specialists is the development of medical technology. Most hospitals with more than 100 beds try to become clinical centers offering medical services in all major specialty fields and, consequently, employ specialists in these fields (Friedenberg 1996). Most insured patients, because they are shielded from the financial burden of health care, have the tendency to turn to physicians who provide them the most up-to-date, sophisticated treatment. Because the population increases at a significantly slower rate than technological advancements, the gap between primary and specialty care workforces continues to expand.

Higher incomes of specialists relative to PCPs have also contributed to an oversupply of specialists. In the last few years, reimbursement systems designed to increase payments to PCPs have been implemented, but wide disparities between the incomes of generalists and specialists continue (Table 4–6).

Specialists not only earn higher incomes, but they also have more predictable work hours and enjoy higher prestige among their colleagues and the public at large (Rosenblatt and Lishner 1991; Samuels and Shi 1993). High status and prestige are accorded to tertiary care and specialties employing high technology. Such considerations influence medical students' career decisions.

The medical education environment in the United States is organized according to specialties and controlled by those who have achieved leadership positions by demonstrating their abilities in narrow scientific or clinical areas. Medical education in the United States emphasizes technology, intensive procedures, and tertiary care settings, which are generally more appealing to medical students than more rudimentary

Table 4–6  Mean Annual Compensation of US Physicians by Specialty, May 2009

| | |
|---|---|
| Anesthesiologists | 211,750 |
| Family and general practitioners | 168,550 |
| Internists, general | 183,990 |
| Obstetricians and gynecologists | 204,470 |
| Pediatricians, general | 161,410 |
| Psychiatrists | 163,660 |
| Surgeons | 219,770 |
| Physicians and surgeons, all other | 173,860 |

*Source:* US Department of Labor, Bureau of Labor Statistics. *Occupational Employment and Wages – May 2009*, published May 14, 2010. http://www.bls.gov/news.release/pdf/ocwage.pdf (accessed November 15, 2010).

primary care (Anonymous 1990; Verby et al. 1991).

The imbalance between generalists and specialists has several undesirable consequences. Having too many specialists has contributed to the high volume of intensive, expensive, and invasive medical services, as well as to the rise in health care costs (Greenfield et al. 1992; Rosenblatt 1992; Schroeder and Sandy 1993; Wennberg et al. 1993). A greater supply of surgeons increases the demand for initial contacts with surgeons (Escarce 1992). In fact, the rate of surgery in the United States grew at twice the rate of the population from 1979 to 1986 (Kramon 1991). Seeking care directly from specialists is often less effective than using primary care because the latter attempts to provide early intervention before complications develop (Starfield 1992; Starfield and Simpson 1993). Higher levels of primary care professionals are associated with lower overall death and lower mortality rates due to diseases of the heart and cancer (Shi 1992, 1994). PCPs have been the major providers of care to minorities, the poor, and people living in underserved areas (Ginzberg 1994; Starr 1982). Hence, the underserved populations suffer the most from shortages of PCPs.

To help alleviate the shortage of PCPs, some medical schools strive to develop students' competencies in skills, values, and attitudes relevant to the practice of primary care. Their curricula are adapted toward issues of special concern to generalists, such as outpatient experience; public health concepts; disease prevention; and cultural, ethnic, and population-specific knowledge. They develop opportunities for students to work with the poor, minorities, and the uninsured and make such opportunities available in rural and other underserved areas (Verby et al. 1991).

The methods of financing medical training, research, and physician services have built-in incentives for specialty-oriented training and disincentives for primary care training (Institute of Medicine 1989; Wennberg et al. 1993). With respect to medical training, the system of graduate medical education payments through Medicare is based on the number of trainees rather than prioritizing medical specialties that are more needed. With respect to research, much of the clinical research, funded by the National Institutes of Health, is carried out under the auspices of specialty departments of medical schools (Ginzberg and Dutka 1989) and the research topics are often very narrowly focused.

With respect to physician payment, current reimbursement structures lack appropriate financial incentives aimed at advancing health promotion, disease prevention, and other primary care services. Incentives are also needed to reinforce primary care-seeking behavior among patients. For example, primary care services should be exempt from deductibles and copayments. Out-of-pocket costs discourage primary care-seeking behavior and, eventually, lead to higher health care expenditures and poorer health outcomes (Lurie et al. 1986).

## International Medical Graduates

The ratio of IMGs to population has steadily grown over time (Figure 4–2) and so has the proportion of IMGs to total active physicians practicing in the United States (Figure 4–4). About 25% of professionally active physicians in the United States are IMGs, also known as foreign medical graduates (Cohen 2006). This translates to more than 150,000 active IMGs in the United States physician

Figure 4–4  IMG Physicians As a Proportion of Total Active Physicians.

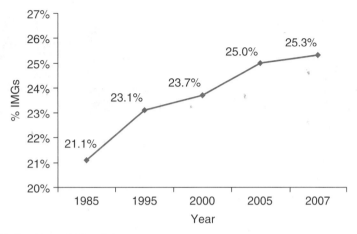

*Source:* Data from *Health, United States, 2009*, p. 376.

workforce (Gastel 2006). An estimated one-fourth of all residency positions are filled by IMGs (Mullan 1999), and an increasing number of IMGs are filling family practice residency slots (Koehn et al. 2002). In 1995, only 6.3% of IMGs entered family practice residencies; by 2003, the number had increased to 15.8% (Boulet et al. 2006).

# Dentists

Dentists diagnose and treat dental problems related to the teeth, gums, and tissues of the mouth. All dentists must be licensed to practice. The licensure requirements include graduation from an accredited dental school that awards a Doctor of Dental Surgery (DDS) or Doctor of Dental Medicine (DMD) degree and successful completion of both written and practical examinations. Some states require dentists to obtain a specialty license before practicing as a specialist in that state (Stanfield et al. 2009). Nine specialty areas are recognized by the

American Dental Association: orthodontics (straightening teeth), oral and maxillofacial surgery (operating on the mouth and jaws), oral and maxillofacial radiology (producing and interpreting images of the mouth and jaws), pediatric dentistry (dental care for children), periodontics (treating gums), prosthodontics (making artificial teeth or dentures), endodontics (root canal therapy), public health dentistry (community dental health), and oral pathology (diseases of the mouth). The growth of dental specialties is influenced by technological advances, including implant dentistry, laser-guided surgery, orthognathic surgery (surgery performed on the bones of the jaw) for the restoration of facial form and function, new metal combinations for use in prosthetic devices, new bone graft materials in "tissue-guided regeneration" techniques, and new materials and instruments.

Many dentists are involved in the prevention of dental decay and gum disease. Dental prevention includes regular cleaning of patients' teeth and educating patients on proper dental hygiene. Dentists also spot symptoms that require treatment by a physician. Dentists employ dental hygienists and assistants to perform many of the preventive and routine care services.

*Dental hygienists* work in dental offices and provide preventive dental care, including cleaning teeth and educating patients on proper dental care. Dental hygienists must be licensed to practice. The licensure requirements include graduation from an accredited school of dental hygiene and successful completion of both a national board written examination and a state or regional clinical examination. Many states require further examination on legal aspects of dental hygiene practice.

*Dental assistants* work for dentists in the preparation, examination, and treatment of patients. Dental assistants do not have to be licensed to work; however, formal training programs that offer a certificate or diploma are available. Dental assistants, typically, work alongside dentists.

Most dentists practice in private offices as solo or group practitioners. As such, dental offices are operated as private businesses, and dentists often perform business tasks, such as staffing, financing, purchasing, leasing, and work scheduling. Some dentists are employed in clinics operated by private companies, retail stores, or franchised dental outlets. Group dental practices, offering lower overhead and increased productivity, have slowly grown. The federal government also employs dentists, mainly in the hospitals and clinics of the Department of Veterans Affairs and the US Public Health Service. Mean annual earnings of salaried dentists were $156,850 in 2009 (US Bureau of Labor Statistics 2010).

The emergence of employer-sponsored dental insurance caused an increased demand for dental care because it enabled a greater segment of the population to afford dental services. The demand for dentists will continue to grow with an increase in populations having high dental needs, such as the elderly, and an increase in public awareness of the importance of dental care toward general health status. Demand will also be affected by the fairly widespread appeal of cosmetic and esthetic dentistry, the prevalence of dental insurance plans, and the inclusion of dental care as part of many public-funded programs, such as Head Start, Medicaid, community and migrant health centers, and maternal and infant care.

## Pharmacists

The traditional role of *pharmacists* has been to dispense medicines prescribed by physicians, dentists, and podiatrists and to provide consultation on the proper selection and use of medicines. All states require a license to practice pharmacy. The licensure requirements include graduation from an accredited pharmacy program that awards a Bachelor of Pharmacy or Doctor of Pharmacy (PharmD) degree, successful completion of a state board examination, and practical experience or completion of a supervised internship (Stanfield et al. 2009). After 2005, the bachelor's degree was phased out, and a PharmD, requiring six years of postsecondary education, became the standard. The mean annual earnings of pharmacists in 2009 were $106,630 (US Bureau of Labor Statistics 2010).

Although most pharmacists are generalists, dispensing drugs and advising providers and patients, some become specialists. Pharmacotherapists specialize in drug therapy and work closely with physicians. Nutrition-support pharmacists determine and prepare drugs needed for nutritional therapy. Radiopharmacists, or nuclear pharmacists, produce radioactive drugs used for patient diagnosis and therapy.

Most pharmacists hold salaried positions and work in community pharmacies that are independently owned or are part of a national drugstore, discount store, or department store chain. Pharmacists are also employed by hospitals, MCOs, home health agencies, clinics, government health services organizations, and pharmaceutical manufacturers.

The role of pharmacists has expanded from primarily preparing and dispensing prescriptions to include drug product education and serving as experts on specific drugs, drug interactions, and generic drug substitution.

Under the Omnibus Budget Reconciliation Act of 1990, pharmacists are required to give consumers information about drugs and their potential misuse. This educating and counseling role of pharmacists is broadly referred to as *pharmaceutical care*. The American Council on Pharmaceutical Education (ACPE) (1992) defined pharmaceutical care as "a mode of pharmacy practice in which the pharmacist takes an active role on behalf of patients, by assisting prescribers in appropriate drug choices, by effecting distribution of medications to patients, and by assuming direct responsibilities collaboratively with other health care professionals and with patients to achieve the desired therapeutic outcome." This concept entails a high level of drug knowledge, clinical skill, and independent judgment and requires that pharmacists share with other health professionals the responsibility for optimizing the outcome of patients' drug therapy, including health status, quality of life, and satisfaction

(Helper and Strand 1990; Schwartz 1994; Strand et al. 1991). Pharmacists are often consulted by physicians to identify and prevent potential drug-related problems and resolve actual drug-related problems (Morley and Strand 1989).

In about half of the states, pharmacists have the authority to initiate or modify drug treatment as long as they have collaborative agreements with physicians. For example, a stroke patient who needs blood thinning medication might walk into the drugstore for an assessment and walk out with a different dosage. Other states are weighing whether to give pharmacists similar authority.

# Other Doctoral-Level Health Professionals

In addition to physicians, dentists, and some pharmacists, other health professionals have doctoral education, including optometrists, psychologists, podiatrists, and chiropractors.

*Optometrists* provide vision care, such as examination, diagnosis, and correction of vision problems. They must be licensed to practice. The licensure requirements include the possession of a Doctor of Optometry (OD) degree and passing a written and clinical state board examination. Most optometrists work in solo or group practices. Some work for the government, optical stores, or vision care centers as salaried employees.

*Psychologists* provide patients with mental health care. They must be licensed or certified to practice. The ultimate recognition is the diplomate in psychology, which requires a Doctor of Philosophy (PhD) or Doctor of Psychology (PsyD) degree, a minimum of 5 years' postdoctoral experience, and the successful completion of an examination by the American Board of Examiners in Professional Psychology. Psychologists may specialize in several areas, such as clinical, counseling, developmental, educational, engineering, personnel, experimental, industrial, psychometric, rehabilitation, school, and social domains (Stanfield et al. 2009).

*Podiatrists* treat patients with diseases or deformities of the feet, including performing surgical operations, prescribing medications and corrective devices, and administering physiotherapy. They must be licensed to practice. Requirements for licensure include completion of an accredited program that awards a Doctor of Podiatric Medicine (DPM) degree and passing a national examination by the National Board of Podiatry. Most podiatrists work in private practice, but some are salaried employees of health service organizations.

*Chiropractors* provide treatment to patients through chiropractic (done by hand) manipulation, physiotherapy, and dietary counseling. They typically help patients with neurological, muscular, and vascular disturbances. Chiropractic care is based on the belief that the body is a self-healing organism. Chiropractors do not prescribe drugs or perform surgery. Chiropractors must be licensed to practice. Requirements for licensure include completion of an accredited program that awards a 4-year Doctor of Chiropractic (DC) degree and passing an examination by the state chiropractic board. Most chiropractors work in private solo or group practice.

## Nurses

Nurses constitute the largest group of health care professionals. The nursing profession developed around hospitals after World War I, primarily attracting women. Before that time, more than 70% of nurses worked in private duty, either in patients' homes or for private-pay patients in hospitals. Hospital-based nursing flourished after the war as the effectiveness of nursing care became apparent. Federal support of nursing education increased after World War II, represented by the Nursing Training Act of 1964, the Health Manpower Act of 1968, and the Nursing Training Act of 1971; however, state funding remains the primary source of financial support for nursing schools.

Nurses are the major caregivers of sick and injured patients, addressing their physical, mental, and emotional needs. All states require nurses to be licensed to practice. Nurses can be licensed in more than one state through examination or endorsement of a license issued by another state. The licensure requirements include graduation from an approved nursing program and successful completion of a national examination. Educational preparation distinguishes between two levels of nurses. *Registered nurses* (RNs) must complete an associate's degree (ADN), a diploma program, or a baccalaureate degree (BSN). ADN programs take about 2 to 3 years and are offered by community and junior colleges. Diploma programs take 2 to 3 years and are still offered by a few hospitals. BSN programs take 4 to 5 years and are offered by colleges and universities (Stanfield et al. 2009). *Licensed practical nurses* (LPNs)—called licensed vocational nurses (LVNs) in some states—must complete a state-approved program in practical nursing and a national written examination. Most practical nursing programs last about one year and include classroom study, as well as supervised clinical practice.

Nurses work in a variety of settings, including hospitals, nursing homes, ambulatory care centers, community and migrant health centers, emergency medical centers, MCOs, certain industries, government agencies, clinics, schools, retirement communities, rehabilitation centers, and as private-duty nurses in patients' homes. Nurses are often classified according to the settings in which they work: hospital nurses, long-term care nurses, public health nurses, private-duty nurses, office nurses, and occupational health or industrial nurses. Head nurses act as supervisors of other nurses. RNs supervise LPNs.

With the remarkable growth in various types of outpatient settings (see Chapter 7), hospitals and nursing homes now treat much sicker patients than before. Hence, the ratio of nurses to patients has increased, and nurses' work has become more intensive. On the other hand, the growth in outpatient settings has created new opportunities for nursing employment in home care, hospice services, assisted living facilities, community health centers, and physicians' clinics. The growing opportunities for RNs in supportive roles, such as case management, utilization review, quality assurance, and prevention counseling, have also expanded the demand for their services. These roles also give RNs greater autonomy to organize their work. The role of nurses has undergone a significant change. To reduce their subservience to physicians, nurses are clarifying their relationship to physicians within the context of clinical decisionmaking.

In 2009, registered nurse was one of the largest occupations in the United States, with approximately 2.6 million RNs earning an average salary of $66,530 per year. Physicians' clinics, home health services, and long-term care facilities are projected to experience increases in employment for RNs (US Bureau of Labor Statistics 2009).

Between 2001 and 2008, the total full-time equivalent (FTE) RN workforce increased by 476,000. During this time period, older RNs accounted for about two-third of the total increase, and about one-third was supplied by foreign-born RNs (Buerhaus et al. 2009). Such composition of the RN workforce has raised issues regarding supply and quality of care. With large "baby-boom" RN cohorts retiring during the next decade, the RN workforce is expected to experience a shortage, although large cohorts born in the 1970s and 1980s may prevent the workforce from shrinking (Buerhaus et al. 2009). Thus, strategies to ensure the long-term supply of younger RNs are warranted. Communication skills of foreign-born RNs have also become an issue pertaining to quality of care and patient safety. Since it is likely that the demand for foreign-educated RNs will increase to meet the growing demand for health care workforce, interventions must take place to improve communication skills among both US-native and foreign-born RNs (Buerhaus et al. 2009).

Projections of the future need for nurses indicate there will be a deficit of 340,000 nurses in 2020 (Auerbach et al. 2007). To make the nursing profession more attractive, health services organizations need to initiate measures, such as creating incentive packages to attract new nurses, increasing pay and benefits of current nurses, introducing more flexible work schedules, awarding tuition reimbursement for continuing education, and providing on-site day care assistance.

## Advanced Practice Nurses

The term *advanced practice nurse* (APN) is a general classification of nurses who have education and clinical experience beyond that required of an RN. APNs include four areas of specialization (Cooper et al. 1998): clinical nurse specialists (CNSs), certified registered nurse anesthetists (CRNAs), nurse practitioners (NPs), and certified nurse midwives (CNMs). NPs and CNMs are also categorized as NPPs and will be discussed in the next section. Besides being direct caregivers, APNs perform other professional activities, such as collaborating and consulting with other health care professionals; educating patients and other nurses; collecting data for clinical research projects; and participating in the development and implementation of total quality management programs, critical pathways, case management, and standards of care (Grossman 1995).

The main difference between CNSs and NPs is that CNSs work in hospitals, whereas NPs work mainly in primary care settings. CNSs can specialize in specific fields, such as oncology, neonatal health, cardiac care, or psychiatric care. Examples of their functions in an acute care hospital include taking social and clinical history at the time of admission, conducting physical assessment after admission, adjusting IV infusion rates, managing pain, managing resuscitation orders, removing intracardiac catheters, and ordering routine laboratory tests and radiographic examinations. They generally do not have the legal authority to prescribe drugs. NPs, on the other hand, may prescribe drugs in most states. CRNAs are trained to manage anesthesia during surgery, and CNMs deliver babies and manage the care of mothers and healthy newborns before, during, and after delivery.

The requirements for becoming an APN vary greatly from state to state. In general, the designation requires a graduate degree in nursing or certification in an advanced practice specialty area.

## Nonphysician Practitioners NPP

The terms *nonphysician practitioners* (NPPs), nonphysician clinicians (NPCs), and midlevel providers (MLPs) refer to clinical professionals who practice in many of the areas similar to those in which physicians practice but who do not have an MD or a DO degree. NPPs receive less advanced training than physicians but more training than RNs. They are also referred to as *physician extenders* because in the delivery of primary care, they can, in many instances, substitute for physicians. However, they do not engage in the entire range of primary care or deal with complex cases requiring the expertise of a physician (Cooper et al. 1998). Hence, NPPs often work in close consultation with physicians. Efforts to formally establish the NPP role began in the late 1960s, in recognition of the fact that they could improve access to primary care, especially in rural areas. NPPs include physician assistants (PAs), NPs, and CNMs.

### Nurse Practitioners

The American Nurses' Association defines *nurse practitioners* as individuals who have completed a program of study leading to competence as RNs in an expanded role. NPs constitute the largest group of NPPs and the group that has undergone the most growth (Cooper et al. 1998). As of 2010, there were approximately 140,000 NPs in the United States (American Academy of Nurse Practitioners 2010).

Close to 6,000 new NPs are trained every year in 325 colleges and universities (American Association of Nurse Practitioners 2007). The training of NPs may be a certificate program (at least 9 months in duration) or a master's degree program (2 years of full-time study). States vary with regard to licensure and accreditation requirements. Most NPs are now trained in graduate or postgraduate nursing programs. In addition, NPs must complete clinical training in direct patient care. Certification examinations are offered by the American Nurses Credentialing Center, the American Academy of Nurse Practitioners, and specialty nursing organizations.

The expanded role of nursing emerged as a viable option to remedy the many facets of the health labor force problem after research showed the clinical skills of NPs were comparable to those of physicians when employed for conditions cared for by both. Patients also seemed to be more satisfied with the care received from NPs than with care received from physicians (Office of Technology Assessment 1986, 1991).

NPs work predominantly in primary care, whereas PAs are evenly divided between primary care and specialty care. Another main difference between the practice orientation of NPs and PAs is that NPs are oriented toward health promotion and education; PAs are oriented more toward a practice model that focuses on disease (Hooker and McCaig 2001). NPs spend extra time with patients to help them understand the need to take responsibility for their own health.

NPs possess the technical skills to practice independently of physicians; however, physicians are consulted when patients' conditions require treatment beyond NPs' expertise. NP specialties include pediatric, family, adult, psychiatric, and geriatric programs. NPs also provide services to geriatric patients in nursing homes (Brody et al. 1976). NPs have statutory prescribing authority in almost all states. NPs can also receive direct reimbursement as providers under the Medicaid and Medicare programs.

## Physician Assistants

The American Academy of Physician Assistants (1986) defines *physician assistants* "as part of the healthcare team . . . [who] work in a dependent relationship with a supervising physician to provide comprehensive care." In 2009, there were approximately 76,900 jobs available for PAs in the United States (US Bureau of Labor Statistics 2010). The number of PA jobs is greater than the number of PAs because about 15% of PAs work more than one job.

PAs are licensed to perform medical procedures only under the supervision of a physician. In the delivery of care by a PA, the supervising physician may be either on-site or off-site. The major services provided by PAs include evaluation, monitoring, diagnostics, therapeutics, counseling, and referral (Fizgerald et al. 1995). As of 2005, 135 accredited PA training programs were operating in the United States, with a steady growth in enrollment (US Bureau of Labor Statistics 2007). PA programs award bachelor's degrees, certificates, associate degrees, or master's degrees. The mean length of the program is 26 months (Hooker and Berlin 2002). PAs are certified by the National Commission on Certification of Physician Assistants. In most states, PAs have the authority to prescribe medications.

## Certified Nurse Midwives

*Certified nurse midwives* are RNs with additional training from a nurse midwifery program, in areas such as maternal and fetal procedures, maternity and child nursing, and patient assessment (Endicott 1976). CNMs deliver babies, provide family planning education, and manage gynecological and obstetric care and can substitute for obstetricians/gynecologists in prenatal and postnatal care. They are certified by the American College of Nurse-Midwives (ACNM) to provide care for normal expectant mothers. They refer abnormal or high-risk patients to obstetricians or jointly manage the care of such patients. There are approximately 45 ACNM accredited nurse-midwifery education programs in the United States (US Bureau of Labor Statistics 2007).

Midwifery has never assumed the central role in the management of pregnancies in the United States that it has in Europe (Wagner 1991). Physicians, mainly obstetricians, attend most deliveries in the United States, but some evidence indicates that, for low-risk pregnancies, CNMs are much less likely to use available technical tools to monitor or modify the course of labor. Patients of CNMs are less likely to be electronically monitored, have induced labor, or receive epidural anesthesia. These differences are associated with lower Caesarean section rates and less resource use, such as hospital stay, operating room costs, and use of anesthesia staff (Rosenblatt et al. 1997).

## Value of NPP Services

Studies have confirmed the efficacy of NPPs as health care providers. NPs and PAs often render care equivalent in quality to that provided by physicians (Office of Technology Assessment 1986). Later studies also demonstrated that NPPs can provide both high-quality and cost-effective medical care (Hooker 2006; Garrard et al. 1990; Ostwald and Abanobi 1986) because they show greater personal interest in patients and cost significantly less (Sellards and Mills 1995). Moreover, NPs have been noted to have better communication and interviewing skills than physicians. These skills are considered particularly important in community and migrant health centers in assessing patients who are predominantly of minority origin and often have little education (Brody et al. 1976). CNMs are considered effective in providing access to obstetrical and prenatal services in rural and poor communities (Institute of Medicine 1985; Rosenbaum 1995). CNMs can manage routine pregnancies as competently as, if not better than, physicians (Office of Technology Assessment 1986). Patients cared for by CNMs have shorter waiting times for visits, have shorter hospitalizations, and are more likely to express satisfaction with their care.

Especially repetitive technical tasks, such as the use of flexible sigmoidoscopy to screen for colon cancer, can be performed effectively and less expensively by specially trained NPPs. NPPs can also manage quick turnover cases in emergency departments, when a patient's life is not in jeopardy. In occupational medicine, such as preemployment physicals, drug testing, and evaluation of workers' compensation cases, an NP can probably handle 80 to 90% of the tasks performed by physicians. Moreover, NPs and PAs cost about 40% of what physicians cost. Hence, utilization of NPPs adds value to the delivery of health care.

Among the issues that need to be resolved before NPPs can be used to their full potential are legal restrictions to practice, reimbursement policies, and relationships with physicians (Samuels and Shi 1993). The lack of autonomy to practice is a great legislative barrier facing midlevel providers. Most states require physician supervision as a condition for practice. In some states, midlevel providers lack prescriptive authority. NPPs also face reimbursement barriers. Reimbursement for their services is generally indirect; that is, payments are made to the physicians with whom they practice. Also, NPPs' opinions are not actively sought in making medical policies and decisions.

## Allied Health Professionals

The term *allied health* is used to loosely categorize several different types of professionals in many health-related technical areas. Among these professionals are technicians, assistants, therapists, and technologists. These professionals receive specialized training, and their clinical interventions complement the work of physicians and nurses. Certain professionals, however, are allowed to practice independently, depending on state law.

In the early part of the 20th century, the health care provider workforce consisted of physicians, nurses, pharmacists, and optometrists. As knowledge in health sciences expanded and medical care became more complex, physicians found it difficult to spend the necessary time with their patients. Time constraints, as well as the limitations in learning new skills, created a need to train other professionals who could serve as adjuncts to or as substitutes for physicians and nurses.

Section 701 of the Public Health Service Act defines an allied health professional as someone who has received a certificate; associate's, bachelor's, or master's degree; doctoral level preparation; or postbaccalaureate training in a science related to health care and has responsibility for the delivery of health or related services. These services may include those associated with the identification, evaluation, and prevention of diseases and disorders, dietary and nutritional services, rehabilitation, or health system management. Further, these professionals are other than those who have received a degree in medicine, dentistry, veterinary medicine, optometry, podiatry, chiropractic, or pharmacy; a graduate degree in health administration; a degree in clinical psychology; or a degree equivalent to one of these.

Allied health professionals can be divided into two broad categories: technicians/assistants and therapists/technologists. The main allied health professions in the United States are listed in Exhibit 4–2. Formal requirements for these professionals range from certificates gained in postsecondary educational programs to postgraduate degrees for some professions.

Typically, technicians and assistants receive less than 2 years of postsecondary education. They require supervision from therapists or technologists to ensure that treatment plans are followed. Technicians and assistants include physical therapy assistants (PTAs), certified occupational therapy assistants (COTAs), medical laboratory technicians, radiologic technicians, and respiratory therapy technicians.

Technologists and therapists receive more advanced training. They evaluate patients, diagnose problems, and develop treatment plans. Many technologists and therapists have independent practices. For example, physical therapy is practiced in most US states without the requirement of a prescription or referral from a physician. Many states also allow occupational therapists and speech therapists to see patients without referral from a physician.

### Therapists

*Physical therapists* (PTs) provide care for patients with movement dysfunction. Educational programs in physical therapy are accredited by the Commission on Accreditation of Physical Therapy Education. Of the

Exhibit 4–2 Examples of Allied Health Professionals

Activities Coordinator
Audiology Technician
Cardiovascular Technician
Cytotechnologist
Dental Assistant
Dietary Food Service Manager
Exercise Physiologist
Histologic Technician
Laboratory Technician
Legal Services
Medical Records Technician
Medical Technologist
Mental Health Worker
Nuclear Medicine
Occupational Therapist
Occupational Therapy Assistant
Optician
Pharmacist
Physical Therapist
Physical Therapy Assistant
Physician Assistant
Radiology Technician
Recreation Therapist
Registered Dietitian
Registered Records Administrator
Respiratory Therapist
Respiratory Therapy Technician
Social Services Coordinator
Social Worker
Speech Therapist
Speech Therapy Assistant

212 physical therapist education programs in the United States, in 2009, 12 awarded master's degrees and 200 awarded doctoral degrees. Currently, only graduate degree physical therapy programs are accredited. Master's degree programs typically are 2 to 2.5 years in length, while doctoral degree programs last 3 years. To obtain a license, PTs must also pass the National Physical Therapy Examination (US Bureau of Labor Statistics 2011).

*Occupational therapists* (OTs) help people of all ages improve their ability to perform tasks in their daily living and working environments. They work with individuals who have conditions that are mentally, physically, developmentally, or emotionally disabling. A master's degree in occupational therapy is the typical minimum requirement for entry into the field. In 2009, 150 master's degree programs or combined bachelor's and master's degree programs were accredited, and 4 doctoral degree programs were accredited by the Accreditation Council for Occupational Therapy Education (US Bureau of Labor Statistics 2011).

Speech–language pathologists treat patients with speech and language problems. Audiologists treat patients with hearing problems. The American Speech-Language-Hearing Association is the credentialing association for audiologists and speech–language pathologists.

## Other Allied Health Professionals

Medical dietetics includes dietitians or nutritionists and dietetic technicians who ensure that institutional foods and diets are prepared in accordance with acceptable nutritional standards. Dietitians are registered by the Commission on Dietetic Registration of the American Dietetic Association. Dispensing opticians fit eyeglasses and contact lenses. They are certified by the American Board of Opticianry and the National

Contact Lens Examiners. Social workers help patients and families cope with problems resulting from long-term illness, injury, and rehabilitation. The Council on Social Work Education accredits baccalaureate and master's degree programs in social work in the United States.

Many programs are accredited by the Committee on Allied Health Education and Accreditation under the American Medical Association, including anesthesiologist assistants, cardiovascular technologists, cytotechnologists (study changes in body cells under a microscope), diagnostic medical sonographers (work with ultrasound diagnostic procedures), electroneurodiagnostic technologists (work with procedures related to the electrical activity of the brain and nervous system), emergency medical technician–paramedics (provide medical emergent care to acutely ill or injured persons in prehospital settings), histologic technicians/technologists (analyze blood, tissue, and fluids), medical assistants (perform a number of administrative and clinical duties in physicians' offices), medical illustrators, medical laboratory technicians, medical record administrators (direct the medical records department), medical record technicians (organize and file medical records), medical technologists (perform clinical laboratory testing), nuclear medicine technologists (operate diagnostic imaging equipment and use radioactive drugs to assist in the diagnosis of illness), ophthalmic medical technicians, perfusionists (operate life support respiratory and circulatory equipment), radiologic technologists (perform diagnostic imaging exams, such as X-rays, computed tomography, magnetic resonance imaging, and mammography), respiratory therapists and technicians (treat patients with breathing disorders), specialists in blood bank technology, surgeon's assistants, and surgical technologists (prepare operating rooms and patients for surgery).

Certain health care workers are not required to be licensed, and they usually learn their skills on the job; however, their roles are limited to assisting other professionals in the provision of services. Examples include dietetic assistants, who assist dietitians or dietetic technicians in the provision of nutritional care; electroencephalogram technologists or technicians, who operate electroencephalographs; electrocardiogram technicians, who operate electrocardiographs; paraoptometrics, including optometric technicians and assistants, who perform basic tasks related to vision care; health educators, who provide individuals and groups with facts on health, illness, and prevention; psychiatric/mental health technicians, who provide care to patients with mental illness or developmental disabilities; and sanitarians, who collect samples for laboratory analysis and inspect facilities for compliance with public health regulations. Increasingly, these practitioners seek their credentials through certifications, registrations, and training programs.

As the number of older people continues to grow and as new developments allow for the treatment of more medical conditions, more allied health professionals will be needed. For example, home health aides will be needed as more individuals seek care outside of traditional institutional settings. Jobs for LPNs, LVNs, and pharmacy technicians are also expected to increase by a substantial number, roughly 155,600 and 99,800, respectively (US Bureau of Labor Statistics 2009).

In an effort to meet the growing demand for allied health professionals, the Patient Protection and Affordable Care Act (ACA) of 2010 has provisions for the forgiveness of existing education loans. The program includes allied health professionals who are employed full-time in a federal, state, local, or tribal public health agency or other qualified employment location, including acute care and ambulatory care facilities, settings located in Health Professional Shortage Areas (HPSAs), or medically underserved areas (Redhead and Williams 2010).

---

## Health Services Administrators

Health services administrators are employed at the top, middle, and entry levels of various types of organizations that deliver health services. Top-level administrators provide leadership and strategic direction, work closely with the governing boards (see Chapter 8), and are responsible for an organization's long-term success. They are responsible for operational, clinical, and financial outcomes of their entire organization. Middle-level administrators may have leadership roles for major service centers, such as outpatient, surgical, and nursing services, or they may be departmental managers in charge of single departments, such as diagnostics, dietary, rehabilitation, social services, environmental services, or medical records. Their jobs involve major planning and coordinating functions, organizing human and physical resources, directing and supervising, operational and financial controls, and decision making. They often have direct responsibility for implementing changes, creating efficiencies, and developing new procedures with respect to changes in the health care delivery system. Entry-level administrators may function as assistants to middle-level managers. They may

supervise a small number of operatives. For example, their main function may be to oversee and assist with operations critical to the efficient operation of a departmental unit.

Today's medical centers and integrated delivery organizations are among the most complex organizations to manage. Leaders in health care delivery face some unique challenges, including changes in financing and payment structures, as well as having to work with reduced levels of reimbursement. Other challenges include pressures to provide uncompensated care, greater responsibility for quality, accountability for community health, separate contingencies imposed by public and private payers, uncertainties created by new policy developments, changing configurations in the competitive environment, and maintaining the integrity of an organization through the highest level of ethical standards.

Health services administration is taught at the bachelor's and master's level in a variety of settings, and the programs lead to several different degrees. The settings for such academic programs include schools of medicine, public health, public administration, business administration, and allied health sciences. Bachelor's degrees prepare students for entry-level positions. Mid- and senior-level positions require a graduate degree. The most common degrees are the Master of Health Administration (MHA) or Master of Health Services Administration (MHSA), Master of Business Administration (MBA, with a health care management emphasis), Master of Public Health (MPH), or Master of Public Administration (or Affairs; MPA) (Pew Health Professions Commission 1993). The schools of public health that are accredited by the Council on Education for Public Health (CEPH) play a key role in training health services administrators in their MHA (or MHSA) and MPH programs (CEPH 2011). The MHA programs, however, compared to the MPH programs, have more course requirements to furnish skills in business management (both theory and applied management) and quantitative/analytical areas, considered crucial for managing today's health services organizations. This disparity has been viewed as a concern that the schools of public health need to address (Singh et al. 1996).

Educational preparation of nursing home administrators is a notable exception to the MHA model. The training of nursing home administrators has largely been influenced by government licensing regulations. Even though licensure of nursing home administrators dates back to the mid-1960s, regulations favoring a formal postsecondary academic degree are more recent. Passing a national examination administered by the National Association of Boards of Examiners of Long-Term Care Administrators (NAB) is a standard requirement; however, educational qualifications needed to obtain a license vary significantly from one state to another. Although about one-third of the states still require less than a bachelor's degree as the minimum academic preparation, an increasing number of practicing nursing home administrators have at least a bachelor's degree. The problem is that most state regulations call for only general levels of education rather than specialized preparation in long-term care administration. General education does not furnish adequate skills in all the domains of practice relevant to nursing home management (Singh et al. 1997). However, various colleges and universities offer specialized programs in nursing home administration.

## Summary

Health services professionals in the United States constitute the largest labor force. The development of these professionals is influenced by demographic trends, advances in research and technology, disease and illness trends, and the changing environment of health care financing and delivery. Physicians play a leading role in the delivery of health services. The United States has an overall surplus of physicians and a maldistribution of physicians both by specialty and by geography. The current shortage of PCPs is likely to continue well into the future. Various policies and programs have been used or proposed to address both physician imbalance and maldistribution, including regulation of health care professions, reimbursement initiatives targeting suitable incentives, targeted programs for underserved areas, changes in medical school curricula, changes in the financing of medical training, and a more rational referral system.

In addition to physicians, many other health services professionals contribute significantly to the delivery of health care, including nurses, dentists, pharmacists, optometrists, psychologists, podiatrists, chiropractors, NPPs, and other allied health professionals. These professionals require different levels of training. They work in a variety of health care settings as complements to or substitutes for physicians. Health services administrators face new challenges in the leadership of health care organizations. These challenges call for some reforms in the educational programs designed to prepare adequately trained managers for the various sectors of the health care industry.

## Test Your Understanding

### Terminology

| | | |
|---|---|---|
| advanced practice nurse | hospitalist | physical therapists |
| allied health | licensed practical nurses | physician assistants |
| allopathic medicine | maldistribution | physician extenders |
| certified nurse midwives | nonphysician practitioners | podiatrists |
| chiropractors | nurse practitioners | primary care |
| comorbidity | occupational therapists | psychologists |
| dental assistants | optometrists | registered nurses |
| dental hygienists | osteopathic medicine | residency |
| dentists | pharmaceutical care | specialist |
| generalist | pharmacists | specialty care |

## Review Questions

1. Describe the major types of health services professionals (physicians, nurses, dentists, pharmacists, physician assistants, nurse practitioners, certified nurse midwives), including their roles, training, practice requirements, and practice settings.

2. What factors are associated with the development of health services professionals in the United States?

3. What are the major distinctions between primary care and specialty care?

4. Why is there a geographic maldistribution of the physician labor force in the United States?

5. Why is there an imbalance between primary care and specialty care in the United States?

6. What measures have been or can be employed to overcome problems related to physician maldistribution and imbalance?

7. Who are nonphysician primary care providers? What are their roles in the delivery of health care?

8. In general, who are allied health professionals? What role do they play in the delivery of health services?

9. Provide a brief description of the roles and responsibilities of health services administrators.

# Appendix 4–A

## List of Professional Associations

American Academy of Nurse Practitioners
American Academy of Physician Assistants
American Art Therapy Association, Inc.
American Association for Practical Nurse
    Education and Service
American Association for Rehabilitation
    Therapy
American Association for Respiratory Care
American Association of Colleges of
    Nursing
American Association of Colleges of Osteo-
    pathic Medicine
American Association of Colleges of
    Pharmacy
American Association of Dental Schools
American Association of Homes and Ser-
    vices for the Aging
American Association of Medical
    Assistants
American Chiropractic Association
American College of Emergency Physicians
American College of Health Care
    Administrators
American College of Healthcare Executives
American College of Nurse Midwives
American Corrective Therapy Association
American Council on Pharmaceutical
    Education
American Dance Therapy Association
American Dental Assistants Association
American Dental Association
American Dental Association SELECT
    Program
American Dental Hygienists' Association

American Dietetic Association
American Health Care Association
American Hospital Association
American Medical Association
American Medical Technologists
American Nurses' Association
American Occupational Therapy
    Association
American Optometry Association
American Organization of Nurse Executives
American Osteopathic Association
American Pharmaceutical Association
American Physical Therapy Association
American Psychiatric Association
American Psychological Association
American Public Health Association
American Registry of Radiologic
    Technologists
American School Health Association
American Society of Clinical Pathologists
American Society of Hospital Pharmacists
American Society of Radiologic
    Technologists
American Speech-Language-Hearing
    Association
American Therapeutic Recreation
    Association
Association of American Medical Colleges
Association of Physician Assistant
    Programs
Association of Schools and Colleges of
    Optometry
Association of Schools of Public Health
Association of Surgical Technologists

Association of University Programs in Health Administration

Council on Podiatry Education

Council on Social Work Education

Dental Assisting National Board, Inc.

Environmental Management Association

Healthcare Financial Management Association

International Society for Clinical Laboratory Technology

National Academy of Opticianry

National Association for Music Therapy

National Association of Boards of Pharmacy

National Association of Chain Drug Stores, Inc.

National Association of Emergency Medical Technicians

National Association of Social Workers

National Board for Respiratory Care, Inc.

National Board of Podiatry

National Certification Agency for Medical Laboratory Personnel

National Commission for Health Certifying Agencies

National Council for Therapeutic Recreational Certification

National Council for Therapy and Rehabilitation through Horticulture

National Environmental Health Association

National League for Nursing

National Nursing Centers' Consortium

National Registry of Emergency Medical Technicians

National Society of Cardiovascular Technology

National Society of Pulmonary Technology

National Therapeutic Recreation Association

Opticians' Association of America

Society of Nuclear Medicine

# REFERENCES

Agency for Healthcare Research and Quality (AHRQ). 2005. *Health care disparities in rural areas: Selected findings from the 2004 National Healthcare Disparities Report.* Available at: http:// www.ahrq.gov/research/ruraldisp/ruraldispar.htm. Accessed October 2010.

American Academy of Nurse Practitioners. 2010. *AANP annual report.* Available at: http:// www.aanp.org/NR/ roonlyres/AID9B4BD-ACSE-45BF-9EB0-DEFCA1123204/4271 /FAQsWhatisanNP83110.pdf. Accessed November 2010.

American Academy of Physician Assistants. 1986. *PA fact sheet.* Arlington, VA:

American Association of Colleges of Osteopathic Medicine. 2007. Available at: http://www.aacom .org/om.html. Accessed January 2007.

American Association of Nurse Practitioners. 2007. Available at: http://www.aanp.org/default.asp. Accessed February 2007.

American Council on Pharmaceutical Education. 1992. *The proposed revision of accreditation standards and guidelines.* Chicago: National Association of Boards on Pharmacy.

American Physical Therapy Association. 1998. Pew Commission urges increased action to cut US physician supply. *PT Bulletin* November 10, no. 10.

Anonymous. 1990. Medical education may deter grads from choosing primary care careers. *AAMC Weekly Rep* March 15, no. 4: 1.

Auerbach, D.I. et al. 2007. Better late than never: Workforce supply implications of later entry into nursing. *Health Affairs* 26, no. 1: 178–185.

Boulet, J.R. et al. 2006. The international medical graduate pipeline: Recent trends in certification and residency training. *Health Affairs* 25, no. 6: 469–477.

Brody, S.J. et al. 1976. The geriatric nurse practitioner: A new medical resource in the skilled nursing home. *Journal of Chronic Diseases* 29, no. 8: 537–543.

Buerhaus, P.I. et al. 2009. The recent surge in nurse employment: Causes and implications. *Health Affairs* 28, no.4: w657–w668.

Bylsma, W.H. et al. 2010. Where have all the general internists gone? *Journal of General Internal Medicine* 25, no. 10: 1020–1023.

Cohen, J.J. 1993. Transforming the size and composition of the physician work force to meet the demands of health care reform. *New England Journal of Medicine* 329, no. 24: 1810–1812.

Cohen, J.J. 2006. The role and contribution of IMGs: A US perspective. *Academic Medicine* 81, no. 12 (suppl): S17–S21.

Cooper, R.A. 1994. Seeking a balanced physician workforce for the 21st century. *Journal of the American Medical Association* 272, no. 9: 680–687.

Cooper, R.A. et al. 1998. Current and projected workforce of nonphysician clinicians. *Journal of the American Medical Association* 280, no. 9: 788–794.

Council on Education for Public Health (CEPH). 2011. *ASPH graduate training programs.* Available at: http://www.asph.org/document.cfm?page=752. Accessed January 2011.

Crandall, L.A. et al. 1990. Recruitment and retention of rural physicians: Issues from the 1990s. *Journal of Rural Health* 6, no. 1: 19–38.

Eisenberg, J.M. 1985. Physician utilization: The state of research about physician's practice patterns. *Medical Care* 23, no. 5: 461–483.

Endicott, K.M. 1976. Health and health manpower. In: *Health in America: 1776–1976*. Health Resources Administration, US Public Health Service. DHEW Pub. No. 76616. Washington, DC: US Department of Health, Education, and Welfare: pp. 138–165.

Escarce, J.J. 1992. Explaining the association between surgeon supply and utilization. *Inquiry* 29, no. 4: 403–415.

Field, M.J., and K.N. Lohr. 1992. *Guidelines for clinical practice. Institute of Medicine*. Washington, DC: National Academy Press.

Fizgerald, M.A. et al. 1995. The midlevel provider: Colleague or competitor? *Patient Care* 29, no. 1: 20.

Freed D.H. 2004. Hospitalists: Evolution, evidence, and eventualities. *The Health Care Manager* 23, no. 3: 238–256.

Friedenberg, R.M. 1996. Future physician requirements: Generalists and specialists, shortage or surplus. *Radiology* 200, no. 1: 45A–47A.

Garber, A.M. 2005. Evidence-based guidelines as a foundation for performance incentives. *Health Affairs* 24, no.1: 174–179.

Garrard, J.L. et al. 1990. Impact of geriatric nurse practitioners on nursing home residents' functional status, satisfaction, and discharge outcome. *Medical Care* 28, no. 3: 271–283.

Gastel, B. 2006. Concurrent sessions: Exploring issues relating to international medical graduates. *Academic Medicine* 81, no. 12 (suppl): S63–S68.

General Accounting Office. 2003. *Physician workforce: Physician supply increased in metropolitan and nonmetropolitan areas but geographic disparities persisted*. Available at: http://www.gao.gov/new.items/d04124.pdf. Accessed October 2010.

Ginzberg, E. 1994. Improving health care for the poor. *Journal of the American Medical Association* 271, no. 6: 464–467.

Ginzberg, E., and A.L. Dutka. 1989. *The financing of biomedical research*. Baltimore, MD: Johns Hopkins University.

Greenfield, S. et al. 1992. Variation in resource utilization among medical specialties and systems of care. *Journal of the American Medical Association* 267, no. 12: 1624–1630.

Grossman, D. 1995. APNs: Pioneers in patient care. *American Journal of Nursing* 95, no. 8: 54–56.

Health Resources and Services Administration (HRSA). 1996. Council on Graduate Medical Education: *Patient care supply and requirements: Testing CHGME recommendations*. 8th report to Congress and the Health and Human Services Secretary. Rockville, MD: Health Resources and Services Administration.

Health Resources and Services Administration, Bureau of Health Professions HRSA/BHP). 2006. *Physician supply and demand: Projections to 2020*. Available at: ftp://ftp.hrsa.gov/bhpr/workforce/PhysicianForecastingPaperfinal.pdf. Accessed January 2007.

Helper, C., and L. Strand. 1990. Opportunities and responsibilities in pharmaceutical care. *American Journal of Hospital Pharmacy* 47, no. 3: 533–543.

Hibbard, H., and P.A. Nutting. 1991. Research in primary care: A national priority. In: *AHCPR conference proceedings: Primary care research: Theory and methods*. M.L. Grady, ed. Washington, DC: Department of Health and Human Services. pp. 1–4.

Hooker, R.S. 2006. Physician assistants and nurse practitioners: The US experience. *Medical Journal of Australia* 185, no. 1: 4–7.

Hooker, R.S., and L.E. Berlin. 2002. Trends in the supply of physician assistants and nurse practitioners in the United States. *Health Affairs* 21, no. 5: 174–181.

Hooker, R.S., and L.F. McCaig. 2001. Use of physician assistants and nurse practitioners in primary care, 1995–1999. *Health Affairs* 20, no. 4: 231–238.

Institute of Medicine. 1985. *Preventing low birthweight: Summary.* Washington, DC: National Academy Press.

Institute of Medicine. 1989. *Primary care physicians: Financing their GME in ambulatory settings.* Washington, DC: National Academy Press.

Kahn, N.B. et al. 1994. AAFP constructs definitions related to primary care. *American Family Physician* 50, no. 6: 1211–1215.

Kindig, D., and G. Yan. 1993. Physician supply in rural areas with large minority populations. *Health Affairs* 12, no. 2: 177–184.

Koehn, N.N. et al. 2002. The increase in international medical graduates in family practice residency programs. *Family Medicine* 34, no. 6: 429–435.

Kohler, P.O. 1994. Specialists/primary care professionals: Striking a balance. *Inquiry* 31, no. 3: 289–295.

Kramon, G. 1991. Medical second-guessing—In advance. *New York Times.* February 24: 12.

Lurie, N. et al. 1986. Termination of medical benefits: A follow-up study one year later. *New England Journal of Medicine* 314, no. 9: 1266–1268.

Martin, A. et al. 2010. Recession contributes to slowest annual rate of increase in health spending in five decades. *Health Affairs* 30, no. 1: 11–22.

Morley, P., and L. Strand. 1989. Critical reflections of therapeutic drug monitoring. *Journal of Clinical Pharmacy* 2, no. 3: 327–334.

Mullan, F. 1999. The muscular Samaritan: The National Health Service Corps in the new century. *Health Affairs* 18, no. 2: 168–175.

Office of Technology Assessment. 1986. *Nurse practitioners, physician assistants, and certified nurse midwives: A policy analysis.* Health technology case study 37. Washington, DC: US Government Printing Office.

Office of Technology Assessment. 1991. *Health care in rural America. OTA-H-434.* Washington, DC: US Government Printing Office.

Ostwald, S.K., and O.C. Abanobi. 1986. Nurse practitioners in a crowded marketplace: 1965–1985. *Journal of Community Health Nursing* 3, no. 3: 145–156.

Pew Health Professions Commission. 1993. *Health professions education for the future: Schools in service to the nation.* San Francisco, CA: Pew Health Professions Commission.

Phillips, R.L. et al. 2005. COGME's 16th report to Congress: Too many physicians could be worse than wasted. *Annals of Family Medicine* 3, no. 3: 268–270.

Pugno, P.A. et al. 2001. Results of the 2001 national resident matching program: Family practice. *Family Medicine* 33, no. 8: 594–601.

Redhead, C.S., and E.D. Williams. 2010. *Public health, workforce, quality, and related provisions in PPACA: Summary and timeline.* Congressional Research Service.

Rich, E.C. et al. 1994. Preparing generalist physicians: The organizational and policy context. *Journal of General Internal Medicine* 9 (suppl 1): S115–S122.

Rosenbaum, S. 1995. *The Children's Defense Fund's adolescent pregnancy prevention/prenatal care campaign.* Washington, DC: The Children's Defense Fund.

Rosenblatt, R.A. 1992. Specialists or generalists: On whom should we base the American health care system? *Journal of the American Medical Association* 267, no. 12: 1665–1666.

Rosenblatt, R.A., and D.M. Lishner. 1991. Surplus or shortage? Unraveling the physician supply conundrum. *Western Journal of Medicine* 154, no. 1: 43–50.

Rosenblatt, R.A. et al. 1997. Interspecialty differences in the obstetric care of low-risk women. *American Journal of Public Health* 87, no. 3: 344–351.

Samuels, M.E., and L. Shi. 1993. *Physician recruitment and retention: A guide for rural medical group practice.* Englewood, CO: Medical Group Management Press.

Schneller, E.S. 2006. The hospitalist movement in the United States: Agency and common agency issues. *Health Care Management Review* 31, no. 4: 308–316.

Schroeder, S., and L.G. Sandy. 1993. Specialty distribution of U.S. physicians: The invisible driver of health care costs. *New England Journal of Medicine* 328, no. 13: 961–963.

Schroeder, S.A. 1992. Physician supply and the U.S. medical marketplace. *Health Affairs* 11, no. 1: 235–243.

Schwartz, M. 1994. Creating pharmacy's future. *American Pharmacy* NS34: 44–45, 59.

Sehgal, N.J., and R.M. Wachter. 2006. The expanding role of hospitalists in the United States. *Swiss Medical Weekly* 136: 591–596.

Sellards, S., and M.E. Mills. 1995. Administrative issues for use of nurse practitioners. *Journal of Nursing Administration* 25, no. 5: 64–70.

Shi, L. 1992. The relation between primary care and life chances. *Journal of Health Care for the Poor and Underserved* 3, no. 2: 321–335.

Shi, L. 1994. Primary care, specialty care, and life chances. *International Journal of Health Services* 24, no. 3: 431–458.

Singh, D.A. et al. 1996. A comparison of academic curricula in the MPH and the MHA-type degrees in health administration at the accredited schools of public health. *The Journal of Health Administration Education* 14, no. 4: 401–414.

Singh, D.A. et al. 1997. How well trained are nursing home administrators? *Hospital and Health Services Administration* 42, no. 1: 101–115.

Stanfield, P.S. et al. 2009. *Introduction to the health professions.* 2nd ed. Boston: Jones & Bartlett Publishers.

Starfield, B. 1992. *Primary care: Concepts, evaluation, and policy.* New York: Oxford University Press.

Starfield, B., and L. Simpson. 1993. Primary care as part of US health services reform. *Journal of the American Medical Association* 269, no. 24: 3136–3139.

Starr, P. 1982. *The social transformation of American medicine: The rise of a sovereign profession and the making of a vast industry.* New York: Basic Books.

Strand, L.R. et al. 1991. Levels of pharmaceutical care: A needs-based approach. *American Journal of Hospital Pharmacy* 48, no. 3: 547–550.

US Bureau of Labor Statistics. 2007. *Occupational outlook handbook, 2006–2007.* Available at: http://www.bls.gov/oco/home.htm. Accessed January 2007.

US Bureau of Labor Statistics. 2009. *Occupational employment and wages.* Available at: www.bls .gov/oes/2009/may/figure1.pdf. Accessed December 2010.

US Bureau of Labor Statistics. 2010. *Occupational employment and wages – May 2009.* Available at: http://www.bls.gov/news,release/pdf/ocwage.pdf. Accessed November 2010.

US Bureau of Labor Statistics. 2011. *Occupational outlook handbook, 2010–11.* Available at: http:// www.bls.gov/oco/home.htm. Accessed January 2011.

US Census Bureau. 2010. *Statistical abstract of the United States, 2011.* Washington, DC: US Census Bureau.

Verby, J.E. et al. 1991. Changing the medical school curriculum to improve patient access to primary care. *Journal of the American Medical Association* 266, no. 1: 110–113.

Wachter, R.M. 2004. Hospitalists in the United States—Mission accomplished or work in progress? *New England Journal of Medicine* 350, no. 19: 1935–1936.

Wagner, M. 1991. Maternal and child health services in the United States. *Journal of Public Health Policy* 12, no. 4: 443–449.

Weiner, J.P. 1993. The demand for physician services in a changing health care system: A synthesis. *Medical Care Review* 50, no. 4: 411–449.

Wennberg, J.E. et al. 1993. Finding equilibrium in U.S. physician supply. *Health Affairs* 12, no. 2: 89–103.

Williams, S.J. 1994. Ambulatory health care services. In: *Introduction to health services.* 4th ed. S.J. Williams and P.R. Torrens, eds. Albany, NY: Delmar Publishers. pp. 108–133.

# Chapter 5

---

# Medical Technology

## Learning Objectives

- To understand the meaning and role of medical technology in health care delivery
- To appreciate the growing role of information technology and informatics in the delivery of health care
- To survey the factors influencing the creation, dissemination, and utilization of technology
- To discuss the government's role in technology diffusion
- To examine the impact of technology on various aspects of domestic and global delivery of health care
- To study the various facets of technology assessment
- To discuss the current and future directions in health technology assessment
- To become familiar with provisions in the Patient Protection and Affordable Care Act of 2010 that pertain to medical technology

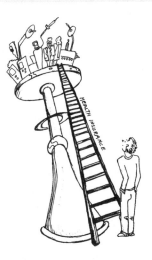

*"This must be high technology."*

# Introduction

Drake and colleagues (1993) labeled technology as "the boon and bane of medicine." In one respect, medical technology has been a great blessing to modern civilization. Sophisticated diagnostic procedures have reduced complications and disability, new medical cures have increased longevity, and new drugs have helped stabilize chronic conditions. However, most new technology comes at a price that society must ultimately pay. A tremendous amount of costly research is necessary to produce most modern breakthroughs. Once technology is developed and put into use, even more costs are generated through staff training, increased need for skilled professionals, facility upgrading, and demand from both consumers and providers for the utilization of new technology. As total health care spending continues to rise, debates have emerged as to whether unrestrained development and use of new technology is worth the cost.

Chapter 3 pointed out that developments in science and technology were instrumental in drastically changing the nature of health care delivery during the postindustrial era. Since then, the ever-increasing proliferation of new technology has continued to profoundly alter many facets of health care delivery. Technology has triggered several main changes: (1) Technology has raised consumer expectations that the latest may also be the best. These expectations have led to increased demand and utilization of new technology once it becomes available. (2) Technology has changed the organization of medical services. Specialized services that previously could be offered only in hospitals are now available in outpatient settings. (3) Technology has driven the scope and content of medical training and the practice of medicine, fueling specialization in medicine. (4) Technology has influenced the way status is imputed to various medical workers. Specialization is held in higher regard than primary care and public health. (5) Technology has contributed to health care cost inflation. From the consumer's standpoint, the cost of excessive treatment is no concern as long as a third party—either an insurance plan or the government—pays for it. (6) Technology assessment is becoming a growing activity because new drugs, devices, and procedures are not always useful or safe. Their effectiveness and potential negative consequences must be evaluated using scientific methods. (7) Technology has raised complex social and ethical concerns that defy straightforward solutions. Perplexing social and ethical controversies raised by modern innovations and promises of "miracle cures" include such questions as Who should be subjected to the experimental evaluations of technological breakthroughs to determine their safety? Who should and who should not receive high-tech interventions? To what extent should life-supporting procedures be continued? Is it moral to use human embryos in biomedical research?

The phenomenon of economic globalization has also enveloped biomedical knowledge and technology. In both developed and developing nations, physicians have access to the same scientific knowledge through medical journals and the Internet. Most drugs and medical devices available in the United States are also available in almost all parts of the world. However, depending on the extent of supply-side rationing (see Chapter 2), the timing of adoption and subsequent diffusion of new technology often differ widely from one country to another. Thus, even in developed nations, people do not necessarily have adequate access to the latest high-tech therapies. Conversely, in almost all parts of the world, people who possess adequate means can gain access to the latest and best in medicine regardless of the type of health care delivery system in their country.

From an economic standpoint, technology includes all inputs, both human and nonhuman, used in the production and management of medical goods and services (Warner 1982). This chapter discusses technology and related issues within this broad context. Highlights from the American Recovery and Reinvestment Act of 2009 and the Patient Protection and Affordability Act of 2010 are also incorporated.

## What Is Medical Technology?

At a fundamental level, *medical technology* is the practical application of the scientific body of knowledge for the purpose of improving health and creating efficiencies in the delivery of health care. Medical science benefited from rapid developments in other applied sciences, such as chemistry, physics, engineering, and pharmacology. For example, advances in organic chemistry made it possible to identify and extract the active ingredients in plants to produce drugs and anesthetics, which then became available in purer forms that were better adapted to controlled dosages than their earlier botanical forms. Developments in electrical and mechanical engineering led to such medical advances as radiology, cardiology, and encephalography (Bronzino et al. 1990). Magnetic resonance imaging (MRI), a technology that had its origins in basic research on the structure of the atom, was later transformed into a major diagnostic tool (Gelijns

and Rosenberg 1994). The disciplines of computer science and communication systems find their application in information technology and telemedicine (Tan 1995).

A broad concept of technology includes not just sophisticated machines and ultramodern facilities but also pharmaceuticals and biologicals, medical and surgical procedures used in rendering medical care, organizational support systems through which care is delivered (Riley and Brehm 1989), and the use of computer-supported information systems. For example, computers used to facilitate billing and other systems used to operate and manage health services organizations are part of health care technology (Rakich et al. 1992). Table 5–1 shows some of the main categories of medical technologies.

## Information Technology and Informatics

*Information technology* (IT) deals with the transformation of data into useful information. IT involves determining data needs, gathering appropriate data, storing and analyzing the data, and reporting the information generated in a user-friendly format. Different types of information are made available for specific uses by health care professionals, managers, payers, and patients. Today, many health care organizations have IT departments and managers to handle the continually increasing flow of information (Tan 1995). IT departments play a critical role in decisions to adopt new information technologies that improve health care delivery and organizational efficiency. These technologies include medical records systems to collect, transcribe, and store clinical data; radiology and clinical laboratory reporting systems; pharmacy

• • • • • • • • • • • • • • • • • • • • • • • • • • • • • • •

Table 5–1  Types of Medical Technologies

| Type | Examples |
| --- | --- |
| Diagnostic | CAT scanner |
| | Fetal monitor |
| | Computerized electrocardiography |
| | Automated clinical laboratories |
| | Magnetic resonance imaging |
| | Ambulatory blood pressure monitor |
| Survival (life saving) | Intensive care unit (ICU) |
| | Cardiopulmonary resuscitation (CPR) |
| | Bone marrow transplant |
| | Liver transplant |
| | Autologous bone marrow transplant |
| Illness management | Renal dialysis |
| | Pacemaker |
| | PTCA (angioplasty) |
| | Stereotactic cingulotomy |
| | (pyschosurgery) |
| Cure | Hip joint replacement |
| | Organ transplant |
| | Lithotripter |
| Prevention | Implantable automatic |
| | cardioverter defibrillator |
| | Pediatric orthopaedic repair |
| | Diet control for phenylketonuria |
| | Vaccines for immunization |
| System management | Medical information systems |
| | Telemedicine |
| Facilities and clinical settings | Hospital satellite centers |
| | Clinical laboratories |
| | Subacute care units |
| | Modern home health |
| Organizational delivery structure | Managed care |
| | Integrated delivery networks |

*Sources:* Adapted from Rosenthal, G. *Anticipating the costs and benefits of new technology: A typology for policy. Medical technology: The culprit behind health care costs?* Washington, DC: Department of Health and Human Services, 1979.

• • • • • • • • • • • • • • • • • • • • • • • • • • • • • • •

data systems to monitor medication use and avoid errors, adverse reactions, and drug interactions; scheduling systems for patients, space (such as surgery suites), and personnel; and financial systems for billing and collections, materials management, and many other aspects of organizational management (Cohen 2004a).

In health care organizations, IT applications fall into three general categories (Austin 1992):

1. *Clinical information systems* involve the organized processing, storage, and retrieval of information to support patient care delivery. Electronic medical records, for example, provide quick and reliable information necessary to guide clinical decision making and produce timely reports on quality of care delivered. Computerized physician order entry (CPOE) enables physicians to electronically transmit orders from a patient's bedside. The system's design increases efficiency and reduces medical errors. However, because of high costs, only about 5% of hospitals use this technology (Jha et al. 2006).

2. *Administrative information systems* assist in carrying out financial and administrative support activities, such as payroll, patient accounting, billing, materials management, budgeting and cost control, and office automation. For medical clinics, CPOE technology can interface with the billing system to minimize rejected claims by pinpointing errors in billing codes. Administrative information systems are also increasingly used in predictive modeling

applications that use health care claims data to identify patients who are likely to generate significant health care costs and, therefore, would benefit from newer utilization management programs, such as case management (see Chapter 9; Short et al. 2003).

3. *Decision support systems* provide information and analytical tools to support managerial decision making. Such tools are used to forecast patient volume, project staffing requirements, and schedule patients to optimize utilization of patient care and surgical facilities.

Managers, boards of directors, and medical staff increasingly depend on information systems for timely management data in several areas: financial performance, utilization of services, clinical quality, and trends in health care delivery. They use such information for cost control and productivity enhancement, strategic planning, utilization analysis and demand assessment, program planning and evaluation, simplification of external reporting, clinical research, and quality assessment and improvement (Austin 1992).

The field of *health informatics* is broadly defined as the application of information science to improve the efficiency, accuracy, and reliability of health care services. Health informatics requires the use of IT but goes beyond IT by emphasizing the improvement of health care delivery. For example, the use of IT is necessary for designing clinical decision support systems for practitioners, such as those used to improve decision making in cancer treatment. Health informatics is a wide and growing field, which includes, for example, nursing informatics, imaging

informatics, consumer health informatics, public health informatics, clinical research informatics, bioinformatics, and pharmacy informatics. Applications of informatics are also found in electronic health records and telemedicine.

## Electronic Health Records and Systems

*Electronic health records* (EHRs) are IT applications that enable the processing of any electronically stored information pertaining to individual patients for the purpose of delivering health care services (Murphy et al. 1999). EHRs replace the traditional paper medical records, which include a patient's demographic information, problems and diagnoses, plan of care, progress notes, medications, vital signs, past medical history, immunizations, laboratory data, and radiology reports. Information contained in EHRs is used to coordinate care, routinely measure quality, or reduce medical errors, which paper medical records do not allow (Hillestad et al. 2005).

EHR systems make it possible to access individual records online from many separate, interoperable automated systems within an electronic network. Since the overwhelming majority of Americans receive care from more than one caregiver, interoperability makes a patient's medical records portable and available to the different clinicians (Brailer 2005). For example, interoperability makes it possible to share EHRs among physicians, pharmacists, and hospitals. More important, however, EHR systems integrate individual records with evidence-based clinical decision support, which provides reminders and best-practice guidelines for treatment (Hillestad et al. 2005). The system can also interface with quality management and outcomes reporting. According to the Institute of Medicine (2003), a fully developed EHR system includes four key components: (1) collection and storage of health information on individual patients over time, where health information is defined as information pertaining to the health of an individual or health care provided to an individual; (2) immediate electronic access to person and population level information by authorized users; (3) provision of knowledge and decision support that enhances the quality, safety, and efficiency of patient care; and (4) support of efficient processes for health care delivery.

It is generally believed that widespread adoption of EHR systems will lead to major savings in health care costs, reduced medical errors, and improved health (Hillestad et al. 2005). However, the adoption of EHRs has been slow, particularly among physicians. In 2007, only 35% of office-based physicians reported using any EHR system although this represented an increase of 91% since 2001 (Hing and Hsiao 2010). Research suggests that among physicians, overall satisfaction with EHRs after implementation tends to be significantly lower than their preimplementation expectations (Vishwanath et al. 2010). EHR systems require a sizable investment to purchase and implement the technology, which is one major hurdle that many smaller organizations face. For example, group practices with 50 or more physicians are more likely to use EHR technology (Reed and Grossman 2004). Initial acquisition and set-up costs range between $37,000 and $64,000 per physician or nurse practitioner, and annual operating costs average $8,400 per physician or nurse practitioner; however, improved billing and decreased personnel costs do result in savings that can help recoup the investment in less than 3 years (Miller et al. 2005).

To accelerate the adoption of EHRs, some major policy initiatives were launched during the George W. Bush Administration. These initiatives culminated in the enactment of the Health Information Technology Economic and Clinical Health (HITECH) Act, which was part of the American Recovery and Reinvestment Act of 2009—the $787 billion plan to stimulate the economy—passed shortly after the Obama administration took office. This Act earmarked an estimated $19 billion in direct grants and financial incentives to promote the adoption of EHRs. Starting in 2011, Medicare and Medicaid offer financial incentives, over multiple years, of up to $40,000 to $65,000 per physician and up to $11 million per hospital for "meaningful use" of health information technology (Steinbrook 2009a). To demonstrate "meaningful use," health care providers have to meet a range of metrics in areas such as quality, safety, efficiency, reduction of health disparities, patient engagement, care coordination, and security of health information (Halamka 2010). The law also authorized federal dollars to establish Regional Extension Centers to provide technical assistance to primary care providers, health centers, and others to achieve meaningful use. Also envisioned in the law is a Health Information Technology Research Center to conduct research and analysis and disseminate best practices for EHR use (Hogan and Kissam 2010).

In the minds of many providers and patients alike, confidentiality of patient information has been a major concern. The Health Insurance Portability and Accountability Act (HIPAA) of 1996 made it illegal to gain access to personal health information (PHI) for reasons other than health care delivery, operations, and reimbursement. HIPAA legislation mandated strict controls on the transfer of personally identifiable health data between two entities, provisions for disclosure of protected information, and criminal penalties for violation (Clayton 2001).

## The Internet, E-Health, M-Health, and E-Therapy

The Internet has continued to revolutionize certain aspects of health care delivery, and its use will continue to grow. Use of the Internet to obtain health care information is becoming increasingly common. In one consumer survey, 65% of respondents indicated that, before making a decision about their health, they try to find everything they can about the issue (Schur and Berk 2008). Consequently, patients are becoming active participants in their own health care. In many instances, using the right source can provide valid and up-to-date information to both consumers and practitioners. Information empowers patients, which leads to changes in the traditional patient–physician dynamics.

There appears to be a significant difference in the extent of Internet use and reliance on it for health information based on whether users are satisfied or dissatisfied with the care they receive from their physicians. Those satisfied with care tend to rely more on their physician than on the Internet, using the physician as the primary source of health information. Conversely, dissatisfied patients turn to the Internet as their primary source of information, regarding it as a more credible and more authoritative information source than their physicians. Dissatisfied patients may also be less likely to comply with treatments prescribed by their physicians (Tustin 2010).

A number of websites also offer physician consultations, and others sell prescription medications. Patients are also forming online communities to help themselves through e-mail discussion groups and bulletin boards. Patients are interacting with their health care providers through secured specialty websites that cover disease management, personal health records, self-monitoring, and communication (Maheu et al. 2001).

"*E-health* refers to all forms of electronic health care delivered over the Internet, ranging from informational, educational, and commercial 'products' to direct services offered by professionals, nonprofessionals, businesses, or consumers themselves" (Maheu et al. 2001). The proliferation of mobile phones in both developed and developing nations has led to innovative applications of mobile technology. The term mobile health, or *m-health*, has emerged to refer to "the use of wireless communication devices to support public health and clinical practice" (Kahn et al. 2010). These devices facilitate communication among researchers, clinicians, and patients. Yet, evidence for the value of m-health remains scarce, especially for the developing world (Kahn et al. 2010).

E-therapy has emerged as an alternative to face-to-face therapy for behavioral health support and counseling (Skinner and Latchford 2006). Also referred to as online therapy, e-counseling, teletherapy, or cyber-counseling, *e-therapy* refers to any type of professional therapeutic interaction that makes use of the Internet to connect qualified mental health professionals and their clients (Rochlen et al. 2004). Although, at this point, e-therapy is not widely used, many Internet mental health interventions have reported early results that are promising.

Both therapist-led and self-directed online therapies indicate significant alleviation of disorder-related symptomatology (Ybarra and Eaton 2005). Nevertheless, e-therapy remains controversial. Issues and problems potentially best suited for online therapy include personal growth and fulfillment; adult children of alcoholics; anxiety disorders, including agoraphobia and social phobias; and body image and shame/guilt issues. Clients not appropriate for online therapy include those who have suicidal ideation, thought disorders, borderline personality disorder, or unmonitored medical issues (Stofle 2001).

The Internet is also used to register patients, direct them to alternative care sites, and order pharmaceuticals and other products. Using Web-based access to patient information from their homes or from hospital lounges, physicians can get a head start on their hospital rounds (Morrissey 2002). Another emerging application is *virtual physician visits*, which are online clinical encounters between a patient and physician. OptumHealth, a division of United Health Group, the nation's largest insurer, plans to offer NowClinic, a service that connects patients and doctors using video chat. The program is being introduced state by state, starting with Texas, but not without resistance from state medical associations (Miller 2009).

## Telemedicine and Telehealth

The terms "telemedicine" and "telehealth" are often used interchangeably. Both employ telecommunication systems for the purpose of promoting health, but there is a technical difference between the two. *Telemedicine*, or distance medicine, employs the use of telecommunications technology for medical diagnosis and patient care when the provider and client are separated by distance. It eliminates the requirement for face-to-face contact between the examining physician and the patient. It also enables a generalist to consult a specialist when a patient's illness and diagnosis are complex. The term *telehealth* is broader in scope. It encompasses telemedicine, as traditionally known, and educational, research, and administrative uses, as well as clinical applications that involve a variety of caregivers, such as physicians, nurses, psychologists, and pharmacists (Field and Grigsby 2002).

Telemedicine can be synchronous or asynchronous. *Synchronous technology* allows telecommunication to occur in real time. For example, interactive videoconferencing allows two or more professionals to see and hear each other and even share documents in real time. The technology allows a specialist located at a distance to directly interview and examine a patient. *Asynchronous technology* employs store-and-forward technology that allows users to review the information later. It allows greater flexibility because it does not depend on the simultaneous presence of parties at the sending and receiving ends (Maheu et al. 2001). Examples of telemedicine services include teleradiology, the transmission of radiographic images and scans; telepathology, the viewing of tissue specimens via videomicroscopy; telesurgery, controlling robots from a distance to perform surgical procedures; and clinical consultation provided by a wide range of specialists.

Telemedicine and telehealth have found many actual and potential uses. The adoption of these technologies has been slow, but their use is growing. Newer applications are in the delivery of mental health services and telemonitoring patients receiving home health care. Vital signs, blood pressure, and blood glucose levels can be monitored remotely, using video technology, which has been shown to be effective, well received by patients, and capable of maintaining quality of care and to have the potential for cost savings (Johnston et al. 2000). The Veterans Health Administration has demonstrated the effectiveness of telehealth in the delivery of psychotherapy and mental health care for other psychiatric conditions, such as obsessive-compulsive disorder, panic disorder, and anger management (Gros et al. 2010). Rural populations, in particular, face various types of barriers in access to quality health care. Barriers, such as shortage of providers, long travel distances, physical and social isolation, and weather-related difficulties can be overcome with appropriate telehealth services.

The largest barrier to telemedicine adoption is the lack of a reimbursement model, according to a survey of 75 health care executives (Smith 2010). Also, the cost effectiveness of most telemedicine applications remains unsubstantiated. Conversely, diagnostic and consultative teleradiology is almost universally reimbursed and has been proven cost effective (Field and Grigsby 2002). The American Recovery and Reinvestment Act of 2009 provides funding for not only improving the IT infrastructure in health care institutions but also for implementing telehealth networks designed to serve patients in rural areas and to integrate telehealth into the delivery of home health care (Singh et al. 2010).

## Innovation, Diffusion, and Utilization of Medical Technology

In the context of medical technology, innovation is the creation of a product, technique, or service perceived to be new

by members of a society. The spread of technology into society once it is developed is referred to as *technology diffusion* (Luce 1993). Rapid diffusion of a technology occurs when the innovation is perceived to be of benefit that can be evaluated or measured, is compatible with the adopter's values and needs, and is covered through third-party payment. Once technology is acquired, its use is almost ensured. Hence, the diffusion and utilization of technology are closely intertwined. The desire to have state-of-the-art technology available and to use it despite its cost or established health benefit is called the *technological imperative.*

High-tech procedures are more readily available in the United States than in most other countries, and little is done to limit the expansion of new medical technology. Compared to most European hospitals, American hospitals perform a far greater number of catheterizations, angioplasties, and bypass heart surgeries. The United States also has more high-tech equipment, such as magnetic resonance imaging (MRI) and computed tomography (CT) scanners, available to its population than most countries (Kim et al. 2001). By contrast, almost all other nations have tried to limit, mainly through central planning, the diffusion and utilization of high-tech procedures to control medical costs. The British government, for instance, established the National Institute for Health and Clinical Excellence (NICE) in 1999 to decide whether the National Health Service should make select health technologies available (Milewa 2006). Thanks to central control, compared to the United States, Canada had 76% fewer MRI machines and performed 72% fewer coronary bypass procedures per 100,000 population; Great Britain also had 55% fewer MRIs and performed 82% fewer coronary bypass surgeries (Anderson and Hussey 2001). Only Japan and Switzerland were estimated to have more MRI machines per 100,000 population than the United States.

Even though the United States has made tremendous strides in medical innovation, corresponding innovations in the health care delivery system have lagged behind. Investments in information technology have particularly lagged behind (Institute of Medicine 2002). For example, smart cards—credit card-like devices with an embedded computer chip and memory are already in use in Europe for health care services. *Smart cards* hold personal medical information that can be accessed and updated at hospitals or physicians' offices (Ellis 2000). Mainly due to privacy concerns, the United States is behind in using this technology.

## Factors That Drive Innovation and Diffusion

The rate and pattern by which a technology diffuses is often governed by multiple forces (Cohen 2004b). For example, public and private financing for research and development (R&D) can promote or inhibit innovation; government regulations, such as the Food and Drug Administration (FDA) approval process, can promote or hinder the availability of new drugs and devices; marketing and promotion by the manufacturers can have an impact on the decisions of both providers and consumers about the adoption and use of technology.

Some of the main forces that have shaped the innovation, diffusion, and utilization of technology in the United States are:

- Cultural beliefs and values
- Medical specialization

- Financing and payment
- Competition
- Expenditures on research and development
- Supply-side controls
- Government policy

## Cultural Beliefs and Values

Studies have shown that, when technology becomes available for a particular indication, it is used at significantly different intensities in various countries and among regions within countries (Wennberg 1988). American beliefs and values have been instrumental in determining the nature of health care delivery in the United States (discussed in Chapter 2). Based on these beliefs and values, Americans have much higher expectations of what medical technology can do to cure illness than, for instance, Canadians and Germans. In an opinion survey, a significantly higher number of Americans (35%) than Germans (21%) indicated that it was absolutely essential for them to be able to get the most advanced tests, drugs, medical procedures, and equipment (Kim et al. 2001). In another survey, 91% of Americans indicated that their ability to get the most advanced tests, drugs, medical equipment, and procedures is very important to improving the quality of health care (Schur and Berk 2008). In a national telephone random poll, 58% of Americans indicated that increased funding for medical and health research is essential for their future health and economic prosperity, and 63% expressed their willingness to pay a modest amount in additional taxes to fund medical research (Research America 2006).

The primacy of technology can also be traced to the medical model that has dominated medical practice in the United States (see Chapter 2). American beliefs and values reinforce delivery of health care according to the medical model. Consequently, the emphasis on specialty care, rather than primary care and preventive services, raises the expectations of both physicians and patients for the use of all available technology. Similarly, cultural beliefs and values have influenced the training of health care providers, the financing of services, and the structure of medical care delivery in the United States. Each of these domains reflects the premium that US society places on high technology, and, consequently, the United States leads the world in the development of new technology.

## Medical Specialization

Evidence of the technological imperative is most apparent in acute care hospitals, especially those affiliated with medical schools, because they are the main centers for specialty residency training programs in which physicians are trained to use the latest medical advances. Broad exposure to technology early in training affects not only clinical preferences but also future professional behavior and practice patterns (Cohen 2004c). Both patients and practitioners also equate high-quality care with high-intensity care. Patient demand for direct access to specialists has grown in the United States, which reflects the population's insatiable appetite for high-technology medicine (Spann 2001). Specialty training and the inclination of specialists to use the technology they have been trained to use fuel the demand for new technology. Since medical specialization revolves around technology, an oversupply of specialists in the United States (discussed in Chapter 4) has compounded the rate of technology diffusion.

## Financing and Payment

Evidence from several countries suggests that fixed provider payments, such as salaried physicians, and strong limits on payments to hospitals, such as stringent use of global budgets, curtail the incentive to use high-tech procedures. Hence, payment incentives can place limitations on how quickly and widely new treatments are diffused into medical practice (McClellan and Kessler 1999).

Traditionally, the US health care delivery system has lacked internal checks and balances to determine when high-cost services are appropriate. Financing of health care through private insurance promotes the phenomenon referred to as moral hazard and provider-induced demand (introduced in Chapter 1). Insurance insulates both patients and providers from any personal accountability for the utilization of high-cost services. As long as out-of-pocket costs are of little concern, patients expect their physicians to provide all that medical science has to offer. Knowing that insurance covers the services demanded by their patients, providers also show little hesitation to provide the services.

There is likely a two-way relationship between technology diffusion and insurance coverage. Increasingly generous insurance coverage causes increases in spending for new products. Conversely, the development of beneficial but costly new technology puts pressure on insurers to cover those costs (Danzon and Pauly 2001).

The rate of innovation is sensitive to changes in the level of reimbursement set for new interventions. Under the Medicare prospective payment system (discussed in Chapter 6), a higher level of reimbursement than the cost of the procedure itself stimulated rapid adoption of percutaneous transluminal coronary angioplasty (PTCA) and a high degree of innovation in PTCA catheters. By contrast, only a fraction of the cost of cochlear implants was covered. The result was not only underdiffusion but also a markedly reduced subsequent investment in research and development by the manufacturers of cochlear implants (Gelijns and Rosenberg 1994).

## Competition

As pointed out in Chapter 1, the health care delivery system in the United States is not characterized by true market conditions in which competition is prompted by patients who shop around for the best *value*, that is, the most benefits possible for the price they are willing to pay. Providers of health care services do compete. Paradoxically, however, competition in health care often increases costs. Hospitals, as well as outpatient centers, compete to attract insured patients. Well-insured patients look for quality, and institutions create perceptions of higher quality by acquiring and advertising state-of-the-art technology. Specialists have also been responsible for stimulating competition. Many physicians, for example, have opened highly specialized hospitals, diagnostic imaging facilities stocked with next-generation scanners, and same-day surgery centers that have hotel-like facilities—these developments have fueled a de facto medical arms race. In response, hospitals are adding new service lines—such as cancer, heart, and brain centers—and are acquiring costly CT scanners and high-field MRI machines (Kher 2006). To recruit specialists, medical care centers often have to obtain new technology and offer high-tech procedures. When hospitals develop new services

and invest heavily in modernization programs, other hospitals in the area are often forced to do the same. Such practices result in a tremendous amount of duplication of services and equipment.

Investment interests by physicians in various types of facilities prompted Congress to pass regulations against *self-referrals*. These laws prohibit physicians from sending patients to facilities in which the referring physician or a family member has an ownership interest. The Ethics in Patient Referrals Act of 1989 (commonly known as Stark I after Representative Pete Stark, author of the original bill) prohibited the referral of Medicare patients to laboratories in which the referring physician had an ownership interest. Provisions of this law expanded under the Omnibus Budget Reconciliation Act of 1993 (OBRA-93). Commonly referred to as Stark II, the statute covers both Medicare and Medicaid referrals. It also expanded the categories of services to include clinical laboratory services; physical therapy, occupational therapy, and speech pathology services; radiology services, including MRI, computerized axial tomography (CAT) scans, and ultrasound services; radiation therapy services and supplies; durable medical equipment and supplies; prosthetics, orthotics, and prosthetic devices and supplies; home health services; outpatient prescription drugs; and inpatient and outpatient hospitalization services. There are some exceptions, however, such as in-office ancillary services (Wachler and Avery 2011).

## Expenditures on Research and Development

Innovation is driven by expenditures in research and development. Since the early

1980s, total expenditures in biomedical sciences have exceeded those in engineering and the physical sciences (US Census Bureau 1999). It is estimated that, in 2007, both government and private sources of funding for biomedical research in the United States amounted to $101.1 billion, or approximately 4.5% of the total health care expenditures. This actually represents a slowing of expenditures, after they had doubled (on an inflation-adjusted basis) between 1994 and 2003 (Dorsey et al. 2010). In 2007, private sources accounted for 62% of the funding; the remaining came from government sources. Between 2003 and 2007, the government's share of funding declined from 42.6 to 37.8%. Figure 5–1 illustrates the sources of funding in 2007.

The American Recovery and Reinvestment Act of 2009 allocated $10.4 billion in new funding to the National Institutes of Health (NIH). Of this amount, $8.2 billion (78.8%) is allocated to support research (Steinbrook 2009b). It is safe to assume that, compared to other countries, the United States spends the most on medical research.

## Supply-Side Controls

Americans resist supply-side controls. Most other countries employ supply-side rationing (discussed in Chapter 2), also referred to as central planning, to limit the diffusion of medical technology. It curtails costs, but it also restricts access to critically needed care. Canada, which restricts specialist services

Figure 5–1  Sources of Funding for Biomedical Research, 2007.

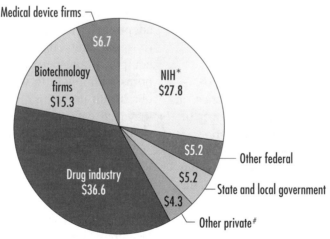

Medical device firms — $6.7

Biotechnology firms $15.3

NIH* $27.8

$5.2 — Other federal

$5.2 — State and local government

Drug industry $36.6

$4.3 — Other private#

**Amounts are in billions of dollars**
*National Institutes of Health
#Foundations, charities, and other private funds

*Source:* Data from Dorsey, E.R. et al. 2010. Funding of US biomedical research, 2003–2008. *Journal of the American Medical Association* 303, no. 2: 137–143.

and limits expensive medical equipment to control health care spending, is a case in point. According to a 2006 study by the Fraser Institute, Canadians have to wait, on average, 8.8 weeks to see a specialist and another 9.0 weeks to obtain specialty treatment. The same study also found that median waiting times across Canada were 4.3 weeks for a CT scan, 10.3 weeks for an MRI, and 3.8 weeks for an ultrasound (Esmail and Walker 2006). Access to care in Canada has actually been deteriorating. The total average waiting time for specialty care increased from 13.1 weeks in 1999 to 17.8 weeks in 2006. Because of unreasonable waits for non-emergency services, as many as 72% of Canadians expressed that they experience worry, stress, or anxiety, and one-half reported experiencing pain while waiting for specialized services (Statistics Canada 2004). Waiting lists for health care in Canada have even resulted in deaths, for example, due to delayed heart surgery (Tuffnell and Kirby 1994; Steinbrook 2006).

## Government Policy

Unlike most other developed countries, in the United States, direct controls over the innovation, diffusion, and utilization of technology through government policy have not been possible. Nevertheless, public policy does play a significant role in deciding which drugs and devices are made available to Americans. The US government is also one of the largest sources of funding for biomedical research. By controlling the amount of funding, public policy indirectly influences medical innovation. A more extensive discussion of the government's role is covered in the subsequent section, "The Government's Role in Technology Diffusion."

## Managed Care and Technology Diffusion

The growth of managed care has drawn considerable attention to the question of how managed care may have affected the services delivered to patients enrolled in these plans. An essential aspect of this question relates to the effects of managed care on the availability and use of medical technologies. Research literature that addresses the issue of managed care's impact on technology adoption is relatively small and generally supports the view that managed care has contributed to slowing the adoption of high-cost technologies (Baker 2002). For example, a study based on all 3,705 MRI sites across the United States provides some preliminary evidence that high levels of market penetration by health maintenance organizations (HMOs) were associated with reduced levels of availability and use of MRI (Baker and Wheeler 1998). In another study that examined the relationship between managed care penetration and the adoption of neonatal intensive care units (hospital units that organize a range of equipment and personnel to care for newborns with low birth weight and other serious health problems), it was observed that managed care did not affect the diffusion of the most advanced high-level units. A slower adoption of midlevel units, however, was observed (Baker and Phibbs 2002). The authors of this study concluded that health outcomes for seriously ill newborns are better in higher-level units and that slower growth of midlevel units could actually be beneficial due to a greater likelihood that seriously ill newborns would receive care in higher-level units.

Earlier, it was believed that not only managed care was slowing the rate of technology diffusion but that there could also potentially be harmful effects for patients. Extant literature, however, does not find any negative effects on patient care and outcomes because of slower rates of technology diffusion. Conversely, there was clear evidence that excessive technology use had occurred during the fee-for-service era before managed care (Brook 1989). Overuse of technology, in fact, needs to be curtailed because it not only wastes economic resources but can also result in adverse health outcomes. Limitations on the adoption and use of technology do not necessarily correlate with negative health status of a population, as evidence from other industrialized countries demonstrates. Despite the intensive use of high technology in the United States, Americans actually trail behind people in other industrialized nations on broad measures of health. The critical issue is not whether the use of technology is curtailed but whether its appropriate use is curtailed. The issue of appropriateness is discussed later in this chapter (see "The Assessment of Medical Technology").

# The Government's Role in Technology Diffusion

The growth of technology has been accompanied by issues of cost, safety, benefits, and risks. Federal legislation has primarily aimed at addressing these concerns. Acquisition of new technology and building construction programs (both construction of new facilities and expansion of existing facilities) used to be regulated under the certificate-of-need (CON) legislation but have more recently been left to the discipline of the marketplace. As previously indicated, the government is also an important source of funding for biomedical research.

## Regulation of Drugs and Devices

The FDA is an agency of the US Department of Health and Human Services (DHHS) that is responsible for ensuring that drugs and medical devices are safe and effective for their intended use. It also controls access to drugs by deciding whether a certain drug will be available by prescription only or as an over-the-counter purchase. The FDA may also stipulate standards on how certain over-the-counter products may be purchased and sold. For example, under the Patriot Act signed by President Bush in March 2006, certain cold and allergy medicines containing pseudoephedrine were required to be kept behind pharmacy counters and sold in only limited quantities to consumers, who must show identification and sign a logbook. This action was taken because pseudoephedrine is used in making methamphetamine—a highly addictive drug—in home laboratories.

The FDA's regulatory functions have evolved over time (Table 5–2). The first piece of drug legislation in the United States was the Food and Drugs Act of 1906. The purpose of the law was to prevent the manufacture, sale, or transportation of adulterated, misbranded, poisonous, or deleterious foods, drugs, medicines, and liquors (FDA 2009). It authorized the Bureau of Chemistry (predecessor of the FDA) to take action only after drugs had been marketed to consumers. It was assumed that the manufacturer would conduct safety tests before marketing the product. If innocent consumers were harmed, however, the Bureau of Chemistry could act only after such harm had been done (Bronzino et al. 1990). The drug law was strengthened by the passage of the Federal Food, Drug, and Cosmetic Act of 1938 (FD&C Act) in response to the infamous

Table 5–2  Summary of FDA Legislation

1906    Food and Drugs Act
        The FDA was authorized to take action only after drugs sold to consumers caused harm.

1938    Food, Drug, and Cosmetic Act
        Required premarket notification to the FDA so the agency could assess the safety of a new drug or device.

1962    Kefauver-Harris Amendments
        Premarket notification was inadequate. The FDA took charge of reviewing the efficacy and safety of new drugs, which could be marketed only once approval was granted.

1976    Medical Devices Amendments
        Authorized premarket review of medical devices, and classified devices into three classes.

1983    Orphan Drug Act
        Drug manufacturers were given incentives to produce new drugs for rare diseases.

1990    Safe Medical Devices Act
        Health care facilities must report serious or potentially serious device-related injuries, illness, or death of patients and/or employees.

1992    Prescription Drug User Fee Act
        The FDA received authority to collect application fees from drug companies to provide addition resources to shorten the drug approval process.

1997    Food and Drug Administration Modernization Act
        Provides for fast-track approvals for life-saving drugs when expected benefits exceed those of current therapies.

Elixir Sulfanilamide disaster, which caused almost 100 deaths in Tennessee due to poisoning from a toxic solvent used in the liquid preparation (Flannery 1986). According to the revised law, a new drug could not be marketed without first notifying the FDA and allowing the agency time to assess the drug's safety (Merrill 1994).

The drug approval system was further transformed by the drug amendments of 1962, after thalidomide (a sleeping pill that was distributed in the United States as an experimental drug but had been widely marketed in Europe) was shown to cause birth defects (Flannery 1986). The 1962 amendments (Kefauver-Harris Drug Amendments) essentially stated that premarket notification was inadequate. The amendments put a premarket approval system in force, giving the FDA authority to review the effectiveness and safety of a new drug before it could be marketed. Its consumer protection role enabled the FDA to prevent harm before it occurred. However, the drug approval process was criticized for slowing down the introduction of new drugs and, consequently, denying patients early benefit of the latest treatments. Drug manufacturers essentially "became prisoners of the agency's [FDA's] indecision, its preoccupation with other issues, or its lack of resources" (Merrill 1994).

The Orphan Drug Act of 1983 and subsequent amendments were passed to provide incentives for pharmaceutical firms to develop new drugs for rare diseases and conditions. Incentives, such as grant funding to defray the expenses of clinical testing and exclusive marketing rights for 7 years, were necessary because a relatively small number of people are afflicted by rare conditions, creating a relatively small market. As a result of the Orphan Drug Act, certain new drug therapies, called *orphan drugs*, have become available for conditions that affect fewer than 200,000 people in the United States.

In the late 1980s, pressure on the FDA from those wanting rapid access to new drugs for the treatment of the human immunodeficiency virus (HIV) infection called for a reconsideration of the drug review process (Rakich et al. 1992). For example, Saquinavir, a protease inhibitor indicated for patients with advanced HIV infection, received accelerated approval in late 1995; however, its manufacturer, Roche Laboratories, was required to, subsequently, show that the drug prolonged survival or slowed clinical progression of HIV.

In 1992, Congress passed the Prescription Drug User Fee Act, which authorized the FDA to collect fees from biotechnical and pharmaceutical companies to review their drug applications. The additional funds provided needed resources, and, according to the General Accounting Office (GAO), the fees allowed the FDA to make new drugs available more quickly. From 1993 to 2001, the median approval time for standard new drugs dropped from 21 months to approximately 14 months. In 2004, the approval time dropped even further to 12.9 months. Although critics allege that faster reviews have allowed unsafe drugs to be brought to market, studies have found no evidence to support such claims (Agres 2005).

In 1997, Congress passed the Food and Drug Administration Modernization Act. The law provides for increased patient access to experimental drugs and medical devices. It provides for "fast-track" approvals when the potential benefits of new drugs for serious or life-threatening conditions are considered significantly greater than those for current therapies. In 1997, the FDA approved Prandin and Rezulin for Type II diabetes, Evista for the prevention of osteoporosis, and Plavix for atherosclerosis—all within 7 months (Neumann and Sandberg 1998). In addition, the law provides for an expanded database on clinical trials, which is accessible to the public. Under a separate provision, when a manufacturer plans to discontinue a drug, patients who are heavily dependent on the drug receive advance notice.

The FDA first received jurisdiction over medical devices under the FD&C Act of 1938. However, such jurisdiction was confined to the sale of products believed to be unsafe or that made misleading claims of effectiveness (Merrill 1994). In the 1970s, several deaths and miscarriages were attributed to the Dalkon Shield, which had been marketed as a safe and effective contraceptive device (Flannery 1986). In 1976, the Medical Device Amendments extended the FDA's authority to include premarket review of medical devices divided into three classes. Devices in Class I are subject to general controls regarding misbranding, that is, fraudulent claims regarding the therapeutic effects of certain devices. Class II devices are subject to special requirements for labeling, performance standards, and postmarket surveillance. The most stringent requirements of premarket approval regarding safety and effectiveness apply to Class III devices that support life, prevent health impairment, or present an unreasonable risk of illness or injury. For most Class III devices, premarket approval is required to ensure their safety and effectiveness. The Safe Medical Devices Act of 1990 strengthened the FDA's hand in controlling entry of new products and in monitoring use of marketed products (Merrill 1994). Under this Act, health care facilities must report serious or potentially serious device-related injuries or illness of patients and/or employees to the manufacturer of the device and, if death is involved, to the FDA as well. In essence, the Act is intended to serve as an "early warning" system through which the FDA can obtain important information on device problems.

The Patient Protection and Affordable Care Act (ACA) of 2010 places some restrictions on the licensing of new biological products. If a product is shown to be biosimilar or interchangeable with an existing licensed biological product, referred to as a reference product, the FDA is not allowed to approve such a product until 12 years from the date on which the reference product was first approved.

## Certificate of Need

The National Health Planning and Resources Development Act of 1974 designated a regional network of health systems agencies (HSAs) for the planning and allocation of health resources, including technology. States were required to enact CON laws to obtain federal funds for planning functions under this Act. These activities were intended to influence the diffusion of technology by requiring hospitals to seek state approval before acquiring major equipment or embarking on new construction or modernization projects (Iglehart 1982). In 1986, the federal government terminated funding for HSAs. Although some states have abandoned CON requirements, approximately 36 states retain some control over planning and construction of new health care facilities (National Conference of State Legislatures 2011).

Various reasons have been cited to explain why the federal government relinquished support of health planning:

- The assumption that providing quality health care did not require extensive use of technology conflicted with societal expectations that all available technology should be used (Rakich et al. 1992).

- The CON emphasis on high-cost technologies was considered misdirected because high-volume utilization of low-cost technologies could also have a significant effect on health care costs (Rakich et al. 1992).

- The CON regulations fell victim to the shift away from regulatory controls over health care providers in favor of a competitive market approach to cost containment (Haglund and Dowling 1993). In fact, the CON regulations were blamed for unfair interference with the ability of hospitals to compete based on which services they could offer.

- As technology became increasingly portable, freestanding facilities could acquire the same technology that hospitals had been prohibited from acquiring. Because these freestanding facilities were not subject to CON review (Rakich et al. 1992), the state approval process was regarded as unfair toward hospitals.

As previously noted in this chapter, the proliferation of specialty hospitals and duplication of services have, perhaps, resulted in unnecessary and costly diffusion of technology. It has been noted that virtually all of the specialty hospitals that opened since 1990 are located in states that have minimal or no CON requirements (Zimmerman 2006).

## Research on Technology

The Agency for Healthcare Research and Quality (AHRQ) was established in 1989 under the Omnibus Budget Reconciliation Act of 1989 (Public Law 101–239) and was originally the Agency for Health Care Policy and Research. AHRQ, a division of the DHHS, is the lead federal agency charged with supporting research that focuses on improving the quality of health care, reducing health care cost, and improving access to essential services. For instance, the agency's Center for Outcomes and Evidence (formerly the Center for Outcomes and Effectiveness Research) conducts and supports studies of the outcomes and effectiveness of diagnostic, therapeutic, and preventive health services and procedures. The agency's technology assessments are available to medical practitioners, consumers, and other health care purchasers.

## Funding for Research

The federal government is a major provider of financial support for biomedical research. The NIH—a division of the DHHS—both conducts and supports basic and applied biomedical research in the United States. Funding through NIH provided much of the impetus for medical schools to undertake research in the medical subspecialties, which

led to the growth of specialty departments within academic medical centers (Rakich et al. 1992). These institutions have produced many specialists, which is reflected in the sustained imbalance between the number of general practitioners, compared to specialists.

## The Impact of Medical Technology

Health care technology involves the practical application of scientific discoveries in many disciplines. The deployment of scientific knowledge has had far-reaching and pervasive effects, as the various categories in Table 5–1 indicate. The effects of technology often overlap, making it difficult to pinpoint technology's impact on the delivery of health care.

## Impact on Quality of Care

When advanced techniques can provide more precise medical diagnoses than before, quicker and more complete cures than previously available, or reduce risks in a cost-effective manner, the result is improved quality. Technology can provide new remedies where none existed. Technology continuously offers more effective, less invasive, and safer therapeutic and preventive remedies. Increased longevity and decreased morbidity are often the outcomes.

Numerous examples illustrate the role of technology in enhancing the quality of care. Coronary angioplasty has become a common procedure for opening blocked or narrowed coronary arteries. More than a million people receive this treatment every year in the United States. Before this treatment became available, patients suffering a heart attack were prescribed prolonged bed rest and treated with morphine and nitroglycerin (CBO 2008). Angioplasty has reduced the need for open-heart bypass surgery. In 2005, the FDA approved the total artificial heart (TAH) for implantation in patients with end-stage heart failure. This device is a life saver for those awaiting heart transplantation. Implantable cardioverter defibrillators can save lives in people who have life-threatening irregular heartbeats.

Laser technology permits surgery with less trauma; it also shortens the period for postsurgical recovery. Laser applications are widely used in most medical specialties for both medical and cosmetic procedures. For example, advanced laser procedures are available for high-precision eye surgery. In the cosmetic arena, facial resurfacing, wrinkle removal, and many other treatments are performed using lasers, which deliver a specific wavelength of light to the area to be treated.

Robot-assisted surgeries have gained significant momentum in areas such as urology. For example, in the United States, more than 70% of all radical prostatectomies are performed using the da Vinci robot (Rassweiler et al. 2010). The robotic approach allows improved dexterity and precision of the instruments.

Advanced bioimaging methods have opened new ways to see the body's inner workings, while minimizing invasive procedures. Modern imaging technologies include MRI, positron emission tomography (PET), single-photon emission computed tomography (SPECT), computed tomography (CT), and fluorescence imaging. PET has important applications both for research and for clinical purposes in cardiology, neurology, and oncology. PET can show abnormal processes, such as those associated with cancers and metabolic dysfunction. It can spot tumors and other problems that may

not be detectable with traditional MRI or CT scans. SPECT is of great value in imaging the brain. SPECT imaging could also reduce inappropriate use of invasive procedures through a more accurate diagnosis of coronary artery disease (Shaw et al. 2000). Integrated PET/CT is increasingly becoming an established imaging technique in the management of many cancers (Devaraj et al. 2007).

Molecular and cell biology has opened a new era in clinical medicine. Screening for genetic disorders, gene therapy, and powerful new drugs for cancer and heart disease promise to radically improve the quality of medical care. Genetic research might even help overcome the critical shortage of transplantable organs. Certain farm animals have been successfully cloned, which holds the promise of transplanting animal organs into humans, technically referred to as *xenografting* (or xenotransplantation). On a parallel track, regenerative medicine and tissue engineering hold the promise of creating other biological and bioartificial substitutes that will restore and maintain normal function in a variety of diseased and injured tissues. Products such as bioartificial kidneys, artificial implantable livers, and insulin-producing cells to replace damaged pancreatic cells are examples of what biomedical science might be able to accomplish. Treatment of disease using stem cells that can be derived from discarded human embryos (human embryonic stem cells), fetal tissue, or adult sources (bone marrow, fat, or skin) is another example of regenerative medicine.

Amid all the enthusiasm emerging technologies might generate, some degree of caution must prevail. Experience shows that greater proliferation of technology may not necessarily equal higher quality. Unless the effect of each individual technology is appropriately assessed, some innovations may be wasteful and others may be harmful.

## Impact on Quality of Life

Thanks to new scientific developments, thousands of people are able to live normal lives, which otherwise would not be possible. People with disabling conditions have been able to overcome their limitations in speech, hearing, vision, and movement. Long-term maintenance therapies have enabled people suffering from conditions such as diabetes and end-stage renal disease to engage in activities that they otherwise would not be able to do. Major pharmaceutical breakthroughs enable people suffering from heart disease, cancer, acquired immune deficiency syndrome (AIDS), and preterm birth to have a much longer life expectancy and improved health (Kleinke 2001).

Modern technology has also been instrumental in relieving pain and suffering, and pain management is being recognized as a new subspecialty in medicine. For example, for cancer pain management, new opioids have been developed for transdermal, nasal, and nebulized administration, which allow needleless means of controlling pain (Davis 2006). Apart from new drugs, patient-controlled analgesia allows patients to determine when and how much medication they receive, which gives patients more independence and control. HIV/AIDS was recognized as a killer disease in the early 1980s, but modern treatments, such as protease inhibitors and nonnucleoside reverse transcriptase inhibitors (known as antiretroviral agents), have suppressed the disease's ability to proliferate and damage organs. Thanks to these treatments, HIV/AIDS has become a chronic disease, not a

death sentence (Komaroff 2005). Clinical trials have been under way to evaluate the effectiveness and safety of inhaled and oral administration of insulin for patients with Type II diabetes. A substitute for injectable insulin could greatly enhance the quality of life for diabetic patients, particularly the elderly, who require assistance with insulin injections.

## Impact on Health Care Costs

Technological innovations have been the single most important factor in medical cost inflation over the second half of the 20th century. They have accounted for about one-half of the total rise in real (after eliminating the effects of general inflation) health care spending during the past several decades (Institute of Medicine 2002; CBO 2008).

Technology in the health care field demonstrates a unique characteristic. In virtually all other industries, new technology has the effect of reducing labor force and production costs, and price considerations often play an important role in the adoption of new technologies. In health care, however, new technology has increased both labor and capital costs (Iglehart 1982). First, there is the cost of acquiring the new technology and equipment. Second, specially trained physicians and technicians are often needed to operate the equipment and to analyze the results, which often leads to increases in labor costs. Third, new technology may require special housing and setting requirements, resulting in facility costs (McGregor 1989).

Littell and Strongin (1996) argued that technology's purchase price itself has a minimal effect on system-wide health care costs. The total purchase price of medical products represents only a small fraction,

estimated to be a little over 5%, of total annual US health care expenditures. Costs associated with utilization of technology, once
it becomes available, may be more important
because a technology's clinical performance
is often evaluated on the basis of its effectiveness—no matter how small—and ease
of operation rather than on its cost reduction (Gelijns and Rosenberg 1994). For example, each additional MRI unit incurs approximately 733 additional MRI procedures
(Baker et al. 2008). Also, many of the most
notable medical advances in recent decades
involve ongoing treatments for the management of chronic conditions, such as diabetes
and coronary artery disease (CBO 2008).

Although it is true that many new technologies increase costs, some have been
found to reduce costs. For example, antiretroviral therapies have been largely credited
with the dramatic reduction in hospitalization of AIDS patients (Centers for Disease
Control and Prevention 1999). Thanks to
technology, the initially estimated cost burden of the AIDS epidemic has not materialized. Technology should also be credited for
an overall reduction in the average length of
inpatient hospital stays. Many services that
previously could be provided only in hospitals can now be delivered in less costly
home and outpatient settings without adversely affecting health outcomes. Whereas
many new technologies may increase labor
costs, some actually produce labor cost savings. For example, when Northwestern University Medical Center in Chicago automated its lab, it dropped the human handling
steps from 14 to 1.5, and the turnaround
time from 8 hours to 90 minutes. Largely
because of a significant drop in labor costs,
a saving of 30% was realized. Not only that,
but the error rate dropped to zero since the
system was installed (Flower 2006).

Instead of focusing solely on the excessive costs that new technologies may produce, increasing attention is being given to
the value or worth of the advances in medical care. In a groundbreaking study, Cutler
and colleagues (2006) addressed this issue
by examining how medical spending has
translated into additional years of life saved,
based on the assumption that 50% of the improvements in life expectancy have resulted
from medical care. These researchers concluded that the increases in medical spending in the 1960 to 2000 period, in terms of
increased life expectancy, have rendered
reasonable value for the money spent.
For example, for a 45-year-old American
who has a remaining life expectancy of
30 years, the value of remaining life is more
than $200,000 per year (Murphy and To-
pel 2003). For this 45-year-old person, the
average annual spending in health care for
each year of life gained was $53,700 (Cutler
et al. 2006).

## Impact on Access

Geography is an important factor in access to technology. If a technology is not
physically available to a patient population,
access is limited. Geographic access can
improve for many technologies by providing mobile equipment or by employing new
communications technologies to allow remote access to centralized equipment and
specialized personnel. For example, GPS
(global positioning system) technology
significantly improves emergency medical
services response time to the scene of motor vehicle crashes and other emergencies
(Gonzalez et al. 2009).

Mobile equipment can be transported
to rural and remote sites, making it accessible to those populations. Mobile cardiac

catheterization laboratories, for example, can provide high technology in rural settings. Such services not only provide needed health care to the community, but they also protect a patient base from migrating to tertiary referral centers (Lewis 1989). Access to specialized medical care for rural and other hard-to-reach populations has transformed through innovations in telemedicine, which eliminates the requirement for face-to-face contact between the examining physician and the patient.

## Impact on the Structure and Processes of Health Care Delivery

Modern technology has turned hospitals into capital-intensive institutions (Iglehart 1982). Large urban hospitals have been transformed into medical centers, where the latest diagnostic and therapeutic remedies are offered. Recent growth in alternative settings (home health and outpatient) has also been made possible primarily by technology. Financial pressures may have prompted the use of outpatient and home settings for health care delivery, but without technological innovations, extensive adaptations of modern treatments to these alternative sites may not have been possible. Lithotripsy (a noninvasive procedure for crushing kidney and bile stones by using shockwaves) and MRI have become increasingly available in outpatient settings. More patients, who would have required lengthy hospital stays, are now undergoing outpatient surgery. Extensive home health services have brought many hospital and nursing home services to the patient's home. Monitoring devices can permit cardiac implants to transmit vital information over telephone lines; respirators maintain breathing in the home; and kidney dialyzers are commonly used at home, as

is parenteral feeding—an intravenous technology used to provide full nutritional supplements to help feed patients who cannot swallow or digest food (Luce 1993).

Certain technologies adopted from other industries have improved health care delivery. For example, the bar-coding system has found several new applications in hospitals, including automation of drug dispensing, which drastically reduces medication errors. Scanning of information on nurses' badges, patients' wristbands, and drugs administered ensures that the right drug is given in the right dose to the right patient (Nicol and Huminski 2006). In some applications, radio frequency identification (RFID) has started to replace bar-coding technology in the areas of patient identification, equipment management, inventory control, and automatic supply and equipment billing (Roark and Miguel 2006).

Telecommunications technology used in telemedicine is also used for administrative teleconferencing and continuing medical education. For example, interactive compressed videoconferencing allows for an almost face-to-face meeting in which vendors can demonstrate new products or services and discuss their utilization, costs, and delivery schedules. Eliminating airfares, hotel expenses, and other travel-related costs can achieve significant savings. Interactive videoconferencing is also used for continuing education in the United States and abroad, with a high degree of satisfaction from participants. This technology is particularly helpful to rural health practitioners in overcoming barriers of distance to keep their knowledge and skills up to date (Klein et al. 2005). Recently, videoconferencing applications have been tried to provide language interpretation to translate physician orders and medication regimens for patients who have limited English proficiency (Hamblen 2006).

Managed care has been instrumental in transforming the way in which health services are delivered in the United States. Simpson (1994) observed that, without technology, managed care would not be possible because it is based on managing information and managing information requires technology. For example, information management is the backbone needed for monitoring cost effectiveness and quality and for tracking referrals to specialized services.

## Impact on Global Medical Practice

Technology developed in the United States has significantly impacted the practice of medicine worldwide. Many nations wait for the United States to develop new technologies, which can then be introduced into their systems in a more controlled and manageable fashion. This process gives them access to high-technology medical care with less national investment. If technology development were slowed by a modest amount in the United States, it would likely have serious health consequences globally (Massaro 1990). Telemedicine has also made clinical care, distance education, and medical research possible in parts of the world traditionally unexposed to such advances (Umar 2003).

## Impact on Bioethics

Increasingly, technological change is raising serious ethical and moral issues. For example, when in vitro fertilization is applied in medical practice and leads to the production of spare embryos, the moral question is what to do with these embryos. Gene mapping of humans, genetic cloning, stem cell research, and other areas of growing interest to scientists may hold potential benefits, but they also present serious ethical dilemmas. Life support technology raises serious ethical issues, especially in medical decisions regarding continuation or cessation of mechanical support, particularly when a patient exists in a permanent vegetative state.

## The Assessment of Medical Technology

Technology assessment, or more specifically, *health technology assessment* (HTA), refers to "any process of examining and reporting properties of a medical technology used in health care, such as safety, effectiveness, feasibility, and indications for use, cost, and cost-effectiveness, as well as social, economic, and ethical consequences, whether intended or unintended" (Institute of Medicine 1985). HTA seeks to contribute to clinical decision making by providing evidence about the efficacy, safety, and cost effectiveness of medical technologies. It also informs decision makers, clinicians, patients, and the public about the ethical, legal, and social implications of medical technologies (Lehoux et al. 2009).

Technology assessment can play a critical role in distinguishing between services that are appropriate and those that are not. According to the Congressional Budget Office, roughly $700 billion each year goes to health care spending that cannot show improved health outcomes (Orszag 2008). The amount of $700 billion is 32% of total expenditures on health services and supplies ($2181 billion; Hartman et al. 2010) in 2008. Hence, HTA presents a tremendous opportunity to reduce waste and improve health outcomes. Questions related to the adoption of new technology and decisions to control its diffusion should be governed by HTA (Garber 1994).

Efficacy and safety are the basic starting points in evaluating the overall utility of medical technology. Cost effectiveness and cost benefit go a step further in evaluating the safety and efficacy in relation to the cost of using technology. Efficacy and safety are evaluated through clinical trials. A *clinical trial* is a carefully designed research study in which human subjects participate under controlled observations. Clinical trials are carried out over three or four phases, starting with a small number of subjects to evaluate the safety, dosage range, and side effects of new treatments. Subsequent studies using larger groups of people are carried out to confirm effectiveness and further evaluate safety. Compliance with rigid standards is required under HIPAA to protect the rights of study participants and to ensure that the experimentation protocols are ethical. Every institution that conducts or supports biomedical or behavioral research involving human subjects must establish an Institutional Review Board (IRB), which initially approves and periodically reviews the research.

## Efficacy

Determination of efficacy is based on the premise that, if a technology is not efficacious, it should not be used. Without the information on efficacy, it is almost impossible to know a technology's usefulness.

In a broad sense, *efficacy* is defined simply as health benefit derived from the use of technology. Some authors see a technical distinction between efficacy and *effectiveness* (see Wan 1995). Although such a distinction may be important in the actual process of assessment, in a general sense, efficacy is synonymous with effectiveness. If a product or service actually produces some health benefit, it can be considered efficacious or effective. Decisions about efficacy require that one ask the right questions. For example, is the current diagnosis satisfactory? What is the likelihood that a different procedure would result in a better diagnosis? If the problem is more accurately diagnosed, what is the likelihood of a better cure? The question of benefit is not as simple as it first seems because health outcomes have traditionally been measured in terms of mortality and morbidity. However, improvement in one's quality of life is an important outcome. Reliable measures of improvement in quality of life, however, are difficult to obtain. They are not nearly as objective as mortality rates and are subject to bias (Fuchs 2004). Moreover, the same technology employed by different caregivers can sometimes yield different results, although such variations can be minimized by education and training.

## Safety

Safety considerations are designed to protect patients against unnecessary harm from technology. As a primary benchmark, benefits must outweigh any negative consequences; however, negative consequences cannot always be foreseen. Hence, clinical trials involving patients who may stand to gain the most from a technology are employed to obtain a reasonable consensus on safety. Subsequently, outcomes from the wider use of the technology are closely monitored to identify any problems related to safety.

## Cost Effectiveness

An evaluation of efficacy and safety alone is not sufficient. *Cost efficiency* (or cost effectiveness) is a step beyond the determination of efficacy. Whereas efficacy is concerned only with the benefit derived from the technology, cost effectiveness evaluates the additional (marginal) benefits derived in relation to the additional (marginal) costs incurred. Thus, cost efficiency weighs benefits against costs. A new technology may be clinically effective, that is, it may provide some benefit, but it is not cost effective if the benefit is small and the cost is high.

As shown in Figure 5–2, at the start of medical treatment, each unit of technology utilization is likely to provide benefits in excess of its costs. At some point (Point A in Figure 5–2), an additional unit of technology utilization would result in parity between benefits and costs. This is where the slopes of the benefit and cost lines are equal, as illustrated by the parallel lines. From an economic standpoint, this is the optimum point of health resource inputs. From this point on, it is highly unlikely that additional technological interventions would result in benefits equal to or in excess of the additional costs. As costs continue to increase, the health benefit curve becomes flatter. At Point B (Figure 5–2), the marginal benefits from additional care approach zero, which is referred to as the *flat of the curve*.

A considerable amount of the care delivered in the United States is at the flat of the curve, referring to a level of intensity of care that provides no incremental health benefit (Fuchs 2004). Hence, high-intensity care is often wasteful. In general, differences in intensity of care play, at most, a minor role in explaining cross-section differences in health outcomes, which are primarily determined by nonmedical factors: the physical and psychosocial environments,

Figure 5–2  Cost Effectiveness and Flat of the Curve.

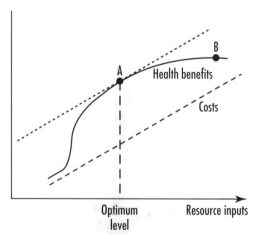

*Source:* Adapted from T.A. Massaro, Impact of New Technologies on Health Care Costs and on the Nation's Health, *Clinical Chemistry*, Vol. 36, no. 8B, p. 1612, © 1990, The American Association for Clinical Chemistry, Inc.

socioeconomic factors, personal behavior, and genetics (See Blum's model in Chapter 2; Fuchs 2004).

A more expensive procedure may actually be more cost efficient when used appropriately. For instance, CAT scans are more expensive than traditional X-ray images, but the use of CAT scans has markedly reduced the need for exploratory surgery (Nitzkin 1996). When CAT scan use is warranted, the benefits can outweigh their cost. Their use also bypasses the risks associated with exploratory surgery that may otherwise be necessary.

A *cost-effectiveness analysis* incorporates the elements of both costs and benefits, especially when the costs and benefits are not expressed in terms of dollars (Wan 1995). In this case, costs may or may not be calculated in monetary terms. If costs cannot be monetarily measured, they may be evaluated in terms of resource inputs, such as staff time, number of service units, space requirements, and degree of specialization needed (specialist versus generalist, physician versus allied health professional). Benefits, evaluated in terms of health outcomes, include elements such as efficacy of treatment, prognosis or expected outcomes, number of cases of a certain disease averted, years of life saved, increase in life expectancy, hospitalization and sick days avoided, early return to work, patient satisfaction, and quality of life. Benefits are then evaluated in relation to dollar costs or resource inputs.

Risk is another type of nonmonetary cost. Most medical procedures are not totally safe. They may have the potential for significant benefits, but they are also accompanied by certain risks. Sometimes, these risks are small; at other times, the risks can be significant. The process of medical care can result in undesired side effects, iatrogenic illnesses, medical complications, injuries, or death, all of which carry a cost that is often difficult to measure. Hence, the effectiveness of medical interventions should be evaluated not only in terms of costs but also in terms of risks. Thus, Figure 5–2 can also be used to determine the optimum point at which the benefits equal the risks. Beyond that point, the risks from additional technological interventions are likely to exceed the benefits. An example is overutilization of imaging procedures, such as CT scans, which carry potentially harmful radiation exposure. When used for the wrong reason, such as whole body CT scans for asymptomatic patients, they contribute to unnecessary costs and potential harm (Roberts and Keene 2008).

Cost (and risk) and benefit evaluations are not precise or objective determinations. Such assessments are based on professional judgments and expert opinions. However, standardization of clinical guidelines based on clinical evidence or expert medical consensus is a step toward making this process more objective.

## Cost Benefit

In contrast to cost-effectiveness analysis, *cost-benefit analysis* evaluates benefits in relation to costs, when both are expressed in dollar terms (Seidel et al. 1995; Wan 1995). Hence, cost-benefit analysis is subject to a more rigorous quantitative analysis compared to cost-effectiveness analysis. Cost-benefit analysis is based on four main assumptions: (1) The problem or health condition can be identified or diagnosed. (2) The problem can be controlled or eradicated using an appropriate intervention. (3) The benefit or outcome can be assigned a dollar value. (4) The cost of intervention can be determined in dollars.

The same principles that apply to cost effectiveness are also used for assessing cost benefit. If the estimated benefits exceed costs, the additional spending on medical care is worth the extra costs. The *quality-adjusted life year* (QALY) is commonly used as a measure of health benefit. Analyses that include the use of QALYs are referred to as *cost-utility analyses* (Neumann and Weinstein 2010). QALY is defined as the value of one year of high-quality life. Cutler and McClellan (2001) assigned a value of $100,000 per QALY and demonstrated that, at least in the case of four selected conditions, namely, heart attacks, low-birth-weight infants, depression, and cataracts, the estimated benefit of technological change was much greater than the cost. For breast cancer treatment, the costs and benefits were found to be equal in magnitude. The value of $100,000 per QALY is debatable. Others have proposed $200,000 per year of life (Murphy and Topel 2003).

# Current and Future Directions in Health Technology Assessment

## Private Sector Initiatives

In the United States, HTA is conducted predominantly in the private sector, unlike nations such as Sweden, the Netherlands, and Canada, which have centralized technology assessment agencies (Neumann and Sandberg 1998). In the public sector, the Department of Veterans Affairs and the Department of Defense mainly conduct the clinical trials and other evaluations of technology. Hence, much of the talent needed to assess medical technology is also located, organized, and

financed in the private sector. Pharmaceutical firms, for example, have developed pharmacoeconomics departments concerned with internal analysis of the cost effectiveness of new products (Rettig 1994). Before new drugs are introduced, their economic evaluation has become almost as important as the clinical trials used to determine their safety and efficacy. Private agencies, among them the Blue Cross and Blue Shield Association, Kaiser Permanente, the AMA, and other professional societies, have undertaken technology assessment.

## Need for Coordinated Effort

At present, efforts in HTA remain fragmented and poorly funded, with little or no coordination between public or private sector groups to deliberately address the assessment and diffusion of technologies. Also, information garnered from HTA studies is not efficiently shared among medical organizations, health care systems, and policy makers. The response has been a demand for broad regional and national HTA programs that would study the effects of health care technology more systematically and involve providers, policy makers, patient advocacy groups, and government representatives (Bozic et al. 2004). Provisions under the Medicare Prescription Drug Improvement and Modernization Act of 2003 provide for increased funding for the AHRQ to support clinical effectiveness and cost-effectiveness research on new medical technology (Wechsler 2004).

## Need for Standardization

Future efforts in HTA will require greater transparency of methods employed and standardization, which would allow comparison of efficacy and cost-effectiveness results across studies. In 1996, the Panel on Cost-Effectiveness in Health and Medicine—a panel of physicians, health economists, ethicists, and other health policy experts commissioned by the US Public Health Service—recommended the use of QALYs as a standard measure of health benefits from various interventions. The use of QALYs provides a common measure of health effects across studies (Siegel et al. 1997). As a standard measure, QALYs enable comparisons of varied interventions across diverse diseases and conditions. However, the Patient Protection and Affordable Care Act of 2010 prohibits the use of cost-per-QALY thresholds by the Patient-Centered Outcomes Research Institute created under the Act (Neumann and Weinstein 2010).

## Balance Between Clinical Efficacy and Economic Worth

American consumers often want all available medical resources utilized regardless of how little health benefit is received in relation to costs. Physicians often find themselves in a precarious situation when they are required to withhold treatment because of its known cost inefficiency. Payers are blamed as uncaring profit mongers when they intervene in the delivery of medical care based on costs. Even US policy makers are not at ease with bringing cost effectiveness into the equation of health care delivery. Consequently, cost effectiveness has not taken central stage in the United States, and its application is not openly discussed in health care decision making. In contrast, European countries, Canada, and Australia use cost effectiveness openly and explicitly in their centralized health planning decisions (Neumann and Sullivan 2006).

Current research has highlighted the value or worth of medical care spending in terms of gains in life expectancy in the United States (see Cutler et al. 2006). Although such findings may suggest current levels of expenditures for health care are acceptable, rising health care costs in the United States and excessive spending, according to international comparisons, are of growing concern to most Americans. Policy makers are likely to respond to any public outcry over health care expenditures. Hence, cost-effectiveness analysis is likely to play a larger role in the approval process for drugs and devices, and regulatory initiatives to contain future costs are likely to demand greater emphases on the economic worth of individual technologies.

## Clinical Practice Guidelines

*Clinical practice guidelines* (or medical practice guidelines) are systematically developed protocols to assist practitioners in delivering appropriate health care for specific clinical circumstances (Field and Lohr 1990). The goal is to assist practitioners in adopting a "best practice" approach in delivering care to a given patient population with a given condition (Ramsey 2002). Practice guidelines result from an evaluation of medical procedures, regarding their effectiveness, appropriateness, and safety and the integration of these assessments into clinical practice. Such evidence-based guidelines provide a mechanism for standardizing the practice of medicine and improving the quality of care. The benchmark practice patterns become norms governing what is and is not appropriate in clinical practice. However, cost-effectiveness information is not commonly incorporated in the development of clinical practice guidelines

(Wallace et al. 2002). Ramsey (2002) suggested that this disconnect between practice guidelines and economic analyses emanates mainly from clinicians' inclination to treat patients until there is no more health benefit to be gained (the flat of the curve, discussed earlier). Conversely, economic analyses weigh treatments based on their incremental health value at a given cost, and they provide a reference point at which additional medical interventions must be discontinued to achieve maximum value in the delivery of medical care. In view of the escalating health care expenditures and the ongoing development and diffusion of expensive new technology, the concept of value—improved benefits at lower costs—will become increasingly important to both public and private payers of health care.

## Ethical Issues

With the rapid pace of innovation, concerns in HTA transcend the traditional questions about safety, effectiveness, and economic value. New technologies also raise social, ethical, and legal concerns. These issues raise complex questions but provide few answers. Yet, in an era of resource constraints, HTA will have to take into account social, ethical, economic, and legal concerns.

Health care budgets are under constraint not only in the United States but in other developed countries as well. How to provide the latest and best in health care within limited resource parameters has become a major concern for all developed countries. Insurers, pharmaceutical companies, medical device manufacturers, MCOs, and physician advocacy institutions often act and advocate out of their own self-interests. For example, physicians' representatives, such as medical associations, and the medical device and pharmaceutical industries frequently argue in favor of increasing resource inputs in delivering health care (Wild 2005). They often claim that quality would deteriorate and/or harm would ensue unless new innovations are funded. Since these same groups have also assumed major roles in HTA, the probability of circulating biased results is high. Biases might also arise in studies funded by sources that have a financial stake in the results. Such concerns have stimulated interest in developing standards for assessments, perhaps under the aegis of a governmental body.

Within social, ethical, and legal constraints, public and private insurers face the problem of deciding whether to cover novel treatments. Recent challenges include, for example, decisions about new reproductive techniques, such as intracytoplasmic sperm injection in vitro fertilization (ICSI IVF), new molecular genetic predictive tests for hereditary breast cancer, and new drugs such as sildenafil (Viagra) for erectile dysfunction (Giacomini 2005). The question arises as to whether society should even bear the cost of infertility treatments, genetic tests, and lifestyle remedies that do not affect people's health and longevity.

Therapies classified as experimental are, generally, not covered by insurance. When new treatments promise previously unattainable health benefits, decisions about assessment of such treatments are often surrounded by controversy. Critical to the debate, but defying easy answers, are questions regarding the adequacy of studies used to determine whether a certain treatment should be considered experimental, ethical questions regarding the needs of patients who could possibly benefit from the treatment, and financial questions concerning the responsibility of payers (Reiser 1994). Concerns about withholding treatment from patients are not easily juxtaposed against equally valid concerns about exposing these same patients to unjustified risk.

Ethical issues also surround the conduct of clinical research. Emanuel and colleagues (2000) contended that ethical clinical research must fulfill seven requirements: (1) The research must have social or scientific value for improving health or enhancing knowledge. (2) The study must be scientifically valid and methodologically rigorous. (3) The selection of subjects in clinical trials must be fair. (4) The potential benefits to patients and the knowledge gained for further scientific work must outweigh the risks. (5) Independent review of the research methods and findings must be conducted by unaffiliated individuals. (6) Informed, voluntary consent must be obtained from subjects. (7) The privacy of enrolled subjects must be protected, they must be offered the opportunity to withdraw, and their well-being must be maintained throughout the trial.

## Summary

Medical technology is the practical application of scientific knowledge produced by biomedical research and the adaptation of scientific advances from other fields to the delivery of health care. The application of information technology and informatics is becoming indispensable in efficient delivery of care and in the effective management of modern health care organizations. With the growth of Internet applications, e-health is becoming a growing field in health care delivery. Telemedicine and telehealth are used in both synchronous and asynchronous applications to deliver medical care, when the provider and client are separated by distance.

Medical technology has greatly enhanced the capabilities of the delivery system to provide more effective and less invasive treatments. The problem is that the development and diffusion of technology are closely intertwined with its use. The United States is foremost in the world in developing new technology, but the uncontrolled use of technology has prompted deep concerns about rising costs. Several factors have influenced the growth of technology: beliefs and values in the American culture, medical specialization, financing, competition, and expenditures in research and development. Most other developed countries apply supply-side controls to limit technology diffusion and its use. It curtails cost, but it also restricts access to care. Such direct controls over the innovation, diffusion, and utilization of technology through government policy have not been possible in the United States. However, health policy does play a role through the FDA's drug and device approval process and government funding for biomedical research.

Technology has had a tremendous impact on the delivery of health care. It has positively influenced the quality of care, enhanced the quality of life, and improved access in remote areas. Many large institutional providers and MCOs cannot function efficiently without computer-based information systems. Because much of the technology developed in the United States is either purchased or reproduced by other countries, technology development in the United States also has a profound effect on the practice of medicine globally. Advances in genetics and many other areas have the potential to provide unprecedented benefits, but they also raise critical ethical issues.

Given the costs and risks associated with the use of technology, its assessment has become an area of growing interest. Current thought in technology assessment calls for a balance between benefits (efficacy) and costs/risks. Additional interventions, beyond the point where costs and/or risks begin to exceed the benefits, are considered inappropriate, but the assessment of cost effectiveness is not an exact science. Evidence-based clinical practice guidelines are paving the way toward standardizing medical practice. However, there is a disconnect between practice guidelines and economic analysis. As escalating health care expenditures reach a critical point, appropriateness of medical treatments may have to be based on their incremental health value at a given cost.

Use of technology is not without controversy. Critical moral dilemmas arise from the use of experimental therapies, delays in the assessment and approval process, life-sustaining treatments, and waste of resources when interventions are not cost effective.

## Terminology

administrative information
    systems
asynchronous technology
clinical information systems
clinical practice guidelines
clinical trial
cost-benefit analysis
cost-effectiveness analysis
cost efficiency
cost-utility analysis
decision support systems
effectiveness

efficacy
e-health
electronic health records
e-therapy
flat of the curve
health informatics
health technology
    assessment
information technology
medical technology
m-health
orphan drugs

quality-adjusted life year
    (QALY)
self-referrals
smart cards
synchronous technology
technological imperative
technology diffusion
telehealth
telemedicine
value
virtual physician visits
xenografting

## Test Your Understanding

## Review Questions

1. Medical technology encompasses more than just sophisticated equipment. Discuss.
2. What role does an information systems (IS) department play in a modern health care organization?
3. Provide brief descriptions of clinical information systems, administrative information systems, and decision support systems in health care delivery.
4. Distinguish between information technology (IT) and health informatics.

5. According to the Institute of Medicine, what are the four main components of a fully developed electronic health records (EHR) system?

6. Why have EHR systems not been widely adopted in the United States?

7. What are the main provisions of HIPAA with regard to the protection of personal medical information?

8. What is telemedicine? How do the synchronous and asynchronous forms of telemedicine differ in their applications?

9. Which factors have been responsible for the low diffusion and low use of telemedicine?

10. Generally speaking, why is medical technology more readily available in the United States than in other countries?

11. How does competition lead to greater levels of technology diffusion? How does technological diffusion, in turn, lead to greater competition?

12. Summarize the government's role in technology diffusion.

13. What was the effect of Kefauver-Harris Drug Amendments of 1962? Why was the law criticized?

14. Provide a brief overview of how technology influences the quality of medical care and quality of life.

15. Discuss the relationship between technological innovation and health care expenditures.

16. What impact has technology had on access to medical care?

17. Discuss the roles of efficacy, safety, and cost effectiveness in the context of technology assessment.

18. Why is it important to achieve a balance between clinical efficacy and economic worth (cost effectiveness) of medical treatments?

19. What purpose do clinical practice guidelines serve in health care delivery? What main shortcoming exists in the practice guidelines currently in use?

20. What are some of the ethical issues surrounding the development and use of medical technology?

## REFERENCES

Agres, T. 2005. Trouble with drug debuts. *Drug Discovery & Development* 8, no. 11: 14–16.

Anderson, G., and P.S. Hussey. 2001. Comparing health system performance in OECD countries. *Health Affairs* 20, no. 3: 219–232.

Austin, C.J. 1992. *Information systems for health services administration.* 4th ed. Ann Arbor, MI: AUPHA Press/Health Administration Press.

Baker, L. 2002. Managed care, medical technology, and the well-being of society. *Topics in Magnetic Resonance Imaging* 13, no. 2: 107–113.

Baker, L.C., and C.S. Phibbs. 2002. Managed care, technology adoption, and health care: The adoption of neonatal intensive care. *RAND Journal of Economics* 33, no. 3: 524–548.

Baker, L.C., and S.K. Wheeler. 1998. Managed care and technology diffusion: The case of MRI. *Health Affairs* 17, no. 5: 195–207.

Baker, L.C. et al. 2008. Expanded use of imaging technology and the challenge of measuring value. *Health Affairs* 27, no. 6: 1467–1478.

Bozic, K.J. et al. 2004. Health care technology assessment: Basic principles and clinical applications. *The Journal of Bone and Joint Surgery* 86A, no. 6: 1305–1314.

Brailer, D.J. 2005. Interoperability: The key to the future health care system. *Health Affairs: Web Exclusive* 24 (Suppl 1): w5-19–w5-21.

Bronzino, J.D. et al. 1990. *Medical technology and society: An interdisciplinary perspective.* Cambridge, MA: MIT Press.

Brook, R.H. 1989. Practice guidelines and practicing medicine: Are they compatible? *Journal of the American Medical Association* 262: 3027–3030.

Centers for Disease Control and Prevention. 1999. *New data show AIDS patients less likely to be hospitalized.* Available at: http://www.cdc.gov/od/oc/media/pressrel/r990608.htm. Accessed June 1999.

Clayton, P.D. 2001. Confidentiality and medical information. *Annals of Emergency Medicine* 38, no. 3: 312–316.

Cohen, A.B. 2004a. The adoption and use of medical technology in health care organizations. In: *Technology in American healthcare: Policy directions for effective evaluation and management.* A.B. Cohen and R.S. Hanft, eds. Ann Arbor, MI: The University of Michigan Press. pp. 105–147.

Cohen, A.B. 2004b. Critical questions regarding medical technology and its effects. In: *Technology in American healthcare: Policy directions for effective evaluation and management.* A.B. Cohen and R.S. Hanft, eds. Ann Arbor, MI: The University of Michigan Press. pp. 15–42.

Cohen, A.B. 2004c. The diffusion of new medical technology. In: *Technology in American healthcare: Policy directions for effective evaluation and management.* A.B. Cohen and R.S. Hanft, eds. Ann Arbor, MI: The University of Michigan Press. pp. 79–104.

Congressional Budget Office (CBO). 2008. *Technological change and the growth of health care spending.* Washington, DC: Congressional Budget Office.

Cutler, D.M., and M. McClellan. 2001. Is technological change in medicine worth it? *Health Affairs* 20, no. 5: 11–29.

Cutler, D.M. et al. 2006. The value of medical spending in the United States, 1960–2000. *The New England Journal of Medicine* 355, no. 9: 920–927.

Danzon, P.M., and M.V. Pauly. 2001. Insurance and new technology: From hospital to drugstore. *Health Affairs* 20, no. 5: 86–100.

Davis, M.P. 2006. Management of cancer pain: Focus on new opioid analgesic formulations. *American Journal of Cancer* 5, no. 3: 171–182.

Devaraj, A. et al. 2007. PET/CT in non-small cell lung cancer staging—promises and problems. *Clinical Radiology* 62, no. 2: 97–108.

Dorsey, E.R. et al. 2010. Funding of US biomedical research, 2003–2008. *Journal of the American Medical Association* 303, no. 2: 137–143.

Drake, D. et al. 1993. *Hard choices: Health care at what cost?* Kansas City, MO: Andrews and McMeel.

Ellis, D. 2000. *Technology and the future of health care: Preparing for the next 30 years.* San Francisco, CA: Jossey-Bass Publishers.

Emanuel, E.J. et al. (2000). What makes clinical research ethical? *Journal of the American Medical Association* 283, no. 20: 2701–2711.

Esmail, N., and G. Walker. 2006. *Waiting your turn: Hospital waiting lists in Canada.* 16th ed. Vancouver, British Columbia: The Fraser Institute.

Field, M.J., and J. Grigsby. 2002. Telemedicine and remote patient monitoring. *Journal of the American Medical Association* 288, no. 4: 423–425.

Field, M.J., and K.N. Lohr, eds. 1990. *Clinical practice guidelines: Directions for a new agency.* Washington, DC: National Academy Press.

Flannery, E.J. 1986. Should it be easier or harder to use unapproved drugs and devices? *Hastings Center Report* 16, no. 1: 17–23.

Flower, J. 2006. Imagining the future of health care. *The Physician Executive* 32, no. 1: 64–66.

Food and Drug Administration (FDA). 2009. *Federal Food and Drugs Act of 1906.* Available at: http://www.fda.gov/regulatoryinformation/legislation/ucm148690.htm. Accessed January 2010.

Fuchs, V.R. 2004. More variation in use of care, more flat-of-the-curve medicine. *Health Affairs* 23 (Variations Suppl): 104–107.

Garber, A.M. 1994. Can technology assessment control health spending? *Health Affairs* 13, no. 3: 115–126.

Gelijns, A., and N. Rosenberg. 1994. The dynamics of technological change in medicine. *Health Affairs* 13, no. 3: 28–46.

Giacomini, M. 2005. One of these things is not like the others: The idea of precedence in health technology assessment and coverage decisions. *The Milbank Quarterly* 83, no. 2: 193–223.

Gonzalez, R.P. et al. 2009. Improving rural emergency medical service response time with global positioning system navigation. *The Journal of Trauma* 67, no. 5: 899–902.

Gros, D.F. et al. 2010. Telehealth technologies for the delivery of mental health services. *Forum* (updated November 2010): p. 6.

Haglund, C.L., and W.L. Dowling. 1993. The hospital. In: *Introduction to health services.* 4th ed. S.J. Williams and P.R. Torrens, eds. Albany, NY: Delmar Publishers. pp. 135–176.

Halamka, J.D. 2010. Making the most of federal health information technology regulations. *Health Affairs* 29, no. 4: 596–600.

Hamblen, M. 2006. Hospitals expand videoconferencing. *Computerworld* 40, no. 23: 21.

Hartman, M. et al. 2010. Health spending growth at a historic low in 2008. *Health Affairs* 29, no. 1: 147–155.

Hillestad, R. et al. 2005. Can electronic medical record systems transform health care? Potential health benefits, savings, and costs. *Health Affairs* 24, no. 5: 1103–1117.

Hing, E., and C.J. Hsiao. 2010. Electronic medical record use by office-based physicians and their practices: United States, 2007. *National Health Statistics Reports* 23: 1–11.

Hogan, S.O., and S.M. Kissam. 2010. Measuring meaningful use. *Health Affairs* 29, no. 4: 601–606.

Iglehart, J.K. 1982. The cost and regulation of medical technology: Future policy directions. In: *Technology and the future of health care*. J.B. McKinlay, ed. Cambridge, MA: MIT Press. pp. 69–103.

Institute of Medicine. 1985. *Assessing medical technologies*. Washington, DC: National Academy Press.

Institute of Medicine. 2002. *Medical innovation in the changing healthcare marketplace*. Washington, DC: National Academy Press.

Institute of Medicine. 2003. *Key capabilities of an electronic health records system*. Washington, DC: National Academy Press.

Jha, A.K. et al. 2006. How common are electronic health records in the United States? A summary of the evidence. *Health Affairs* 25, no. 6: w496–w507.

Johnston, B. et al. 2000. Outcomes of the Kaiser Permanente tele-home health research project. *Archives of Family Medicine* 9: 40–45.

Kahn, J.G. et al. 2010. "Mobile" health needs and opportunities in developing countries. *Health Affairs* 29, no. 2: 252–258.

Kher, U. 2006. The hospital wars. *Time* 168, no. 24: 64–68.

Kim, M. et al. 2001. How interested are Americans in New Medical Technologies? A multicountry comparison. *Health Affairs* 20, no. 5: 194–201.

Klein, D. et al. 2005. Videoconferencing for rural physicians' continuing health education. *Journal of Telemedicine and Telecare* 11 (Suppl. 1): 97–99.

Kleinke, J.D. 2001. The price of progress: Prescription drugs in the health care market. *Health Affairs* 20, no. 5: 43–60.

Komaroff, A.L. 2005. Beyond the horizon. *Newsweek* 146, no. 24: 82–84.

Lehoux, P. et al. 2009. What medical specialists like and dislike about health technology assessment reports. *Journal of Health Services Research & Policy* 14, no. 4: 197–203.

Lewis, S. 1989. Mobile cardiac catheterization services: Invasive diagnostic for small hospitals in the 1990s. *Hospital Technology Series Special Report* 8, no. 29.

Littell, C.L., and R.J. Strongin. 1996. The truth about technology and health care costs. *IEEE Technology and Society Magazine* 15, no. 3: 10–14.

Luce, B.R. 1993. Medical technology and its assessment. In: *Introduction to health services*. 4th ed. S.J. Williams and P.R. Torrens, eds. Albany, NY: Delmar Publishers. pp. 245–268.

Maheu, M.M. et al. 2001. *E-health, telehealth, and telemedicine: A guide to start-up and success*. San Francisco, CA: Jossey-Bass.

Massaro, T.A. 1990. Impact of new technologies on health care costs and on the nation's health. *Clinical Chemistry* 36, no. 8B: 1612–1616.

McClellan, M., and D. Kessler. 1999. A global analysis of technological change in health care: The case of heart attacks. *Health Affairs* 18, no. 3: 250–257.

McGregor, M. 1989. Technology and the allocation of resources. *The New England Journal of Medicine* 320, no. 2: 118–120.

Merrill, R.A. 1994. Regulation of drugs and devices: An evolution. *Health Affairs* 13, no. 3: 47–69.

Milewa, T. 2006. Health technology adoption and the politics of governance in the UK. *Social Science and Medicine* 63, no. 12: 3102–3112.

Miller, C.C. 2009. The virtual visit may expand access to doctors. *The New York Times* December 21: 4.

Miller, R.H. et al. 2005. The value of electronic health records in solo or small group practices. *Health Affairs* 24, no. 5: 1127–1137.

Morrissey, J. 2002. Hospitals offer remote control. *Modern Healthcare* 32, no. 51: 32–35.

Murphy, G.F. et al. 1999. EHR vision, definition, and characteristics. In: *Electronic health records: Changing the vision*. G.F. Murphy, M.A. Hanken, and K.A. Waters, eds. Philadelphia, PA: Saunders. pp. 3–26.

Murphy, K.M., and R.H. Topel. 2003. The economic value of medical research. In: *Measuring the gains from medical research: An economic approach*. K.M. Murphy and R.H. Topel, eds. Chicago: University of Chicago Press. pp. 41–73.

National Conference of State Legislatures. 2011. *Certificate of need: State health laws and programs*. Available at: http://www.ncsl.org/default.aspx?tabid=14373. Accessed January 2011.

Neumann, P.J., and E.A. Sandberg. 1998. Trends in health care R&D and technology innovation. *Health Affairs* 17, no. 6: 111–119.

Neumann, P.J., and S.D. Sullivan. 2006. Economic evaluation in the US: What is the missing link? *Pharmacoeconomics* 24, no. 11: 1163–1168.

Neumann, P.J., and M.C. Weinstein. 2010. Legislation against use of cost-effectiveness information. *The New England Journal of Medicine* 363, no. 16: 1495–1497.

Nicol, N., and L. Huminski. 2006. How we cut drug errors. *Modern Healthcare* 36, no. 34: 38.

Nitzkin, J.L. 1996. Technology and health care—Driving costs up, not down. *IEEE Technology and Society Magazine* 15, no. 3: 40–45.

Orszag, P.R. 2008. *Opportunities to increase efficiency in health care*. Washington, DC: Congressional Budget Office.

Rakich, J.S. et al. 1992. *Managing health services organizations*. Baltimore, MD: Health Professions Press.

Ramsey, S.D. 2002. Economic analyses and clinical practice guidelines: Why not a match made in heaven? *Journal of General Internal Medicine* 17, no. 3: 235–237.

Rassweiler, J. et al. 2010. The role of laparoscopic radical prostatectomy in the era of robotic surgery. *European Urology Supplements* 9, no. 3: 379–387.

Reed, M.C., and J.M. Grossman. 2004. *Limited information technology for patient care in physician offices*. Issue Brief 89 (September 2004). Washington, DC: Center for Studying Health System Change.

Reiser, S.J. 1994. Criteria for standard versus experimental therapy. *Health Affairs* 13, no. 3: 127–136.

Research America. 2006. *National survey, 2006*. Available at: http://www.researchamerica.org /polldata/2006/NationalPoll2006.pdf. Accessed January 2007.

Rettig, R.A. 1994. Medical innovation duels cost containment. *Health Affairs* 13, no. 3: 7–27.

Riley, J.G., and H.P. Brehm. 1989. Technological innovations and their impact on care delivery. In: *Health care, technology, and the competitive environment*. H.P. Brehm and R.M. Mullner, eds. New York: Praeger Publishers. pp. 21–39.

Roark, D.C., and K. Miguel. 2006. Replacing bar coding: Radio frequency identification. *Nursing* 36, no. 12: 30.

Roberts, J., and S. Keene. 2008. Asymptomatic CT scans: A health assessment or a health risk? *Internet Journal of Radiology* 9, no. 1: 18.

Rochlen, A.B. et al. 2004. Online therapy: Review of relevant definitions, debates, and current empirical support. *Journal of Clinical Psychology* 60, no. 3: 269–283.

Schur, C.L., and M.L. Berk. 2008. Views on health care technology: Americans consider the risks and sources of information. *Health Affairs* 27, no. 6: 1654–1664.

Seidel, L.F. et al. 1995. *Applied quantitative methods for health services management*. Baltimore, MD: Health Professions Press.

Shaw, L.J. et al. 2000. Clinical and economic outcomes assessment in nuclear cardiology. *Quarterly Journal of Nuclear Medicine* 44, no. 2: 138–152.

Short, A.C. et al. 2003. *Disease management: A leap of faith to lower-cost, higher-quality health care*. Issue Brief No. 69 (October 2003). Washington, DC: Center for Studying Health System Change.

Siegel, J.E. et al. 1997. Guidelines for pharmacoeconomic studies. Recommendations from the panel on cost effectiveness in health and medicine. Panel on Cost Effectiveness in Health and Medicine. *Pharmacoeconomics* 11, no. 2: 159–168.

Simpson, R.L. 1994. The role of technology in a managed care environment. *Nursing Management* 25, no. 2: 26–28.

Singh, R. et al. 2010. Sustainable rural telehealth innovation: A public health case study. *Health Services Research* 45, no. 4: 985–1004.

Skinner, A.E.G., and G. Latchford. 2006. Attitudes to counselling via the Internet: A comparison between in-person counselling client and Internet support group users. *Counseling and Psychotherapy Research* 6, no. 3: 92–97.

Smith, B.D. 2010. Reimbursement, implementation seen as barriers to telemedicine. *PT in Motion* 2, no. 10: 41–42.

Spann, S.J. 2001. The future of family medicine: Clinical practice. *Journal of Family Practice* 50, no. 7: 584–585.

Statistics Canada. 2004. *Access to health care services in Canada, 2003*. Ottawa, Ontario: Statistics Canada.

Steinbrook, R. 2006. Private health care in Canada. *The New England Journal of Medicine* 354, no. 16: 1661–1664.

Steinbrook, R. 2009a. Health care and the American Recovery and Reinvestment Act. *The New England Journal of Medicine* 360, no. 11: 1057–1060.

Steinbrook, R. 2009b. The NIH stimulus—The Recovery Act and biomedical research. *The New England Journal of Medicine* 360, no. 15: 1479–1481.

Stofle, G.S. 2001. *Choosing an online therapist*. Harrisburg, PA: White Hat Communications.

Tan, J.K.H. 1995. *Health management information systems: Theories, methods, and applications.* Gaithersburg, MD: Aspen Publishers, Inc.

Tuffnell, S., and J. Kirby. 1994. *Price controls and global budgets: Lessons from Canada*. Brief Analysis No. 104. Washington, DC: National Center for Policy Analysis.

Tustin, N. 2010. The role of patient satisfaction on online health information seeking. *Journal of Health Communication* 15, no. 1: 3–17.

Umar, K. 2003. *Telemedicine works: Quality, access, and cost impacts cited.* Closing the Gap (January/February). Washington, DC: Office of Minority Health Resource Center, Department of Health and Human Services.

US Census Bureau. 1999. *Statistical abstract of the United States*. Washington, DC: US Census Bureau.

Vishwanath, A. et al. 2010. The impact of electronic medical record systems on outpatient work-flows: A longitudinal evaluation of its workflow effects. *International Journal of Medical Informatics* 79, no. 11: 778–791.

Wachler, A.B., and P.A. Avery. 2011. *Stark II proposed regulations: Rule offers additional guidance while regulators seek more input from health care community*. Available at: http://www.wachler.com/CM/Publications/Publications17.asp. Accessed January 2011.

Wallace, J.F. et al. 2002. The limited incorporation of economic analyses in clinical practice guide-lines. *Journal of General Internal Medicine* 17, no. 3: 210–220.

Wan, T.T.H. 1995. *Analysis and evaluation of health care systems: An integrated approach to managerial decision making*. Baltimore, MD: Health Professions Press.

Warner, K.E. 1982. Effects of hospital cost containment on the development and use of medical technology. In: *Technology and the future of health care*. J.B. McKinlay, ed. Cambridge, MA: MIT Press. pp. 41–65.

Wechsler, J. 2004. Streamlining clinical research oversight. *Applied Clinical Trials* 13, no. 6: 24–26.

Wennberg, J.E. 1988. Improving the medical decision-making process. *Health Affairs* 7, no. 1: 99–106.

Wild, C. 2005. Ethics of resource allocation: Instruments for rational decision making in support of a sustainable health care. *Poiesis & Praxis* 3, no. 4: 296–309.

Ybarra, M.L., and W.W. Eaton. 2005. Internet-based mental health interventions. *Mental Health Services Research* 7, no. 2: 75–87.

Zimmerman, E. 2006. The implications of reimbursement changes for specialty hospitals. *Health-care Financial Management* 60, no. 7: 42–45.

# Chapter 6

# Health Services Financing

## Learning Objectives

- To study the role of health care financing and its impact on the delivery of health care
- To understand the basic concept of insurance and how general insurance terminology applies to health insurance
- To differentiate between the concepts of group insurance, self-insurance, individual health insurance, and managed care
- To examine the distinctive features of public programs, such as Medicare, Medicaid, Department of Defense, Veterans Administration, CHIP, and PACE
- To understand the various methods of reimbursement
- To discuss national health care and personal health care expenditures
- To become familiar with the requirements of the Patient Protection and Affordable Care Act of 2010 as they pertain to financing and insurance
- To get acquainted with the key trends, problems, and issues in health care financing

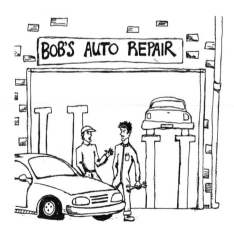

*"I have comprehensive insurance."*

# Introduction

Complexity of financing is one of the primary characteristics of medical care delivery in the United States. Both private and public resources are used to purchase health care services through a multitude of programs and health plans. The actual payment to providers of care is also handled in numerous ways. Patients themselves pay for some services directly, but most services are paid for indirectly through a variety of insurance plans, managed care organizations (MCOs), and government programs. The government and some large employers use the services of third-party administrators (TPAs) to process payment claims from providers.

The financing mechanisms are commonly referred to as health insurance. People who are not covered by either private or government-sponsored health insurance programs are referred to as uninsured (see Chapter 1). In the mid-1960s, the US government created the Medicare and Medicaid programs to extend public health insurance to the most vulnerable Americans. Since then, public outlays for health care financing have steadily increased, while private financing has decreased.

Chapter 1 characterized the structure of health services delivery in terms of its four main functions: financing, insurance, delivery, and payment. Because the dollars to fund health insurance come primarily from employers and the government, these entities are the financiers of health services delivery. Unless these financiers assume the basic financing function, the burden for health care expenses falls on the individual consumers of health care, the patients. However, when discussing financing in broad terms, as in this chapter, the concepts of financing, insurance, and payment are generally included. This does not mean, however, that the three functions are structurally integrated. For example, the government-financed programs, Medicare and Medicaid, integrate the functions of financing and insurance, but contracted TPAs make the actual payments to the providers after services have been delivered. Commercial insurance companies integrate the functions of insurance and payment, whereas employers largely constitute the source of financing. Managed care has gone one step further in integrating all four functions.

This chapter focuses on the financing mechanisms in both private and public programs and discusses national health care spending, which continues to be a matter of concern. Provisions of the Patient Protection and Afford Care Act (ACA) of 2010 are incorporated as applicable to the topics covered in this chapter and are also summarized in Exhibit 6–7. The chapter concludes with current trends and directions in financing, as well as points out some of the main problems and issues in financing health care services.

# The Role and Scope of Health Services Financing

As its central role, health services financing pays for health insurance premiums to cover individuals and families. Health insurance is the primary mechanism that enables people to obtain health care services. Hence, the insurance function is often regarded as a key component of health care financing in its broad sense. Providers often rely on the patients' insurance status to be assured that they will receive payment for the services they deliver. The various methods used to determine how much providers should be paid (i.e., reimbursement) for their services are also closely intertwined with the broad financing function.

Financing often determines who has access to health care and who does not. Thus, the demand for health care is directly related to its financing. Health insurance increases the demand for covered services; the demand would be less if those same services were noncovered. Increased demand means greater utilization of health services, given adequate supply. According to economic theory, insurance lowers the out-of-pocket cost of medical care to consumers; hence, they will consume more health services than if they had to pay the entire price out of their own pockets. Consumer behavior that leads to a higher utilization of health care services when the services are covered by insurance is referred to as *moral hazard* (Feldstein 1993).

Financing also exerts powerful influences on supply-side factors, such as how much health care is produced. New programs and services proliferate when private insurance plans or Medicare start paying for them. Indeed, financing has given rise to new subindustries within the health care delivery system. Subacute care and home health care are two such examples. Similarly, when new technologies are covered by health plans, their diffusion and utilization increase, as discussed in Chapter 5. When reimbursement is constrained, supply of services curtails accordingly.

Issues pertaining to reimbursement for services are critical in health services management decision making. Demand-side factors, including reimbursement, typically guide health services managers in evaluating the type and extent of services to offer. The amount of reimbursement needed to recoup capital costs over time also heavily influences management decisions, such as acquisition of new equipment, renovation or expansion of facilities, and launching of new programs.

Financing can also influence the supply and distribution of health care delivery professionals. Employer financing for dental insurance has spawned the growth of dentists and dental hygienists. Mechanisms for reimbursing physicians, such as the resource-based relative value scale (RBRVS) used by Medicare, directly affect physicians' incomes. One of the main intents of RBRVS, implemented in 1992, was to entice more medical residents into general practice by increasing the reimbursement for services provided by generalists. Due to other factors, however, the imbalance between generalists and specialists continues (see Chapter 4).

Financing eventually affects, directly as well as indirectly, the total health care expenditures (also referred to as health care costs or health care spending) incurred by a health care delivery system. The level of health care spending and the rise of these expenditures in the United States has been a matter of ongoing concern. The subsequent section discusses the relationship between financing and health care expenditures and provides a general framework for controlling health care costs.

## Financing and Cost Control

Health care financing and cost control are closely intertwined. As Figure 6–1 illustrates, in the US health care delivery system, insurance is the main factor that determines the level of demand for health services. Restricting financing for health insurance (see demand-side rationing in

Figure 6–1  Influence of Financing on the Delivery of Health Services.

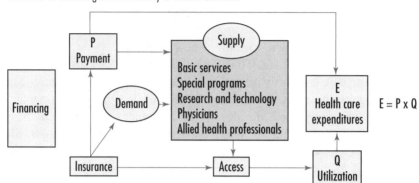

Chapter 2) eventually controls total health care expenditures. Conversely, extension of health insurance to the uninsured, without other restrictions, will increase total health care expenditures (E). Apart from the extent of insurance coverage, the cost of health insurance also affects system-wide health care expenditures.

Insurance, along with payment (i.e., price = P), influences the supply or availability of health services. Reducing reimbursement for providers has a direct influence on E, as well as an indirect influence through shrinkage in supply. Cuts in reimbursement have been used in the United States, as well as in other countries, to contain the growth of health care expenditures.

As discussed in Chapter 5, diffusion of technology and other types of services can be directly restricted through health planning to limit supply (see supply-side rationing in Chapter 2). When supply of technology is rationed, people may be insured but do not have free access to those services. Reduced utilization of expensive technology results in direct savings. This approach to cost containment is common in national health care programs. In addition to the direct savings realized by rationing technology, nations

that have national health care achieve indirect savings by having fewer specialist physicians and specialized technicians and by spending less on research and development (R&D).

Insurance and supply of health care services together determine access and, eventually, the utilization of services (i.e., quantity of services consumed = Q). Utilization can also be directly controlled. For example, private health plans, as well as Medicare and Medicaid, contain utilization by specifying which services are noncovered. Managed care directly controls utilization using various mechanisms (discussed in Chapter 9).

Because E = P × Q, rising health care costs can be controlled by managing the numerous factors that influence P and Q. Many of these factors are external to the health care delivery system. P, for example, includes general economy-wide inflation, as well as medical inflation that exceeds general inflation. In addition to the intrinsic factors discussed in this section, Q is also a function of changes in the size and demographic composition (i.e., age, sex, and racial mix) of the population (Levit et al. 1994). Chapter 12 discusses these factors more extensively.

# The Insurance Function

*Insurance* is a mechanism for protection against risk; that is its primary purpose. In this context, *risk* refers to the possibility of a substantial financial loss from an event of which the probability of occurrence is relatively small (at least in a given individual's case). For example, even though auto accidents are common in the United States, the likelihood is quite small that a specific individual will have an auto accident in a given year. Even though the risk is small, people buy insurance to protect their assets against catastrophic loss.

The insuring agency that assumes risk is called the *insurer*, or underwriter. *Underwriting* is a systematic technique for evaluating, selecting (or rejecting), classifying, and rating risks. Four fundamental principles underlie the concept of insurance (Health Insurance Institute 1969; Vaughn and Elliott 1987): (1) Risk is unpredictable for the individual insured. (2) Risk can be predicted with a reasonable degree of accuracy for a group or a population. (3) Insurance provides a mechanism for transferring or shifting risk from the individual to the group through the pooling of resources. (4) All members of the insured group share actual losses on some equitable basis.

Technically, health services for all Americans 65 and over are provided through Medicare. For those below the age of 65, private insurance is the predominant avenue for receiving health care. Medicaid and Children's Health Insurance Program cover many of the poor, including children in low-income households. Other public programs cover a small number of people, such as the Department of Veterans Affairs (VA) and the military health system. The remainder, without any coverage, are the uninsured.

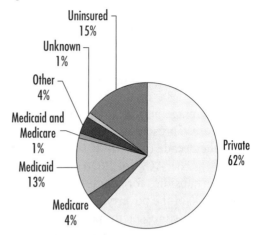

Figure 6–2  Sources of US Health Insurance, 2009.

*Source:* Data from *Summary health statistics for the U.S. population: National health interview survey, 2009.* National Center for Health Statistics, Table 18.

Sources for health insurance for all Americans appear in Figure 6–2.

## Some Health Insurance Concepts

### The Insured

The *insured*, also called a *beneficiary*, is anyone covered under a particular health insurance plan. Two types of employer-sponsored plans are single coverage plans and family coverage plans. The latter cover the spouse and dependent children of the working employee. Medicare and Medicaid plans recognize only individual beneficiaries. In the case of married couples, for instance, Medicare and Medicaid recognize each spouse as an independent beneficiary.

### Premiums

A *premium* is the amount charged by the insurer to insure against specified risks.

The average cost of premiums in 2010 was $5,049 per year for single coverage and $13,770 per year for family coverage (Claxton et al. 2010). For most job-based health insurance, the employee is asked to share in the cost of premiums. In 2010, workers contributed 19% of the premium cost for single coverage and 30% for family coverage. These represent the highest cost sharing in the decade of 2001–2010 (Claxton et al. 2010). The ACA of 2010 provides for premium subsidies for people with incomes up to 400% of the poverty level.

Premiums are determined by the actuarial assessment of risk. Two methods have been commonly used to determine premiums: The first, called *experience rating*, is based on a group's own medical claims experience. Under this method, premiums differ from group to group because different groups have different risks. For example, people working in various industries are exposed to various levels and types of hazards, people in certain occupations are more susceptible to certain illnesses or injuries, and older groups represent higher risks than younger groups. High-risk groups are expected to incur high utilization of medical care services, so these groups are charged higher premiums compared to preferred or favorable risk groups. Experience rating was the common method adopted by insurance companies (HIAA 1991), but several states have passed legislation that requires insurers to price their premiums according to community rating or modified community rating. *Community rating* spreads the risk among members of a larger community and establishes premiums based on the utilization experience of the whole community. Under pure community rating, the same rate applies to everyone regardless

of age, gender, occupation, or any other indicator of health risk (Goodman and Musgrave 1992). For example, a person who has AIDS would pay the same premium as someone who does not. Under "modified" community rating, price differences could be based on age and gender, while ignoring other risk factors. When premiums are based on community rating, the good risks (i.e., healthy people) actually subsidize the insurance cost for the poor risks (Somers and Somers 1977). In other words, costs shift from people in poor health to people in good health and make health insurance less affordable for those who are healthy.

## Cost Sharing

In addition to paying a share of the cost of premiums through payroll deductions, insured individuals, as well as those participating in certain public insurance programs, pay a portion of the actual cost of medical services out of their own pockets. These out-of-pocket expenses are in the form of deductibles and copayments and are incurred only if and when medical services are used. A *deductible* is the amount the insured must first pay before any benefits are payable by the plan. Commonly, the deductible must be paid on an annual basis. For example, suppose a plan requires the insured to pay a $500 deductible. When the insured receives medical care, the plan starts paying only after the cost of medical services received by the insured has exceeded $500 in a given year. The insured must pay the first $500 out of pocket each year. Not all health plans have a deductible. Most HMO plans, for example, do not have deductibles.

The second type of out-of-pocket cost is *copayment*, which most health plans have.

It is the amount the insured must pay each time health services are received. A copayment is set either as a dollar amount or as a proportion of the medical costs incurred. In the latter case, copayment is established in the form of what is referred to as *coinsurance*. As an example, for an office visit, the copayment amount could be $30, or a plan may require 80/20% coinsurance. In the latter case, once the deductible requirement has been met, the plan starts paying 80% of all covered medical expenditures; the insured pays the remaining 20%. Most plans include a *stop-loss* provision, which is the maximum out-of-pocket liability an insured could incur in a given year. In case of a catastrophic illness or injury, the copayment amount can add up to a substantial sum. The purpose of the stop-loss provision is to limit the total out-of-pocket costs to a certain amount, such as $2,000. This means that once the deductible and copayments have totaled $2,000 in a given year, no further copayments are required and the plan pays 100% of any additional expenses. Some plans have set lifetime benefits limits of $1 to $2 million; others have no limits. The ACA of 2010 prohibits the use of lifetime limits in all health plans and insurance policies issued or renewed on or after September 23, 2010.

The rationale for cost sharing is to control utilization of health care services. Since insurance creates moral hazard by insulating the insured against the cost of health care, making the insured pay part of the cost promotes more responsible behavior in health care consumption. A comprehensive study employing a controlled experimental design conducted in the 1970s, commonly referred to as the Rand Health Insurance Experiment, demonstrated that cost sharing had a material impact on lowering utilization, without any significant negative health consequences.

Over the years, employers have shifted an increasing amount of the cost of health care to their employees. For example, the percentage of workers enrolled in single-coverage non-HDHPs (high-deductible health plans) carrying deductibles that exceed $1,000 increased from 10% in 2006 to 27% in 2010 (Claxton et al. 2010).

## Indemnity and Service Plans

Technically, health insurance plans can be classified as either "indemnity" or "service" plans. Most health insurance plans are service plans. An *indemnity plan* provides reimbursement to the insured, without regard to the expenses actually incurred (Health Insurance Institute 1969). For example, a predetermined cash amount is paid to the beneficiary per procedure or per day in the hospital. The insured is responsible for paying the provider. There is no relationship between the insurer and the provider of services. If the actual expense is more than the indemnity amount, the balance becomes an out-of-pocket expense. A *service plan* provides specified services to the insured. The plan pays the hospital or physician directly, except for the deductible and copayments for which the insured is responsible. The insured does not get a bill from the providers, except for the out-of-pocket portion of the charges. Traditionally, private insurance companies offered indemnity plans, whereas Blue Cross/Blue Shield offered service plans (HIAA 1991). Plans offered by MCOs are also regarded as service plans. Even though, technically, the term "indemnity plan" carries a specific meaning, all traditional health insurance plans, other than managed care plans, are now loosely referred to as indemnity plans.

## Covered Services

Services covered by an insurance plan are referred to as *benefits*. Each health insurance plan spells out the type of medical services it covers. It also specifically lists services that are not covered. A contract outlines the covered and noncovered services, and a copy is provided to the insured. A typical disclaimer included in most contracts states that only "medically necessary" health services are covered regardless of whether or not such services are provided by a physician. Most plans include medical and surgical services, hospitalizations, emergency services, prescriptions, maternity care, and delivery of a baby. Within specified limits, most plans also provide mental health services, substance abuse services, home health care, skilled nursing care, rehabilitation, supplies, and equipment. Services, such as eyeglasses and dental care, may or may not be covered. Services most commonly excluded are those not ordered by a physician, such as self-care and over-the-counter products. Other services commonly excluded from health insurance coverage are cosmetic and reconstructive surgery, work-related illness and injury (covered under workers' compensation), rest cures, genetic counseling, and the like. Many plans had excluded coverage of preexisting medical conditions for new enrollees until a certain time had elapsed. HIPAA of 1996 made this practice illegal in case of employees who had health insurance coverage in their previous job. Starting July 2010, the ACA of 2010 has enabled people with a *preexisting condition*—a health problem that a person

has prior to obtaining health insurance—to enroll in a Pre-Existing Condition Insurance Plan (PCIP), which is a temporary federal program. This program offers insurance without medical underwriting to people who have been unable to get it because of a preexisting condition. In 2014, when the law is scheduled to be fully implemented, insurers will be legally required to cover people with preexisting health conditions.

Some managed care plans, especially health maintenance organizations (HMOs), exclude certain services unless the insured's primary care physician (PCP) prescribes them or refers the insured to them. Other plans may require preauthorization (also called precertification) or second opinions for certain surgical procedures or hospitalizations.

Dental insurance is often a separate plan, independent of major medical plans. Dental insurance generally covers oral examinations, routine cleanings, X-rays, fillings, extractions, inlays, bridgework, dentures, root canal therapy, and orthodontia (Health Insurance Institute 1969).

## Private Financing

Private health insurance, also referred to as "voluntary health insurance," is not mandatory. The modern health insurance industry is pluralistic. Private insurance includes many different types of health plan providers, such as commercial insurance companies (e.g., Aetna, Cigna, Metropolitan Life, and Prudential), Blue Cross/Blue Shield, self-insured employers, and MCOs. The nonprofit Blue Cross and Blue Shield Associations are similar to private health insurance companies.

## Types of Private Insurance

### Group Insurance

Group insurance can be obtained through an employer, a union, or a professional organization. A *group insurance* program anticipates that a substantial number of people in the group will purchase insurance through its sponsor. Risk, and often the cost of insurance, is spread out among the insured individuals. As discussed in Chapter 3, health insurance became an attractive fringe benefit to workers when wages were frozen during World War II. Around that time, fringe benefits also received favorable tax treatment. Unlike monetary wages, health insurance benefits are not subject to income tax. Consequently, a dollar of health insurance received from the employer is worth more than the same amount received in taxable wages or an after-tax dollar spent out of pocket for medical care. The tax policy has provided an incentive to obtain health insurance as a benefit paid by the employer. Such a nontaxable benefit leads to the purchase of excessive health insurance coverage—more than what people may actually need. These same people would likely purchase less generous health insurance plans if they had to pay all the premiums out of pocket.

Early health insurance policies were often inadequate to cover extended illnesses or long hospital stays. With the rapid growth of health insurance as a fringe benefit, which expanded competition among insurance companies, major medical insurance became common, starting in the 1950s. *Major medical* was designed to cover catastrophic situations that could subject families to substantial financial hardships, such as hospitalization, extended illness, and expensive surgery. Blue Cross/Blue Shield followed the lead of insurance companies and offered similar plans. The most common type of health insurance coverage available in the 1950s and 1960s included hospital care, surgical fees, and related physicians' expenses. Since the 1970s, health insurance plans have commonly combined major medical coverage with all-inclusive comprehensive coverage, which includes basic and routine physician office visits and diagnostic services (HIAA 1991). The term "major medical" is no longer limited to a single type of expense but rather applies broadly to almost all types of medical care (Somers and Somers 1977).

### Self-Insurance

Some big employers have a large enough and well-diversified workforce in terms of risk, which enables them to safely predict their medical expenditures from year to year. In a *self-insured plan*, the employer acts as its own insurer. Rather than pay insurers a dividend to bear the risk, large employers can simply assume the risk by budgeting a certain amount to pay medical claims incurred by their employees. Self-insured employers can protect themselves against any potential risk of high losses by purchasing *reinsurance* from a private insurance company. Being self-insured also gives such employers a greater degree of control, and costs are contained through a slower rise in premiums during periods of rapid inflation (Gabel et al. 2003).

Self-insurance was spurred by government policies. Self-insured employers were exempt from a premium tax that insurance companies had to pay, the cost of which was passed on to customers through higher premiums. Further, the Employee Retirement Income Security Act (ERISA) of 1974 exempts self-insured plans from certain mandatory benefits that regular health insurance plans are required to provide in many states. Self-insured plans also avoid other types of state insurance regulations, such as reserve requirements and consumer protection requirements. Premium taxes and other regulatory requirements would increase the cost of health insurance. Thus, employers that are large enough to make it feasible for themselves have viewed self-insurance as a better economic alternative. In 2008, 55% of all covered workers in private firms were covered by a self-insured plan; 89% of workers employed in firms with 5,000 or more employees were in self-insured plans (Fronstin 2009).

## Individual Private Health Insurance

Individually purchased private health insurance (nongroup plans) is an important source of coverage for some Americans. The family farmer, the early retiree, the self-employed, and the employee of a business that does not offer health insurance make up most of those relying on individual health insurance. Unlike group insurance, which spreads risk over the entire group, individual private insurance determines premium price and eligibility based on the risk indicated by each individual's health status and demographics (GAO 1996). Consequently, high-risk individuals are often unable to obtain privately purchased health insurance. For those who can obtain coverage, premiums are much higher than for those in group plans, and deductibles and copayments are often high. It is estimated that, in 2009, approximately 27 million Americans (14% of all privately insured individuals, 9% of all Americans)

were covered under private, nongroup plans (DeNavas-Walt et al. 2010). Not surprising, there is a strong association between income level and purchase of nongroup insurance (The Henry J. Kaiser Family Foundation 2008). Premiums vary considerably by state, reflecting a variety of factors that include differences in underwriting rules, health care costs, demographics, and consumer benefit preferences (AHIP Center for Policy and Research 2009).

## Managed Care Plans

MCOs, such as HMOs and preferred provider organizations (PPOs), emerged in response to the rapid escalation of health care costs. Managed care plans are a type of health insurance because they assume risk in exchange for an insurance premium. The full range of functions of MCOs, however, extends beyond the simple insurance function. In a nutshell, MCOs provide a broad range of services, generally emphasizing primary and preventive care. Services are provided through the MCOs' own internally employed professionals, through contractual arrangements with external providers, or through a combination of the two. MCOs also use a variety of mechanisms to monitor utilization. Chapter 9 presents a detailed discussion on managed care.

## High-Deductible Health Plans

High-deductible health plans (HDHPs) have been gaining popularity. In 2010, 15% of firms offering health benefits offered such a plan, up from 4% in 2005 (Claxton et al. 2010). HDHPs combine health insurance with a savings option. A savings account linked to the health plan is used to pay for routine health care expenses; the health plan covers expenses after the annual deductible has been met. This arrangement gives consumers greater control over how to use the funds. Hence, these plans are also referred to as *consumer-driven health plans*. Both employers and employees share in the cost of premiums. The employee's portion of premium costs can range between 11% and 30% (Claxton et al. 2010). Because of the high-deductible feature, premiums are lower than in other types of insurance plans. Depending on the type of plan, annual deductibles can range between $1,000 and $3,000 or more (Claxton et al. 2010). There are two types of HDHP arrangements:

The first type includes a health reimbursement arrangement (HRA). The HRA is funded solely by the employer; employees are prohibited from contributing. The funds are used to reimburse the insured for qualified medical expenses, which include premiums for HDHP and premiums for long-term care insurance if purchased. Employees do not pay taxes on withdrawals from the HRAs. An employer may decide to pay for medical expenses from the remaining balance in the HRA after the employee's retirement or termination from employment.

The second type of arrangement combines a health savings account (HSA) with a HDHP (HDHP/HSA) that meets federal standards and is referred to as a "qualified health plan." For example, federal regulations require reasonable caps on out-of-pocket expenses. HSAs were authorized under the Medicare Prescription Drug, Improvement, and Modernization Act (MMA), 2003. Under the law, HSA holders must have an HDHP, which is not mandated for an HRA. Employers may contribute but are not required to do so. About 65% of the workers covered under these plans receive employer contributions to their HSAs (Claxton et al.

2010). Funds belong to the account holder and can accumulate without limit. Hence, upon termination of employment, the employee carries the remaining funds. HSAs have significant tax advantages. Contributions are tax deductible, withdrawals used to pay for medical expenses are exempt from federal income taxes, and account earnings are tax exempt.

## State of Employment-Based Insurance

Because the majority of health insurance in the United States is job based, changes in insurance coverage follow the patterns of economic growth and decline. Economic downturns affect not only the level of employment but also health insurance coverage. Certain small employers may drop coverage altogether. The US economy experienced a recession from 2000 to 2004, a modest economic growth from 2004 to 2007, and a severe recession from 2007 to 2009. Thus, throughout 2000 to 2004, 4.1 million Americans lost employer-based coverage. Coverage increased by 1.2 million from 2004 to 2007, and it declined by 8.3 million from 2007 to 2009. In 2009, 50 million nonelderly Americans were uninsured, compared to 38.2 million in 2000 (Holahan 2011). The proportion of all firms, small and large, offering health insurance benefits dropped to its lowest level in 2005, when only 60% of firms offered health insurance, down from 69% in 2000. By 2010, however, health insurance offered by firms regained the 2000 levels of 69%. Most of this variation occurred in small firms that employ between 3 and 24 workers. Health insurance coverage offered by large firms that employ 200 or more workers has remained relatively unchanged (at over 98%) during good and bad economic times. Smaller firms of

200 employees or fewer, however, employ nearly 40% of workers who are more likely to be affected by economic trends (Claxton et al. 2010).

Layoffs and plant closures negatively affect people's ability to have health insurance. Between December 2000 and December 2009, the unemployment rate in the United States rose from 3.9 to 9.9%, according to the Bureau of Labor Statistics. By 2009, 9.7 million fewer Americans were covered by employer-based health insurance, a drop of 5.4% from 2000 (DeNavas-Walt et al. 2010).

The ability to have continuous health insurance coverage has long been an issue when changing jobs or waiting out periods of unemployment. In response, Congress passed the Consolidated Omnibus Budget Reconciliation Act of 1985 (COBRA), which allows employees to pay for continued group coverage for 18 months after leaving a job. The individuals are required to pay 102% of the group rate to continue health benefits, but without employer subsidy, the high cost of premiums prevents many from keeping their health insurance during periods of unemployment. HIPAA of 1996 provided for continued coverage beyond the original COBRA provisions. Extended coverage of up to 29 months is available if the insured or a family member is determined by the Social Security Administration to be disabled at any time during the first 60 days of COBRA coverage. Extended coverage of up to 36 months is available to the spouse and dependent children if the former employee dies, enrolls in Medicare, or gets divorced or legally separated. The extension is also available to a dependent child when that child stops being eligible under the plan as a dependent. The ACA of 2010 requires health plans to cover dependent children up to the age of 26 under their parents' health plans.

# Public Financing

Since 1965, government financing has played a significant role in expanding services, particularly to those who otherwise would not be able to afford them. Today, a significant proportion of health services in the United States is supported through public programs. In 2009, more than 18% of the US population was covered under various public insurance programs (see Figure 6–2). Chapter 3 discussed the inception of Medicare and Medicaid programs. This section discusses the financing, eligibility requirements, and services covered under the major public health insurance programs.

Public financing supports *categorical programs*, each designed to benefit a certain category of people. Examples are Medicare for the elderly and certain disabled individuals, Medicaid for the indigent, Defense Department programs for active service people, and VA programs for former armed forces personnel. The government finances Medicare and Medicaid, but services are purchased from providers in the private sector. Similarly, in two other government programs, TriCare (formerly called CHAMPUS—Civilian Health and Medical Program of the Uniformed Services)—(see The Military Health Services System later in this chapter) and CHAMPVA (Civilian Health and Medical Program of the Department of Veterans Affairs), the government provides the financing, but insurance and health care services are obtained through the private sector. In contrast, the government finances health care services for the uniformed armed forces and veterans, and delivery of services, with few exceptions, is also through the public sector.

## Medicare

The Medicare program, also referred to as Title 18 of the Social Security Act, finances medical care for three groups of people: (1) persons 65 years and older, (2) disabled individuals who are entitled to Social Security benefits, and (3) people who have end-stage renal disease (permanent kidney failure, requiring dialysis or a kidney transplant). People in these three categories can enroll regardless of income status. Among Medicare enrollees, 83% are 65 years and older, 12% are 85 years and older, 47% have income levels below 200% of the federal poverty level (FPL),* 29% have a cognitive/ mental impairment, and 28% are in fair to poor health (The Henry J. Kaiser Family Foundation 2010a).

Medicare is a federal program operated under the administrative oversight of the Centers for Medicare and Medicaid Services (CMS, formerly Health Care Financing Administration [HCFA]), a branch of the US Department of Health and Human Services (DHHS). Being a federal program, eligibility criteria and benefits are consistent throughout the United States.

Shortly after creation of the program, it had 19.5 million enrollees in 1967. In 2009, Medicare enrollees totaled 46.3 million in all US states, the District of Columbia, and US territories (CMS 2010a).

The Balanced Budget Act of 1997 established an independent federal agency, the Medicare Payment Advisory Commission (MedPAC), to advise the US Congress on various issues affecting the Medicare program. MedPAC's statutory mandate extends beyond payments to private health care providers participating in Medicare. The Commission is also tasked with analyzing access to care, quality of care, and other issues affecting Medicare.

For almost 30 years after its inception, Medicare had a dual structure comprising two separate insurance programs referred to as Part A and Part B. It subsequently became a four-part program.

### Part A (Hospital Insurance)

Part A, the Hospital Insurance (HI) portion of Medicare, is financed primarily by special payroll taxes. The employer and employee share equally in financing the Hospital Insurance trust fund. All working individuals, including those who are self-employed, pay the mandatory taxes. Prior to 1994, a maximum taxable ceiling was set each year. The Omnibus Budget Reconciliation Act of 1993 (OBRA-93) eliminated the maximum taxable earnings base, and all earnings became subject to Medicare tax (Davis and Burner 1995).

Part A covers hospital inpatient services, care in a skilled nursing facility (SNF), home health visits, and hospice care. Following is an overview of the type of benefits:

1. A maximum of 90 days of inpatient hospital care is allowed per benefit period. Once the 90 days are exhausted, a lifetime reserve of 60 additional hospital inpatient days remains. A *benefit period* is a spell of illness beginning with hospitalization and ending when a beneficiary has not been an inpatient in a hospital or an SNF for 60 consecutive days. The number of benefit periods is unlimited.

---

*FPL for 2011: Annual income of $22,050 for a family of four ($25,360 in Hawaii and $27,570 in Alaska).

2. Medicare pays for up to 100 days of care in a Medicare-certified SNF, subsequent to inpatient hospitalization for at least 3 consecutive days, not including the day of discharge. Admission to the SNF must occur within 30 days of hospital discharge.

3. Medicare pays for home health care when a person is homebound and requires intermittent or part-time skilled nursing care or rehabilitation care.

4. For terminally ill patients, Medicare pays for care provided by a Medicare-certified hospice.

The Part A program requires beneficiaries to pay a deductible (except for home health and hospice) for each benefit period and to make copayments based on the duration of services (except for home health). Most people 65 years of age or older do not have to pay a premium if they paid Medicare taxes while working. Some who do not meet the Social Security Administration's qualifications for premium-free coverage can get Part A by paying a monthly premium. Exhibit 6–1 gives details on the Part A program.

## Part B (Supplementary Medical Insurance)

Part B, the supplementary medical insurance (SMI) portion of Medicare, is a voluntary program financed partly by general tax revenues and partly by required premium contributions. Effective 2007, CMS implemented income-based Part B premiums as mandated by the MMA of 2003. Those whose incomes exceed a threshold amount pay a higher income-based premium. For 2011, the income threshold that triggers higher premiums is $85,000 per year ($170,000 per couple).

The intent of this legislation is to reduce tax-financed premium subsidies for higher-income individuals. Hence, for example, an individual earning more than $214,000 in 2011 will pay $369.10 in monthly premiums, whereas someone earning less than or equal to $85,000 will pay $115.40.

Almost all persons entitled to HI also choose to enroll in SMI because they cannot get similar coverage at the same price from private insurers. The main services covered by SMI are physician services; hospital outpatient services, such as outpatient surgery, diagnostic tests, radiology, and pathology services; emergency department visits; ambulance services; outpatient rehabilitation services; renal dialysis; radiation treatment; tissue transplants; prostheses; and medical equipment and supplies. Part B also covers limited home health services that are not associated with a hospital or SNF stay. The ACA of 2010 provides for an annual physical exam (called a Wellness Exam) for all Part B enrollees, effective January 2011. The physical exam is exempt from deductibles and copayments. Part B also covers a number of preventive and screening services, such as bone mass measurement, cardiovascular screening, screening for colorectal and prostate cancer, diabetes screening, glaucoma screening, Pap smears, screening mammography, flu shots, vaccinations against pneumonia, and smoking cessation counseling. Medicare does not cover services such as routine dental care, dentures, acupuncture, hearing aids, and eyeglasses (except after cataract surgery). Exhibit 6–2 provides a summary of the Part B program.

## Part C (Medicare Advantage)

Part C is, in reality, not a new program because it does not add specifically defined

Exhibit 6–1   Medicare Part A Financing, Benefits, Deductible, and Copayments for 2011

### Financing

The Hospital Insurance trust fund is financed by a payroll tax of 1.45 percent from the employee and 1.45 percent from the employer. All income is taxed.

| | |
|---|---|
| Premiums | None<br>(Those who do not qualify for premium-free coverage can buy coverage at a monthly premium of $450) |
| Deductible | $1,132 per benefit period |

| Benefits | Copayments |
|---|---|
| Inpatient hospital (room, meals, nursing care, operating room services, blood transfusions, special care units, drugs and medical supplies, laboratory tests, rehabilitation therapies, and medical social services) | None for the first 60 days [benefit period]<br>$283 per day for days 61–90 [benefit period]<br>$566 per day for days 91–150 [nonrenewable lifetime reserve days]<br>100% of costs after 150 days |
| Skilled nursing facility (after a 3-day hospital stay) | None for the first 20 days [benefit period]<br>$141.50 per day for days 21–100 [benefit period] |
| Home health services (part-time skilled nursing care, home health aide, rehabilitation therapies, medical equipment, social services, and medical supplies) | None for home health visits<br>20% of approved amount for medical equipment |
| Hospice care | A small copayment for drugs |
| Inpatient psychiatric care (190 days lifetime limit) | Same as for inpatient hospital |

### Noncovered Services

Long-term care

Custodial services

Personal convenience services (televisions, telephones, private-duty nurses, private rooms when not medically necessary)

*Source:* Data from Centers for Medicare and Medicaid Services.

new services. It merely provides some additional choices of health plans, with the objective of channeling a greater number of beneficiaries into managed care plans. The Balanced Budget Act (BBA) of 1997 authorized the Medicare+Choice program, which took effect on January 1, 1998. The law expanded the role of private health plans, such as HMOs, PPOs, provider-sponsored organizations (PSOs), and private fee-for-service (PFFS) plans to serve Medicare beneficiaries, who could either choose to

Exhibit 6–2  Medicare Part B Financing, Benefits, Deductible, and Coinsurance for 2011

### Financing

The general tax revenues of the federal government support approximately 75 percent of the program costs. The remaining 25 percent is financed through monthly premiums paid by persons enrolled in Part B.

| | |
|---|---|
| Standard premium | $115.40 per month |
| Income-adjusted premium* | $161.50 to $369.10 annually |
| Deductible | $162 annually |
| Coinsurance | 80/20 (50/50 for outpatient mental health) |

### Main Benefits

Physician services
Emergency department services
Outpatient surgery
Diagnostic tests and laboratory services
Outpatient physical therapy, occupational therapy, and speech therapy
Outpatient mental health services
Part-time home health care
Ambulance
Renal dialysis
Artificial limbs and braces
Blood transfusions and blood components
Organ transplants
Medical equipment and supplies
Rural health clinic services
Annual physical exam
Preventive services, such as Pap smears, mammography, colorectal and prostate cancer screening, glaucoma screening, flu shots, etc.

### Noncovered Services

Dental services
Hearing aids
Eyeglasses (except after cataract surgery)
Services not related to treatment or injury

*Source:* Data from Centers for Medicare and Medicaid Services.

*For single beneficiaries whose annual incomes exceed $85,000.

enroll in Medicare+Choice or remain in the original Medicare fee-for-service program. Medicare+Choice was renamed Medicare Advantage through the passage of the MMA of 2003. In 2010, nearly one-quarter of the total Medicare beneficiaries (11.8 million) were enrolled in a Medicare Advantage plan. Virtually all beneficiaries will continue to have access to at least one plan, and the vast majority will have access to more than 10 plans in 2011 (Gold et al. 2010).

Medicare Advantage plans offer additional benefits that are not available in the original Medicare Plan. Part C enrollees also have lower out-of-pocket costs. Hence, it is a good option, particularly for lower-income Medicare beneficiaries.

The MMA of 2003 required that Medicare Advantage include special needs plans. These plans were first offered in 2005 to meet the special needs of people who were institutionalized, enrolled in both Medicare and Medicaid, or had chronic or disabling conditions. Medicare Advantage Special Needs Plans (MA-SNP) are available in limited areas. The program is designed to benefit people who have special needs and to coordinate services between Medicare and Medicaid for those enrolled in both programs.

## Part D (Prescription Drug Coverage)

Like Part B, the prescription drug program is voluntary because it requires payment of a monthly premium by those who want the coverage. The program is available to anyone, regardless of income, who has coverage under Part A or Part B. Part D was added to the existing Medicare program under the MMA of 2003 and was fully implemented in January 2006. Coverage is offered through two types of private plans approved by Medicare: (1) Stand-alone Prescription

Drug Plans that offer only drug coverage are available to those who want to stay in the original Medicare fee-for-service program. (2) Medicare Advantage Prescription Drug Plans are available to those who want to obtain all health care services through MCOs participating in Part C. Monthly premiums vary according to the beneficiaries' income and the type of plan, except that Medicare Advantage plans do not charge additional premiums for prescription drugs. The average monthly premium expected for 2011 was $40.70, an increase of 10% from $36.90 in 2010 (Hoadley et al. 2010).

The Part D program requires payment of a deductible, following which a basic level of coverage becomes available. After that, there is a coverage gap or "doughnut hole," which requires the beneficiary to pay the full cost of drugs until a defined level of spending is reached. The gap is then followed by a catastrophic level of coverage (see Exhibit 6–3). Special provisions in the program are designed to help low-income enrollees by keeping their out-of-pocket costs to a minimum.

Effective 2011, under the ACA of 2010, all Part D drugs must be covered under a manufacturer discount agreement with the CMS. Under the provisions of the new law, beneficiaries are to receive discounts on drugs while in the coverage gap. The discounts amount to 50% on brand name drugs and 7% on generic drugs. The law also requires a phaseout of the coverage gap by 2020.

## Medicare Financing and Spending

Medicare represents 13% of the federal budget and accounts for 22% of national health expenditures. Data on the sources of financing appear in Figure 6–3. Medicare

Exhibit 6–3   Medicare Part D Benefits and Individual Out-of-Pocket Costs for 2011

| | |
|---|---|
| Premiums | $40.72 per month (estimated national average)* |
| Deductible | $310 annually |

Three levels of benefits and out-of-pocket costs beyond the $250 deductible:

| | |
|---|---|
| Basic level | Medicare pays 75% of the cost of drugs until the combined total payments by the plan and the beneficiary reach $2,840 |
| Coverage gap | The beneficiary gets 50% discount on brand name drugs, 7% on generics. Coverage gap ends when the beneficiary has spent $4,550 out of pocket |
| Catastrophic level | Beneficiary pays 5% or a small copayment for the rest of the year |

**The Extra Help program**
A special part of the Medicare drug coverage program called Extra Help is designed to serve people who have low incomes and savings. This group of beneficiaries includes those who receive Medicaid or Supplemental Security Income. For those who qualify, the out-of-pocket costs are minimal.

*Actual premium varies according to income and the plan selected by the beneficiary
*Source:* Data from Centers for Medicare and Medicaid Services

Figure 6–3    Estimated Sources of Financing Medicare, 2010

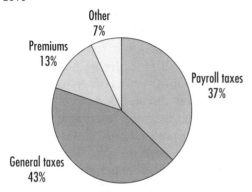

*Source:* Data from The Henry J. Kaiser Foundation, *Medicare Spending and Financing,* August 2010.

Table 6–1  Status of HI and SMI Trust Funds, 2009 (billions of dollars)

|  | HI | SMI |
| --- | --- | --- |
| Assets at the end of 2008 | $321.3 | $60.3 |
| Income | 225.4 | 282.8 |
| Disbursements | 242.5 | 266.5 |
| Net increase in assets | –17.1 | 16.3 |
| Assets at the end of 2009 | 304.2 | 76.6 |

*Source:* Social Security Administration. 2010. *A summary of the 2010 annual reports: Social Security and Medicare Board of Trustees.* Available at: http://www.ssa.gov/OACT/TRSUM/index.html.

has established two main trust funds: The HI trust fund provides the money pool for Part A services, and the SMI trust fund provides the money pool for Parts B and D. Each trust fund accounts for incomes and disbursements. Taxes, premiums, and other incomes are credited to the respective trust funds, and benefit payments and administrative costs are the only purposes for which disbursements from the funds can be made. The excess of revenues over expenditures generates interest income that stays in each fund (Social Security Administration 2010). Table 6–1 shows the trust fund results for 2010.

Projected depletion of the trust funds has been a matter of concern for quite some time. A combination of three main factors raises such concerns: (1) The cost of delivering health care continues to grow at a rate faster than the rate of inflation in the general economy. (2) An aging population will consume a greater quantity of health care services. (3) The workforce is shrinking, and wage increases to support tax revenues are smaller than the rise in medical inflation.

The HI trust fund fails to meet the tests for both short-range and long-range financial adequacy. By 2029, the fund is expected to cover just 85% of the HI costs. The SMI trust fund, on the other hand, is expected to remain adequately financed into the indefinite future (Social Security Administration 2010).

The distribution of Medicare payments to various providers under HI and SMI funding is shown in Figure 6–4. Data on enrolled population and expenditures are given in Exhibit 6–4. Data for 2007 reflect the increased proportion of national health expenditures consumed by Medicare because of Part D. This trend appears to be on the rise. More recent data suggest that, in 2009, total Medicare expenditures amounted to $502.3 billion, which is 20.2% of national health expenditures (Martin et al. 2011). The ACA of 2010 provides for a new Independent Payment Advisory Board to be responsible for containing the growth in Medicare spending. The new law also established the Center for Medicare and Medicaid Innovation and provided $10 billion over

Figure 6–4　Percentage Distribution of Medicare Payments, 2007

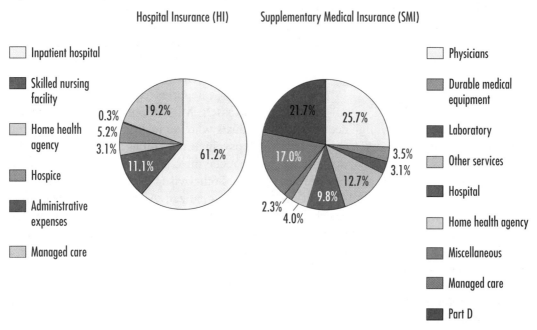

Source: Data from *Health, United States, 2009*, pp. 426–27, National Center for Health Statistics.
Note: The "other services" category under SMI includes freestanding surgery centers, freestanding dialysis centers, ambulance services, outpatient rehabilitation facilities, psychiatric facilities, rural health clinics, and community health centers.

Exhibit 6–4　Medicare: Enrolled Population and Expenditures in Selected Years

| Population Covered (in millions) | | | | |
|---|---|---|---|---|
| 1970 | 1980 | 1990 | 2000 | 2007 |
| 20.4 | 28.4 | 34.3 | 39.7 | 44.3 |
| Expenditures (in billions) | | | | |
| $7.5 | $36.8 | $111.00 | $221.8 | $431.7 |
| Proportion of Total US Health Care Expenditures | | | | |
| 10.0% | 14.5% | 15.5% | 16.4% | 19.3% |

Source: Data from *Health, United States, 2000*, pp. 325, 348; *Health, United States, 2009*, pp. 396, 426. National Center for Health Statistics.

10 years for the center to test innovative payment and service delivery models to reduce program expenditures, while preserving or enhancing the quality of care furnished to Medicare and Medicaid beneficiaries.

## Medicare Out-of-Pocket Costs

Medicare carries relatively high deductibles, copayments, and premiums (see Exhibits 6–1, 6–2, and 6–3). Eyeglasses, dental care, and many long-term care services are not covered, and there is no limit on out-of-pocket expenses, except that about half of Medicare Advantage plans have such limits. Hence, most Medicare beneficiaries are left with high out-of-pocket costs. Medicaid (provided the beneficiary qualifies), employer retirement benefits, and purchase of private supplemental insurance are some ways to pay for some of these out-of-pocket costs. Still, in 2005, Medicare beneficiaries spent an average of $4,394 of their own money; 10% of the beneficiaries spent more than $8,000 (Nonnemaker and Sinclair 2009). The median out-of-pocket spending amounts to 16.2% of the beneficiaries' income (The Henry J. Kaiser Family Foundation 2010a).

## Medicaid

Medicaid, also referred to as Title 19 of the Social Security Act, finances health care services for the indigent; however, Medicaid does not provide medical assistance for all poor persons. Certain categories of people are automatically eligible under federal guidelines: (1) Families with children receiving support under the Temporary Assistance for Needy Families (TANF) program. (2) People receiving Supplemental Security Income (SSI), which includes many of the elderly, the blind, and the disabled with low incomes. (3) Children and pregnant women whose family income is at or below 133% of the FPL. (4) Other categories defined by federal law. In addition, most states, at their discretion, have defined other "medically needy" categories based on people's income and assets. Most important of these are individuals who are institutionalized in nursing or psychiatric facilities and individuals who are receiving community-based services but would otherwise be eligible for Medicaid if institutionalized. All of these people have to qualify based on assets and income, which must be below the threshold levels established by each state. Hence, Medicaid is a *means-tested program*.

The ACA of 2010 requires US states to greatly expand Medicaid eligibility by removing many of the existing restrictions. Beginning 2014, when the law is expected to be fully implemented, states must cover everyone under age 65 with income up to 133% of FPL. Hence, the law envisions Medicaid to become the coverage pathway for low-income people in the national framework for universal health insurance (The Henry J. Kaiser Family Foundation 2010b). The law also requires states to deliver integrated "health home" services in which a Medicaid beneficiary who has chronic conditions can designate a provider as a health home.

All US states; the District of Columbia; and US territories, such as Guam, Puerto Rico, American Samoa, and the Virgin Islands, operate Medicaid plans. Each state administers its own Medicaid program. Hence, eligibility criteria, covered services, and payments to providers vary considerably from state to state. However, for a state to receive federal matching funds, federal law mandates that every state provide some specific basic health services (see Exhibit 6–5).

**Exhibit 6–5** Federally Mandated Services for State Medicaid Programs

- Inpatient hospital services
- Hospital outpatient services
- Physician services
- Federally qualified health center services
- Rural health clinic services
- Outpatient laboratory and X-ray services
- Nursing facility services for beneficiaries age 21 and older
- Home health services for those eligible for nursing facility services, including medical supplies and equipment
- Certified pediatric and family nurse practitioner services (when licensed to practice under state law)
- Nurse–midwife services
- Medical and surgical services of a dentist
- Preventive, diagnosis, and treatment services (including vaccinations) for children
- Family planning services and supplies
- Pregnancy-related services, including postpartum care for 60 days

*Source:* Adapted from Smith, G.A. 2007. *A primer on how to use Medicaid to assist persons who are homeless to access medical, behavioral health and support services.* Baltimore, MD: Centers for Medicare and Medicaid Services.

In addition, states may also receive federal matching funds for providing certain optional services, such as prescription drugs and prostheses, optometrist services and eyeglasses, transportation services, rehabilitation, home and community-based care for people with chronic impairments, and services in intermediate care facilities for the mentally retarded (ICF/MR). States may impose nominal deductibles and copayments on some Medicaid recipients for certain services, but some exclusions exist. Emergency services, family planning services and supplies, and hospice care are exempt from copayments.

Changes to Medicaid benefits were legislated under the Deficit Reduction Act of 2005. The law required states to institute premium and cost sharing based on income.

## Medicaid Financing and Spending

The federal and state governments jointly finance the Medicaid program. The federal government provides matching funds to the states based on the per capita income in each state. By law, federal matching—known as the Federal Medical Assistance Percentage (FMAP)—cannot be less than 50% nor greater than 83% of total state Medicaid program costs. Wealthier states have a smaller share of their costs reimbursed by the federal government. For the federal fiscal year 2011, Congress established the FMAPs from 50% for approximately 14 states to 74.7% for Mississippi (Federal Register 2009).

The Medicaid program serves approximately 60 million low-income Americans. Figure 6–5 presents the main characteristics of people covered by Medicaid. The pie chart on the left gives the proportion of recipients in each classification; the one on the right gives the proportion of payments made to health care providers on behalf of each category of recipient. Notice that children under 21 years of age, who constitute a little less than half of all Medicaid recipients, incur almost 19% of total expenditures. The blind and disabled constitute approximately 14% of the recipients but incur 43% of all expenditures. Also, the elderly, who constitute less than 8% of all recipients, incur nearly 22%

Figure 6–5  Medicaid Recipients and Medical Vendor Payments According to Basis of Eligibility, 2006 Data.

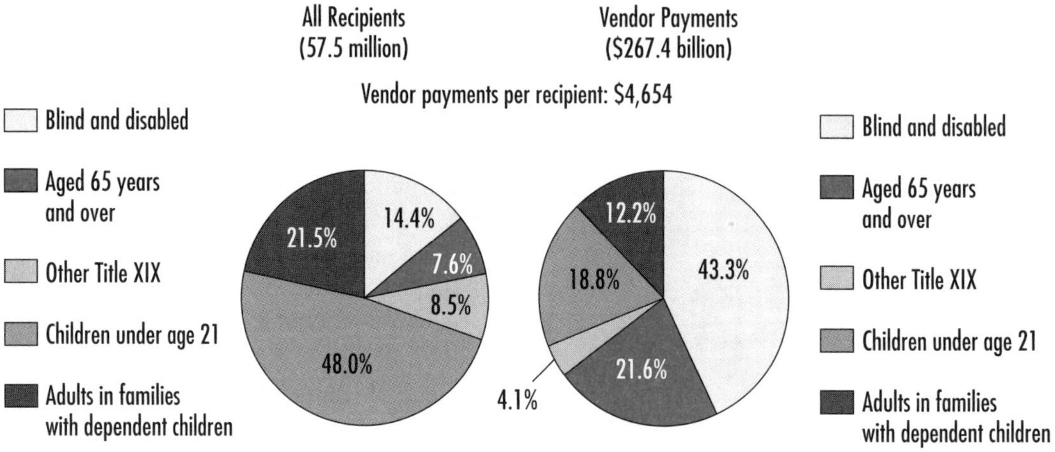

**All Recipients**
**(57.5 million)**

**Vendor Payments**
**($267.4 billion)**

Vendor payments per recipient: $4,654

- Blind and disabled
- Aged 65 years and over
- Other Title XIX
- Children under age 21
- Adults in families with dependent children

All Recipients pie: 14.4%, 7.6%, 8.5%, 48.0%, 4.1%, 21.5%

Vendor Payments pie: 12.2%, 43.3%, 21.6%, 18.8%

- Blind and disabled
- Aged 65 years and over
- Other Title XIX
- Children under age 21
- Adults in families with dependent children

*Source:* Data from *Health, United States, 2009*, p. 431, National Center for Health Statistics.

of the expenses. Medicaid paid almost 44% of all expenses for nursing home care, a service mostly used by the elderly (National Center for Health Statistics 2010).

Medicaid enrollment and spending vary according to the state of the US economy. For example, the level of spending rose at an annual rate of 12% between 2000 and 2002 and moderated down to 7.6% from 2002 to 2004 as the economy improved following the 2001 recession (The Kaiser Commission on Medicaid and the Uninsured 2006). From 2008 to 2009, amid rising unemployment and a severe recession, the rate of growth in Medicaid spending increased from 4.9% to 9.0% (Martin et al. 2011).

Managed care enrollment has been increasingly used to control costs. According to data from the CMS, in 2009, almost 72% of the beneficiaries were enrolled in managed care. In 2009, at least 10 states had 90% or more of their Medicaid recipients enrolled in managed care plans.

Exhibit 6–6 provides data on enrolled population, including children under the age of 21, and expenditures. Table 6–2 shows proportional payments to the various types of vendors providing services to Medicaid recipients. The shift toward the delivery of medical services through managed care is clearly seen. There also has been a shift from nursing home care to delivery of services through community-based long-term care programs.

## Main Distinctions and Relationships Between Medicare and Medicaid

Although Medicare and Medicaid may both be loosely referred to as entitlement programs, technically, there is an important distinction between the two. Similar to Social Security, Medicare is an *entitlement* program. Because people have contributed to Medicare through taxes, they are "entitled" to the benefits regardless of the amount of

Exhibit 6–6  Medicaid: Population Covered and Expenditures in Selected Years

| Population Covered (in millions) | | | | |
|---|---|---|---|---|
| 1970 | 1980 | 1990 | 2000 | 2006 |
| 17.6 | 21.6 | 25.3 | 42.8 | 57.5 |
| Number of Under Age 21 Children Covered (in millions) | | | | |
| | 9.3 | 11.2 | 19.7 | 27.6 |
| Expenditures (in billions) | | | | |
| $5.4 | $26.4 | $74.8 | $204.8 | $319.0 |
| Proportion of Total US Health Care Expenditures | | | | |
| 7.2% | 10.7% | 10.5% | 15.1% | 15.1% |

*Source:* Data from *Health, United States, 1998*, pp. 346, 348, 369; *Health, United States, 2009*, pp. 396, 411, 431. National Center for Health Statistics.

income and assets they may have. Medicare beneficiaries are, specifically, given the legal right to enforce in federal courts, if necessary, their eligibility and access to services (Jost 2003). Medicaid, on the other hand, is a welfare program to assist the indigent with their medical needs. Unlike Medicare, individual Medicaid beneficiaries cannot enforce their rights through legal action.

Medicare beneficiaries who have low incomes and limited resources may also receive help from the Medicaid program. For the elderly and disabled who qualify for Medicaid, the program pays their Medicare premiums, deductibles, and copayments. For such dually covered persons, Medicaid is the payer of last resort, that is, the Medicare program pays for any services covered under Medicare before Medicaid kicks in. In 2007, beneficiaries with dual eligibility accounted for 15% of Medicaid enrollment (Rousseau

et al. 2010). Dual-eligible beneficiaries are covered under two separate programs. Under the Qualified Medicare Beneficiary (QMB) program, Medicaid picks up Medicare Part A and Part B premiums, as well as all deductibles and copayments. Depending on the state's Medicaid guidelines, beneficiaries may also qualify for full Medicaid benefits, which about half actually do. The QMB program covers individuals whose incomes are at, or below, the FPL. The second program, Specified Low-Income Medicare Beneficiary (SLMB) program, pays only the Part B premiums for people whose incomes are higher than the Medicaid threshold but no more than 120% of the FPL. Two additional, but less important, programs are also available to low-income or disabled people. The qualified individual (QI) program provides states with block grants to pay Medicare premiums for individuals with incomes

Table 6–2  Proportional Medicaid Vendor Payments, Selected Years

|  | 1995 | 2000 | 2006 |
| --- | --- | --- | --- |
| Nursing facilities | 24.2 | 20.5 | 17.0 |
| Managed care and other prepaid care | ... | 14.5 | 18.8 |
| Inpatient hospital | 21.9 | 14.4 | 13.5 |
| Prescribed drugs | 8.1 | 11.9 | 10.4 |
| Personal support | ... | 6.9 | 8.0 |
| Intermediate care facilities/ Mentally retarded | 8.6 | 5.6 | 4.4 |
| Outpatient hospital services | 5.5 | 4.2 | 3.8 |
| Physicians | 6.1 | 4.0 | 3.9 |
| Clinic | 3.6 | 3.7 | 3.2 |
| Home health | 7.8 | 1.9 | 2.2 |
| Mental health facility | 2.1 | 1.1 | 0.9 |
| Dental | 0.8 | 0.8 | 1.2 |
| Miscellaneous | 11.1 | 10.1 | 12.7 |

Total payments: 1995    $120.1 billion
                2000    168.3 billion
                2006    267.4 billion

*Source:* Data from *Health, United States, 2009,* p. 432, and National Center for Health Statistics.

between 120 and 135% of the FPL. Under this program, qualified people are served on a first-come first-served basis until the available funds are exhausted. Under the Qualified Disabled and Working Individual (QDWI) program, states are required to pay Part A premiums for certain low-income people who qualified for Medicare because of disability but were able to return to work and lost the entitlement.

## Public Programs Initiated Under the Balanced Budget Act of 1997

### PACE

A program that spans both Medicare and Medicaid is the Program of All-Inclusive Care for the Elderly (PACE), but it is not available in all states. PACE provides community-based care for persons aged 55 years or older who otherwise qualify for placement in a nursing facility. The care is provided in day-care centers, homes, hospitals, and nursing homes. Chapter 10 provides further details.

### CHIP

The Children's Health Insurance Program (CHIP), codified as Title 21 of the Social Security Act, is another program enacted under the BBA of 1997. The program was initiated in response to the plight of uninsured children, who were estimated to number 10.1 million (nearly one-quarter of all uninsured) in 1996 and whose families' incomes exceeded the Medicaid threshold levels, which made them ineligible for Medicaid coverage.

The program offers federal funds in the form of set block grants to states. To cover children up to 18 years of age, a state can expand its existing Medicaid program, establish a separate program for children, or use a combined approach. Federal law requires that ineligibility for Medicaid be established before approval for CHIP coverage. Within federal guidelines, each state establishes eligibility criteria for CHIP. Most states cover children in families with incomes up to or above 200% of the FPL, provided the children are not covered under another private or public health insurance program. CHIP does not cover parents or adults.

Research has shown that CHIP has had a significant impact in reducing uninsurance among children (Hudson 2005). CHIP has also been credited with improved access, continuity of care, and quality of care for all racial/ethnic groups, as well as a reduction in preexisting racial/ethnic disparities in access, unmet need, and continuity of care (Shone et al. 2005).

The ACA of 2010 extends the authorization of CHIP through September 30, 2015. The law requires states to maintain current income eligibility levels through September 30, 2019. States are prohibited from implementing eligibility standards, methodologies, or procedures that are more restrictive than those in place as of March 23, 2010, with the exception of waiting lists for enrolling children in CHIP.

## The Military Health Services System

The United States Department of Defense operates a substantial program to provide medical services to active duty and retired members of the armed forces, their dependents, and their survivors through the Military Health Services System (MHSS). The MHSS is equipped to provide medical care worldwide. It operates 59 hospitals and 364 clinics to serve an eligible population of 9.6 million at an annual budget of $50 billion, according to the Department of Defense. These hospitals and clinics are mainly for active-duty service members, but dependents of service members, retirees and their dependents, and survivors of deceased members can also obtain services at military facilities if space is available. Otherwise, they can receive medical care under a program known as TriCare (previously called CHAMPUS).

The TriCare program was developed in response to the growing health care needs of military personnel, an increasing number of whom are retirees. Closing of military bases and other downsizing efforts in the mid-1990s during the Clinton Administration, resulted in the closure of 35% of the military hospitals that existed in the United States in 1987. Yet, the total number of people seeking health care through the MHSS dropped by only 9%. Consequently, military facilities no longer had the capacity to meet the demand for health care (Department of Defense 1996).

TriCare has three main features: (1) It is regionally managed to facilitate administration of the program; (2) it is structured after managed care; and (3) it brings together the medical resources of the army, navy, and air force and supplements them with networks of civilian health care professionals and facilities. There are 11 TriCare regions in the United States, plus TriCare Europe, TriCare Latin America, and TriCare Pacific.

For elderly beneficiaries enrolled in Medicare Part B, TriCare for Life (TFL) serves as a second payer to Medicare, paying out-of-pocket costs for services covered under Medicare. The program also provides benefits not covered by Medicare but covered by TriCare (Best 2005).

## Veterans Health Administration

Formerly called Veterans Administration, VA is an executive department of the US government. Veterans Health Administration (VHA), the health services branch of the VA, operates the largest integrated health services system in the United States, with approximately 153 hospitals, 956 outpatient clinics, 134 community living centers (nursing homes), and various other facilities. In all, the VHA provides care to nearly 6 million veterans through more than 1400 sites throughout the nation. VHA employs a staff of 255,000 and maintains affiliations with 107 academic health systems. More than 65% of all physicians in the United States have received their training in VA facilities (Department of Veterans Affairs 2010).

The VA health care system was originally established to treat veterans with war-related injuries and to help rehabilitate past service members with war-related disabilities. This original mission was expanded, and nonservice-related conditions account for the bulk of the care provided because poor veterans with medical conditions unrelated to military combat services increasingly use the system. Almost 60% of the veterans served by VHA have no service-connected disabilities (National Center for Health Statistics 2010). However, Congress requires VHA to provide services on a priority basis to veterans with service-connected illnesses and disabilities, low incomes, or special health care needs. Eligible veterans are classified into one of eight priority groups upon enrollment. Priority Group 1 receives the highest priority: these veterans have service-connected disabilities rated as 50% or more disabling. Apart from delivering health care services, the VHA system also actively participates in medical education and research.

In 2009, the veteran population was over 23 million. The median age of all veterans was 61 years (Department of Veterans Affairs 2010). Each year, a growing number of veterans use VA medical services.

The VA is a tax-financed agency that, for the most part, delivers care directly through salaried physicians and government-owned facilities. Funding for the VHA program is appropriated in the annual presidential budget approved by Congress. The structure of VA funding is patterned after the global budget model in which budget appropriations are determined in advance for the entire system. The VHA then distributes the funds to its organizational units having oversight for the delivery of health care.

The VHA administers the delivery of health services through 21 geographically distributed Veterans Integrated Service Networks (VISNs). Each VISN is responsible for coordinating the activities of the hospitals, outpatient clinics, nursing homes, and other facilities located within its jurisdiction. Each VISN is also responsible for allocating resources among the facilities in its prescribed geographic area to ensure care and equitable access within the network. Another role of the VISNs is to improve efficiency by reducing duplicate services and consolidating medical facilities and programs. Since 1995, when the system was organized according to VISNs, the VHA has gradually moved to an outpatient model of care in which more than 1400 sites deliver services in communities where the veterans live. The system focuses on health promotion and disease prevention and on meeting the chronic care needs of an aging veteran population (Department of Veterans Affairs 2010). Despite its many successes, however, the system suffers from capacity and financing constraints, which result in lack of access and timely care for many veterans.

The VA also operates a health care benefits program for the eligible dependents of veterans. The program is called CHAMP-VA, which covers (1) dependents of permanently disabled veterans and (2) survivors of veterans who died in the line of duty, died from service-related conditions, or were permanently disabled at the time of death.

## Indian Health Service

The federal program administered by the Indian Health Service (IHS), a division of the DHHS, provides comprehensive health care services directly to members of federally recognized American Indian and Alaska Native Tribes and their descendants. American Indians and Alaska Natives, as citizens of the United States, are eligible to participate in all public, private, and state health programs available to the general population. However, for many Indians, IHS-supported programs are the only source of health care because no alternative sources of medical care are available, especially in isolated areas. IHS programs serve 1.9 million American Indians and Alaska Natives residing on or near reservations and in rural communities. The 2010 budget for services was over $4 billion.

Besides medical and dental care, services include health promotion and disease prevention and programs in substance abuse, maternal and child health, sanitation, and nutrition. The IHS system includes 29 hospitals, 59 health centers, and 28 health stations. Additional services are contracted from tribally operated health programs and private providers (IHS 2010). Additional details on IHS are presented in Chapter 11.

## Miscellaneous Private and Public Programs

### Medigap

As previously mentioned, Medicare beneficiaries incur high out-of-pocket expenses. Beneficiaries who do not have other options to cover these expenses can purchase a private supplemental plan called *Medigap.*

Medigap policies cover all or a portion of Medicare deductibles and copayments, and they may pay for services not covered by Medicare. To protect consumer interests and to simplify plan selection, the Omnibus Budget Reconciliation Act of 1990 mandated that Medicare designate standardized plan categories containing uniform benefits from which consumers could choose. There are 11 standard plans that are available in most states. These plans are labeled A through G and K through N. The most common out-of-pocket costs covered by most plans include hospital copayments, hospital deductibles, and skilled nursing facility copayments. Premiums vary according to the plan selected and the insurance company selling the plan.

### Workers' Compensation

The theory underlying workers' compensation is that all accidents that occur during the course of employment and all illnesses directly attributable to the workplace must be regarded as risks of industry. In other words, the employer is financially liable for the full cost of such injuries and illnesses regardless of who is at fault. Since workers' compensation is a state-administered program, financing and benefits vary among states. There are four categories of benefits: (1) cash payment for lost wages, (2) payment for medical treatment, (3) indemnification for loss of occupational capacity and skills, and (4) survivors' death benefits. Employers finance these benefits through one of three mechanisms: private insurance, a state fund to which the employers contribute, or self-insurance.

Federal programs cover only specific categories of workers. The Federal Employees' Compensation Act, administered by the Office of Workers' Compensation Programs, covers civilian employees of the federal government. The Longshore and Harbor Workers' Compensation Act provides benefits to approximately 500,000 workers when they are injured, disabled, or contract an occupational disease occurring on the navigable waters of the United States. The Black Lung Benefits program covers coal miners who are totally disabled from black lung disease (pneumoconiosis) (US Department of Labor 2006).

Workers' compensation is not a regular health insurance program, although it provides a significant amount of medical benefits. The medical component may account for 50% or more of workers' compensation costs (Harty 2005). Nearly all standard employer-sponsored health insurance programs contain provisions that exclude coverage for medical care for work-related accidents and illnesses to avoid duplicate payments by both the medical plan and workers' compensation (Whitted 1993). Managed care and physician networks specializing in workers' compensation are increasingly used to contain medical costs for worker's compensation beneficiaries.

## Other Public Programs

In addition to Medicaid, Medicare, MHSS, TriCare, VHA, CHAMPVA, and IHS programs, the government acts as financier and provider for other types of services. Such programs are administered mainly by state and local governments and are limited in scope. Notable among these programs are state mental hospitals, general hospitals operated by county and municipal governments (discussed in Chapter 8), and community health centers and public health services (discussed in Chapter 7).

## The Payment Function

Insurance companies, MCOs, Blue Cross/Blue Shield, and the government (for Medicare and Medicaid) are referred to as *third-party payers*, the other two parties being the patient and the provider. The payment function has two main facets: (1) the determination of the methods and amounts of reimbursement for the delivery of services and (2) the actual payment after services have been rendered. The set fee for a service is commonly referred to as a charge or rate. Technically, a *charge* is a fee set by the provider, which is akin to price in general commerce. A *rate* is a price set by a third-party payer. An index of charges listing individual fees for each type of service is referred to as a *fee schedule*. In general, to receive payment for services rendered, the provider must file a *claim* with the third-party payer. For the sake of simplicity, in this section, we refer to the determination of rates as "reimbursement" and to the payment of claims as "disbursement."

## Reimbursement Methods

Various methods for determining how much providers should be paid are in use. Traditionally, providers have preferred the fee-for-service method, which has fallen out of favor with payers because of cost escalations. Private payers, as well as the government, have devised various methods aimed at limiting the amount of reimbursement, but the main thrust for devising innovative reimbursement methods has come from Medicare. The reimbursement methods subsequently discussed are all in use, depending on the nature of service. Physicians, dentists, optometrists, therapists, hospitals, nursing facilities, and so on may be paid according to different reimbursement mechanisms. For many providers, however, methods adopted by managed care and prospective payment methods have become more common.

## Fee for Service

Fee-for-service reimbursement is based on the assumption that health care is provided in a set of identifiable and individually distinct units of services, such as examination, X-ray, urinalysis, and a tetanus shot, in the case of physician services. For surgery, such individual services may include an admission kit, numerous medical supplies each accounted for separately, surgeon's fees, anesthesia, anesthesiologist's fees, recovery room charges, and so forth. Each of these services is separately itemized on one bill, and there can be more than one bill. For example, the hospital, the surgeon, the pathologist, and the anesthesiologist bill for their services separately.

Initially, providers set fee-for-service charges, and insurers passively paid the claims. Later, insurers started to limit reimbursement to a usual, customary, and reasonable (UCR) amount. Each insurer determined on its own what the UCR charge should be, through community or statewide surveys of what providers were charging. If the actual charges exceeded the UCR amount, then reimbursement from insurers was limited to the UCR amount. Providers then *balance billed*, that is, asked the patients to pay the difference between the actual charges and the payments received from insurers.

The main problem under fee-for-service arrangements is that providers have an incentive to deliver additional services that are not essential. Providers can increase their incomes by increasing the volume of services. However, dentists, therapists, and some physicians continue to receive payment according to fee for service.

## Bundled Charges (Package Pricing)

Fee for service essentially pays for unbundled services. Bundled-fee, or package pricing, includes a number of related services in one price. For example, optometrists sometimes advertise package prices that include the charges for eye exams, frames for eyeglasses, and corrective lenses. The various prospective payment systems of reimbursement are also examples of payments for bundled services.

## Resource-Based Relative Value Scale

Under the Omnibus Budget Reconciliation Act of 1989 (OBRA-89), Medicare developed a new initiative to reimburse physicians according to a "relative value" assigned to each physician service. The resource-based relative value scale (RBRVS) was implemented in 1992. Prior to this date, physician services under Part B were reimbursed according to fee for service. Over the years, third-party payers other than Medicare have also adopted variations of RBRVS.

RBRVS incorporates *relative value units* (RVUs) based on the time, skill, and intensity (physician work) it takes to provide a service. Hence, RVUs reflect resource inputs—time, effort, and expertise—to deliver a service. RVUs are established for different types of services that are identified by their *Current Procedural Terminology* (CPT) codes—a standard coding system for physician services developed by the AMA. For each CPT, in addition to RVUs associated with physician work, separate RVUs are included for the cost of practice (overhead costs) and for malpractice insurance. Because of geographic cost variations, each of the RVU categories is multiplied by its own geographic adjustment factor (Geographic Practice Cost Index). Finally, for each year's Medicare budget for physician payments, a conversion factor (CF) is established. The payment for each CPT equals its RVU × CF. Medicare establishes a national *Medicare Physician Fee Schedule* (MPFS), a price list for physician services, based on which individual payments are made when physicians file their claims.

## Managed Care Approaches

MCOs have concentrated on three main approaches. The first is the preferred-provider approach, which may be regarded as a variation of fee for service. The main distinction is that an MCO establishes fee schedules based on discounts negotiated with providers. The second mechanism for reimbursing providers is called *capitation*. The provider is paid a set monthly fee per enrollee (sometimes referred to as per member per month, or PMPM, rate). The fixed monthly fee (PMPM rate × number of enrollees) is paid to the provider regardless of how often the enrollees receive medical services from the provider. Capitation removes the incentive for providers to increase the volume of services to generate additional revenues. It also makes providers prudent in providing only necessary services. Salary is the third method used by some MCOs that employ their own physicians.

## Cost-Plus Reimbursement

Cost-plus was the traditional method used by Medicare and Medicaid to establish *per diem* (daily) rates for inpatient stays in hospitals, nursing homes, and other institutions. Home health services were also reimbursed based on cost. Under the cost-plus method, reimbursement rates for institutions are based on the total costs incurred in operating the institution. The institution is required to submit a cost report to the third-party payer. Complex formulas are developed, designating certain costs as "nonallowable" and placing cost ceilings in other areas. The formulas are used to calculate the *per diem* reimbursement rate, also referred to as a per-patient-day (PPD) rate. The method is called *cost-plus* because, in addition to the total operating costs, the reimbursement formula also allows a portion of the capital costs in arriving at the PPD rate. Because the reimbursement methodology sets rates after evaluating the costs retrospectively, this mechanism is broadly referred to as *retrospective reimbursement*.

Under the cost-plus system, total reimbursement is directly related to length of stay, services rendered, and cost of providing the services. Providers have an incentive to provide services indiscriminately, thus increasing costs. There is little motivation for efficiency and cost containment in the delivery of services. Paradoxically, health care institutions could increase their profits by increasing costs. Because of the perverse financial incentives inherent in retrospective cost-based reimbursement, it has been largely replaced by various prospective reimbursement methods, except the federal critical access hospital program continues to allow certain rural hospitals to be paid under the cost-plus reimbursement system.

## Prospective Reimbursement

In contrast to retrospective reimbursement, where historical costs are used to determine the amount to be paid, *prospective reimbursement* uses certain established criteria to determine the amount of reimbursement in advance, before services are delivered. Prospective reimbursement not only minimizes some of the abuses inherent in cost-plus approaches, but it also enables providers, such as Medicare, to better predict future health care spending.

Medicare has been using the prospective payment system (PPS) to reimburse inpatient hospital acute care services under Medicare Part A since 1983. Subsequently, the BBA of 1997 mandated implementation of a PPS for hospital outpatient services and postacute care providers, such as SNFs, home health agencies, and inpatient rehabilitation facilities.

Depending on the type of service setting, the three main prospective reimbursement methods, discussed in the subsequent sections, are based on diagnosis-related groups (DRGs), ambulatory payment classification (APC), case-mix methods, and home health resource groups (HHRGs).

In January 2005, Medicare implemented a prospective payment system, using a modified DRG approach, for inpatient psychiatric facilities that had previously been paid according to the cost-plus methodology. The initiative was authorized under the Balanced Budget Refinement Act of 1999. The change affected all of the nearly 2000 freestanding psychiatric hospitals and certified psychiatric units located in general hospitals. The program, phased over a 3-year period, was implemented in 2008.

## Diagnosis-Related Groups

The PPS for hospital inpatient reimbursement was enacted under the Social Security Amendments of 1983. The predetermined reimbursement amount is set according to DRGs. Each DRG groups together principal diagnoses that have similar hospital resource use. The approximately 500 DRGs correspond to the most prevalent diagnoses among patients using acute-care inpatient services. The amount of payment is set per discharge rather than *per diem*. Hence, reimbursement rates are established for bundled services. The bundle of services consists of whatever medical care the patient requires for a given principal diagnosis at the time of admission to an acute-care hospital. The hospital receives the predetermined fixed rate for the particular DRG classification.

The primary factor governing the amount of reimbursement is the type of case, but additional factors can create differences in reimbursement for the same DRG. Such factors include differences in wage levels in various geographic areas; location of the hospital in urban versus rural areas; whether or not the institution is a teaching hospital, that is, it has residency programs for medical graduates (adjustments in reimbursement are based on the intensity of teaching); and whether a location treats a disproportionately large share of low-income patients (HCFA 1996). The latter provision was authorized by Congress under the Consolidated Omnibus Budget Reconciliation Act of 1985 (COBRA) to support "safety net" hospitals (also called disproportionate share hospitals) in inner cities and rural areas, many of which would otherwise have been forced to close, leaving underserved and uninsured persons without access to hospital care (Davis and Burner 1995). Additional payments are made for cases that involve extremely long hospital stays or are extremely expensive, which are referred to as *outliers*.

Inpatient psychiatric facilities receive a *per diem* rate rather than a case-specific rate, based on psychiatric DRGs. The program also includes a stop-loss provision to protect psychiatric hospitals against significant losses. In other respects, the factors considered in arriving at reimbursement rates are similar to those used for reimbursing acute-care hospitals. In 2003, long-term care hospitals (hospitals serving complex postacute cases) were brought under PPS reimbursement.

The prospective rate-setting methodology enabled Medicare to control the growth in Part A hospital expenditures. By keeping the actual costs of services below the fixed reimbursement amount, a hospital gets to keep the difference as profit. A hospital loses money when its costs exceed the prospective reimbursement rate. Initially, concerns were voiced that hospitals may discharge patients too early or underprovide necessary services. However, an interplay of several factors, such as competition among hospitals to attract patients, quality improvement initiatives, internal ethics committees, external peer review organizations, and emergence of postacute care services, such as home health and subacute care for post-discharge continuity of care, mitigated such concerns.

## Outpatient Prospective Payment System

In August 2000, the Medicare's Outpatient Prospective Payment System (OPPS) was implemented to pay for services provided by hospital outpatient departments. Main services included in OPPS are outpatient surgeries, radiology and other diagnostic procedures, clinic visits, and emergency services. Ambulatory payment classification (APC) divides all outpatient services into more than 300 procedural groups. The services within each group are clinically similar and require comparable resources.

Each APC is assigned a relative payment weight based on the median cost of services within the APC. The reimbursement rates are adjusted for geographic variation in wages. APC reimbursement is a bundled rate that includes services such as anesthesia, certain drugs, supplies, and recovery room charges in a packaged price established by Medicare.

In January 2008, Medicare implemented the OPPS to pay for facility services, such as nursing, recovery care, anesthetics, drugs, and other supplies, in freestanding (i.e., nonhospital) ambulatory surgery centers. The most common procedures performed in these centers are eye procedures, such as cataract removal and lens replacement, and colonoscopy. Physician services are reimbursed separately under the Physician Fee Schedule based on RBRVS (MedPAC 2009).

## Case-Mix Methods

*Case mix* is an aggregate of the severity of conditions requiring clinical intervention. Case-mix categories are mutually exclusive and differentiate patients according to the extent of resource use. On a case-mix index, higher score categories comprise patients who have more severe conditions than those in lower score categories. A comprehensive assessment of each patient's condition determines the case mix for an inpatient facility. Patients who require similar levels of services are then categorized into groups that are relatively uniform according to resource consumption.

### Resource Utilization Groups    The Medicare program has adopted a case-mix method to

reimburse SNFs, replacing the old cost-based reimbursement method. Implemented in July 1998, the PPS provides for a *per diem* prospective rate based on the intensity of care needed by patients in an SNF. The case mix is determined through a comprehensive assessment of each patient, using an assessment instrument called the Minimum Data Set (MDS). The MDS consists of a core set of screening elements used to assess the clinical, functional, and psychosocial needs of each patient admitted to an SNF. Using MDS data, a classification system, called resource utilization groups, version 3 (RUG-III), was designed to differentiate patients by their levels of resource use (an updated version, RUG-IV, was scheduled for implementation in 2011). Among the variables used to differentiate resource utilization are patient characteristics, such as principal diagnosis, functional limitations, cognitive patterns, psychological condition, skin problems, bladder and bowel function, nutritional status, and special treatments and procedures needed. RUG-III classifies patients into 53 categories according to their health care needs. The aim of RUG-III–based PPS is to ensure that Medicare payments are related to the care requirements of the patient and are made equitably to SNFs with different patient caseloads. The *per diem* rate is all-inclusive, meaning it includes payment for all covered SNF services provided in a nursing facility. Adjustments to the PPS rate are made for differences in wages prevailing in various geographic areas and for facility location in urban versus rural areas.

Case-Mix Groups    As of January 2002, inpatient rehabilitation facilities (rehabilitation hospitals and distinctly certified rehabilitation units in general hospitals) are reimbursed according to case-mix groups (CMGs). Each patient must undergo a patient assessment at admission and discharge. Based on information from the assessment, the patient is assigned to one of the intensive rehabilitation categories, based on the primary reason for rehabilitation, such as stroke or burns, age, functional level, cognitive impairment, etc. Patients are further categorized into one of four tiers, based on any comorbidities (multiple health problems). Each tier has a specific reimbursement rate associated with it. Length of stay is also taken into account in determining the level of reimbursement (MedPAC 2008a).

## Home Health Resource Groups

Implemented in October 2000, the PPS for home health pays a fixed, predetermined rate for each 60-day episode of care regardless of the specific services delivered. Thus, all services provided by a home health agency are bundled under one payment made on a per-patient basis, except the costs of any durable medical equipment (DME) are not included in the bundled rate. To capture the expected resource use, patients are assigned to 1 of the 153 HHRGs, based on clinical and functional status and service use, which is measured by the Outcome and Assessment Information Set (OASIS). The HHRGs range from groups of relatively uncomplicated patients to those who have severe medical conditions, severe functional limitations, or need extensive therapy. If a patient received fewer than five visits during a 60-day episode, the home health agency is paid per visit based on the type of visit (MedPAC 2008b).

## Disbursement of Funds

After services have been delivered, some agency has to perform the administrative task of verifying and paying the claims received from the providers or, in some cases, indemnifying the patients. Disbursement of funds (claims processing) is carried out in accordance with the reimbursement policy adopted by the particular program. Commercial insurance companies and MCOs have their own claims departments to process payments to providers. Self-insured employers typically contract the services of a *third-party administrator* (TPA) to process and pay claims. The TPA may also monitor utilization and perform other oversight functions. The government contracts with third parties in the private sector to process Medicare and Medicaid claims. These contractors include Blue Cross/Blue Shield and commercial insurance companies. While *fiscal intermediaries* process Part A claims, Medicare refers to claims processors for Part B services as *carriers*. These are also Blue Cross/Blue Shield and commercial insurance companies. Even though Medicare makes a technical distinction between the two, fundamentally, fiscal intermediaries and carriers are the same.

## National Health Care Expenditures

In 2009, national health expenditures (NHE), also referred to as health care spending, in the United States amounted to almost $2.5 trillion, or an average per capita spending of $8,086 for each American. It represented 17.6% of the gross domestic product (GDP; Table 6–3). The *GDP* is the total value of goods and services produced in the United States and is an indicator of total economic production (or total consumption). Hence, 17.6% of GDP refers to the share of the total economic output consumed by health care products and services. Total spending grew at an average annual rate of 6.7% from 1990 to 2000, and at 6.8% from 2000 to 2009. According to projections by the CMS, average annual growth in NHE for 2009 through 2019 is expected to be 6.3%, 0.2 percentage point faster than estimates without the effects of the ACA of 2010. Spending as a share of GDP is expected to be 19.6% in 2019 (CMS 2010b). At this rate of growth, total health care spending in 2019 would reach more than $4.5 trillion. Chapter 12 discusses the reasons for the growth in health care spending, international comparisons, and cost-containment measures.

## Difference Between National and Personal Health Expenditures

*National health expenditures* are an aggregate of the amount the nation spends for all

Table 6–3  US National Health Expenditures, Selected Years

| Year | Amount (in billions) | % of GDP | Amount per capita |
|------|---------------------|----------|-------------------|
| 1960 | $27.3 | 5.2 | $147 |
| 1970 | 74.8 | 7.2 | 356 |
| 1980 | 255.7 | 9.2 | 1,110 |
| 1990 | 724.0 | 12.5 | 2,853 |
| 2000 | 1,378.0 | 13.8 | 4,878 |
| 2009 | 2,486.3 | 17.6 | 8,086 |

*Source:* CMS, Office of the Actuary.

health services and supplies, public health services, health-related research, administrative costs, and investment in structures and equipment during a calendar year. The proportional distribution of NHE into the various categories of health services appears in Table 6–4.

National health expenditures are distinct from *personal health expenditures*. The latter are for services and goods related directly to patient care. More specifically,

personal health expenditures constitute the amount remaining after subtracting from NHE, spending for research, structures (construction, additions, alterations, etc.) and equipment; administrative expenses incurred in private and public health insurance programs; and costs of government public health activities. In 2009, 84.1% of the total health spending was for the various services classified under personal health expenditures (see Table 6–4).

· · · · · · · · · · · · · · · · · · · · · · · · · · · · · · ·

Table 6–4   Percentage Distribution of US National Health Expenditures, 2009

| NHE | 100.0 |
|---|---|
| **Personal health care** | **84.1** |
|   hospital care | 30.5 |
|   physician and clinical services | 20.3 |
|   dental services | 4.1 |
|   nursing home care | 5.5 |
|   other professional services | 2.7 |
|   home health | 2.7 |
|   prescription drugs | 10.1 |
|   other personal health care | 4.9 |
|   other medical products | 3.1 |
| **Govt administration and net cost of private health insurance** | **6.6** |
| **Govt public health activities** | **3.1** |
| **Investment** | **6.3** |
|   noncommercial research | 1.8 |
|   structures & equipment | 4.5 |
| Total NHE: | $2,486.3 billion |
| Personal health expenditures: | $2,089.9 billion |

*Source:* CMS, Office of the Actuary.

· · · · · · · · · · · · · · · · · · · · · · · · · · · · · · ·

## Public and Private Share of Health Care Expenditures

Figure 6–6 illustrates the shift from private financing to public financing since 1960. In 1960, private funds, including out-of-pocket payments, private health insurance premiums, and other private funds, paid for three-quarters of all health care. The introduction of Medicare and Medicaid in 1966 transferred a large portion of the private expenditures to the public sector, while increasing access for many who previously could not afford the growing costs of health care. A few years later, in 1972, when Medicare began coverage of the disabled population, the proportion of health care expenditures from private sources declined to 62%. The share of private funds reached its lowest point in 1997 when 53.6% of the nation's health dollars came from private sources and 46.4% came from public sources. In recent years, the ratio of private to public financing has been relatively stable, with a slower shift of expenditures from the private to the public sector.

Figure 6–7 summarizes the sources of financing and the proportionate consumption of health care dollars by various services. Of the combined private health insurance and out-of-pocket expenses, households paid

Figure 6–6  Proportional Distribution of US Private and Public Shares of National Health Expenditures.

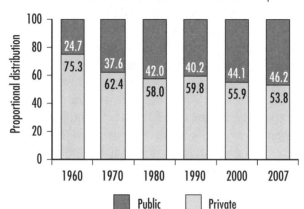

*Source:* Data from *Health, United States, 2009*, p. 393. National Center for Health Statistics.

57.5% and private businesses paid 42.1%. Businesses paid 61.6% of the cost of health insurance. Of the total public share of NHE, 62.6% was borne by the federal government; state and local governments paid the remainder (CMS, Office of the Actuary).

# Trends, Problems, and Issues in Insurance and Financing

## Health Insurance Issues and Reform

That not all Americans have health insurance coverage, and consequently encounter uneven access, has been well documented. An examination of the 1998–2000 National Expenditure Panel Survey data by Klein and colleagues (2005) revealed that 69% of the nonelderly population is always insured, 9% is always uninsured, and the remaining 22% experience health insurance *churning*, a phenomenon in which people gain and lose coverage multiple times. Economic cycles, shifts in the industrial makeup of the economy caused by factors such as globalization and other factors that may affect people's

employment status and ability to maintain job-based health insurance can result in churning. The ACA of 2010 was a sweeping reform effort to extend health insurance coverage to uninsured Americans.

As previously discussed in this chapter, some provisions of the ACA of 2010 have gone into effect. The main provisions of the Act that address the issue of uninsurance, however, do not go into effect until 2014. On the other hand, given the political and legal obstacles the law faces, its implementation is still uncertain (see Chapter 14 for further details). The legislation proposes to reduce the number of uninsured, mainly through individual mandates to purchase health insurance from exchanges to be set up by the government, employer mandates to enroll workers in their employer-sponsored health insurance benefits, and expansion of Medicaid. The Congressional Budget Office and the Joint Committee on Taxation have estimated that by 2019 the legislation will reduce the number of nonelderly people who are uninsured by about 32 million, still leaving approximately 23 million nonelderly residents uninsured. One-third

Figure 6–7  The Nation's Health Dollar: 2009.

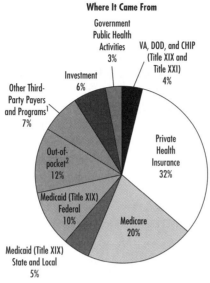

**Where It Came From**

Government Public Health Activities 3%

VA, DOD, and CHIP (Title XIX and Title XXI) 4%

Investment 6%

Other Third-Party Payers and Programs[1] 7%

Out-of-pocket[2] 12%

Medicaid (Title XIX) Federal 10%

Medicaid (Title XIX) State and Local 5%

Medicare 20%

Private Health Insurance 32%

[1] Includes work-site health care, other private revenues, Indian Health Service, workers' compensation, general assistance, maternal and child health, vocational rehabilitation, Substance Abuse and Mental Health Services Administration, school health, and other federal and state local programs.

[2]Includes copayments, deductibles, and any amounts not covered by health insurance.

*Note:* Sum of pieces may not equal 100% due to rounding.

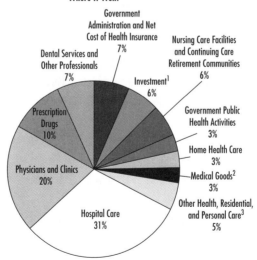

**Where It Went**

Government Administration and Net Cost of Health Insurance 7%

Nursing Care Facilities and Continuing Care Retirement Communities 6%

Dental Services and Other Professionals 7%

Investment[1] 6%

Government Public Health Activities 3%

Prescription Drugs 10%

Home Health Care 3%

Physicians and Clinics 20%

Medical Goods[2] 3%

Other Health, Residential, and Personal Care[3] 5%

Hospital Care 31%

[1] Includes research (2%) and structures and equipment (4%).

[2] Includes durable (1%) and nondurable (2%) goods.

[3] Includes expenditures for residential care facilities, ambulance providers, medical care delivered in nontraditional settings (such as community centers, senior citizens centers, schools, and military field stations), and expenditures for Home and Community Waiver programs under Medicaid.

*Note:* Sum of pieces may not equal 100% due to rounding.

**Total Health Spending = $2,486.3 billion**

of the uninsured will be illegal immigrants (CBO 2010).

The Office of the Actuary estimated the cost of insurance coverage alone would be $150 billion in 2016 after the coverage provisions of the law are fully phased in. If certain proposed cuts are taken into account, mainly in the Medicare program (estimated to be $70 billion), the country will still be left with a cost increase of $71.4 billion. Even after backing out proposed revenues from tax increases, during 2012 and 2013, the United States would still be saddled with a cost of $279.5 billion for the decade of 2010–2019 (Foster 2010). Even though these estimates represent only about 2 to 3% of the NHE, moral hazard and provider-induced demand could substantially raise the actual costs. Various types of supply-side approaches to ration health care would have to be employed to restrain cost escalations, as shown by the experiences of other nations that have national health care programs. Exhibit 6–7 contains a summary of

Exhibit 6–7  Main Provisions of the Patient Protection and Affordable Care Act of 2010

- Individuals will be mandated to purchase health insurance.
- Premium subsidies for people with incomes up to 400% of the poverty level, when they purchase health insurance through health insurance exchanges.
- Employers with more than 50 employees who do not offer health insurance will pay a "free rider" tax. Small businesses with fewer than 25 workers will be eligible for a sliding scale tax credit, based on the employer's contribution to health insurance premiums.
- Lifetime benefit limits eliminated in all health plans and insurance policies issued or renewed on or after September 23, 2010.
- A temporary federal program, starting July 2010, to enroll people with preexisting conditions. In 2014, when the law is scheduled to be fully implemented, insurers must cover people with preexisting conditions.
- Health plans must cover dependent children up to the age of 26 under their parents' health plans.
- States will establish health insurance exchanges to facilitate the purchase of health insurance. Insurers will be required to participate in the exchanges.
- Expansion of Medicaid to cover people at or below 133% of the federal poverty level.
- No change in income eligibility levels for CHIP enrollment until 2019.
- An annual physical exam (called a Wellness Exam) for all Part B enrollees is effective January 2011. No deductible or copayment applies.
- Effective 2011, all Part D drugs must be covered under a manufacturer discount agreement with the CMS. While in the coverage gap (doughnut hole), beneficiaries are to receive discounts amounting to 50% on brand name drugs and 7% on generic drugs. The coverage gap is to be phased out by 2020.
- A new Independent Payment Advisory Board to be responsible for containing the growth in Medicare spending and allocation of $10 billion to establish a Center for Medicare and Medicaid Innovation to test innovative payment and service delivery models, with the aim of reducing program expenditures.

the ACA of 2010 as it pertains to financing and insurance.

## Pay-for-Performance

Payers and policy makers are increasingly turning to *pay-for-performance* (P4P) and other value-based purchasing strategies (Nicholas et al. 2011). The objective of P4P initiatives is to link reimbursement to quality and efficiency as an incentive to improve the quality of health care, as well as reduce systemwide costs. Government agencies and private health plans are establishing programs that encourage hospitals, physicians, and other providers to meet quality standards. Providers who can demonstrate improvement in care and more efficient performance stand to reap financial rewards (Wechsler 2006). With approximately 30% of all health care spending going to hospitals, payers have particularly targeted hospitals to reduce costs. Chapter 12 further discusses P4P and its effects.

## Adverse Selection

*Adverse selection* occurs when high-risk individuals, that is, people who are likely to use more health care services than others because of their poor health status, enroll in health insurance plans in greater numbers, compared to people who are healthy. Consequently, premiums have to be raised for everyone, which makes health insurance less affordable for those in good health.

It is estimated that about one-third of the uninsured who would be eligible to receive premium subsidies under the ACA of 2010 are in good health. Unless they are enrolled in the government exchanges and made to purchase health insurance, premium costs would be higher than expected because of adverse selection (Cunningham 2010).

## Favorable Risk Selection

Favorable risk selection, or, simply, *risk selection*, occurs when healthy people disproportionately enroll into a health plan. It amounts to "cream skimming." For example, health plans may selectively enroll healthier people and avoid sicker people, or health plans may induce risk selection through selective advertising. Since patients with chronic health problems are likely to consume more services, insurers can risk select to avoid these patients to increase their profitability. It has been estimated that the most expensive, very sick 1% of the population, accounts for 30% of all health spending and the least expensive, healthy 50% of the population, accounts for only 3% of health spending. These estimates have been shown to stay stable over time (Berk and Monheit 2001). This disparity is the reason insurers may go to extra lengths to identify and select below-average risks and to avoid high-risk populations (Blumberg and Nichols 1996). Provisions of the MMA of 2003 are designed to deter risk selection, but there is concern that these provisions will be insufficient. Private plan choices in Medicare Part D are likely to provide new opportunities to risk select through advertising (Mehrotra et al. 2006). There is also some evidence that favorable risk selection may occur with pay-for-performance contracting in some settings (Shen 2003).

Although adverse selection and risk selection are regarded as unfair, practices that are more likely to reflect actual risk have also been criticized. Adjusting premiums to reflect health status and making potential high-cost enrollees pay more, a practice called *risk rating*, are also criticized on equity grounds. It has also been politically unacceptable to have the sick pay higher costs for coverage, particularly because ill health may also have reduced one's ability to work. Also, very high-risk individuals may be unable to obtain coverage at affordable rates (Pauly et al. 1992).

## Cost Shifting

When the amount of reimbursement from some payer source becomes inadequate or when uncompensated services are rendered, cost shifting is a mechanism used to make up for revenue shortfalls. Providers resort to *cost shifting* by charging extra to payers who do not exercise strict cost controls. Uninsured families are able to pay less than half of their outpatient care costs, but only 7% of hospital costs (Institute of Medicine 2003). Hence, cross-subsidization by those who bear the burden of cost shifting has been the traditional way to provide needed health care services to the uninsured. However, most payers use some form of cost-containment mechanisms. Capitation and prospective reimbursement methods, in particular, have eroded the margins for cost shifting. Consequently, providers have less ability to provide uncompensated care through cost shifting than was previously possible.

## Fraud and Abuse

Health care fraud and program abuse are troubling aspects of health care financing. The full extent of health care fraud is almost impossible to measure. However, the Federal Bureau of Investigation (FBI) estimates that fraudulent billings to public and private insurance amount to 3 to 10% of total health care spending (Morris 2009). Fraud is difficult to detect because it lacks routine monitoring and control procedures. Fiscal intermediaries who process and pay claims presume that claims are submitted for medically necessary services, and there is limited verification that services are actually provided (Morris 2009).

HIPAA of 1996 established a national Health Care Fraud and Abuse Control Program designed to coordinate federal, state, and local law enforcement activities with respect to health care fraud and abuse. This collaborative approach has resulted in identifying and prosecuting the most egregious instances of health care fraud. During the fiscal year 2010, the federal government recovered approximately $2.5 billion in health care fraud judgments and settlements. The Medicare trust funds have recovered over $18.0 billion since the inception of the program in 1997 (DHHS and the Department of Justice 2011).

## Summary

Financing is the lifeblood of any health care delivery system. At a basic level, it determines who pays for health care services for whom. Access to continuous and comprehensive services hinges on coverage through a health insurance program. Thus, demand for health care is directly linked to financing. Financing also indirectly determines how much and what type of health care services are produced.

Health care financing in the United States is a patchwork of mechanisms that are largely uncoordinated, adding to the complexity of the health care delivery system. Employment-based group health insurance provides most health care in the United

States. As a general rule, employees are required to share the costs. Many large employers are self-insured. Managed care has become the predominant avenue for providing insurance and delivery of services in an integrated fashion. Medicare and Medicaid are the major public insurance programs for a significant segment of the civilian population not covered under private health insurance plans. The Department of Defense and VA also operate large health care delivery systems to care for armed forces personnel and their dependents, military retirees, veterans, and survivors of deceased military personnel. Over the years, the share of public financing, relative to private financing, has gradually increased but seems to have leveled off.

Insurers, TPAs, and fiscal intermediaries handle most payment functions. Fee for service has been the traditional method for reimbursing providers. However, cost pressures have led to the development of innovative approaches designed to realign incentives to provide services more efficiently and at lower cost. Bundling of charges, resource-based relative value scale,

and prospective payment mechanisms are some examples. Prospective reimbursement for hospitals is based on diagnosis-related groups. Reimbursement based on case mix is another prospective payment method adopted for paying nursing homes and inpatient rehabilitation facilities.

The United States has experienced a dramatic growth in national health expenditures. These expenditures have surpassed growth rates in the gross domestic product, as well as the rise in general inflation. Controlling health care costs will be a major challenge in the years ahead.

The Patient Protection and Affordable Care Act became law in 2010, with the main objective of expanding health insurance coverage. Some aspects of the law have been implemented, but the main provisions to extend coverage to the uninsured do not become effective until 2014. The law is facing major political and legal hurdles, and its final implementation is uncertain. Other trends, problems, and issues in financing include pay-for-performance initiatives, adverse selection, favorable risk selection, cost shifting, and fraud and abuse.

## Test Your Understanding

### Terminology

| | | |
|---|---|---|
| adverse selection | claim | entitlement |
| balance bill | coinsurance | experience rating |
| beneficiary | community rating | fee schedule |
| benefit period | consumer-driven health | fiscal intermediaries |
| benefits | plan | GDP |
| capitation | copayment | group insurance |
| carriers | cost-plus | indemnity plan |
| case mix | cost shifting | insurance |
| categorical programs | Current Procedural | insured |
| charge | Terminology | insurer |
| churning | deductible | major medical |

| | | |
|---|---|---|
| *means-tested program* | *personal health* | *risk* |
| *Medicare Physician Fee* | *expenditures* | *risk rating* |
| *Schedule* | *preexisting condition* | *risk selection* |
| *Medigap* | *premium* | *self-insured plan* |
| *moral hazard* | *prospective reimbursement* | *service plan* |
| *national health* | *rate* | *stop-loss* |
| *expenditures* | *reinsurance* | *third-party administrator* |
| *outliers* | *relative value units* | *third-party payers* |
| *pay-for-performance* | *retrospective reimbursement* | *underwriting* |

## Review Questions

1. What is meant by health care financing in its broad sense? What impact does financing have on the health care delivery system?

2. Discuss the general concepts of insurance. Describe the various types of private health insurance options, pointing out the differences among them.

3. Discuss how the concepts of premium, covered services, and cost sharing apply to health insurance.

4. What is the difference between experience rating and community rating?

5. What is Medicare Part A? Discuss the financing and cost-sharing features of Medicare Part A. What benefits does Part A cover? What benefits are not covered?

6. What is Medicare Part B? Discuss the financing and cost-sharing features of Medicare Part B. What main benefits are covered under Part B? What services are not covered?

7. Briefly describe the Medicare Advantage program.

8. Briefly explain the prescription drug program under Medicare Part D.

9. Discuss the financing, eligibility, and covered benefits for the Medicaid program.

10. What provisions has the federal government made for providing health care to military personnel and to veterans of the US armed forces?

11. What are the major methods of reimbursement for outpatient services?

12. What are the differences between the retrospective and prospective methods of reimbursement?

13. Discuss the prospective payment system under DRGs.

14. Distinguish between national health expenditures and personal health expenditures.

15. What is pay-for-performance? What is its main objective?

16. What is adverse selection? What are its consequences?

17. What incentive do insurers have to engage in risk selection?

18. What is risk rating? Why is it criticized?

19. What is the relationship between uncompensated care and cost shifting? Why do providers now have limited ability to shift costs?

## REFERENCES

AHIP Center for Policy and Research. 2009. *Individual health insurance in 2009: A comprehensive survey of premiums, availability, and benefits*. Washington, DC: America's Health Insurance Plans.

Berk, M.L., and A.C. Monheit. 2001. The concentration of health expenditures, revisited. *Health Affairs* 20, no. 2: 9–18.

Best, R.A. 2005. *Military medical care services: Questions and answers*. Congressional Research Service. Available at: http://www.fas.org/sgp/crs/misc/IB93103.pdf. Accessed January 2011.

Blumberg, L.J., and L.M. Nichols. 1996. First, do no harm: Developing health insurance market reform packages. *Health Affairs* 15, no. 3: 35–54.

Centers for Medicare and Medicaid Services (CMS). 2010a. *2010 Annual report of the boards of trustees of the federal hospital insurance and federal supplementary medical insurance trust funds*. Available at: https://www.cms.gov/ReportsTrustFunds/downloads/tr2010.pdf. Accessed January 2011.

Centers for Medicare and Medicaid Services (CMS). 2010b. *National health expenditure projections 2009–2019*. Available at: https://www.cms.gov/NationalHealthExpendData/downloads/NHEProjections2009to2019.pdf. Accessed January 2011.

Claxton, G. et al. 2010. *Employer health benefits: 2010 annual survey*. Menlo Park, CA: The Kaiser Family Foundation.

Congressional Budget Office (CBO). 2010. *Selected CBO publications related to health care legislation, 2009–2010*. Washington, DC: Congressional Budget Office.

Cunningham, P.J. 2010. *Who are the uninsured eligible for premium subsidies in the health insurance exchanges?* Research Brief No. 18 (December 2010). Washington, DC: Center for Studying Health System Change.

Davis, M.H., and S.T. Burner. 1995. Three decades of Medicare: What the numbers tell us. *Health Affairs* 14, no. 4: 231–243.

DeNavas-Walt, C. et al. 2010. *Income, poverty, and health insurance coverage in the United States: 2009*. Washington, DC: US Census Bureau.

Department of Defense. 1996. *Your military health plan: TriCare*. Falls Church, VA: Department of Defense.

Department of Health and Human Services (DHHS) and the Department of Justice. 2011. *Health care fraud and abuse control program annual report for fiscal year 2010*. Available at: http://oig.hhs.gov/publications/docs/hcfac/hcfacreport2010.pdf. Accessed January 2011.

Department of Veterans Affairs. 2010. *2010 organizational briefing book*. Available at: http://www.va.gov/ofcadmin/docs/vaorgbb.pdf. Accessed January 2011.

Federal Register. 2009. From the Federal Register online via GPO access. Available at: http://aspe .hhs.gov/health/fmap11.htm. Accessed January 2011.

Feldstein, P.J. 1993. *Health care economics.* 4th ed. New York: Delmar Publishers.

Foster, R.S. 2010. *Estimated financial effects of the "Patient Protection and Affordable Care Act," as Passed by the Senate on December 24, 2009.* Memo from Richard S. Foster, Office of the Actuary, dated January 8, 2010. Available at: https://www.cms.gov/ActuarialStudies /Downloads/S_PPACA_2010-01-08.pdf. Accessed January 2011.

Fronstin, P. 2009. *Capping the tax exclusion for employment-based health coverage: Implications for employers and workers.* Issue Brief No. 325. Washington, DC: Employee Benefit Research Institute.

Gabel, J.R. et al. 2003. Self-insurance in times of growing and retreating managed care. *Health Affairs* 22, no. 2: 202–210.

General Accounting Office (GAO). 1996. *Private health insurance: Millions relying on individual market coverage face cost and coverage trade-offs.* Washington, DC: General Accounting Office.

Gold, M. et al. 2010. *Medicare Advantage 2011 data spotlight: Plan availability and premiums.* Available at: http://www.kff.org/medicare/upload/8117.pdf. Accessed January 2011.

Goodman, J.C., and G.L. Musgrave. 1992. *Patient power: Solving America's health care crisis.* Washington, DC: CATO Institute.

Harty, S. 2005. Health insurers try to bring managed care to workers comp. *Business Insurance* 39, no. 31: 11–13.

Health Care Financing Administration (HCFA). 1996. *Medicare and Medicaid statistical supplement, 1996.* Pub. No. 03386. Baltimore, MD: Department of Health and Human Services.

Health Insurance Association of America (HIAA). 1991. *Source book of health insurance data.* Washington, DC: Health Insurance Association of America.

Health Insurance Institute. 1969. *Modern health insurance.* New York: Health Insurance Institute.

The Henry J. Kaiser Family Foundation. 2008. *How non-group health coverage varies with income.* Menlo Park, CA: Kaiser Family Foundation.

The Henry J. Kaiser Family Foundation. 2010a. *Medicaid and the uninsured: The Medicaid program at a glance.* Available at: http://www.kff.org/medicaid/upload/7235-04.pdf. Accessed January 2011.

The Henry J. Kaiser Family Foundation. 2010b. *Medicare fact sheet: Medicare at a glance, September 2010.* Available at: http://www.kff.org/medicare/upload/1066-13.pdf. Accessed January 2011.

Hoadley, J. et al. 2010. *Medicare Part D spotlight: Part D plan availability in 2011 and key changes since 2006.* Available at: http://www.kff.org/medicare/upload/8107.pdf. Accessed January 2011.

Holahan, J. 2011. The 2007–09 recession and health insurance coverage. *Health Affairs* 30, no. 1: 145–152.

Hudson, J.L. 2005. The impact of SCHIP on insurance coverage of children. *Inquiry* 42, no. 3: 232–254.

Indian Health Service (IHS). 2010. *IHS fact sheets.* Available at: http://info.ihs.gov/index.asp. Accessed January 2011.

Institute of Medicine. 2003. *A shared destiny: Effects of uninsurance on individuals, families, and communities.* Washington, DC: National Academies Press.

Jost, T.S. 2003. The tenuous nature of the Medicaid entitlement. *Health Affairs* 22, no. 1: 145–153.

The Kaiser Commission on Medicaid and the Uninsured. 2006. *Medicaid facts.* The Henry J. Kaiser Family Foundation. Available at: http://www.kff.org. Accessed February 2007.

Klein, K. et al. 2005. *Entrances and exits: Health insurance churning, 1998–2000.* New York, NY: The Commonwealth Fund.

Levit, K.R. et al. 1994. National health spending trends, 1960–1993. *Health Affairs* 13, no. 5: 14–31.

Martin, A. et al. 2011. Recession contributes to slowest annual rate of increase in health spending in five decades. *Health Affairs* 30, no. 1: 11–22.

MedPAC. 2008a. *Rehabilitation facilities (inpatient) payment system.* Available at: http://www.medpac.gov/documents/MedPAC_Payment_Basics_08_IRF.pdf. Accessed January 2011.

MedPAC. 2008b. *Home health care services payment system.* Available at: http://www.medpac.gov/documents/MedPAC_Payment_Basics_08_HHA.pdf. Accessed January 2011.

MedPAC. 2009. *Ambulatory surgical centers payment system.* Available at: http://www.medpac.gov/documents/MedPAC_Payment_Basics_09_ASC.pdf. Accessed January 2011.

Mehrotra A. et al. 2006. The relationship between health plan advertising and market incentives: Evidence of risk-selective behavior. *Health Affairs* 25, no. 3: 759–765.

Morris, L. 2009. Combating fraud in health care: An essential component of any cost containment strategy. *Health Affairs* 28, no. 5: 1351–1356.

National Center for Health Statistics. 2010. *Health, United States, 2009.* Hyattsville, MD: US Department of Health and Human Services.

Nicholas, L.H. et al. 2011. Do hospitals alter patient care effort allocations under pay-for-performance? *Health Services Research* 46, no. 1: 61–81.

Nonnemaker, L., and S.A. Sinclair. 2009. *Medicare beneficiaries' out-of-pocket spending for health care services: Insight on the issues, June 2009.* Available at: http://assets.aarp.org/rgcenter/health/i30_oop.pdf. Accessed January 2011.

Pauly, M.V. et al. 1992. *Responsible national health insurance.* Washington, DC: AEI Press.

Rousseau, D. et al. 2010. *Dual eligibles: Medicaid enrollment and spending for Medicare beneficiaries in 2007.* Available at: http://www.kff.org/medicaid/upload/7846-02.pdf. Accessed January 2011.

Shen Y. 2003. Selection incentives in a performance-based contracting system. *Health Services Research* 38, no. 2: 535–552.

Shone, L.P. et al. 2005. Reduction in racial and ethnic disparities after enrollment in the State Children's Health Insurance Program. *Pediatrics* 115, no. 6: e697–e705.

Social Security Administration. 2010. *A summary of the 2010 annual reports: Social Security and Medicare Board of Trustees.* Available at: http://www.ssa.gov/OACT/TRSUM/index.html. Accessed January 2011.

Somers, A.R., and H.M. Somers. 1977. *Health and health care: Policies in perspective.* Germantown, MD: Aspen Systems.

US Department of Labor. 2006. *Workers' compensation programs: Fact sheets.* Available at: http://www.dol.gov/esa/regs/compliance/owcp/owcpfact.htm. Accessed February 2007.

Vaughn, E.J., and C.M. Elliott. 1987. *Fundamentals of risk and insurance.* New York: John Wiley & Sons.

Wechsler, J. 2006. Pay for performance. *Managed Healthcare Executive* 16, no. 8: 30–32.

Whitted, G. 1993. Private health insurance and employee benefits. In: *Introduction to health services.* 4th ed. S.J. Williams and P.R. Torrens, eds. Albany, NY: Delmar Publishers. pp. 332–360.

# PART III

## System Processes

# Chapter 7

# Outpatient and Primary Care Services

## Learning Objectives

- To understand the meanings of outpatient, ambulatory, and primary care
- To identify why there has been a dramatic growth in outpatient services
- To develop an understanding of the various types of outpatient settings and services
- To appreciate the role of complementary and alternative medicine in health care

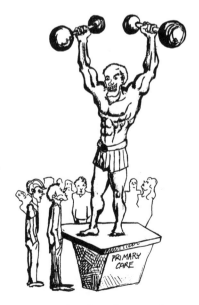

*"I suppose a system based on primary care is more robust."*

## Introduction

Outpatient health care services originated with the healing arts themselves (Williams 1993) and have been in existence for a long time. Historically, outpatient care has been independent from services provided in health care institutions. In earlier days, physicians saw patients in their clinics, and most physicians also made home visits to treat patients. Given the limitations of medical science in those days, physicians provided the full spectrum of medical services, including diagnosis, treatment, surgery, and dispensing of medications. Institutions for inpatient care, such as hospitals and nursing homes, developed later. With advances in medical science, the locus of health care delivery concentrated around the institutional core of community hospitals. As the range of services that could be provided on an outpatient basis continued to expand, hospitals gradually became the dominant players in providing the vast majority of outpatient care as well, with the exception of cognitive and basic diagnostic care provided in physicians' offices (Barr and Breindel 1995). Hospitals were better equipped to provide such services because they increasingly capitalized on technological innovation. Hospital laboratories and diagnostic units, for example, were better equipped to perform most tests and diagnostic procedures. Independent providers, on the other hand, faced capital constraints and competitive pressures in the health care marketplace. To better cope with the changing realities of the new marketplace, most solo practitioners consolidated into group practices.

Various changes in the health care delivery system, both financial and social, have led to new alignments in the delivery of outpatient services. The process of health care delivery, in a broad sense, has increasingly shifted outside of expensive acute care hospitals, and the trend is likely to continue. Although basic primary care has traditionally been the foundation of outpatient services, certain intensive procedures are increasingly being performed on an outpatient basis. Consumer demand has fueled the growth of complementary and alternative medicine, on a self-pay basis.

Delivery of outpatient care by public agencies has been limited in scope and detached from the dominant private system of health services delivery. State and local government agencies sponsor limited outpatient services to meet the needs of underserved populations, mainly indigent patients who lack personal resources to obtain health care in the private sector. Examples include public health clinics and dispensaries. As discussed in Chapter 3, public health functions, in most cases, have been limited to child immunizations, care of mothers and infants, health screening in public schools, monitoring for certain contagious diseases like tuberculosis, family planning, and prevention of sexually transmitted diseases. Community health centers depend on federal and state funds, and provide a wide array of outpatient services to a number of rural and inner city areas.

The terms "outpatient" and "ambulatory" have been used interchangeably, as they are in this book, but the term "outpatient" is more comprehensive. It better describes the range of services now being referred to as "ambulatory." Apart from that, there is little distinction between the two.

## What Is Outpatient Care?

Outpatient services do not require an overnight inpatient stay in an institution of health care delivery, such as a hospital or long-term care facility, although certain outpatient services may be offered by a hospital or nursing home. Many hospitals, for instance, have emergency departments (EDs) and other outpatient service centers, such as outpatient surgery, rehabilitation, and specialized clinics.

Outpatient services are also referred to as *ambulatory care*. Strictly speaking, ambulatory care constitutes diagnostic and therapeutic services and treatments provided to the "walking" (ambulatory) patient. Hence, in a restricted sense, the term "ambulatory care" refers to care rendered to patients who come to physicians' offices, hospital outpatient departments, and health centers to receive care. The term is also used synonymously with "community medicine" (Wilson and Neuhauser 1985) because the geographic location of ambulatory services is intended to serve the surrounding community, providing convenience and easy accessibility.

Patients do not always walk to the service centers to receive ambulatory care, however. For example, in a hospital ED, patients may arrive by land or air ambulance. EDs, in most cases, are equipped mainly to provide secondary and tertiary care services rather than primary care. In other instances, such as mobile diagnostic units and home health care, services are transported to the patient, instead of the patient coming to receive the services. Hence, the terms "outpatient" and "inpatient" are more precise, and the term *outpatient services* refers to any health care services that are not provided on the basis of an overnight stay in which room and board costs are incurred.

## The Scope of Outpatient Services

Since the 1980s, extraordinary growth has occurred in the volume of outpatient services and the emergence of new settings in which outpatient services are delivered.

The most basic outpatient services, such as physical exams and minor treatments, are still delivered in a physician's office. Advanced outpatient care has traditionally been provided in hospital-based facilities, often in various building complexes surrounding the main hospital. In addition, explosive growth has occurred in the type and ownership of nonhospital-based facilities offering ambulatory care (see examples in Table 7–1).

Since the 1980s, as hospital occupancy rates continued to decline, hospital executives were forced to view ambulatory care as an essential portion of their overall health care business rather than as a supplemental product line (Barr and Breindel 1995). Over time, many hospitals have established a firm position in the ambulatory care market to ensure continued survival of their organizations.

The growth of nonhospital-based ambulatory services has intensified competition for outpatient services between hospitals and community-based providers. Examples of such competition include home health care, freestanding clinics for routine and urgent care, and outpatient surgery. Other services, such as dental care and optometric services, remain independent of other types of health care services. Financing is the main reason dental and optometric services have not been integrated with other outpatient medical services. Traditionally, medical insurance plans have been separate from dental and vision care plans. Philosophical and technical differences account for other variations. Chiropractic care, for instance, is generally covered by most health plans but remains isolated from the mainstream practice of medicine. Complementary and alternative therapies and self-care are not covered by insurance, yet continue to experience remarkable growth.

Table 7–1   Owners, Providers, and Settings for Ambulatory Care Services

| Past | Present |
|---|---|
| Owners/Providers | |
| • Independent physician practitioners | • Independent physician practitioners |
| • Hospitals | • Hospitals |
| • Community health agencies | • Community health agencies |
| • Home health agencies | • Managed care organizations |
| | • Insurance companies |
| | • Corporate employers |
| | • Group practices |
| | • National physician chains |
| | • Home health companies |
| | • National diversified health care companies |
| Service Settings | |
| • Hospital outpatient departments | • Physicians' offices |
| • Physicians' offices | • Walk-in clinics/Urgent care centers |
| • Outpatient surgery centers | • Outpatient surgery centers |
| • Hospital emergency departments | • Chemotherapy and radiation therapy centers |
| • Home health agencies | • Dialysis centers |
| • Neighborhood health centers | • Community health centers |
| | • Diagnostic imaging centers |
| | • Mobile imaging centers |
| | • Fitness/wellness centers |
| | • Occupational health centers |
| | • Psychiatric outpatient centers |
| | • Rehabilitation centers |
| | • Sports medicine clinics |
| | • Hand injury rehab clinics |
| | • Women's health clinics |
| | • Wound care centers |

*Source:* Data from Barr, K.W.- and C.L. Breindel. 1995. Ambulatory care. In: *Health care administration: Principles, practices, structure, and delivery.* Gaithersburg, MD: Aspen Publishers, Inc.

Primary care is the foundation for ambulatory health services, but not all ambulatory care is primary care. For example, hospital ED services are not intended to be primary in nature. Conversely, services other than primary care have now become an integral part of outpatient services. Thanks to the technological advances in medicine, many secondary and tertiary treatments are now provided in ambulatory care settings. Examples include conditions requiring urgent treatment, outpatient surgery, rehabilitative therapies, and tertiary treatments, such as renal dialysis and chemotherapy.

# Primary Care

Primary care plays a central role in a health care delivery system (see Chapter 4). Other essential levels of care include secondary and tertiary care (distinct from primary, secondary, and tertiary prevention discussed in Chapter 2). Compared to primary care, secondary and tertiary care services are more complex and specialized. Primary care is distinguished from secondary and tertiary care according to its duration, frequency, and level of intensity. *Secondary care* is usually short term, involving sporadic consultation from a specialist to provide expert opinion and/or surgical or other advanced interventions that primary care physicians (PCPs) are not equipped to perform. Secondary care thus includes hospitalization, routine surgery, specialty consultation, and rehabilitation. *Tertiary care* is the most complex level of care, needed for conditions that are relatively uncommon. Typically, tertiary care is institution based, highly specialized, and technology driven. Much of tertiary care is rendered in large teaching hospitals, especially university hospitals.

Examples include trauma care, burn treatment, neonatal intensive care, tissue transplants, and open heart surgery. In some instances, tertiary treatment may be extended, and the tertiary care physician may assume long-term responsibility for the bulk of the patient's care. It has been estimated that 75 to 85% of people in a general population require only primary care services in a given year, 10 to 12% require referrals to short-term secondary care services, and 5 to 10% use tertiary care specialists (Starfield 1994). These proportions vary in populations with special health care needs.

Specialization is oriented toward treating disease. Hence, delivery of health care with a central focus on specialization cannot maximize health because preventing illness and promoting optimal health require a broader perspective than can be achieved by the disease specialist (Starfield 1992).

Definitions of primary care often focus on the type or level of services, such as prevention, diagnostic and therapeutic services, health education and counseling, and minor surgery. Although primary care specifically emphasizes these services, many specialists also provide the same spectrum of services. For example, the practice of most ophthalmologists has a large element of prevention, as well as diagnosis, treatment, follow-up, and minor surgery. Similarly, most cardiologists are engaged in health education and counseling. Hence, primary care should be more appropriately viewed as an approach to providing health care rather than as a set of specific services (Starfield 1994).

## World Health Organization Definition

Traditionally, primary care has been the cornerstone of ambulatory care services.

The World Health Organization (WHO) describes primary health care as:

> Essential health care based on practical, scientifically sound, and socially acceptable methods and technology made universally accessible to individuals and families in the community by means acceptable to them and at a cost that the community and the country can afford to maintain at every stage of their development in a spirit of self-reliance and self-determination. It forms an integral part of both the country's health system of which it is the central function and the main focus of the overall social and economic development of the community. It is the first level of contact of individuals, the family, and the community with the national health system, bringing health care as close as possible to where people live and work and constitutes the first element of a continuing health care process (WHO 1978).

Three elements in this definition are particularly noteworthy for an understanding of primary care: point of entry, coordination of care, and essential care.

## Point of Entry

Primary care is the point of entry into the health services system in which health care delivery is organized around primary care (Starfield 1992). Primary care is the first contact a patient makes with the health care delivery system. This first contact feature is closely associated with the "gatekeeper" role of the primary care practitioner. *Gatekeeping* implies that patients do not visit specialists and are not admitted to a hospital without being referred by their PCPs. On the surface, gatekeeping may appear to be a controlling mechanism for denying needed care. In most cases, however, the interposition of primary care protects patients from unnecessary procedures and overtreatment (Franks et al. 1992) because specialists use medical tests and procedures to a much greater extent than primary care providers and such interventions carry a definite risk of *iatrogenic* (caused by the process of health care) complications (Starfield 1994).

One of the goals of primary care is to bring health care as close as possible to where people live and work. In other words, true primary care is community based. It represents convenience and easy accessibility. To make such services widely available to communities in urban, suburban, and rural areas, the nature of primary care services must remain basic, routine, and inexpensive. Yet, appropriate technology must be incorporated into the delivery of primary care so that costly referrals to other components of the health delivery system are made only when necessary.

The British National Health Service (NHS) is an example of a health care delivery system founded on the principles of gatekeeping. In the NHS, primary care is the single portal of entry to secondary care and acts as a filter so that 90% of care is provided outside hospitals in ambulatory care settings (Orton 1994). General practitioners (GPs) are primary care gatekeepers in the British system. In the United States, under certain managed care gatekeeping arrangements, patients initiate care with their PCPs and obtain authorization when specialized services are needed.

## Coordination of Care

One of the main functions of primary care is to coordinate the delivery of health services between the patient and the myriad of delivery components of the system. Hence, in addition to providing basic services, primary care professionals serve as patient advisors, advocates, and system gatekeepers. In this coordinating role, the provider refers patients to sources of specialized care, gives advice regarding various diagnoses and therapies, discusses treatment options, and provides continuing care for chronic conditions (Williams 1993). Coordination of an individual's total health care needs is meant to ensure continuity and comprehensiveness. These desirable goals of primary care are best achieved when the patient and provider have formed a close mutual relationship over time. Primary care can be regarded as the hub of the health care delivery system wheel. The various components of the health care delivery system are located around the rim, and the spokes signify the coordination of continuous and comprehensive care (see Figure 7–1).

Figure 7–1 The Coordination Role of Primary Care in Health Care Delivery.

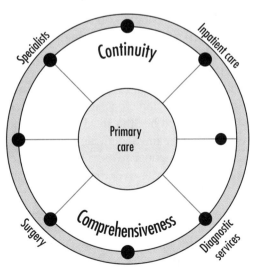

Countries whose health systems are oriented more toward primary care achieve better health levels, higher satisfaction with health services among the populations, and lower expenditures in the overall delivery of health care (Starfield 1994, 1998). Countries with weak primary care infrastructures incur poorer health outcomes and higher health care costs. Even in the United States, better health outcomes are achieved in states with higher ratios of PCPs and better availability of primary care (Shi 1994; Shi and Starfield 2000, 2001; Shi et al. 2002). Higher ratios of family and general physicians in the population are also associated with lower hospitalization rates for conditions treatable with good primary care (Parchman and Culler 1994). Having a regular source of primary care also leads to lower ED visits and inappropriate specialty consults. It also provides a setting to manage chronic conditions so individuals can stay healthier over time (Sepulveda et al. 2008). Research has also shown that primary care may play an important role in mitigating the adverse health effects of income inequality (Shi et al. 1999). Adults who have PCPs as their regular source of care experience lower mortality and incur lower health care costs (Franks et al. 1998). A higher proportion of PCPs in a given area has been shown to lead to lower spending on health care (Chernew et al. 2009).

An ideal system of health care delivery is based on primary care that is closely interlinked to adequate and timely specialized services. Continuous and coordinated care requires secondary and tertiary services to be integrated with primary care through appropriate interaction and consultation among physicians. Coordination of health care has certain definite advantages. Studies have shown that both the appropriateness and the outcomes of health care interventions are better when PCPs refer patients to specialists, as opposed to being self-referred (Bakwin 1945; Roos 1979).

## Essential Care

Primary health care is regarded as essential health care. The goal of the health care delivery system is to optimize population health, not just the health of individuals who have the means to access health services. Achieving this goal requires that disparities across population subgroups be minimized to ensure equal access. Because financing of health care is a key element in determining access, universal access to primary care services is better achieved under a national health care program. For this reason, lack of access to primary care for countless millions remains a nagging concern in the United States.

Most Western nations have adopted programs based on universal coverage financed through general tax revenues. As a result, primary care has been an integral part of the national health policy of these nations and is fundamental to the structure of their national health care systems. In the United States, the amalgam of public and private financing has created a fragmented system in which primary care does not form the organizing hub for continuous and coordinated health services.

## Institute of Medicine Definition

The Institute of Medicine (IOM) Committee on the Future of Primary Care recommended that primary care be the usual and preferred, but not the only, route of entry into the health care system. As part of this emphasis, the IOM defined primary care as "The provision of integrated, accessible health care services by clinicians who are accountable for addressing a large majority of personal health care needs, developing a sustained partnership with patients, and practicing in the context of family and community" (Vanselow et al. 1995, 192).

The term "integrated" embodies the concepts of comprehensive, coordinated, and continuous services that provide a seamless process of care. Primary care is *comprehensive* because it addresses any health problem at any given stage of a patient's life cycle. *Coordination* ensures the provision of a combination of health services to best meet the patient's needs. *Continuity* refers to care over time by a single provider or a team of health care professionals. The IOM definition goes further to emphasize accessibility and accountability as key characteristics of primary care. *Accessibility* refers to the ease with which a patient can initiate an interaction with a clinician for any health problem. It includes efforts to eliminate barriers, such as those posed by geography, financing, culture, race, and language. The IOM Committee recognizes that both clinicians and patients have **accountability**. The clinical system is accountable for providing quality care, producing patient satisfaction, using resources efficiently, and behaving in an ethical manner. On the other hand, patients are responsible for their own health to the extent that they can influence it. Patients are also responsible for judicious use of resources when they need health care. Partnership between a patient and a clinician does not necessarily imply equal roles. The role played by each party varies over time and from case to case. Mutual trust, respect, and responsibility are the hallmarks of this partnership.

The IOM Committee has proposed that primary care clinicians possess the knowledge and skills necessary to manage most of the physical, mental, social, and emotional concerns that affect patients' health. Primary care clinicians must use their best judgment to involve other practitioners in diagnosis, treatment, or both when it is appropriate to do so. The IOM Committee also believes that primary care clinicians should be able to address most personal health needs, including health promotion and disease prevention. The definition recognizes that primary care clinicians must consider the influence of the family on a patient's health status and be aware of the patient's living conditions, family dynamics, and cultural background. Finally, exemplary primary care requires an understanding of and a responsibility for the community's health (Vanselow et al. 1995).

# Models of Patient-Centered Primary Care

The two models presented in this section are still in their infancy in the United States. Chapter 14 outlines some ideas about moving from theoretical concepts to practical applications of these models.

## Medical Home

The medical home concept is directly related to the practice of good primary care. The term "medical home" was first coined in 1967 and established for special-needs children whose health care needs required constant coordination. The medical home began to evolve in the primary care realm after the Declaration of Alma-Ata as managed care programs began to use primary care providers to coordinate patient care.

A *medical home* consists of an interdisciplinary team of physicians and allied health professionals who partner with patients and their families, taking responsibility for ongoing patient care using a team approach, technology, and evidence-based protocols to coordinate and provide care. PCPs serve as advocates for patients across the care continuum, ensuring that the patient's values, wishes, and directives are honored (Caudill et al. 2011). If established properly, medical homes carry the potential to fix problems found in the current organization of primary care. They could provide patient-centered care to the community, providing patients with a "home" that is accessible and will coordinate their care.

A cross-national survey of seven countries with medical homes showed positive feedback from patients. The medical home could be a better setting to manage chronic care, especially if the chronic care model (CCM) is used within the home. CCM is based on the idea that chronic conditions are best managed with multidisciplinary practice-based teams in productive interaction with an informed and motivated patient. The model has proven to be effective within a demonstrative context and in research. Despite all this potential, the idea of a medical home is still met with much hesitancy even from physicians, who are skeptical of change because the fee-for-service structure still pays them more for acute care than preventive care (Berenson et al. 2008).

## Community-Oriented Primary Care

The 1978 International Conference on Primary Health Care (held at Alma-Ata in the former Soviet Union, under the auspices of WHO) concluded that people throughout the world had very little control over their own health care and that emphasis should be placed on attaining health through a response from the community to their health problems (WHO

1978). More positive outcomes occur when people have a greater sense of ownership of health programs that address their needs. It requires a partnership between health care providers and the communities in which they serve. It has been suggested that collective action by communities may enhance their competence in mitigating risk factors and thereby reduce their vulnerability to social problems and disease (Minkler 1992).

Current thoughts about primary care delivery have extended beyond the traditional biomedical paradigm, which focuses on medical care for the individual in an encounter-based system. The broader biopsychosocial paradigm emphasizes the health of the population, as well as that of the individual (Lee 1994). *Community-oriented primary care* (COPC) is based on the concept of "ecology of medical care," which emphasizes the relations between the population and community, on the one hand, and personal health care, on the other (Van Weel et al. 2008). COPC incorporates the elements of good primary care delivery and adds a population-based approach to identifying and addressing community health problems.

## Primary Care Providers

Specialization focuses on a specific disease or organ system, and specialists may provide the most appropriate care for particular illnesses within their area of competence. A generalist is needed, however, to integrate care for the variety of health problems that individuals experience over time (Starfield 1992).

Physicians in general practice are most commonly the providers of primary care in Europe. In the United States, primary care practitioners are not restricted to physicians trained in general and family practice.

Providers of primary care include physicians trained in internal medicine, pediatrics, and obstetrics and gynecology. One cannot assume, however, that these various types of practitioners are equally skilled in rendering primary care services (Starfield 1994). Unless a medical training program is dedicated to providing instruction in primary care, significant differences are likely to exist (Noble et al. 1992). In fact, some controversy and competition have arisen among practitioners as to which specialists should be providing primary care. The specialty of family practice, in particular, represents a challenge to internal medicine in providing adult primary care and to pediatrics in providing child primary care.

As discussed in Chapter 4, it is also important to note the expanded role that nonphysician practitioners (NPPs) play in the delivery of primary care. In view of the increasing emphasis on health care cost containment, NPPs, such as nurse practitioners (NPs), physician assistants (PAs), and certified nurse midwives (CNMs), are in great demand in primary care delivery settings, particularly in medically underserved areas. In addition to more effective health care, evidence suggests that a high proportion of primary care professionals in a population results in lower health care expenditures (Welch et al. 1993). Data from Medicaid MCOs demonstrate that patients receiving care from NPs at nurse-managed health centers experience significantly fewer emergency room visits, hospital inpatient days, and specialist visits and are at a significantly lower risk of giving birth to low-birth-weight infants, compared to patients in conventional health care (National Nursing Centers Consortium 2003).

Two key factors determine the proportion of primary care personnel to specialists needed for the adequate provision of primary care. The first is how rigidly a health care delivery system employs the concept of gatekeeping. The NHS, for instance, employs this concept more rigidly than the Canadian health system. Consequently, the proportion of PCPs is approximately 50% in Canada, compared to 70 to 72% in Britain (Hodge 1994). In the United States, emphasis on gatekeeping in some managed care plans increased demand for PCPs. For instance, a growth of 54% in family practice residency programs between 1993 and 2000 (Colwill and Cultice 2003) coincided with the rapid expansion of managed care. The second factor driving the need for primary care providers is the propensity of people in a given population to use primary care services. Utilization of primary care is greater in national health care systems.

After a healthy trend in the growth of medical school graduates who chose careers in primary care, a reversal has occurred. Block and colleagues (1996) concluded that the culture, values, and educational practices prevailing in the academic medical community are poorly aligned with the goals of enhancing the education and environment for primary care practice. One reason cited is the numerical dominance of specialists and subspecialists on the clinical faculties of medical schools, which is reflected in a negative cultural bias toward primary care. The situation is perhaps difficult to rectify without substantial changes in the composition of medical school faculties, including an infusion of community-based generalists who can serve as teachers, role models, and advocates for primary care (Petersdorf 1993; Roos and Roos 1980). Moreover, current reimbursement systems must realign to create financial incentives for people to enter primary care (Reuben 2007). At a

time when the United States needs a robust system built on the foundation of primary care, it is unfortunate that the values of traditional biomedicine and medical education continue to emphasize specialization as opposed to breadth of knowledge and training, biological factors as opposed to social and emotional factors in health, and inpatient as opposed to outpatient care and training.

## Growth in Outpatient Services

As previously mentioned, outpatient care now includes much more than primary care services. Duffy and Farley (1995) studied the 150 most frequently performed procedures in hospitals in 1980. By 1987, 37 of the 150 procedures had declined in use by more than 40% (Figure 7–2). Some of these procedures have been replaced by more advanced procedures, and a few have been largely abandoned as ineffective. The most prominent reason for the decline (for 33 of the 37 procedures), however, was that most of these procedures were shifted to outpatient settings, especially for patients who did not need to be hospitalized for other health reasons. Patients who did receive 1 of the 37 procedures in 1987 on an inpatient basis tended to be more severely ill, compared to those in 1980. By 1990, more than one-half of all surgeries performed by hospitals took place in an outpatient setting. The proportion of total surgeries performed in outpatient departments of community hospitals increased from 16.3% in 1980 to 62.7% in 2007 (Figure 7–2). The fact that it is not a simple trade-off is of some concern. The decline in inpatient procedures has actually been outweighed by the growth of ambulatory procedures. Also, for patients older than 65 years of age, the rate of inpatient

Figure 7–2 Percentage of Total Surgeries Performed in Outpatient Departments of US Community Hospitals, 1980–2005.

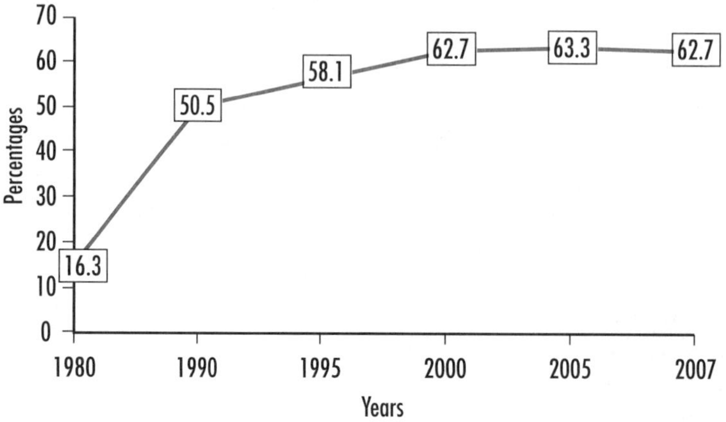

*Source:* Data from *Health, United States, 2009*, p. 372, National Center for Health Statistics, US Department of Health and Human Services.

surgeries has not decreased (Kozak et al. 1999). According to Russo et al. (2010), the 10 most common ambulatory surgeries performed in community hospitals in 28 states were colonoscopy and biopsy (18.1% of all ambulatory surgeries); upper gastrointestinal endoscopy; biopsy (10.8%), lens and cataract procedures (5.5%), diagnostic cardiac catheterization; coronary arteriography (3.8%), debridement of wound, infection, or burn (2.6%); excision of semilunar cartilage of knee (2.5%); cholecystectomy and common duct exploration (2.5%); tonsillectomy and/or adenoidectomy (2.5%); inguinal and femoral hernia repair (2.1%); and other excisions of the cervix and uterus (2.1%).

# Reasons for the Growth in Outpatient Services

Over the years, several noteworthy changes have occurred in the health care delivery system and in the social environment in which health services are delivered. As a result of these changes, many hospital admissions are regarded as unwarranted. A Rand Corporation study based on a sample of hospital records from 1974 to 1982 concluded that 17% of the admissions could have been avoided through the use of outpatient surgery (Siu et al. 1986). Several key changes have been instrumental in shifting the balance between inpatient and outpatient services. These factors can be broadly classified as reimbursement, technological factors, utilization control factors, physician practice factors, and social factors.

## Reimbursement

Until the 1980s, health insurance coverage was usually more generous for inpatient services than for outpatient services. For years, many interventions that could have been performed safely and effectively on an outpatient basis remained inpatient procedures, because third-party reimbursement for outpatient care was limited. These payment policies began to change during the 1980s. In response to the changes in financial incentives, hospitals aggressively developed outpatient services to offset declining inpatient income.

In the mid-1980s, Medicare substituted a prospective payment system (PPS) for the cost-plus system to reimburse inpatient hospital services (see Chapter 6). PPS reimbursement based on diagnosis-related groups (DRGs) provides fixed case-based payment to hospitals. The outpatient sector, on the other hand, had no payment restrictions. Hospitals, therefore, had a strong incentive to minimize inpatient lengths of stay and to provide continued treatment in outpatient settings. To contain costs in the mushrooming outpatient sector, in 2000, Medicare implemented prospective reimbursement mechanisms, such as the Medicare Outpatient Prospective Payment System (OPPS) for services provided in hospital outpatient departments and home health resource groups (HHRGs) for home health care (see Chapter 6). Cost-containment strategies adopted by managed care also stress lower inpatient use, with a corresponding emphasis on outpatient services.

## Technological Factors

Development of new diagnostic and treatment procedures and less invasive surgical methods has made it possible to provide services in outpatient settings that previously required hospital stays. Shorter-acting anesthetics are now available. The diffusion of arthroscopes, laparoscopes, lasers, and other minimally invasive technologies has made many surgical procedures less traumatic. These modern procedures have dramatically curtailed recuperation time,

which has made same-day surgical procedures very common. Many office-based physicians have expanded their capacity to perform outpatient diagnostic, treatment, and surgical services because acquisition of technology has become more feasible and cost effective.

## Utilization Control Factors

Various payers have strongly discouraged hospital stays. Prior authorization for inpatient admission, as well as close monitoring during hospitalization, has been actively pursued, with the objective of minimizing length of stay. Chapter 9 discusses the common utilization control methods.

## Physician Practice Factors

The growth of managed care and the consolidation by large hospital-centered institutions weakened physician autonomy and professional control over the delivery of medical care. Physicians also lost income. To counter these forces, an increasing number of physicians have broken their ties with hospitals and started their own specialized care centers, such as ambulatory surgery centers and cardiac care centers. In specialized ambulatory care centers, physicians find that they can perform more procedures in less time and earn higher incomes (Jackson 2002). As one would expect to find in the industrial mass-production model, in a study of hospital outpatient procedures, a higher case volume for the same procedures resulted in significant reduction in average cost per procedure (Center for Healthcare Industry Performance Studies 1997). Higher volumes may also be associated with better quality. Such factors may be behind the growth in specialized centers of excellence for cataract and hernia surgeries and cardiac procedures.

## Social Factors

Patients have a strong preference for receiving health care in home- and community-based settings. Unless absolutely necessary, most patients do not want to be institutionalized. Staying in their own homes gives people a strong sense of independence and control over their lives, elements considered important for quality of life.

Large hospitals have traditionally been located in congested urban centers. Increasing numbers of suburbanites have perceived these locations as inconvenient. Hence, many freestanding outpatient centers and satellite clinics operated by inner city hospitals are now located in the suburbs.

# Types of Outpatient Care Settings and Methods of Delivery

The myriad of outpatient care and community-based services now operating sometimes makes it difficult to adequately differentiate between the structural settings in which these services are provided. For example, agencies providing home health services can be freestanding, hospital based, or nursing home based. Many physician group practices are merging with hospitals; hospitals and freestanding surgical clinics often compete for various types of surgical procedures. Therefore, the classifications used in this section are only illustrative because many exceptions exist. Also, in this constantly evolving system, new settings and methods are likely to emerge. The various settings for outpatient service delivery

found in the US health care delivery system can be grouped as

- private practice
- hospital-based services
- freestanding facilities
- mobile medical, diagnostic, and screening services
- home health care
- hospice services
- ambulatory long-term care services
- public health services
- public and voluntary clinics
- telephone access
- complementary and alternative medicine

## Private Practice

Physicians, as office-based practitioners, are the backbone of ambulatory care and constitute the vast majority of primary care services. Most visits entail relatively limited examination and testing, and encounters with the physician are generally brief. Office waiting time is typically longer than the actual time spent with the physician.

In the past, the solo practice of medicine and small partnerships attracted the most practitioners. Self-employment offered a degree of independence not generally available in large organizational settings. Today, most physicians are affiliated with group practices or institutions, such as hospitals and MCOs. Several factors account for this shift, including uncertainties created by rapid changes in the health care delivery system, contracting by MCOs with consolidated rather than solo entities, competition from large health care delivery organizations, high cost of operating a solo practice, complexity of billings and collections in a multiple-payer system, and increased external controls over the private practice of medicine. Group practice and other organizational arrangements offer the benefits of a patient referral network; negotiating leverage with MCOs; sharing overhead expenses; ease of obtaining coverage from colleagues for personal time off; and, in a growing number of instances, attractive starting salaries, with benefits and profit-sharing plans.

Group practice of medicine in the United States has experienced a sharp increase (Figure 7–3). An estimated one-fourth of all US physicians now practice in a group clinic (SMG Solutions 2000). Most of these groups are small, with about 69% having no more than 6 physicians. Of these, 27% have 7 to 25 physicians. Only 4% have 26 or more physicians; however, nearly one-half of all

physicians working in group practices have 26 or more partners. In other words, roughly 4% of group practices employ nearly one-half of all physicians.

Group practice clinics also offer important advantages to patients. In many instances, patients can receive up-to-date diagnostic, treatment, pharmaceutical, and certain surgical services. All but the most advanced secondary and tertiary procedures can be performed within these large clinics. Patients also often see cross-referrals among partner physicians located near each other as an added convenience.

Apart from physicians, other private practitioners often work in solo or group practice settings, for example, dentists; optometrists; podiatrists; psychologists; and physical, occupational, and speech therapists. Group practice among these health care providers is becoming increasingly common, generally for the same reasons as for physicians.

Figure 7–4 shows the distribution of total ambulatory visits among physicians' offices, hospital-based outpatient departments, and hospital EDs. In 2007, approximately 82.9% of all ambulatory care visits occurred in physicians' offices. It is interesting to note that hospitals have made substantial strides gaining market share for outpatient services.

Figure 7–3 Growth in the Number of Medical Group Practices.

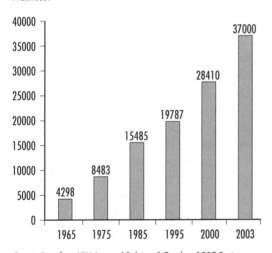

Source: Data from VHA Inc. and Deloitte & Touche, *1997 Environmental assessment: Redesigning health care for the millennium,* Irving, TX: VHA Inc.; SMG Solutions, *2000 Report and directory: Medical group practices,* Chicago, IL: SMG Solutions; Medical Group Management Association. Medical Group Fast Facts. http://www.mgma.com /press/default.aspx?id=1434, accessed 11-15-10.

## Hospital-Based Outpatient Services

Only a couple of decades ago, hospital professionals regarded outpatient departments of urban hospitals with certain contempt. The outpatient department was often viewed as the stepchild of the institution and the least popular area of the hospital in which to work. Hospital outpatient clinics, which were mainly operated by city and county government hospitals and located in urban

Figure 7–4  Ambulatory Care Visits in the United States.

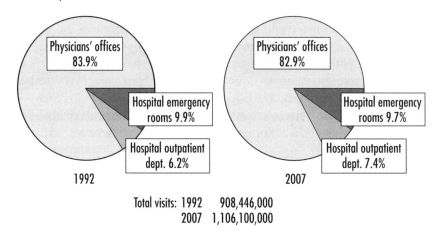

Total visits:  1992    908,446,000
               2007  1,106,100,000

*Source:* Data from National Center for Health Statistics, United States Department of Health and Human Services. *Statistical Abstracts of United States,* 2001, p. 108; and *Statistical Abstracts of United States,* 2010, p. 113.

centers, served primarily indigent populations because these people lacked access to private medical care (Sultz and Young 1997). Even today, many hospital outpatient clinics, particularly those in inner city areas, function as the community's safety net, providing primary care to medically indigent and uninsured populations. Some of the early nonprofit community hospitals also had outpatient departments. For example, in the mid-1970s, the Pennsylvania Hospital in Philadelphia treated almost 200 patients a year in its outpatient department (Raffel and Raffel 1994). However, these hospitals preferred to serve paying patients.

Outpatient services are now a key source of profit for hospitals. Consequently, hospitals have expanded their outpatient departments, and utilization has grown (see Figure 7–4). This trend is the result of fierce competition in the health care industry in which MCOs emphasizing preventive and outpatient care have waged a relentless drive to cut costs. As hospitals have seen inpatient revenues steadily erode, they have begun sprucing up and expanding outpatient services. In doing so, they are competing for privately insured patients who favor private physicians' offices. Beth Israel Hospital of New York City has struggled over the years to compete for patients with the city's more prestigious academic medical centers. In 1996, the hospital opened the Phillips Ambulatory Care Center in a gleaming building that looks like a medical mall. Inside are cozy offices, plush glass-walled waiting rooms looking out on an atrium with a waterfall, and state-of-the-art examining rooms (Fein 1996). The center provides a full range of outpatient services, from primary care to over 50 different on-site diagnostic services, a cancer center, ambulatory surgery, a spine institute, and a wellness library (Phillips Ambulatory Care Center 2000).

A continuum of inpatient and outpatient services developed by a hospital offers opportunities for cross-referral among services to keep patients within the same delivery system. A hospital providing both inpatient and outpatient services can enhance its revenues by referring postsurgical cases to its affiliated units for rehabilitation and home care follow-up. Patients receiving various types of outpatient services constitute an important source of referrals back to hospitals for inpatient care. A hospital can thus expand its patient base.

Prior to 1985, outpatient care had less than 15% of the total gross patient revenue for all US hospitals. This ratio has now grown to nearly 40% (AHA 2006). Between 1996 and 2000, hospital outpatient revenues grew by approximately 54.4%, whereas the growth of inpatient revenues was merely 32% (Health Forum 2002). Given the growing competition in the delivery of outpatient services, hospitals and hospital systems have launched specialized services, such as sports medicine, women's health, and renal dialysis. Many hospitals have also developed health promotion/disease prevention and health fitness programs as outreaches to the communities they serve.

Most hospital-based outpatient services can be broadly classified into five main types: clinical, surgical, emergency, home health, and women's health.

## Clinical Services

Acquisition of group practices has enabled hospitals to increase their market share for outpatient care. Downstream referrals for inpatient, surgical, and other specialized services have generated additional revenues for these hospitals. Both public and private nonprofit hospitals located in inner city locations provide uncompensated care to patients who do not have access to private practitioners' offices for routine care, mainly because they are uninsured. Teaching

hospitals operate various clinics, offering highly specialized, research-based services.

## Surgical Services

Hospital-based ambulatory surgery centers originated in Washington, DC; Los Angeles; and other large cities. They provide same-day surgical care; patients are sent home after a few hours of recovery time following surgery. Follow-up care generally continues in the physician's office. Although most procedures are still performed on an inpatient basis, in outpatient medical procedures, hospitals also have the upper hand over freestanding centers (see Figure 7–5).

## Emergency Services

The ED has been a vital outpatient component of many community hospitals. The main purpose of this department is to

Figure 7–5 Medical Procedures by Location.

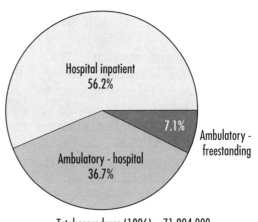

Total procedures (1996) = 71,904,000

*Source:* Data from *Vital and Health Statistics: Ambulatory and Inpatient Procedures in the United States, 1996*, p. 25, November 1998, National Center for Health Statistics, US Department of Health and Human Services.

have services available around the clock for patients who are acutely ill or injured, particularly those with serious or life-threatening conditions requiring immediate attention. When deemed medically appropriate, prompt hospitalization can occur directly from the ED. The department is commonly staffed by physicians who have specialized training in emergency medicine. In small hospitals, the staff may be members of the regular medical staff in rotation (Wilson and Neuhauser 1985). Another option is to contract ED staffing to physician groups specializing in emergency medicine.

Weinerman and colleagues (1966) defined three categories of conditions for which patients present themselves to the ED: *emergent conditions* are critical and require immediate medical attention, time delay is harmful to the patient, and the disorder is acute and potentially threatening to life or function. *Urgent conditions* require medical attention within a few hours, a longer delay presents possible danger to the patient, and the disorder is acute but not severe enough to be life threatening. *Nonurgent conditions* do not require the resources of an emergency service, and the disorder is nonacute or minor in severity.

It has been well documented that, in the United States, EDs are overused for nonurgent or routine care that could be more appropriately addressed in a primary care setting (Glick and Thompson 1997). Actually, fewer than one-half of the visits are for emergency conditions (McCaig and Burt 2002). For many of the uninsured lacking access to routine primary care, the ED has become the family physician, especially at night and on weekends (Raffel and Raffel 1994). Reasons for nonurgent use of the ED include unavailability of primary care, erroneous self-assessment of severity of

ailment or injury, the 24-hour open-door policy, convenience, socioeconomic stress, psychiatric comorbidities, and a lack of social support (Liggins 1993; Padgett and Brodsky 1992). The uninsured and people on Medicaid use disproportionately more ED services than those who have private insurance coverage (McCaig and Burt 2002). Many private physicians do not provide services to Medicaid enrollees because of low reimbursement, which leaves people on Medicaid without a regular source of primary care (McNamara et al. 1993). Conversely, people who have a source of ongoing primary care are less likely to use EDs (Rosenblatt et al. 2000).

The Emergency Medical Treatment and Labor Act of 1986 (EMTALA) requires screening and evaluation of every patient, necessary stabilizing treatment, and admitting when necessary, regardless of ability to pay. Hence, Medicaid patients and the uninsured often use EDs for primary care treatments. Thus, EDs often function as a public "safety net."

Crowding in EDs has also been exacerbated by hospital and ED closings nationwide. In 1992, approximately 6,000 hospitals had EDs. Less than 4,000 remain today. Yet, the demand for ED visits has increased considerably, as reflected by the growth in the annual number of ED visits from 93.4 million to 110.2 million between 1994 and 2004 (McCaig and Newar 2006). Causes of ED overcrowding include hospital bed shortages in some areas, high medical acuity of patients, increasing patient volume, too few examination spaces, and a shortage of registered nurses (Derlet and Richards 2002). Because of overcrowding, EDs must use triage mechanisms to screen patients for the level of severity and for the referral of nonemergency cases to PCPs.

Because EDs require sophisticated facilities and highly trained personnel and must be accessible 24 hours a day, costs are high and services are not designed for nonurgent care (Williams 1993). Inappropriate use of emergency services wastes precious resources. Hence, alternatives to the ED for nonurgent and routine care are critically needed, especially for Medicaid and uninsured patients. Freestanding walk-in clinics and urgent care centers provide extended hours, but their services are mainly available to insured patients. Because of competition from such freestanding clinics, some hospitals now offer extended evening and weekend hours at their own outpatient centers. After-hours telephone access to trained professionals is another alternative that is both economical and convenient.

## Home Health Care

Many hospitals have opened separate home health departments, which provide mainly postacute care and rehabilitation therapies. Hospitals have entered the home health business to keep discharged patients within the hospital system. Hospitals operate about 24% of all Medicare-certified home health agencies in the United States (National Association for Home Care and Hospice 2004).

Home health care is discussed in detail later in this chapter.

## Women's Health Centers

Emerging recognition in the 1980s of the prominence of women as a major health market led medical institutions to develop specialized women's health centers in hospital-based and/or hospital-affiliated settings. Women's health is discussed in greater detail in Chapter 11. Following are some of the reasons behind the growth of women's centers:

- Women are the major users of health care. They seek health care more often than men do. Morbidity is greater among women than among men, even after childbearing-related conditions are factored out (see Chapter 11).

- A change in philosophy in American culture toward women, including gender equality.

- A recognition that the female majority in the United States will continue to grow, as the aging population includes more females. Table 7–2 shows current population trends.

Hospital-sponsored women's health centers have a variety of service provision models

Table 7–2  Growth in Female US Resident Population by Age Groups Between 1980 and 2007 (in thousands)

| | Age Groups | | | | | | |
|---|---|---|---|---|---|---|---|
| | <15 | 15 to 44 | 45 to 64 | 65 to 74 | 75 to 84 | 85+ | Total |
| 1980 | 25,073 | 52,833 | 23,342 | 8,824 | 4,862 | 1,559 | 116,493 |
| 2007 | 29,736 | 62,097 | 39,217 | 10,465 | 7,711 | 3,735 | 152,961 |
| Growth | 4,663 | 9,264 | 15,875 | 1,641 | 2,849 | 2,176 | 36,468 |

*Source:* Data from *Health, United States, 2009,* p. 147.

on a continuum that includes telephone information and referral, educational programs, health screening and diagnostics, comprehensive primary care for women, and mental health services. In addition to services in obstetrics, gynecology, and primary care, women's health centers offer mammography, ultrasound, osteoporosis screening, and other health screenings. Specialized inpatient programs for women, such as special units, pavilions, and women's hospitals, are also in operation (Looker 1993).

## Freestanding Facilities

Freestanding medical clinics include walk-in clinics; urgent care centers; surgicenters; and other outpatient facilities, such as outpatient rehabilitation centers, optometric centers, and dental clinics. These clinics, which are often owned or controlled by private corporations, commonly employ practitioners on salary. The growing number of ambulatory centers might be expected to reduce the use of hospital EDs for nonurgent care. However, because these centers cater mainly to insured patients, the use of hospital EDs by the uninsured is likely to continue unless other alternatives are developed to meet the routine medical needs of the uninsured population.

*Walk-in clinics* provide ambulatory services, ranging from basic primary care to urgent care, but they are used on a nonroutine, episodic basis. The main advantages of these clinics are convenience of location, evening and weekend hours, and availability of services on a "walk-in" (no appointment) basis. *Urgent care centers* offer extended hours; many are open 24 hours a day, 7 days a week and accept patients with no appointments. These centers offer a wide range of routine services for basic and acute conditions on a first-come first-served basis, but they are not comparable to hospital EDs. *Surgicenters* are freestanding ambulatory surgery centers independent of hospitals. They usually provide a full range of services for the types of surgery that can be performed on an outpatient basis and do not require overnight hospitalization. On the other hand, office-based specialists still use their own offices for routine procedures, such as oral surgery, plastic surgery, and ophthalmology.

Outpatient rehabilitation centers provide physical therapy, occupational therapy, and speech pathology services. In the past, generous Medicare reimbursement attracted various operators to open outpatient rehabilitation centers, but caps were instituted under the Balanced Budget Act of 1997. Therapy caps are determined on a calendar year basis. For physical therapy and speech–language pathology services combined, the annual cap per patient is $1,870 for 2011. For occupational therapy services, the cap is $1,870 for 2011. Deductible and coinsurance amounts applied to therapy services count toward the amount accrued before a cap is reached (CMS 2011).

Neighborhood optical centers providing vision services have become quite popular in recent years, replacing many office-based opticians. Other freestanding facilities include audiology clinics, dental centers, hemodialysis centers, pharmacies, and suppliers of *durable medical equipment* (DME). DME suppliers furnish ostomy supplies, hospital beds, oxygen tanks, walkers, wheelchairs, and many other types of supplies and equipment. A growing number of the various types of freestanding facilities are part of large regional and nationwide chains, which are opening new facilities at an unprecedented rate in new geographic locations.

## Mobile Medical, Diagnostic, and Screening Services

Mobile health care services are transported to patients. Ambulance service and first aid treatment provided to the victims of severe illness, accidents, and disasters by trained emergency medical technicians (EMTs) are the most commonly encountered mobile medical services. Such services are also referred to as prehospital medicine. Early attention following traumatic injury is often lifesaving. EMTs are specially trained to provide such attention at the site and in transit to the hospital. Most ambulance personnel have a Basic-EMT rating. Advanced training can lead to EMT-Paramedic certification. Paramedics are trained to administer emergency drugs and provide advanced life support emergency medical services. Examples include intravenous administration of fluids and drugs, treatment for shock, electrocardiograms, electrical interventions to support cardiac function, and endotracheal intubation (insertion of a tube as an air passage through the trachea).

To provide a speedy response to emergencies, most urban centers have developed formal emergency medical systems that incorporate all area hospital EDs, along with transportation and communication systems. Most such communities have established 911 emergency phone lines to provide immediate access to those needing emergency care. An ambulance is dispatched by a central communications center, which also identifies and alerts the hospital most appropriately equipped to deal with the type of emergency and located closest to the site where the emergency has occurred. Specialized ambulance services or advanced life support ambulances include mobile coronary care units, shock-trauma vans, and disaster relief vans. They are staffed by paramedics and EMTs who have advanced training.

Mobile medical services also constitute an efficient and convenient way to provide certain types of routine health services. Mobile eye care, podiatric care, and dental care units, for example, can be brought to a nursing home site where they can efficiently serve many patients residing in the facility. They are a convenient service for the patients, many of whom are frail elderly, who can then avoid an often difficult and tiring trip to a regular clinic.

Mobile diagnostic services include mammography and magnetic resonance imaging (MRI). Such mobile units take advanced diagnostic services to small towns and rural communities. They offer the advantages of convenience to patients and cost efficiency in the delivery of diagnostic care. Other screening services are more basic in nature. Screening vans, staffed by volunteers who are trained professionals and operated by various nonprofit organizations, are often seen at malls and fair sites. Various types of health education and health promotion services and screening checks, such as blood pressure and cholesterol screening, are commonly performed for anyone who walks in.

## Home Health Care

For most ambulatory care, patients must voluntarily leave their homes to go to the settings where such care is delivered. In *home health care*, services are brought to patients in their own homes. Without home services, the only alternative for most such patients would be institutionalization in a hospital or nursing home. Home health is consistent with the philosophy of maintaining people in the least restrictive environment possible. Most people express a strong preference for receiving health services at home rather than in an institution.

Before the home health boom, the Visiting Nurse Associations (VNAs) provided nursing and other services in patients' homes. The first VNAs were established in Buffalo, Boston, and Philadelphia in 1885 and 1886 (Wilson and Neuhauser 1985). VNAs now account for only 6% of all Medicare-certified agencies (National Association for Home Care and Hospice 2004).

Following a lawsuit in 1989, Medicare rules for home health care were clarified, making it easier for Medicare beneficiaries to receive home health services. Patients are eligible to receive these services under Medicare if they are homebound, have a plan of treatment and a periodic review by a physician, and require intermittent or part-time skilled nursing and/or rehabilitation therapies (Waid 1998).

Home health services typically include nursing care, such as changing dressings, monitoring medications, and providing help with bathing, and short-term rehabilitation, such as physical therapy, occupational therapy, and speech therapy. Other services include homemaker services, such as meal preparation, shopping, transportation, and some specific household chores. Not every home health agency provides all of these services, however. For example, home health agencies often assume responsibility for arranging for DME, but private DME companies actually furnish the equipment.

Under Medicare, home health benefits do not include full-time nursing care, food, blood, and drugs. Since the early 1980s, specialized high-technology home therapies have also proliferated. Before that, those services could only be delivered in hospitals. Such specialized services include intravenous antibiotics, oncology therapy, hemodialysis, parenteral and enteral nutrition, and

ventilator care (Evashwick 1993). For specialized services, home health care is cost effective and enhances the patient's quality of life. For example, home hemodialysis costs about one-third of what in-center dialysis costs. Especially for younger patients, the option of dialyzing at home provides greater independence and flexibility, such as the ability to dialyze at night. It has enabled people to maintain employment and, in many cases, saved hours of time spent traveling to and from dialysis centers (Stahl 1997). Overall costs were reduced, on average, by more than $13,000 per patient when a pulmonary specialty team managed the in-home health care of patients suffering from advanced chronic obstructive pulmonary disease (COPD) because of decreased use of hospital, emergency department, and skilled nursing facility resources (Steinel and Madigan 2003).

Figure 7–6 shows the demographic characteristics of home health care patients in 2000. According to the 2007 National Home and Hospice Care Survey, 1.46 million home health care patients were in the United States (National Center for Health Statistics 2010). Home health care patients tended to be aged 65 and over (69%), female (64%), and white (82%). Because of variations in data sources, national expenditures for home health care are difficult to calculate. However, estimates from the Centers for Medicare & Medicaid Services (2006) indicate that total expenditures for home health were $43.2 billion in 2004. Medicare is the largest single payer for home care services. It financed approximately $16.4 billion of home health care expenditures in 2004, compared to $13.7 billion for Medicaid, $5.2 billion for private insurance, and $4.9 billion for out-of-pocket payments (CMS 2006). Payments to home health agencies were sharply cut under the Balanced Budget Act of 1997. As a result,

Figure 7–6 Demographic Characteristics of US Home Health Patients, 2000.

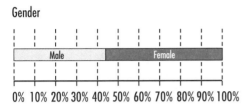

Gender

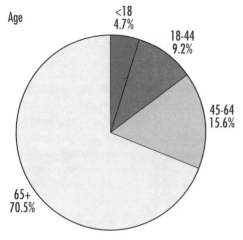

Age

*Source:* Data from National Center for Health Statistics, *2000 National Home and Hospice Care Survey.*

home health expenditures accounted for 4% of total Medicare spending in 2004, compared to 9% in 1997 (National Association for Home Care and Hospice 2004).

Medicaid payments for home care are divided into three main categories: the traditional home health benefit, which is a federally mandated service provided by all states, and two optional programs—the personal care option and home and community-based waivers. Together, these three home health services represent a relatively small but growing portion of total Medicaid payments.

Various private payers also prefer to minimize the high costs associated with hospital inpatient care and opt for home health services wherever possible. Private home

health care is increasingly financed through MCOs. Hence, home health care is no longer synonymous with long-term, home-based care for the elderly, although the elderly are the largest users of home health care.

Reimbursement cuts implemented under the Balanced Budget Act had a marked impact on the home health industry. Between 1997 and 2000, the number of home health agencies in the United States declined from 15,069 to 13,067 (Hoechst Marion Roussel 1999; Aventis Pharmaceuticals 2001). This trend continued through 2007 (CDC 2011). Thirty percent of Medicare-certified agencies are hospital based, 40% are proprietary, and the remaining 24% have other types of ownership. Figure 7–7 shows sources of revenue and average distribution of revenues from these sources for home health care. Tables 7–3 and 7–4 provide additional statistics.

Figure 7–7 Estimated Payments for Home Care by Payment Source, 2009.

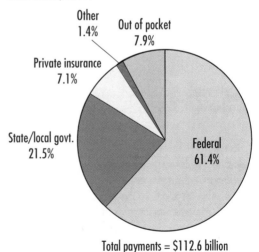

Total payments = $112.6 billion

*Source:* Data from Centers for Medicare & Medicaid Services, Office of the Actuary, *National Health Expenditures Projections: 2009–2019.* https://www.cms.gov/NationalHealthExpendData/downloads/proj2009.pdf, accessed 11-24-10.

Table 7–3  Selected Organizational Characteristics of US Home Health and Hospice Care Agencies: United States, 2007

| Characteristic | Home Health Care[1] | Hospice Care[1] |
|---|---|---|
| | Number (standard error) | |
| All agencies[2] ........................................ | 12,300 (746) | 3,700 (250) |
| | Percent distributions (standard error) | |
| All agencies[2] ........................................ | 100.0 ... | 100.0 ... |
| Ownership | | |
| Proprietary .......................................... | 69.7 (3.2) | 34.0 (3.9) |
| Voluntary nonprofit ................................... | 23.5 (2.9) | 55.5 (4.0) |
| Government and other .................................. | 6.9 (1.2) | 10.6 (2.9) |
| Chain affiliation | | |
| Part of a chain....................................... | 30.5 (3.8) | 23.7 (3.3) |
| Not part of a chain................................... | 69.5 (3.8) | 76.3 (3.3) |
| Medicare certification status | | |
| Certified as home health care agency .................. | 81.6 (4.0) | ... ... |
| Certified as hospice care agency...................... | ... ... | 93.4 (2.9) |
| Medicaid certification status | | |
| Certified as home health care agency .................. | 80.7 (3.9) | ... ... |
| Certified as hospice care agency...................... | ... ... | 86.4 (3.4) |
| Geographic region | | |
| Northeast............................................. | 13.5 (3.3) | 14.8 (2.5) |
| Midwest............................................... | 22.1 (3.2) | 22.6 (2.5) |
| South................................................. | 50.3 (4.2) | 44.5 (4.0) |
| West.................................................. | 14.1 (2.6) | 18.2 (3.3) |
| Location | | |
| Metropolitan statistical area (MSA)[3]................. | 73.6 (1.9) | 66.8 (2.5) |
| Micropolitan statistical area[4] ...................... | 13.8 (1.2) | 19.5 (1.7) |
| Neither............................................... | 12.6 (1.2) | 13.7 (1.2) |

...Category not applicable.

[1]Include agencies that provide both home health and hospice care services (mixed).

[2]Include agencies that provide home health care services, hospice care services, or both types of services and currently or recently served home health and/or hospice care patients. Agencies that provided only homemaker services or housekeeping services, assistance with instrumental activities of daily living (IADLs), or durable medical equipment and supplies were excluded from the survey.

[3]A metropolitan statistical area is a county or group of contiguous counties that contains at least one urbanized area of 50,000 or more population. May also contain other counties that are economically and socially integrated with the central county as measured by commuting.

[4]A micropolitan statistical area is a nonmetropolitan county or group of contiguous nonmetropolitan counties that contains an urban cluster of 10,000 to 49,999 persons. May include surrounding counties if there are strong  economic ties among the counties, based on commuting patterns.

*Note:* Numbers may not add to totals because of rounding and/or because estimates and percent distributions include a category of unknowns not reported in the table. Percentages are based on the unrounded numbers.

*Source:* CDC/NCHS, National Home and Hospice Care Survey, 2007.

Table 7–4  Home Health and Hospice Care Patients Served at the Time of the Interview, by Agency Type and Number of Patients: United States, 2007.

| Number of Patients | Home Health Care Only | Home Health and Hospice Care (Mixed) |
|---|---|---|
| | Mean (standard error) | |
| Number of home health care patients . . . . . . . . . . . . . . . . . . . . . | 109.0 (9.2) | 177.7 (17.7) |
| | Percent distributions (standard error) | |
| Total | 100.0 . . . | 100.0 . . . |
| 0–25 . . . . . . . . . . . . . . . . . . . . . . . . . . . . . . . . . . . . . . | †16.0 (4.3) | †9.8 (2.4) |
| 26–50 . . . . . . . . . . . . . . . . . . . . . . . . . . . . . . . . . . . . . | †21.3 (4.2) | †25.1 (6.4) |
| 51–100 . . . . . . . . . . . . . . . . . . . . . . . . . . . . . . . . . . . . | 29.0 (4.0) | 18.4 (3.1) |
| 101–150 . . . . . . . . . . . . . . . . . . . . . . . . . . . . . . . . . . . | †10.8 (2.3) | †9.4 (1.9) |
| 151 or more. . . . . . . . . . . . . . . . . . . . . . . . . . . . . . . . . . | 23.0 (3.5) | 37.4 (4.8) |

| Number of Patients | Hospice Care Only | Home Health and Hospice Care (Mixed) |
|---|---|---|
| | Mean (standard error) | |
| Number of hospice care patients . . . . . . . . . . . . . . . . . . . . . . | 78.1 (6.4) | 39.1 (5.7) |
| | Percent distributions (standard error) | |
| Total . . . . . . . . . . . . . . . . . . . . . . . . . . . . . . . . . . . . . . . | 100.0 . . . | 100.0 . . . |
| 0–25 . . . . . . . . . . . . . . . . . . . . . . . . . . . . . . . . . . . . . . | 29.5 (5.4) | 57.6 (5.6) |
| 26–50 . . . . . . . . . . . . . . . . . . . . . . . . . . . . . . . . . . . . . | 22.1 (4.9) | 24.5 (5.9) |
| 51–100 . . . . . . . . . . . . . . . . . . . . . . . . . . . . . . . . . . . . | 21.2 (4.0) | †6.3 (1.4) |
| 101–150 . . . . . . . . . . . . . . . . . . . . . . . . . . . . . . . . . . . | †9.9 (2.5) | *  (*) |
| 151 or more. . . . . . . . . . . . . . . . . . . . . . . . . . . . . . . . . . | †11.6 (2.3) | *  (*) |

. . . Category not applicable.

†Estimate does not meet standards of reliability or precision because the sample size is between 30 and 59 or the sample size is greater than 59 but has a relative standard error of 30 percent or more.

*Estimate does not meet standards of reliability or precision because the sample size is fewer than 30.

*Note:* Unknown are excluded when calculating estimates. There was 1 (unweighted) case with unknown number of home health care patients, while 19 (unweighted) cases with unknown number of hospice care patients. Percentages are based on the unrounded numbers.

*Source:* CDC/NCHS, National Home and Hospice Care Survey, 2007.

## Hospice Services

The term *hospice* refers to a cluster of comprehensive services for the terminally ill with a life expectancy of 6 months or less. Over one-half of the patients are diagnosed with cancer upon admission. Hospice, whose programs provide services that address the special needs of dying persons and their families, is a method of care, not a location, and services are taken to patients and their families wherever they are located. Thus, hospice can be a part of home health care when the services are provided in the patient's home. In other instances, hospice services are taken to patients in nursing homes, retirement centers, or hospitals. Services can be organized out of a hospital, nursing home, freestanding hospice facility, or home health agency. The dollar outlays in these four types of hospice operations give a fair indication of the volume of services provided through each setting (see Figure 7–8).

Hospice regards the patient and family as the unit of care. This special kind of care includes:

- meeting the patient's physical needs, with an emphasis on pain management and comfort;
- meeting the patient's and family's emotional and spiritual needs;
- support for the family members before and after the patient's death; and
- focus on maintaining the quality of life rather than prolonging life (Miller 1996).

The two primary areas of emphasis in hospice care are (1) pain and symptom management, which is referred to as *palliation*, and (2) psychosocial and spiritual support according to the holistic model of care (see Chapter 2). Counseling and spiritual help are made available to relieve anguish and help the patient deal with his or her death. After the patient's death, bereavement counseling is offered to the family. Social services include help with arranging final affairs (Dychtwald et al. 1990). Apart from medical, nursing, and social services staff, hospice organizations rely heavily on volunteers.

The idea of providing comprehensive care to terminally ill patients was first promoted by Dame Cicely Saunders in the 1960s in England. In the United States, the first hospice was established in 1974 by Sylvia Lack in New Haven, Connecticut (Beresford 1989). Hospice organizations expanded after Medicare extended hospice benefits in 1983. Hospice is a cost-effective option for both private and public payers. It is estimated that for every dollar spent on hospice, Medicare saves $1.52 in Part A and Part B expenditures (National Hospice and

Figure 7–8  *Medicare Dollar Outlays by Type of Hospice,* 2003.

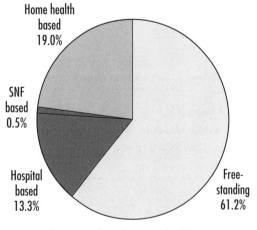

*Source:* Data from Centers for Medicare & Medicaid Services 2005.

Palliative Care Organization 2003). The difference in cost is mainly due to the intensity of services. Many states now provide hospice benefits under Medicaid.

To receive Medicare certification, a hospice must meet these basic conditions:

- Physician certification that the patient's prognosis is for a life expectancy of 6 months or less;
- Make nursing services, physician services, and drugs and biologicals available on a 24-hour basis;
- Provide nursing services under the supervision of a registered nurse;
- Make arrangements for inpatient care when necessary;
- Provide social services by a qualified social worker under the direction of a physician;
- Make counseling services available to both the patient and the family, including bereavement support after the patient's death;
- Provide needed medications, medical supplies, and equipment for pain management and palliation;
- Provide physical, occupational, and speech therapy services when necessary; and
- Provide home health aide and homemaker services when needed.

Under the provisions of the Balanced Budget Act of 1997, Medicare provides for two 90-day benefit periods. Subsequently, an unlimited number of 60-day periods are available, based on recertification by a physician that a patient has 6 months or less to live. Figure 7–9 shows the sources of coverage for hospice services.

Figure 7–9  Coverage of Patients for Hospice Care at the Time of Admission.

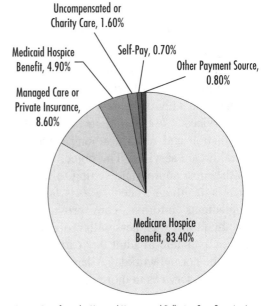

*Source:* Data from the National Hospice and Palliative Care Organization, *NHPCO Facts and Figures, Hospice Care in America.* 2010. http://www.nhpco.org/files/public/Statistics_Research/Hospice_Facts_Figures_Oct-2010.pdf.

In 2009, 1.56 million patients received hospice services, with an average length of services, at 69 days (National Hospice and Palliative Care Organization 2010). The majority of hospice patients were 65 years or older (83%), female (54%), and white (81%). The top diagnoses were cancer (40.1%), debility unspecified (13.1%), heart disease (11.5%), dementia (11.2%), and lung disease (8.2%).

There were approximately 5,000 hospice programs in the United States (National Hospice and Palliative Care Organization 2010). The majority of hospices are independent (57.7%), followed by part of a hospital system (21.4%), part of a home health agency (19.5%), or part of a nursing home (1.4%). Medicare is the largest source of financing for hospice services. Tables 7–3 and 7–4 provide additional statistics.

## Ambulatory Long-Term Care Services

Long-term care has typically been associated with care provided in nursing homes, but two main types of settings—case management and adult day care—deliver outpatient services. *Case management* provides coordination and referral among a variety of health care services. The objective is to find the most appropriate setting to meet a patient's health care needs. *Adult day care* complements informal care provided at home by family members with professional services available in adult day care centers during the normal workday. Chapter 10 discusses both services in more detail.

## Public Health Services

Public health services in the United States are typically provided by local health departments, and the range of services offered varies greatly by locality. Generally, public health programs are limited in scope. They include well-baby care, venereal disease clinics, family planning services, screening and treatment for tuberculosis, and ambulatory mental health. For reasons pointed out in Chapter 3, public health programs offer services that do not directly compete with those provided by private practitioners. Typically, such services are restricted to those areas in which private practitioners have little interest, or they are targeted to serve inner city, poor, uninsured populations. All are *categorical programs* specifically designed to address certain categories of disease or to serve specific categories of persons. School health programs in public schools fall under the public health domain, but they are limited to vision and hearing screening and assistance with dysfunctions that prevent learning. Ambulatory clinics in prisons also fall in the public health domain.

The public school setting is a growing area of practice for physical therapists, occupational therapists, and speech–language pathologists. They help children with special physical and emotional dysfunctions. The Individuals with Disabilities Education Act (IDEA) of 1975 (subject to reauthorization every 3 years) has been instrumental in allowing children with special needs to receive services in public schools so that they can obtain optimum access to education.

## Public and Voluntary Clinics

Examples of public and voluntary clinics include community health centers, free clinics, and others. Most serve mainly underprivileged populations. The combination of these clinics with public health services and some hospitals forms a significant safety net of providers for people who lack private or public health insurance. These clinics also face problems due to inadequate funding and a shortage of primary care providers because of difficulties in recruiting and retaining physicians and other qualified health professionals.

### Community Health Centers

Creation of community health centers (CHCs)—formerly called neighborhood health centers—was authorized during the 1960s, under the Johnson Administration's war on poverty program, mainly to address health care needs in the medically underserved regions of the United States. The federal government determines the *medically underserved* designation to indicate a dearth of primary care providers and delivery settings, as well as poor health indicators for the populace. Such areas are often characterized by economic, geographic, or cultural barriers that limit access to primary health care for a large segment of the population. CHCs are required by law to locate in medically underserved areas and provide services to anyone seeking care, regardless of insurance status or ability to pay. Hence, CHCs are a primary care safety net for the nation's poor and uninsured in both inner city and rural areas.

CHCs operate under the auspices of the Bureau of Primary Health Care (BPHC), US Public Health Service, and US Department of Health and Human Services. Section 330 of the Public Health Service Act provides federal grant funding for CHCs. CHCs are private, nonprofit organizations that nonetheless depend heavily on funding through the Medicaid program and federal grants. Private-pay patients are charged on sliding-fee scales, determined by the patient's income.

CHCs tailor their services to family-oriented primary and preventive health care and dental services (Shi et al. 2007). These centers have developed considerable expertise managing the health care needs of underserved populations. Many have developed systems of care that include outreach programs, case management, transportation, translation services, alcohol and drug abuse screening and treatment, mental health services, health education, and social services.

In 2009, CHCs served 18.8 million patients through 74 million patient visits. The majority of groups that utilize CHCs are vulnerable populations—92% of patients were below the 200% federal poverty level and 38% were uninsured. Among special populations, more than 1 million homeless individuals, 865,000 migrant/seasonal farmworkers, and 165,000 residents from public housing received services under this program (HRSA 2011).

CHCs are governed by an executive director or administrator, have a medical director, and are staffed by multidisciplinary teams of clinicians. The typical CHC employs 6 PCPs, 8 nurses, and 3 NPPs. Also, some clinics have dentists, mental health practitioners, and pharmacists on site. Other members of the team may include case managers and education specialists (Shi et al. 2007).

Studies have shown that CHCs provide accessible, quality care that is cost effective (NACHC 2009a, 2009b, 2009c). Because the majority of the population served belongs to vulnerable groups (i.e., low income, minorities, homeless), studies show potential of health centers in bridging the disparities found in these populations (NACHC 2009d).

Expanding the services of CHCs was a central element of President Bush's plan for expanding health care access to the uninsured and underserved. In 2002, the Bush Administration proposed a $1.5 billion budget to continue a long-term strategy that would add 1,200 new and expanded CHC sites over 5 years and serve an additional 6.1 million patients (Shi et al. 2007). The Obama Administration continued this trend of support. The American Recovery and Reinvestment Act of 2009 allocated $2 billion to CHCs to expand patient population, create new jobs, and meet the demands for primary care services (US DHHS 2011).

Components of the Patient Protection and Affordable Care Act of 2010 that affect CHCs involve payment protections and developing teaching health centers. The law ensures that CHCs are not underpaid for the services they provide and adds preventive services to the Medicare payment rate, while eliminating Medicare payment caps. Additionally, the law allows for a Title VII grant program to develop residency programs in CHCs to teach the next generation of primary care providers (NACHC 2011).

## Free Clinics

Modeled after the 19th century dispensary (see Chapter 3), the *free clinic* is a general ambulatory care center, serving primarily the poor, the homeless, and the uninsured. Free clinics have three main characteristics: (1) services are provided at no charge or at a very nominal charge, (2) they are not directly supported or operated by a government agency or health department, and (3) services are delivered mainly by trained volunteer staff. Free clinics focus on the delivery of primary care. Other services vary, depending on the number and training of their volunteer staff.

A survey of five major US cities disclosed that these clinics are open for limited hours and provide services to about 30 to 200 patients per month. They are funded by churches, hospitals, or private donations (Felt-Lisk et al. 2002). Some of these clinics receive government grants to partially support their operations.

The number of free clinics has continued to grow nationally and is estimated at more than 1,200 (NAFC undated). Although mainly a voluntary effort, it has taken the form of an organized movement. The National Association of Free Clinics (NAFC) focuses on the issues and needs of the free clinics and the people they serve in the United States.

## Other Clinics

Other CHCs that have been developed through federal funding are migrant health centers serving transient farmworkers in agricultural communities and rural health centers in isolated underserved rural areas. The Community Mental Health Center program was established to provide ambulatory mental health services in underserved areas.

## Telephone Access

Telephone access is a means of bringing expert opinion and advice to the patient, especially during the hours when physicians' offices are closed. Referred to as *telephone triage*, this type of access has expanded under managed care. The example of the Park Nicollet Clinic of the Minneapolis-based HealthSystem Minnesota illustrates how such a system functions. The telephone call-in system operates 7 days a week, 24 hours a day. The system is staffed by specially trained nurses who receive patients' calls. Using a computer system, they can access a patient's medical history and view the most recent radiology and laboratory test results. The nurses use standardized protocols to guide them in dealing with the patient's problem and consult with primary care physicians when necessary (Appleby 1995). If necessary, the staff can direct patients to appropriate medical services, such as an ED or a physician's office. The URAC Organization accredits telephone triage and health information programs.

## Complementary and Alternative Medicine

Because of their tremendous growth, the role of complementary and alternative medicine (CAM)—also referred to as "nonconventional therapies," or "natural medicine"—in the delivery of health care cannot be ignored. Although the terms "complementary medicine" and "alternative medicine" are used synonymously, as they are here, technically there is a distinction between the two: Complementary treatments are used together with conventional medicine; alternative interventions are used instead of conventional medicine (Barnes et al. 2008).

In the United States, the dominant health care practice is the biomedicine-based allopathic medicine, which is also referred to as conventional medicine. *Alternative medicine*, or CAM, refers to the broad domain of all health care resources other than those intrinsic to biomedicine (CAM Research Methodology Conference 1997) and covers a heterogeneous spectrum of ancient to new approaches that purport to prevent or treat disease (Barnes et al. 2008).

CAM therapies include a wide range of treatments, such as homeopathy, herbal formulas, use of other natural products as preventive and treatment agents, acupuncture, meditation, yoga exercises, biofeedback, and spiritual guidance or prayer. Chiropractic is also largely regarded as a CAM treatment. The traditional medical establishment has shown growing interest in certain CAM therapies.

No particular settings of health care delivery are involved in CAM treatments. With few exceptions, most therapies are self-administered or at least require active patient participation. The types of trained and licensed health care professionals discussed in Chapter 4 are, generally, not involved in the delivery of unconventional care. Even though the efficacy of most CAM treatments has not been scientifically established, their use has exploded. CAM's growth has happened mainly for these reasons:

- Most people who seek CAM therapies believe that they have already explored conventional Western treatments but have not been helped. Most have chronic disorders, such as persistent pain, for which Western medicine can usually offer only symptomatic relief rather than definitive treatment. According to recent investigations, individuals reporting serious health problems are more likely to use alternative treatments than healthier individuals.

- People are persuaded that at least there is no harm in trying alternative treatments.

- Many fear the harms of iatrogenic effects of modern Western medicine more than any potential dangers inherent in nonconventional therapies.

- Most people feel empowered by access to a vast amount of medical and health-related information available through the Internet and feel in control to pursue what they think is best for their own health.

- Many patients report that they seek alternative therapies and individuals who practice them because they want practitioners to take the time to listen to them, understand them, and deal with their personal life, as well as their pathology. They believe that alternative practitioners will meet those needs (Gordon 1996).

A landmark study by Eisenberg and colleagues (1998) estimated that between 1990 and 1997, the proportion of the US adult population over 18 years of age using alternative therapies increased from 33.8% (60 million) to 42.1% (83 million). Although the estimated number of visits to regular PCPs remained stable, visits to alternative medical practitioners increased by 47% (39 million in 1997 vs. 22 million in 1990). The most common reasons given for seeking alternative therapies were back problems, allergies, fatigue, arthritis, and headaches. In both the 1990 and 1997 surveys, 96% of the respondents who saw a practitioner of alternative therapy for a principal condition also saw a medical doctor, but only a minority discussed these therapies with the conventional physician. Based on conservative estimates, Americans spent $14.6 billion in 1990 and $21.2 billion in 1997 on visits to alternative medicine practitioners. Among people who saw alternative therapy practitioners, 58.3% paid for the services out of pocket in 1997.

Use of CAM has grown in the past decades. In the United States, approximately 38% of adults and 12% of children use at least one type of CAM. Use is most common among women with higher levels of education and income. Among the top 3 CAM therapies are natural products (e.g., fish oil, flaxseed, Echinacea), deep breathing, and meditation (Barnes et al. 2008). Total expenditures on CAM for 2007 were $33.9 billion in out-of-pocket expenses, which constitutes 11.2% of total out-of-pocket expenditures on health care and 1.5% of total health care expenditures. The majority of CAM expenditures are for natural products, at $15.4 billion (Nahin et al. 2009). CAM also appears to be popular in Europe, Canada, and other industrialized countries. Even though most of these countries provide universal access to medical care, a significant number of people try alternative treatments.

Although health insurance coverage for chiropractic has been widely available for some time, only some plans include coverage for other CAM therapies. Chiropractic, and even osteopathy, was once a pariah in medical practice. Doctors of osteopathy now work alongside MDs in medical institutions. Chiropractic, even though largely alienated from mainstream modern

medicine, has been increasingly recognized for its healing values.

Given the growing public demand for complementary medicine and its claims for health promotion, disease prevention, and promise for certain chronic conditions, mainstream medicine is showing a genuine interest in better understanding the value of alternative treatments. On the other hand, skepticism is justifiable because alternative medicine is predominantly unregulated. Also, the efficacy of most treatments and the safety of some have not been scientifically evaluated. The most recent findings on CAM methods are cranberry juice cocktail has no effect on preventing recurrent urinary tract infections (Barbosa-Cesnik et al. 2011); white tea extract has potential anticancer benefit (Mao et al. 2010); and Echinacea does not reduce the duration and severity of the cold (Barrett et al. 2010). Only rigorous scientific inquiry and research-based evidence will bring about a genuine integration of alternative therapies into the conventional practice of medicine.

Nevertheless, some developments are noteworthy. In 1993, Congress established the Office of Alternative Medicine (OAM), which became the National Center for Complementary and Alternative Medicine (NCCAM) in 1998. Budget allocations for the center have increased from $2 million in 1993 to $122.7 million in 2006 (NCCAM 2007). The center has three main objectives: (1) explore complementary and alternative healing practices in the context of rigorous science, (2) train complementary and alternative medicine researchers, and (3) disseminate authoritative information to the public and professionals. A growing number of US medical schools now offer some instruction in alternative medicine.

As cost containment in health care continues to occupy center stage, insurance companies, MCOs, and the government are eager to learn about the cost effectiveness, as well as safety, of alternative therapies. Meanwhile, they are slowly and cautiously proceeding toward accepting the integration of certain unorthodox treatments with traditional medical interventions. At the same time, natural-medicine-based private clinics are emerging across the United States.

## Utilization of Outpatient Services

In 2007, Americans made approximately 994.3 million visits, or three visits per person, to office-based physicians (Table 7–5). Physicians in general and family practice accounted for the largest share of these visits (22.9%), followed by physicians in internal medicine (14.5%), pediatrics (13.2%), and obstetrics and gynecology (7.5%). Doctors of osteopathy accounted for 7.7% of the visits. The South led the nation in the proportion of physician visits (41.7%), followed by the Midwest (20.8%), the West (19.5%), and the Northeast (17.9%). Ambulatory visits per person were the highest in the South (3.8 visits) and lowest in the West (2.8 visits). Most physician office visits (86%) took place in metropolitan areas. Visits per person were also higher in metropolitan areas (3.4), compared to rural areas (2.9), reflecting poorer access to primary care in rural areas of the United States. Some of the conclusions regarding the utilization of primary care services that can be drawn from data in Table 7 include the following: older individuals use more services than younger people; females see doctors more frequently (3.8 visits per year) than males (2.9 visits per year); and whites incur more visits per person (3.5) than blacks (3.2). The latter reflects access barriers for the US African American population.

Table 7–5  US Physician Characteristics

| Physician Characteristics | Number of Visits |
|---|---|
| All visits | 994,321 |
| *Physician specialty[3]* | |
| General and family practice | 227,817 |
| Internal medicine | 143,722 |
| Pediatrics | 130,832 |
| Obstetrics and gynecology | 74,296 |
| Ophthalmology | 58,994 |
| Orthopedic surgery | 51,258 |
| Dermatology | 44,874 |
| Psychiatry | 32,660 |
| Cardiovascular diseases | 32,431 |
| Otolaryngology | 20,204 |
| General surgery | 19,636 |
| Urology | 18,914 |
| Neurology | 17,559 |
| Oncology | 15,581 |
| All other specialties | 105,543 |
| *Professional degree* | |
| Doctor of medicine | 917,359 |
| Doctor of osteopathy | 76,962 |
| *Specialty type[3]* | |
| Primary care | 576,650 |
| Medical specialty | 221,073 |
| Surgical specialty | 196,598 |
| *Geographic region* | |
| Northeast | 178,403 |
| Midwest | 206,546 |
| South | 415,018 |
| West | 194,354 |
| *Metropolitan status* | |
| MSA[6] | 855,224 |
| Non-MSA[6] | 139,097 |

. . . Category not applicable.

[3]Physician specialty and specialty type are defined in the "Technical Notes."

[6]MSA is metropolitan statistical area.

*Note:* Numbers may not add to totals because of rounding.

*Source:* National Health Statistics Reports, Number 27, November 3, 2010. http://www.cdc.gov/nchs/data/nhsr/nhsr027.pdf

Table 7–6 presents the most frequently mentioned principal reasons for visiting a physician in 2007. The top 10 reasons were general medical examination, progress visit, cough, postoperative visit, medication, knee symptoms, other and unspecified test results, routine prenatal examination, symptoms referable to throat, and back symptoms. Table 7–7 shows the most frequent principal diagnoses cared for by office-based physicians.

● ● ● ● ● ● ● ● ● ● ● ● ● ● ● ● ● ● ● ● ● ● ● ● ● ● ● ● ● ● ● ● ● ● ● ● ● ● ● ● ● ● ● ● ● ● ● ● ● ● ● ● ● ● ● ● ● ● ● ● ● ● ● ● ● ● ●

### Table 7–6  Principal Reason for Visit and RVC Code

| Principal Reason for Visit and RVC Code[1] | Number of Visits |
|---|---|
| All visits | 994,321 |
| General medical examination | 74,603 |
| Progress visit, not otherwise specified | 60,901 |
| Cough | 27,881 |
| Postoperative visit | 27,645 |
| Medication, other and unspecified kinds | 21,717 |
| Knee symptoms | 19,038 |
| For other and unspecified test results | 17,765 |
| Prenatal examination, routine | 17,694 |
| Symptoms referable to throat | 16,951 |
| Back symptoms | 14,923 |
| Hypertension | 14,741 |
| Well-baby examination | 14,644 |
| Vision dysfunctions | 13,544 |
| Stomach pain, cramps, and spasms | 13,233 |
| Nasal congestion | 13,162 |
| Gynecological examination | 12,816 |
| Skin rash | 12,511 |
| Fever | 12,358 |
| Earache or ear infection | 12,259 |
| Diabetes mellitus | 11,035 |
| All other reasons | 564,898 |

[1] Based on A Reason for Visit Classification for Ambulatory Care (RVC)

*Note:* Numbers may not add to totals because of rounding.

*Source:* National Health Statistics Reports, Number 27, November 3, 2010. http://www.cdc.gov/nchs/data/nhsr/nhsr027.pdf

● ● ● ● ● ● ● ● ● ● ● ● ● ● ● ● ● ● ● ● ● ● ● ● ● ● ● ● ● ● ● ● ● ● ● ● ● ● ● ● ● ● ● ● ● ● ● ● ● ● ● ● ● ● ● ● ● ● ● ● ● ● ● ● ● ● ●

In a comparative survey, physicians and nurses in the Untied States spent more time with patients (average 25 minutes) than their counterparts in Canada and Germany (average 19 minutes). The differences were found to be statistically significant. Despite receiving more time in face-to-face provider contact, Americans were more inclined

Table 7–7  Primary Diagnosis Group and ICD–9–CM Code(s)

| Primary Diagnosis Group and ICD–9–CM Code(s)[1] | Number of Visits | Percent Distribution |
|---|---|---|
| All visits . . . . . . . . . . . . . . . . . . . . . . . . . . . . . . . . . . . . . . . . | 994,321 | 100.0 |
| Essential hypertension . . . . . . . . . . . . . . . . . . . . . . . . . . . 401 | 42,157 | 4.2 |
| Routine infant or child health check . . . . . . . . . . . . . . . . . . . . .V20.2 | 39,930 | 4.0 |
| Acute upper respiratory infections, excluding pharyngitis . . . . . . . . . . . . . . . . . . . . . . . 460–461,463–466 | 33,614 | 3.4 |
| Arthropathies and related disorders . . . . . . . . . . . . . . . . . .710–719 | 32,671 | 3.3 |
| Spinal disorders . . . . . . . . . . . . . . . . . . . . . . . . . . . . . .720–724 | 26,704 | 2.7 |
| Malignant neoplasms . . . . . . . . . . . . . . . . . . . 140–208,230–234 | 25,220 | 2.5 |
| Diabetes mellitus . . . . . . . . . . . . . . . . . . . . . . . . . . . . . 250 | 24,156 | 2.4 |
| Rheumatism, excluding back . . . . . . . . . . . . . . . . . . .725–729 | 19,417 | 2.0 |
| Specific procedures and aftercare . . . . . . . . . . . . . . . . . V50–V59.9 | 19,351 | 1.9 |
| General medical examination . . . . . . . . . . . . . . . . . . . . . . . . . . V70 | 19,162 | 1.9 |
| Follow-up examination . . . . . . . . . . . . . . . . . . . . . . . . . . . . . . V67 | 18,687 | 1.9 |
| Normal pregnancy . . . . . . . . . . . . . . . . . . . . . . . . . . . . . . . . . V22 | 16,871 | 1.7 |
| Otitis media and eustachian tube disorders . . . . . . . . . . . . .381–382 | 14,771 | 1.5 |
| Asthma . . . . . . . . . . . . . . . . . . . . . . . . . . . . . . . . . . . . . 493 | 13,872 | 1.4 |
| Gynecological examination . . . . . . . . . . . . . . . . . . . . . . . . . . .V72.3 | 13,597 | 1.4 |
| Heart disease, excluding ischemic . . . . . . . . .391–392.0,393– 398,402,404,415–416,420–429 | 13,421 | 1.3 |
| Allergic rhinitis . . . . . . . . . . . . . . . . . . . . . . . . . . . . . . . 477 | 12,871 | 1.3 |
| Ischemic heart disease . . . . . . . . . . . . . . . . . . . . . . . . . . 410–414.9 | 12,378 | 1.2 |
| Glaucoma . . . . . . . . . . . . . . . . . . . . . . . . . . . . . . . . . . . 365 | 11,964 | 1.2 |
| Benign neoplasms . . . . . . . . . . . . . . . . . . . . . 210–229,235–239 | 10,950 | 1.1 |
| All other diagnoses[4] . . . . . . . . . . . . . . . . . . . . . . . . . . . . . . . . | 572,557 | 57.6 |

[1] Based on the International Classification of Diseases, Ninth Revision, Clinical Modification (ICD–9–CM) (10). However, certain codes have been combined in this table to form larger categories that better describe the utilization of ambulatory care services.

[4] Includes all other diagnoses not listed above, as well as unknown and blank diagnoses.

*Note:* Numbers may not add to totals because of rounding.

to think that the amount of time was inadequate. In the same survey, the waiting time in physicians' offices averaged approximately 30 minutes in the United States and Canada, but 36 minutes (statistically significant) in Germany (Donelan et al. 1996).

## Summary

In the history of health care delivery, the main settings for ambulatory services have come full circle. First came a shift from outpatient settings to hospitals. Now, ambulatory services outside the hospital have mushroomed. The reasons for this shift are mainly economic, social, and technological. Thanks to new technology, many physicians have broken their ties with hospitals and have started their own specialized care centers, such as ambulatory surgery centers and cardiac care centers. A variety of general medical and surgical interventions are provided in ambulatory care settings. Thus, ambulatory services now transcend the basic and routine primary care services. Conversely, primary care itself has become "specialized." Primary care is no longer concerned simply with the treatment of colds, sprains, and other simple ailments or with determining who is ill enough to require the attention of a specialist. Primary care physicians must coordinate a plethora of services to maintain the long-term viability of a patient's health. Continuity of care over a period of time is essential not just for individuals but also for an entire community. A health services delivery system that lacks universal access is ill-equipped to meet such an objective. Apart from coordination and continuity, other essential functions served by primary care include point of entry and comprehensiveness. In the United States, the gatekeeping aspect of primary care is sometimes regarded as a threat to free choice, but when a person's comprehensive health care needs are coordinated by a trained primary care professional, it leads to better health outcomes and cost efficiency.

In response to the changing economic incentives within the health care delivery system, numerous types of outpatient services have emerged, and a variety of settings for the delivery of services has developed. In most settings, patients go to the delivery sites to receive services. In other cases, services are brought to the patients. The growing interest in complementary and alternative medicine is largely consumer driven. Compared to our complex health care system, alternative medicine, with its emphasis on self-care, is one area where many patients feel more in control of their own destiny.

Americans, on average, make three visits a year to physician offices. The most common reason is for a general medical examination; however, use of primary care is not consistent across geographic regions and races. There is evidence of barriers to care in rural areas and for racial/ethnic minorities.

## Test Your Understanding

### Terminology

| | | |
|---|---|---|
| accountability | ambulatory care | community-oriented |
| adult day care | case management | primary care |
| alternative medicine | categorical programs | durable medical equipment |

*emergent conditions* *medically underserved* *telephone triage*
*free clinic* *nonurgent conditions* *tertiary care*
*gatekeeping* *outpatient services* *urgent care centers*
*home health care* *palliation* *urgent conditions*
*hospice* *primary health care* *walk-in clinic*
*iatrogenic* *secondary care*
*medical home* *surgicenter*

## Review Questions

1. Describe how some of the changes in the health services delivery system have led to a decline in hospital inpatient days and a growth in ambulatory services.

2. What implications has the decline in hospital occupancy rates had for hospital management?

3. All primary care is ambulatory, but not all ambulatory services represent primary care. Discuss.

4. What are the main characteristics of primary care?

5. Discuss the gatekeeping role of primary care.

6. What is community-oriented primary care? Explain.

7. Discuss the two main factors that determine what should be an adequate mix between generalists and specialists.

8. What are some of the reasons solo practitioners are joining group practices?

9. Why is it important for hospital administrators to regard outpatient care as a key component of their overall business strategy?

10. Discuss the main hospital-based outpatient services.

11. What are some of the social changes that led to the creation of specialized health centers for women?

12. Why is the hospital emergency department sometimes used for nonurgent conditions? What are the consequences?

13. What are mobile health care services? Discuss the various types of mobile services.

14. What is the basic philosophy of home health care? Describe the services it provides.

15. What are the conditions of eligibility for receiving home health services under Medicare?

16. Explain the concept of hospice care and the types of services a hospice provides.

17. What are some of the main requirements for Medicare certification of a hospice program?

18. Describe the scope of public health ambulatory services in the United States.

19. Describe the main public and voluntary outpatient clinics and the main problems they face.

20. Why do both Republican and Democrat presidents support the community health center program?

21. What is alternative medicine? What role does it play in the delivery of health care?

22. Briefly explain how a telephone triage system functions.

## REFERENCES

American Hospital Association (AHA). 2006. *TrendWatch Chartbook*. Washington, DC: AHA.

Appleby, C. 1995. Boxed in? *Hospitals and Health Networks* 69, no. 18: 28–34.

Aventis Pharmaceuticals. 2001. *Managed care digest series, 2001: Institutional highlights digest.* Bridgewater, NJ: Aventis Pharmaceuticals.

Bakwin, H. 1945. Pseudodoxia pediatrica. *New England Journal of Medicine* 232: 691–697.

Barbosa-Cesnik C. et al. 2011. Cranberry juice fails to prevent recurrent urinary tract infection: Results from a randomized placebo-controlled trial. *Clinical Infectious Diseases* 52: 23–30.

Barnes P.M. et al. 2008. *Complementary and alternative medicine use among adults and children: United States, 2007.* Hyattsville, MD: National Center for Health Statistics.

Barr, K.W., and C.L. Breindel. 1995. Ambulatory care. In: *Health care administration: Principles, practices, structure, and delivery*. 2nd ed. L.F. Wolper, ed. Gaithersburg, MD: Aspen Publishers, Inc. pp. 547–573.

Barrett B. et al. 2010. Echinacea for treating the common cold *Annals of Internal Medicine* 153: 769–777.

Berenson, R. et al. 2008. A house is not a home: Keeping patients at the center of practice redesign. *Health Affairs* 27, no. 5: 1219–1230.

Beresford, L. 1989. *History of the National Hospice Organization*. Arlington, VA: The National Hospice Organization.

Block, S.D. et al. 1996. Academia's chilly climate for primary care. *Journal of the American Medical Association* 276, no. 9: 677–682.

Bureau of Primary Health Care (BPHC). 1996. *Community health center program fact sheet.* Bethesda, MD: Bureau of Primary Health Care, US Department of Health and Human Services.

CAM Research Methodology Conference. 1997. Defining and describing complementary and alternative medicine. *Alternative Therapies* 3, no. 2: 49–56.

Caudill, T. et al. 2011. Health care reform and primary care: Training physicians for tomorrow's challenges. *Academic Medicine* 86, no. 2: 158–160.

Center for Healthcare Industry Performance Studies. 1997. Economies of scale in outpatient surgery. *Healthcare Financial Management* 51, no. 9: 105–107.

Centers for Disease Control and Prevention (CDC). 2011. National home and hospice care survey. Available at: http://www.cdc.gov/nchs/nhhcs.htm. Accessed January 2011.

Centers for Medicare & Medicaid Services (CMS). 2006. National health expenditures projections: 2005–2015. Table 10: Home Health Care Expenditures. Available at: http://www.cms.hhs.gov /NationalHealthExpendData/downloads/proj2005.pdf. Accessed January 2007.

Centers for Medicare & Medicaid Services (CMS). 2011. Extension of therapy cap exceptions process. Available at: http://www.cms.gov/TherapyServices. Accessed May 2011.

Chernew, M.E. et al. 2009. Would having more primary care doctors cut health spending growth? *Health Affairs* 28:1327–1335.

Colwill, J.M., and J.M. Cultice. 2003. The future supply of family physicians: Implications for rural America. *Health Affairs* 22, no. 1: 190–198.

Derlet, R.W., and J.R. Richards. 2002. Emergency department crowding in Florida, New York, and Texas. *Southern Medical Journal* 95, no. 8: 846–849.

Donelan, K. et al. 1996. All payer, single payer, managed care, no payer: Patients' perspectives in three nations. *Health Affairs* 15, no. 2: 255–265.

Duffy, S.Q., and D.E. Farley. 1995. Patterns of decline among inpatient procedures. *Public Health Reports* 110, no. 6: 674–681.

Dychtwald, K. et al. 1990. *Implementing eldercare services: Strategies that work.* New York: McGraw-Hill.

Eisenberg, D.M. et al. 1998. Trends in alternative medicine use in the United States, 1990–1997. *Journal of the American Medical Association* 280, no. 18: 1569–1575.

Evashwick, C.J. 1993. The continuum of long-term care. In: *Introduction to health services.* 4th ed. S.J. Williams and P.R. Torrens, eds. Albany, NY: Delmar Publishers. pp. 177–218.

Fein, E.B. 1996. Region's hospitals have seen the future, and it's an outpatient clinic. *The New York Times*, February 19, B1.

Felt-Lisk, S. et al. 2002. Monitoring local safety-net providers: Do they have adequate capacity? *Health Affairs* 21, no. 5: 277–283.

Franks, P. et al. 1992. Gatekeeping revisited: Protecting patients from overtreatment. *New England Journal of Medicine* 327, no. 4: 424–429.

Franks, P. et al. 1998. Primary care physicians and specialists as personal physicians: Health care expenditures and mortality experience. *Journal of Family Practice* 47: 105–109.

Glick, D.F., and K.M. Thompson. 1997. Analysis of emergency room use for primary care needs. *Nursing Economics* 15, no. 1: 42–49.

Gordon, J.S. 1996. Alternative medicine and the family practitioner. *American Family Physician* 54, no. 7: 2205–2212.

Health Forum. 2002. *Hospital Statistics.* Chicago: Health Forum.

Health Resources and Services Administration (HRSA) 2011. Health Center Data. Available at: http://www.hrsa.gov/data-statistics/health-center-data/index.html. Accessed January 2011.

Hodge, R. 1994. The evolving role of the primary care physician. *Physician Executive* 20, no. 10: 15–18.

Hoechst Marion Roussel. 1999. *Managed care digest series 1999: Institutional digest.* Kansas City, MO: Hoechst Marion Roussel, Inc.

Jackson, C. 2002. Cutting into the market: Rise of ambulatory surgery centers. *American Medical News* (April 15). Available at: www.amednews.com/2002/bisa0415. Accessed December 2002.

Kozak, L.J. et al. 1999. Changing patterns of surgical care in the United States, 1980–1995. *Health Care Financing Review* 21, no. 1: 31–49.

Lee, P.R. 1994. Models of excellence. *The Lancet* 344, no. 8935: 1484–1486.

Liggins, K. 1993. Inappropriate attendance at accident and emergency departments: A literature review. *Journal of Advanced Nursing* 18, no. 7: 1141–1145.

Looker, P. 1993. Women's health centers: History and evolution. *Women's Health Issues* 3, no. 2: 95–100.

Mao J.T. et al. 2010. White tea extract induces apoptosis in non-small cell lung cancer cells: The role of peroxisome proliferator-activated receptor-γ and 15-lipoxygenases. *Cancer Prevention Research* 3, no. 9: 1132–1140.

McCaig, L.F., and C.W. Burt. 2002. *National hospital ambulatory medical care survey: 1999 emergency department summary*. Atlanta, GA: Centers for Disease Control and Prevention/National Center for Health Statistics.

McCaig, L.F., and E.W. Newar. 2006. *National hospital ambulatory medical care survey: 2004 emergency department summary*. Atlanta, GA: Centers for Disease Control and Prevention, National Center for Health Statistics.

McNamara, P. et al. 1993. Pathwork access: Primary care in EDs on the rise. *Hospitals* 67, no. 10: 44–46.

Miller, G. 1996. Hospice. In: *The continuum of long-term care: An integrated systems approach*. C.J. Evashwick, ed. Albany, NY: Delmar Publishers. pp. 98–108.

Minkler, M. 1992. Community organizing among the elderly poor in the United States. *International Journal of Health Services* 22, no. 2: 303–316.

Nahin R.L. et al. 2009. *Costs of complementary and alternative medicine (CAM) and frequency of visits to CAM practitioners: United States, 2007*. National health statistics reports no 18. Hyattsville, MD: National Center for Health Statistics.

National Association for Home Care and Hospice. 2004. *Basic statistics about home care*. Available at: http://www.nahc.org/04HC_Stats.pdf. Accessed January 2007.

National Association of Community Health Centers (NACHC). 2009a. *Studies on Health Centers Improving Access to Care*. Available at: http://www.nachc.org/client/documents/HC_access _to_care_studies_11.094.pdf. Accessed January 2011.

National Association of Community Health Centers (NACHC). 2009b. *Studies on Health Centers Quality of Care*. Available at: http://www.nachc.org/client/documents/HC%20Quality%20 Studies%208.09.pdf. Accessed January 2011.

National Association of Community Health Centers (NACHC). 2009c. *Studies on Health Centers Cost Effectiveness*. Available at: http://www.nachc.org/client/documents/HC_Cost _Effectiveness_Studies_11.09.pdf. Accessed January 2011.

National Association of Community Health Centers (NACHC). 2009d. *Studies on Health Centers and Disparities*. Available at: http://www.nachc.org/client/documents/HC_Disparities _Studies_11.091.pdf. Accessed January 2011.

National Association of Community Health Centers (NACHC). 2011. *Community Health Centers and Health Reform*. Available at: http://www.nachc.com/client/Summary%20 of%20Final%20 Health% 20Reform%20Package.pdf. Accessed January 2011.

National Association of Free Clinics (NAFC). Undated. Comparison of safety net providers free clinics to federally funded clinics. Available at: http://www.freeclinics.us. Accessed May 2011.

National Center for Complementary and Alternative Medicine (NCCAM). 2007. Available at: http://nccam.nih.gov/about/appropriations/index.htm.

National Center for Health Statistics. 2010. Home health care patients and hospice care discharges—2007 National home and hospice care survey fact sheet. Available at: http://www.cdc.gov/nchs/data/nhhcs/2007hospicecaredischarge.pdf. Accessed January 2011.

National Hospice and Palliative Care Organization. 2003. *NHPCO facts and figures, January 2003*. Available at: http://www.nhpco.org.

National Hospice and Palliative Care Organization. 2010. *NHPCO facts and figures: Hospice care in America*. Available at: http://www.nhpco.org.

National Nursing Centers Consortium. 2003. *Nurse-managed health centers briefing*. May 2003: 1–4.

Noble, J. et al. 1992. Career differences between primary care and traditional trainees in internal medicine and pediatrics. *Annals of Internal Medicine* 116, no. 7: 482–487.

Orton, P. 1994. Shared care. *The Lancet* 344, no. 8934: 1413–1415.

Padgett D.K., and Brodsky B. 1992. Psychosocial factors influencing non-urgent use of the emergency room: A review of the literature and recommendations for research and improved service delivery. *Social Science & Medicine* 35, no. 9: 1189–1197.

Parchman, M., and S. Culler. 1994. Primary care physicians and avoidable hospitalization. *Journal of Family Practice* 39: 123–128.

Petersdorf, R. 1993. The doctor is in. *Academic Medicine* 68, no. 2: 113–117.

Phillips Ambulatory Care Center. 2000. Available at: http://wehealny.org/patients/pace_description.html.

Raffel, M.W., and N.K. Raffel. 1994. *The US health system: Origins and functions*. 4th ed. Albany, NY: Delmar Publishers.

Reuben, D.B. 2007. Saving primary care. *The American Journal of Medicine* 120, no. 1: 99–102.

Roos, N. 1979. Who should do the surgery? Tonsillectomy and adenoidectomy in one Canadian province. *Inquiry* 16, no. 1: 73–83.

Roos, N.P., and L.L. Roos. 1980. Medical school impact on student career choice: A longitudinal study. *Evaluation and the Health Professions* 3, no. 1: 3–19.

Rosenblatt, R.A. et al. 2000. The effect of the doctor-patient relationship on emergency department use among the elderly. *American Journal of Public Health* 90: 97–102.

Russo A. et al. 2010. Hospital-based ambulatory surgery, 2007. Statistical Brief #86. H-CUP. February 2007. pp. 1–16.

Sepulveda, M.-J. et al. 2008. Primary care: Can it solve employers' health care dilemma? *Health Affairs* 27: 151–158.

Shi, L. 1994. Primary care, specialty care, and life chances. *International Journal of Health Services* 24, no. 3: 431–458.

Shi, L., and B. Starfield. 2000. Primary care, income inequality, and self-related health in the US: Mixed-level analysis. *International Journal of Health Services* 30: 541–555.

Shi, L., and B. Starfield. 2001. Primary care physician supply, income inequality, and racial mortality in US metropolitan areas. *American Journal of Public Health* 91: 1246–1250.

Shi, L. et al. 1999. Income inequality, primary care, and health indicators. *The Journal of Family Practice* 48: 275–284.

Shi, L. et al. 2002. Primary care, self-rated health care, and reduction in social disparities in health. *Health Services Research* 37, no. 3: 529–550.

Shi, L. et al. 2007. Health center financial performance: National trends and state variation, 1998–2004. *Journal of Public Health Management and Practice* 13, no. 2: 133–150.

Siu, A.L. et al. 1986. Inappropriate use of hospitals in a randomized trial of health insurance plans. *New England Journal of Medicine* 315, no. 2: 1259–1266.

SMG Solutions. 2000. *2000 report and directory: Medical group practices.* Chicago, IL: SMG Solutions.

Stahl, C. 1997. Home hemodialysis enjoying a comeback. *ADVANCE for Occupational Therapists* 13, no. 25: 4.

Starfield, B. 1992. *Primary care: Concept, evaluation, and policy.* New York: Oxford University Press.

Starfield, B. 1994. Is primary care essential? *The Lancet* 344, no. 8930: 1129–1133.

Starfield B. 1998. *Primary care: Balancing health needs, services and technology.* New York: Oxford University Press.

Steinel, J.A., and E.A. Madigan. 2003. Resource utilization in home health chronic obstructive pulmonary disease management. *Outcomes Management* 7, no. 1: 23–27.

Sultz, H.A., and K.M. Young. 1997. *Health care USA: Understanding its organization and delivery.* Gaithersburg, MD: Aspen Publishers, Inc.

US Department of Health and Human Services (US DHHS). 2011. Recovery Act (ARRA): Community Health Centers. Available at: http://www.hhs.gov/recovery/hrsa/healthcenter grants .html. Accessed January 2011.

Vanselow, N.A. et al. 1995. From the Institute of Medicine. *Journal of the American Medical Association* 273, no. 3: 192.

Van Weel, C. et al. 2008. Integration of personal and community health care. *Lancet* 372, no. 9642: 871–872.

Waid, M.O. 1998. Overview of the Medicare and Medicaid programs. *Health Care Financing Review: Medicare and Medicaid Statistical Supplement* 1998.

Weinerman, E.R. et al. 1966. Yale studies in ambulatory medical care. V. Determinants of use of hospital emergency services. *American Journal of Public Health* 56, no. 7: 1037–1056.

Welch, W.P. et al. 1993. Geographic variation in expenditure for physicians' service in the United States. *New England Journal of Medicine* 328, no. 9: 621–627.

Williams, S.J. 1993. Ambulatory health care services. In: *Introduction to Health Services.* 4th ed. S.J. Williams and P.R. Torrens, eds. Albany, NY: Delmar Publishers.

Wilson, F.A., and D. Neuhauser. 1985. *Health services in the United States.* 2nd ed. Cambridge, MA: Ballinger Publishing Co.

World Health Organization (WHO). 1978. *Primary health care.* Geneva, Switzerland: WHO.

# Chapter 8

# Inpatient Facilities and Services

## Learning Objectives

- To get a functional perspective on the evolution of hospitals
- To survey the factors that contributed to the growth of hospitals prior to the 1980s
- To understand the reasons for the subsequent decline of hospitals and their utilization
- To learn some key measures pertaining to hospital operations and inpatient utilization
- To differentiate among various types of hospitals
- To become familiar with the requirements of the Patient Protection and Affordable Care Act of 2010 as they pertain to physician-owned and nonprofit hospitals
- To comprehend some basic concepts in hospital governance
- To understand and differentiate licensure, certification, and accreditation and the Magnet Recognition Program of the American Nurses Credentialing Center
- To get a perspective on some key ethical issues

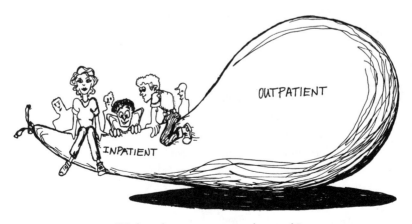

*"We have the inpatient sector under control."*

## Introduction

The term *inpatient* is used in conjunction with an overnight stay in a health care facility, such as a hospital, whereas outpatient refers to services provided while the patient is not lodged in a health care facility. Although the primary function of hospitals is to deliver inpatient acute care services, many hospitals have expanded their scope of services to include nonacute and outpatient care.

According to the American Hospital Association (AHA), a *hospital* is an institution with at least six beds whose primary function is "to deliver patient services, diagnostic and therapeutic, for particular or general medical conditions" (AHA 1994). In addition, a hospital must be licensed, have an organized physician staff, and provide continuous nursing services under the supervision of registered nurses. Other characteristics of a hospital include an identifiable governing body that is legally responsible for the conduct of the hospital, a chief executive with continuous responsibility for the operation of the hospital, maintenance of medical records on each patient, pharmacy services maintained in the institution and supervised by a registered pharmacist, and food service operations to meet the nutritional and therapeutic requirements of the patients (Health Forum 2001). The construction and operation of the modern hospital is governed by federal laws; state health department regulations; city ordinances; standards of the Joint Commission on Accreditation of Healthcare Organizations (JCAHO); and national codes for building, fire protection, and sanitation.

In the past 200 years or so, hospitals have gradually evolved from ordinary institutions of refuge for the homeless and poor to ultramodern facilities providing the latest medical services to the critically ill and injured. The term "medical center" is used by some hospitals, reflecting their high level of specialization and wide scope of services, which may include teaching and research. Growth of multihospital chains, especially those providing a variety of health care services, has led to the nomenclature "hospital system" or "health system."

Hospital care consumes the biggest share of national health care spending (see Figure 6–7). Hence, the hospital inpatient sector was the first targeted by prospective reimbursement methods, during the 1980s. Subsequently, as new technologies emerged to treat patients outside the hospital setting, outpatient services for various types of medical procedures and treatments mushroomed. Managed care also played a significant role in curtailing inpatient utilization.

This chapter describes institutional care delivery with specific reference to acute care—mostly characterized by secondary and tertiary levels of care—in community hospitals. It also discusses various ways to classify hospitals and points out important trends and critical issues that will continue to shape the delivery of inpatient services.

## Hospital Transformation in the United States

From about 1840 to 1900, hospitals underwent a drastic change in purpose, function, and number. From supplying merely food, shelter, and meager medical care to the pauper sick, armies, those infected with contagious diseases, the insane, and those requiring emergency treatment, they began to provide skilled medical and surgical attention and nursing care to all people (Raffel 1980). Subsequently, hospitals became centers of medical training and research. More recent transformations are mainly organizational in nature, as hospitals have consolidated into medical systems, delivering a broad range of health care services. Medical technology has also transformed the delivery of health care and has been a significant factor in shaping the organizational structures within the health care industry. These transformations can be neatly categorized according to five dominant functions in the evolution of hospitals:

1. Primitive institutions of social welfare
2. Distinct institutions of care for the sick
3. Organized institutions of medical practice
4. Advanced institutions of medical training and research
5. Consolidated systems of health services delivery

## Primitive Institutions of Social Welfare

As discussed in Chapter 3, except for a few hospitals that were located in some of the major US cities, municipal almshouses (or poorhouses) and pesthouses existed during the 1800s to provide food and shelter to the destitute. Financed through charitable gifts and local government funds, these institutions essentially served a social welfare function. Medical care, or more proper, nursing care, was only secondary and was quite primitive. Some almshouses had adjoining infirmaries where the sick were isolated. People generally stayed in these institutions for months rather than days.

Pesthouses were used to quarantine people who were sick with contagious diseases, such as smallpox and yellow fever,

so the rest of the community would be protected. Later, hospitals evolved from these almshouses and pesthouses, but even after hospitals developed, people did not want to be admitted to these establishments for treatment because a hospital could do little for them. Most illnesses were treated at home using folk medicine or the services of physicians who made home visits.

## Distinct Institutions of Care for the Sick

Not until the late 1800s did infirmaries or hospital departments of city poorhouses break away to become independent medical care institutions. These were the first public hospitals (Haglund and Dowling 1993), in this case operated by local governments. For example, the Kings County Almshouse and Infirmary, organized in Brooklyn in 1830, later became the Kings County Hospital (Raffel 1980), but such hospitals still served mainly the poor. A few hospitals serving all classes of society and built specifically to care for the sick also emerged during the 19th century. These hospitals were voluntary, or nongovernment.

The founding of *voluntary hospitals*—nonprofit community hospitals financed through local philanthropy as opposed to taxes—was often inspired by influential physicians, with the financial backing of local donors and philanthropists. These hospitals accepted both indigent and paying patients, but to cover their operating expenses, they required charitable contributions from private citizens.

In the United States, most voluntary hospitals had private rather than religious or government sponsorship. In Europe, by contrast, the first hospitals were established predominantly by religious orders. Nurses, who were primarily monks and nuns, attended to the physical, as well as the spiritual, needs of the patients. Later, many of these hospitals became tax-financed public institutions as less church money became available for hospitals and monasteries. In England, private donations and taxes supported the "royal hospitals." Later, hospitals in Britain were voluntary hospitals, which served as a model for such hospitals in the United States (Raffel and Raffel 1994).

The first voluntary hospital in the United States established specifically to care for the sick and patterned after the British voluntary hospitals was the Pennsylvania Hospital in Philadelphia, opened in 1752. The city already had an almshouse. Similar to other seaports, Philadelphia also had pesthouses to isolate people with contagious diseases. However, Dr. Thomas Bond, a London-trained physician, brought to prominence the need for a hospital to care for the sick poor of the city. Benjamin Franklin, who was a friend and advisor of Dr. Bond, was instrumental in promoting the idea and in raising voluntary subscriptions. According to the charter, the contributors had the right to make all laws and regulations relating to the hospital's operation. The contributors also elected members to form the governing board, or the **board of trustees**. Thus, the control of voluntary hospitals was in the hands of influential community laypeople rather than physicians (Raffel and Raffel 1994). The tradition of the voluntary hospital, following this early model, has continued, as the majority of hospitals in the United States have private, nonprofit status.

Other prominent voluntary hospitals included the New York Hospital in New York, which was completed in 1775 but, due to the Revolutionary War, was not opened to civilian patients until 1791. The Massachusetts General Hospital in Boston was incorporated in 1812 and opened in 1821. During this period, the almshouses continued to serve an important function by receiving overflow patients who could not be admitted to the hospitals because of the unavailability of beds or who had to be discharged from hospitals because they were declared incurable (Raffel and Raffel 1994). Later hospitals in the United States were modeled after Pennsylvania, New York, and Massachusetts General.

## Organized Institutions of Medical Practice

Social and demographic change, but above all, the advance of medical science, transformed hospitals into institutions of medical practice. From the latter half of the 19th century, technological progress led to the development of advanced equipment, facilities, and personnel training, all of which became centered in the hospital. Medicine was revolutionized as investigators discovered the causes of disease and developed technological devices for diagnosis and treatment (Raffel 1980). Most notable in terms of their impact on hospitals were (1) the discovery of anesthesia, which significantly aided in advancing new surgical techniques; (2) development of the germ theory of disease, which led to the subsequent discovery of antiseptic and sterilization techniques; and (3) X-ray for diagnostic imaging. Use of antiseptic procedures and, later, introduction of sulfa drugs and penicillin in the mid-20th century produced significant reductions in mortality from infections (Snook 1981). The application of medical science and technology in hospitals also made it necessary for physicians to receive their training and to practice medicine in hospitals.

Drastic improvements in the environmental conditions and the practice of medicine in hospitals made them more acceptable to the middle and upper classes. Hospitals actually began to attract affluent patients who could afford to pay privately. Hospitals also came to be regarded as a necessity because the superior medical services and surgical procedures could not be obtained at home. Thus, the hospital transformed from a charitable institution into one that could generate a profit. In many instances, physicians started opening small hospitals, financed by wealthy and influential sponsors. These facilities were the first proprietary hospitals.

In the early 20th century, the field of hospital administration became a discipline in its own right. Hospitals needed administrators with expertise in financial management and organizational skills to manage them. The administrative structure of the hospital was organized into departments, such as food service, pharmacy, X-ray, and laboratory. It became necessary to employ professional staff to manage the delivery of services. Efficiency began to emerge as an important element in the management of hospitals. The term was defined broadly, encompassing not only economy but also quality and breadth of services, as well as access to care. This early emphasis on efficiency foreshadowed two main issues that continue to affect health policy and hospital management: the pressure on hospitals to introduce new technology while containing cost and the assumption that hospitals should act like businesses (Arndt and Bigelow 2006). With greater pressure for cost containment, hospitals began to limit care to the more acute periods of illness rather than the full course of a disease.

Hospital accreditation was another notable development in the early 20th century. The American College of Surgeons (ACS) began surveying hospitals in 1918 and established the hospital standardization program after it was recommended that a system of standardization of hospital equipment and hospital wards be developed. Until 1951, the ACS single-handedly worked to improve hospital-based medical practice. This effort evolved into the formation of the Joint Commission on Accreditation of Hospitals, a private nonprofit body formed in 1951 with joint effort of the ACS, the American College of Physicians, the AHA, and the American Medical Association (AMA). The organization changed its name in 1987 to the Joint Commission on Accreditation of Healthcare Organizations, which more accurately describes the variety of health facilities it accredits.

## Advanced Institutions of Medical Training and Research

The hospital had a profound influence on medical education in the United States. With the advance of medical science, hospitals became important centers for the dissemination of biomedical knowledge. Hospitals provided the desirable venue for clinical studies. The vast number of clinical records and a large array of medical conditions among patients seeking care in major hospitals provide a wealth of data to conduct investigative studies to advance medical knowledge.

Recognition of the critical role hospitals played in medical education led to collaborations between hospitals and universities. The Pennsylvania Hospital, for example, taught courses required by the College of Philadelphia's medical school, which later became the University of Pennsylvania School of Medicine. Similarly, New York Hospital served as a teaching hospital for medical students of Columbia Medical *b/c not as many inpatient issues*

School, and Massachusetts General Hospital provided practical clinical instruction for Harvard Medical School (Raffel and Raffel 1994). In affiliation with university-based medical schools, many hospitals became centers of medical research, where new discoveries were made, from which the findings were disseminated through publications in medical journals.

*Clin. practice & teaching*

The Johns Hopkins Hospital (opened in 1889), with its adjoining medical school (opened in 1893), inaugurated a new era, combining clinical practice with teaching and the promotion of scientific inquiry in medicine. Patterned after the great European hospitals connected with medical schools, the hospital was to teach students the best methods then known of caring for the sick and to serve as a great laboratory to advance the knowledge of the causes, processes, and treatment of disease (Raffel 1980). From the 1920s, the hospital's teaching role became even more prominent as specialization in medicine led to a proliferation of internships and residencies (Haglund and Dowling 1993).

More recent, the increasing use of non-institutional settings has shifted some aspects of medical education from inpatient to outpatient sectors and to other delivery settings, such as nursing homes, hospices, and community health centers. Nevertheless, the hospital continues to play a central role in the training of physicians. Nursing education has also evolved largely around hospitals, as the role of nursing has become more technically complex. The same is true of many other health care professions (Williams 1995). For both the training and the subsequent employment of virtually the whole spectrum of health professionals, hospitals play a significant role.

## Consolidated Systems of Health Services Delivery

In the late 20th century, hospitals experienced the major impact of radical changes in the health care delivery system because they constituted the institutional nucleus of health care delivery. The most profound changes are seen in the drastic reductions in the length of inpatient stays brought about by prospective and capitated payment methods and aggressive utilization review practices. The declining utilization of acute care beds had left most hospitals with excess capacity, in the form of empty beds. Hence, consolidation of hospitals was particularly intense during the mid-1990s mainly because of economic necessity. As the acute inpatient care sector of health care delivery has become less profitable, hospitals have diversified into nonacute services, such as outpatient centers, home health care, long-term care, subacute care, assisted living, and inpatient and outpatient rehabilitation. Local market pressures have also prompted many hospitals to merge or enter into formal affiliations with other hospitals. The three main types of consolidations, discussed in more detail in Chapter 9, have occurred through mergers and acquisitions, vertical integration, and participation in networks through contractual arrangements. These strategies have offered patients increased access to care across a continuum of services. However, intense consolidation in certain hospital markets has also diluted competition. Research suggests that hospital consolidation in the 1990s raised prices by at least 5% as competition eroded. Evidence also suggests that increasing hospital concentration may also lower quality, but the findings are not robust (Vogt and Town 2006).

# The Expansion Phase: Late 1800s to Mid-1980s

Hospitals grew in numbers when they became a necessary local adjunct of medical practice. Growth in the volume of surgical work especially provided the basis for expansion of hospital beds. The expansion in surgical practice coincided with biomedical discoveries and growth of medical technology.

Profits from surgery enabled physicians to build small hospitals without upper-class sponsorship. The number of hospitals grew from 178 (35,604 beds) in 1872 to 4,359 (421,065 beds) in 1909. By 1929, 6,665 hospitals provided 907,133 beds (Haglund and Dowling 1993). As new beds were built, their availability almost ensured that they would be used. This phenomenon led Milton Roemer (1916–2001) to proclaim, "a built bed is a filled bed," known popularly as Roemer's Law (Roemer 1961).

Haglund and Dowling (1993) pointed to six significant factors in the growth of hospitals: ①advances in medical science, ②development of specialized technology, ③advances in medical education, ④development of professional nursing, ⑤growth of health insurance, and ⑥the role of government. The first three factors were discussed in the previous section; this section covers the last three.

York City), New Haven Hospital (New Haven, Connecticut), and Massachusetts General Hospital (Boston). The benefits of having trained nurses in hospitals became apparent as increased efficacy of treatment and hygiene improved patient recovery (Haglund and Dowling 1993). As a result, hospitals increasingly came to be regarded as places of healing and found acceptance with the middle and upper classes.

## ⑤ Growth of Private Health Insurance

During and after the Great Depression of the 1930s, many hospitals were forced to close, and the financial solvency of many more was threatened. Thus, the number of hospitals in the United States dropped from 6,852 in 1928 to 6,189 in 1937. Subsequently, the growth of private health insurance became a vehicle for enabling people to pay for hospital services, and the flow of insurance funds helped revive the financial stability of hospitals. Insurance also contributed to the increased demand for health services. Historically, insurance plans provided generous coverage for inpatient care. Consequently, there were few restrictions on patients and physicians opting for more expensive hospital services (Feldstein 1971). Note that private health insurance in the United States first began as a hospital insurance plan (see Chapter 3).

## ④ Development of Professional Nursing

During the latter half of the 19th century, Florence Nightingale was instrumental in transforming nursing into a recognized profession in Britain. Following the founding of the Nightingale School of Nursing in England, nursing schools in the United States were established at Bellevue Hospital (New

## ⑥ Role of Government

*— most important role!*

Government funding for hospital construction perhaps played the most important role in the expansion of hospitals. Subsequently, Medicare and Medicaid provided indirect funding to the hospital industry by vastly expanding public-sector health insurance.

*Hill Burton Act.*

## The Hill-Burton Act    1946

Relatively little hospital construction took place during the Great Depression and World War II, so, by the end of the war, the nation was severely short of hospitals. The Hospital Survey and Construction Act of 1946, commonly referred to as the Hill-Burton Act, provided federal grants to states for the construction of new community hospital beds; however, the hospitals would not be under federal control. This legislation required that each state develop and upgrade, annually, a plan for health facility construction—based on bed-to-population ratios—that would serve as a basis for allocation of federal construction grants (Raffel 1980).

In 1946, after the war, 3.2 community hospital beds were available per 1,000 civilian population. The objective of Hill-Burton was to reach 4.5 beds per 1,000 population (Teisberg et al. 1991). The Hill-Burton program assisted in the construction of nearly 40% of the beds in the nation's short-stay general hospitals and was the greatest single factor that increased the nation's bed supply during the 1950s and 1960s (Haglund and Dowling 1993). Hill-Burton made it possible for even small, remote communities to have their own hospitals (Wolfson and Hopes 1994). By 1980, the United States had reached its goal of 4.5 community hospital beds per 1,000 civilian population (DHHS 2002) even though the Hill-Burton program terminated in 1974.

Hill-Burton was also instrumental in promoting the growth of nonprofit community hospitals because it required that hospitals constructed with federal funds must provide a certain amount of uncompensated care. Competition from these new hospitals led to the closure of many smaller proprietary for-profit hospitals. Most of the remaining proprietary hospitals began delivering free or discounted services to those who could not afford to pay (Muller 2003). Thanks to Hill-Burton, nonprofit community hospitals in the United States far outnumber all other types of hospitals.

## Public Health Insurance

The creation of Medicare and Medicaid programs in the mid-1960s also had a significant, although indirect, impact on the increase in the number of hospital beds and their utilization (Feldstein 1993), as government-funded health insurance became available to a large number of elderly and poor Americans. Between 1965 and 1980, the number of community hospitals in the United States increased from 5,736 (741,000 beds) to 5,830 (988,000 beds); total admissions per 1,000 population increased from 130 to 154; and total inpatient days per 1,000 population increased from 1,007 to 1,159. The percentage occupancy also remained relatively stable at around 76% (AHA 1990). Figure 8–1 shows trends from 1940 to 2008 in the number of beds per 1,000 resident population.

## The Downsizing Phase: Mid-1980s Onward

The mid-1980s marked a turning point in the growth and use of hospital beds. After a sharp decline in 1985, the number of community hospitals and the total number of beds have continued to decline (Figure 8–2). The average bed capacity per hospital also declined from 196 beds in 1980 (DHHS 2006) to 161 beds in 2008 (US Census Bureau 2011).

Hill-Burton
—◦ Growth of non-profit hospitals

**Figure 8–1** Trends in the Number of US Community Hospital Beds per 1,000 Resident Population.

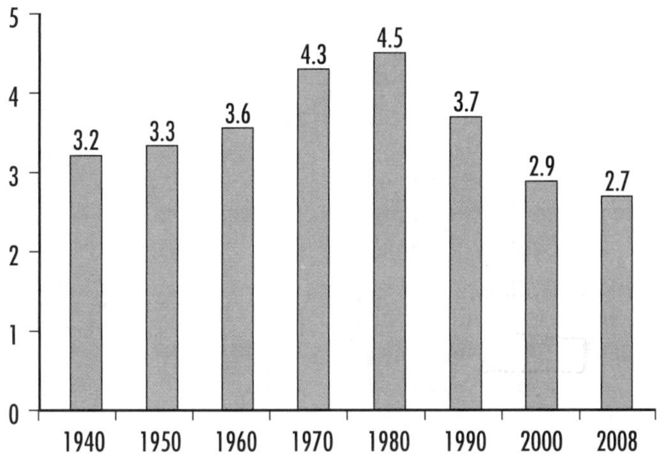

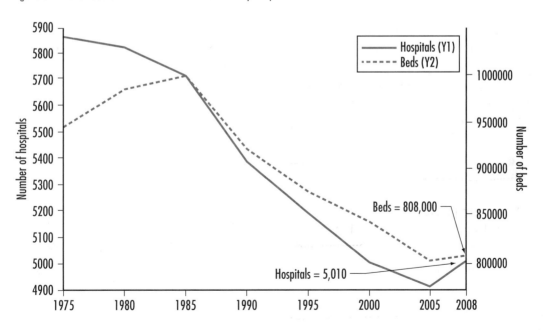

*Source:* Data from *Health, United States, 2002*, p. 281; *Health, United States, 2010*, p. 356; National Center for Health Statistics.

**Figure 8–2** The Decline in the Number of US Community Hospitals and Beds.

*Source:* Data from *Health, United States, 2002*, p. 279; *Statistical Abstract of the United States, 2011*, p. 117.

Even as the numbers of hospitals and capacity have contracted, further declines have occurred in the actual utilization of the shrunken capacity. Occupancy rates (percentage of beds occupied) in community hospitals declined from 75.6% in 1980 to approximately 64% in 2000. Since then, occupancy rates have increased slightly (66.6% in 2007), mainly because capacity (number of available beds) has steadily declined, from 823,560 total community hospital beds in 2000 to 800,892 in 2007. Similarly, the average length of stay (ALOS) in community hospitals has declined from 7.6 days in 1980 to 5.5 days in 2007 (DHHS 2011).

Within hospitals, a tremendous shift from inpatient to outpatient utilization has occurred (as illustrated in Figure 8–3) in the form of increasing ratios between hospital outpatient visits and inpatient days. Along with this shift in the use of hospital services, the share of national expenditures on hospital care continued to decline until 2005. Since then, hospital expenditures compared to all other health care expenditures, have been rising at a slow pace (see Table 8–1).

The downward pressures on hospital utilization have been exerted by three main forces: changes in hospital reimbursement, closure of small rural hospitals, and the impact of managed care. Of these three, hospital reimbursement had the most dramatic effect on hospitals.

*most effect*

① **Changes in Reimbursement** `PPS`

The Tax Equity and Fiscal Responsibility Act (TEFRA) of 1982 required the conversion of hospital Medicare reimbursement from cost-plus to a prospective payment system (PPS) based on diagnosis-related groups (DRGs) (see Chapter 6). Under PPS, hospitals are paid a fixed amount per

Figure 8–3  Ratio of US Hospital Outpatient Visits to Inpatient Days (all hospitals), 1980–2008.

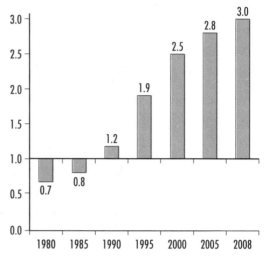

Source: Data from *Statistical Abstract of the United States, 2002,* p. 110; *Statistical Abstract of the United States, 2011,* p. 117.

Table 8–1  US Share of National Expenditures for Hospital Care

|      | NHE    | Hospital | % of NHE |
|------|--------|----------|----------|
| 1980 | 255.7  | 100.5    | 39.3%    |
| 1990 | 724.0  | 250.4    | 34.6%    |
| 2000 | 1378.0 | 415.5    | 30.2%    |
| 2005 | 2021.0 | 606.5    | 30.0%    |
| 2006 | 2152.1 | 648.3    | 30.1%    |
| 2007 | 2283.3 | 686.8    | 30.1%    |
| 2008 | 2391.4 | 722.1    | 30.2%    |
| 2009 | 2486.3 | 759.1    | 30.5%    |

*Note:* Expenditures are in billions of dollars.
*Source:* CMS, Office of the Actuary.

admission according to the patient's principal diagnosis, regardless of how long the patient stays in the hospital. To make a profit, the hospital must keep its costs below the fixed reimbursement amount, which creates an incentive to minimize the patient's length of stay. Following Medicare's lead, several states adopted prospective methods to reimburse hospitals for services provided to their Medicaid enrollees. Private payers also resorted to competitive pricing and discounted fees and closely monitored when patients would be hospitalized and for how long. As PPS reimbursement exerted pressure on hospitals to reduce the length of stay after admission, early discharge from hospitals became practical only as alternative services, such as home health care and subacute long-term care, were developed to provide postacute continuity of care.

The effect of PPS on hospitals was dramatic. In the 1980s, 550 hospitals closed and 159 mergers and acquisitions occurred (Balotsky 2005). Since then, the number of hospitals and beds continued to decline until 2007, but the nation's bed capacity appears to be rising. Between 2007 and 2008, the nation had 107 additional hospitals with almost 6,000 additional beds (DHHS 2011). With the aging of the US population, we can expect to see this trend continue.

## Rural Hospital Closures

During the 1990s, many small rural hospitals had to close because of economic constraints. Hospitals of all sizes throughout the country had to close entire wings or convert those beds for alternative uses, such as psychiatric care or long-term care. To rescue many of the remaining small hospitals from closure, in 1983, the then Health Care Financing Administration (now Centers for

Medicare and Medicaid Services [CMS]) initiated a swing bed program for rural hospitals. *Swing beds* were authorized under the Omnibus Reconciliation Act of 1980. The program is still in place. It allows small rural hospitals to switch the use of hospital beds between acute care and long-term skilled nursing facility (SNF) care as needed. The program enables these hospitals to generate additional revenues. In July 2002, CMS brought hospital swing beds under the existing SNF PPS reimbursement (discussed in Chapter 6), which created further financial pressures for these hospitals.

## Impact of Managed Care

In the 1990s, managed care became a growing force transforming the delivery of health services. Managed care has emphasized cost containment and the efficient delivery of services. Because inpatient care, especially in acute care hospitals, is costly, managed care has emphasized alternative delivery settings, such as outpatient treatments, home health care, and nursing homes whenever appropriate. Such measures have had a tremendous impact on curtailing hospital utilization. It has been demonstrated that market penetration of health maintenance organizations (HMOs) played a significant role in lowering hospital profitability (Clement and Grazier 2001).

## Some Key Utilization Measures and Operational Concepts

### Discharges

The total number of patient discharges per 1,000 population is one indicator of access to hospital inpatient services and of the extent of utilization. Because babies born in the hospital are not included in admissions, discharges provide a more accurate count of inpatients served by a hospital. *Discharge* refers to the total number of patients discharged from a hospital's acute care beds in a given period. Deaths in hospitals are counted as discharges. Discharge rates per 1,000 population (see Table 8–2) are important because all other inpatient use patterns depend on them. Discharges per 1,000

population from community hospitals declined from 122 in 1990 to 114 in 2007 (US Census Bureau 2011), reflecting a lower rate of inpatient hospital utilization.

## Inpatient Days

An *inpatient day* (also called a patient day or a hospital day) is a night spent in the hospital by a patient. The cumulative number of

Table 8–2  Discharges, Days of Care, and Average Length of Stay per 1,000 Population in Nonfederal Short-Stay Hospitals, 2007

| Characteristics | Discharges | Days of Care | Average Length of Stay |
|---|---|---|---|
| **Total** | 114.4 | 553.9 | 4.8 |
| **Age** | | | |
| Under 18 years | 37.7 | 178.5 | 4.7 |
| 18–44 years | 88.9 | 325.8 | 3.7 |
| 45–64 years | 114.4 | 586.8 | 5.1 |
| 65–74 years | 244.0 | 1,327.5 | 5.4 |
| 75–84 years | 398.3 | 2,265.8 | 5.7 |
| 85+ years | 535.9 | 3,012.5 | 5.6 |
| **Gender**[1] | | | |
| Male | 97.4 | 515.7 | 5.3 |
| Female | 128.1 | 568.5 | 4.4 |
| **Geographic Region**[1] | | | |
| Northeast | 127.5 | 728.4 | 5.7 |
| Midwest | 112.6 | 477.5 | 4.2 |
| South | 114.0 | 555.6 | 4.9 |
| West | 96.6 | 418.5 | 4.3 |

[1]Age adjusted.

*Source:* Data from *Health, United States, 2009*, Web update, National Center for Health Statistics. Retrieved February 2011 from http://www.cdc.gov/nchs/data/hus/hus2009tables/Table099.pdf.

patient days over a certain period is known as *days of care*. Days of care per 1,000 population over 1 year reflect access to inpatient services and their utilization. Hospital utilization is highest among people 75 years and older (see Table 8–2). Among younger age groups, children under 1 year of age have the highest utilization. In general, females incur higher use of hospital services than men do, even after childbirth-related utilization is factored out. Hospitalization is higher among blacks than whites. Generally, hospital use is higher among people of lower socioeconomic status than the more affluent because poorer population groups are generally in poorer health and have less access to routine primary care. Consequently, poorer population groups in the United States are more likely to suffer from acute conditions, incurring more frequent hospitalization and longer stays once admitted.

In the western United States, hospital utilization is much lower than in other parts of the country. A high rate of managed care penetration is believed to be primarily responsible for the lower utilization. The utilization patterns also suggest that overall hospital use is higher among Medicare and Medicaid recipients than among the rest of the population.

## Average Length of Stay ALOS

*Average length of stay* (ALOS) is calculated by dividing the total days of care by the total number of discharges. It provides a measure of how many days a patient, on average, spends in the hospital. Hence, this measure, when applied to individuals or specific groups of patients, is an indicator of severity of illness. Figure 8–4 illustrates ALOS trends in community hospitals.

$$ALOS = \frac{\text{total days of care}}{\text{total \# discharges}}$$

Figure 8–4　Trends in Average Length of Stay in Nonfederal Short-Stay Hospitals, Selected Years.

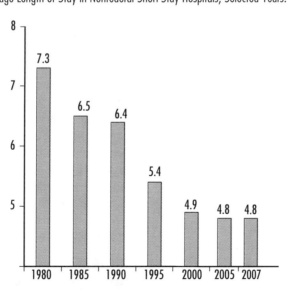

*Source:* Data from *Health, United States, 2009*, Web update, National Center for Health Statistics. Retrieved February 2011 from http://www .cdc.gov/nchs/data/hus/hus2009tables/Table099.pdf.

Figure 8–5  Average Lengths of Stay by US Hospital Ownership: 2000–2008.

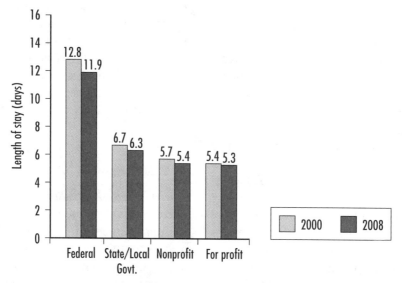

*Source:* Data from *Health, United States, 2010,* p. 344, National Center for Health Statistics.

Figure 8–5 shows trends in ALOS by type of hospital ownership. Government-owned hospitals have higher lengths of stay, compared to private hospitals. Federal hospitals mainly include those in the Veterans Health Administration system, which serve a population that is getting older. State and local government hospitals disproportionately serve the poor and uninsured. ALOS in nonprofit hospitals is slightly higher than in for-profit hospitals.

## Capacity

The number of beds set up and staffed for inpatient use determines the size or capacity of a hospital. Among all community hospitals in the United States, 84% have fewer than 300 beds (see Figure 8–6). The average size of a community hospital was approximately 161 beds in 2008 (DHHS 2011).

## Average Daily Census

The average number of inpatients receiving care each day in a hospital is referred to as *average daily census.* Hence, it is one of the common measures used to define occupancy of inpatient beds in hospitals and other inpatient facilities. The total inpatient days during a given period (days of care) are divided by the number of days in that period to arrive at the average daily census. For example, if the number of total inpatient days for July is 3,131, then the average daily census for July is 101 (3,131/31).

## Occupancy Rate

$$\text{Occupancy Rate} = \frac{ave\ daily\ census}{ave\ \#\ of\ beds}$$

The *occupancy rate* for a given period is derived by dividing the average daily census for that period by the average number of beds (capacity). The fraction is expressed as

Figure 8–6  Breakdown of US Community Hospitals by Size, 2008.

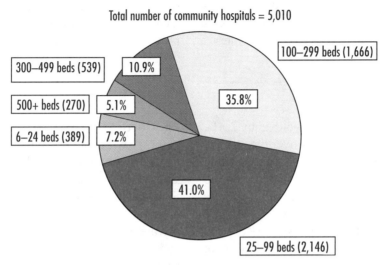

Total number of community hospitals = 5,010

300–499 beds (539)  10.9%

500+ beds (270)  5.1%

6–24 beds (389)  7.2%

100–299 beds (1,666)

35.8%

41.0%

25–99 beds (2,146)

*Source:* Data from *Health, United States, 2010,* p. 354, National Center for Health Statistics.

a percentage (percent of beds occupied). It indicates the proportion of a hospital's total inpatient capacity actually utilized. Occupancy rate is also used for other types of inpatient facilities, such as nursing homes, and

is often used as a measure of performance. Figure 8–7 shows the change in aggregate occupancy rates for US community hospitals from 1960 to 2008. Individual hospitals can compare their own occupancy rates

Figure 8–7  Change in Occupancy Rates (percent of beds occupied) in US Community Hospitals, 1960–2008 (selected years).

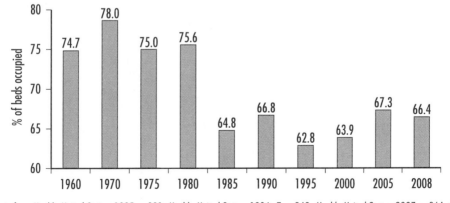

*Source:* Data from *Health, United States, 1995,* p. 231; *Health, United States, 1996–7,* p. 243; *Health, United States, 2007,* p. 364; *Health, United States, 2010,* p. 354, National Center for Health Statistics.

against industry benchmarks. In a competitive environment, facilities with higher occupancy rates are considered more successful than those with lower occupancy rates.

employing an increasing number of personnel (see Figure 8–8). Hospital employment constitutes roughly 4% of all service-providing jobs in the United States.

## Hospital Employment

Employment in hospitals declined by 2.3%, to about 4 million workers over the 1983 to 1986 period when the hospital downsizing trend started. Staff cuts, hiring freezes, and the increased use of contract services were part of a belt-tightening effort in response to declining inpatient admissions (Kahl and Clark 1986). But, as hospitals chased more liberal reimbursement in outpatient markets, employment in hospitals in 1989 rose to 4.3 million workers, an increase of 6.9% from 1986 (Anderson and Wootton 1991). This trend has continued as hospitals have been

## Types of Hospitals

The United States has a variety of institutional forms, with both private and government-owned institutions. Most hospitals are private nonprofit, short-stay, general hospitals. 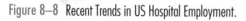 State and local government-owned hospitals are next in predominance. Then come the private for-profit (investor-owned) hospitals and, finally, federal hospitals. Figure 8–9 shows the distribution of hospitals, and Figure 8–10 shows the distribution of beds among various hospital types.

The endless variations in hospital characteristics defy any simple classification. The

Figure 8–8    Recent Trends in US Hospital Employment.

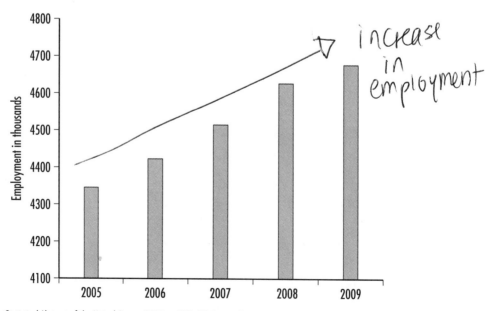

*Source:* Data from *Statistical Abstract of the United States, 2011*, p. 112, US Census Bureau.

Figure 8–9   Proportion of Total US Hospitals by Type of Hospital, 2008.

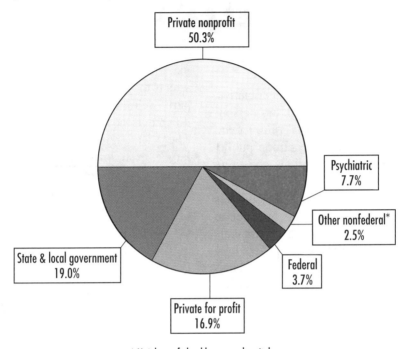

* Mainly nonfederal long-term hospitals.

*Source:* Data from *Statistical Abstract of the United States, 2011*, p. 117, US Census Bureau.

Figure 8–10   Proportion of Total US Hospital Beds by Type of Hospital, 2008.

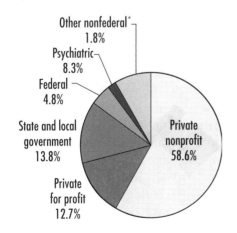

*Mainly nonfederal long-term hospitals.

*Source:* Data from *Statistical Abstract of the United States, 2011*, p. 117, US Census Bureau.

following classification arrangements have been commonly used to differentiate among the various types of hospitals. It is important to keep in mind, however, that these classifications are not mutually exclusive.

## Classification by Ownership

### Public Hospitals → 1st to appear

Public hospitals were the first to appear when almshouses and pesthouses evolved into hospitals providing medical services. *Public hospitals* are owned by agencies of federal, state, or local governments. It should be noted that in health care the word "public" does not carry its ordinary meaning. A public hospital, for instance, is not necessarily a hospital that is open to the

↳ veterans (not for everyone)

general public. In business, a public corporation is one whose stock is publicly traded to attract private investors. In health care, particularly in the United States, the word "public" denotes government ownership.

Federal hospitals are maintained primarily for special groups of federal beneficiaries, such as Native Americans, military personnel, and veterans. As a general rule, federal hospitals do not serve the common public. Veterans Affairs (VA) hospitals constitute the largest group among federal hospitals.

Local governments, such as counties and cities, operate hospitals that are open to the general public. Many of these hospitals are located in large urban areas, where they serve mainly the inner city indigent and disadvantaged populations. Hence, Medicare, Medicaid, and state and local tax dollars pay for a large portion of the services these hospitals provide. Because of increasing financial pressures, many public hospitals had to privatize or close. Out of 1,444 state and local government-owned hospitals in 1990, 1,105 remained in 2008 (US Census Bureau 2011). Most hospitals operated by city and county governments are small to moderate size. Some large public hospitals are affiliated with medical schools; they play a significant role in training physicians and other health care professionals.

Compared to private hospitals, public hospitals incur higher utilization, at least in terms of ALOS (see Figure 8–5). ALOS is the highest in federal hospitals (11.9 days in 2008), and veterans are the biggest users of these hospitals. Of the 23 million veterans living in 2009, 40% were age 65 and older (compared to 13% of the general US population). The number of discharges in VA hospitals increased from 579 thousand in 2000 to 640 thousand in 2009 (DHHS 2011).

## Private Nonprofit Hospitals

Nonprofit hospitals are owned and operated by community associations or other nongovernment organizations. Their primary mission is to benefit the community in which they are located. Patient fees, third-party reimbursement, donations, and endowments cover their operating expenses. The private nonprofit sector constitutes the largest group of hospitals (Figure 8–9), accounting for 50% of all US hospitals and almost 58.5% of all beds in 2008. These hospitals had an average capacity of 190 beds per hospital (DHHS 2011).

## Private For-Profit Hospitals

For-profit *proprietary hospitals*—also referred to as *investor-owned hospitals*—are owned by individuals, partnerships, or corporations. They are operated for the financial benefit of the entity that owns the institution, that is, the stockholders. At the beginning of the 20th century, more than one-half of the nation's hospitals were proprietary. Most of these hospitals were small and were established by physicians who wanted to hospitalize their own patients (Stewart 1973). Later, most of these institutions were closed or acquired by community organizations or hospital corporations, due to population shifts, increased costs, and the necessities of modern clinical practice (Raffel and Raffel 1994). Even though the nonprofit hospital sector has maintained its market dominance, the number of for-profit hospitals and beds has increased (Table 8–3). However, the latter continue to have the lowest occupancy rates (57.8% in 2008, compared to 66.4% for all community hospitals; DHHS 2011).

Table 8–3 Changes in Number of US Community Hospitals, Beds, Average Size, and Occupancy Rates

|  | 2000 | 2008 | Change |
|---|---|---|---|
| **Nonprofit Sector** | | | |
| Number of hospitals | 3,003 | 2,923 | −2.7% |
| Number of beds | 582,988 | 556,651 | −4.5% |
| Average size | 194 | 190 | −1.9% |
| Occupancy rate | 65.5% | 68.4% | 4.4% |
| **For-Profit Sector** | | | |
| Number of hospitals | 749 | 982 | 31.1% |
| Number of beds | 109,883 | 120,887 | 10.0% |
| Average size | 147 | 123 | −16.1% |
| Occupancy rate | 55.9% | 57.8% | 3.4% |

*Source:* Data from *Health, United States*, National Center for Health Statistics.

## Classification by Public Access

Community hospitals are the most common type of hospital in the United States. A *community hospital* is a nonfederal, short-stay hospital, whose facilities and services are available to the general public. Its primary mission is to serve the general community. These hospitals are not restricted to serving a certain category of people. A community hospital may be private for profit, private nonprofit, or owned by the state or local government (but not by the federal government). It may be a general hospital or a specialty hospital. The larger the community served, the larger the hospital, range of specialties, and range of supporting equipment and services (Raffel and Raffel 1994). Noncommunity hospitals include hospitals operated by the federal government, such as VA hospitals to serve veterans; hospital units of institutions, such as prisons and infirmaries in colleges and universities; and long-stay hospitals.

In 2008, of the 5,815 US hospitals, 5,010 (over 86%) were community hospitals (DHHS 2011). Figure 8–11 shows the breakdown of community hospitals by ownership type.

## Classification by Multiunit Affiliation

Hospitals are part of a multihospital chain (referred to as a *multihospital system* [MHS]) when two or more hospitals are owned, leased, sponsored, or contractually managed by a central organization (AHA 1994). Table 8–4 lists the largest of the multihospital chains according to size. In 2008, hospitals affiliated with MHSs accounted for 54.4% of all US hospitals, up from 49% in 2005 and 46% in 2000 (Sanofi-Aventis 2007, 2010). Despite inroads made by

Table 8–4   The Largest US Multihospital Chains, 2008 (Ranked by Staffed Beds)

| Name of Hospital System (Location) | Number of Owned Hospitals | Number of Staffed Beds | Average Occupancy % | ALOS |
|---|---|---|---|---|
| **Nonprofit Chains** | | | | |
| Ascension Health (St. Louis, MO) | 51 | 19,284 | 59.0% | 4.7 |
| Catholic Health Initiatives (Denver, CO) | 70 | 9,491 | 50.4% | 4.5 |
| Catholic Healthcare West (San Francisco, CA) | 38 | 8,847 | 61.7% | 4.8 |
| Kaiser Permanente (Oakland, CA) | 34 | 7,737 | 64.7% | 4.2 |
| Catholic Health East (Newtown, PA) | 19 | 5,256 | 63.9% | 5.5 |
| Trinity Health (Novi, MI) | 30 | 6,266 | 53.1% | 4.1 |
| Adventist Health System (Winter Park, FL) | 35 | 6,134 | 56.1% | 4.6 |
| Christus Health (Irving, TX) | 23 | 5,237 | 56.5% | 4.2 |
| Catholic Healthcare Partners (Cincinnati, OH) | 30 | 4,707 | 54.1% | 4.9 |
| Sutter Health (Sacramento, CA) | 31 | 5,698 | 50.2% | 5.6 |
| Providence Health and Services (Seattle, WA) | 25 | 5,682 | 52.4% | 4.0 |
| UPMC (Pittsburgh, PA) | 15 | 4,619 | 69.8% | 5.2 |
| North Shore — Long Island Jewish Health System (Great Neck, NY) | 10 | 4,230 | 86.8% | 6.3 |
| **For-Profit Chains** | | | | |
| HCA (Nashville, TN) | 156 | 32,140 | 60.5% | 4.7 |
| Tenet Health System (Dallas, TX) | 52 | 12,022 | 60.3% | 5.1 |
| Community Health Systems (Brentwood, TN) | 119 | 16,021 | 51.0% | 4.5 |
| Health Mgmt. Associates (Naples, FL) | 61 | 7,887 | 51.4% | 4.2 |
| Universal Health Services (King of Prussia, PA) | 22 | 4,850 | 60.2% | 4.4 |
| Life Point Hospitals (Brentwood, TN) | 49 | 4,843 | 45.3% | 4.0 |
| **State and Local Government-Owned Chains** | | | | |
| New York City Health and Hospitals Corporation (New York, NY) | 9 | 3,965 | 87.1% | 6.7 |

*Source:* Data from *Managed Care Digest Series: Hospital/Systems Digest*, Sanofi-Aventis, 2010, Bridgewater, NJ: Sanofi-Aventis.

Figure 8–11   Breakdown of US Community Hospitals by Types of Ownership, 2008.

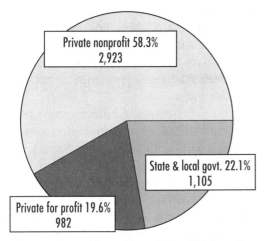

Private nonprofit 58.3%
2,923

State & local govt. 22.1%
1,105

Private for profit 19.6%
982

*Source:* Data from *Health, United States*, 2010, p. 354, National Center for Health Statistics.

investor-owned groups into MHSs, most such systems are operated by nonprofit corporations (Table 8–5). Some of the advantages of multihospital chain affiliation include economies of scale with administrative overhead, the ability to provide a wide spectrum of care, the ability to reach a variety of markets, increased access to capital markets, greater participation in managed care contracting, and access to management resources and expertise.

The VA operates the single largest hospital system in the country, with 153 medical centers owned by the federal government. In fiscal year 2009, VA hospitals had a total of 485,774 acute inpatient medical/surgical hospital discharges and 81,634 acute inpatient psychiatry hospital discharges (Department of Veterans Affairs 2010).

Table 8–5   US Multihospital Health Care Systems: Number of Hospitals and Beds, 2008 (Includes Owned, Leased, Sponsored, and Contract-Managed Hospitals)

| Type of Control | Number of Systems | Hospitals | Beds | % of Beds* |
|---|---|---|---|---|
| Catholic church related | 39 | 556 | 104,581 | 17.2% |
| Other church related | 12 | 102 | 21,990 | 3.6% |
| **Total church related** | **51** | **658** | **126,571** | **20.8%** |
| Other nonprofit | 264 | 1,317 | 285,296 | 46.8% |
| **Total nonprofit** | **315** | **1,975** | **411,867** | **67.6%** |
| Investor owned | 77 | 1,349 | 151,305 | 24.8% |
| Federal government owned | 5 | 212 | 46,311 | 7.6% |
| **Total** | **397** | **3,536** | **609,483** | **100.0%** |

*As percent of all systems

*Source:* Data from AHA Hospital Statistics. 2010. *Health Forum*, p. 199.

## Classification by Type of Service

### General Hospitals

A *general hospital* provides a variety of services, including general and specialized medicine, general and specialized surgery, and obstetrics, to meet the general medical needs of the community it serves. It provides diagnostic, treatment, and surgical services for patients with a variety of medical conditions. Most hospitals in the United States are general hospitals.

It is important to note that the term "general hospital" does not imply that these hospitals are less specialized or that their care is inferior to that of specialty hospitals. The difference lies in the nature of services, not their quality. General hospitals provide a broader range of services for a larger variety of conditions, whereas specialty hospitals provide a narrow range of services for specific medical conditions or patient populations.

### Specialty Hospitals

According to the North American Industry Classification System of the US Census Bureau, *specialty hospitals* are establishments that primarily engage in providing diagnostic and medical treatment to inpatients with a specific type of disease or medical condition, except services for psychiatric care or substance abuse. Specialty hospitals forge a distinct service niche. Traditionally, the two most common specialty hospitals have been rehabilitation hospitals and children's hospitals. With increasing competition, however, other types of specialty hospitals have emerged to provide treatments that are also available in many general hospitals. Examples include orthopedic hospitals, cardiac hospitals, cancer (oncology) hospitals,

and women's hospitals. Physicians find such specialized hospitals more efficient, and in many instances, physicians are full or part owners of these hospitals. Affiliation with such hospitals gives physicians control over hospital operations, flexibility with their time, and opportunity to enhance their incomes.

Physician-owned facilities have raised legal and ethical issues with regard to self-referrals without full disclosure. Stark Laws that prohibit self-referrals (see Chapter 5) do not apply when physicians self-refer to a "whole hospital." Under this exception, physicians may refer patients to a facility if their ownership interest is in the whole hospital rather than a smaller entity (Guterman 2006).

Physician-owned specialty hospitals have been the subject of much controversy, which has invited congressional reviews. In a report to Congress, the Medicare Payment Advisory Commission (MedPAC 2006) pointed out that these hospitals (1) had lower shares of Medicaid patients (2 to 3% of discharges) than community hospitals (13% of discharges) in the same markets; (2) admitted less severe cases that were expected to be more profitable; (3) drew patients from community hospitals, although community hospitals were able to compensate for the revenue loss; and (4) did not have lower costs per severity-adjusted discharge than competing community hospitals in the same markets. Also, the entrance of a physician-owned cardiac hospital was associated with a 6% increase in the number of cardiac surgeries, which suggests that these hospitals may be engaging in creating provider-induced demand. Another issue, emergency care, is at the heart of the controversy between specialty hospitals and community general hospitals. Administrators of general hospitals argue that specialty hospitals are "cream-skimming" insured patients and leaving costly emergency and uncompensated cases to general hospitals (Snyder 2003). Physician-owned specialty hospitals derive approximately 50% of their revenue from Medicare (Weaver 2010).

In 2003, Congress imposed a lengthy moratorium on the construction of new physician-owned hospitals that specialized in cardiac, orthopedic, and certain other areas. The controversial Patient Protection and Affordable Care Act of 2010 closed the door on future physician-owned hospitals effective January 1, 2011. New or existing hospitals had to be certified by December 31, 2010, failing which they would be barred from participating in the Medicare program (Weaver 2010). Existing physician-owned facilities also faced immediate restrictions on expansion. Physician investors lamented that the rules were so strict that virtually none of their hospitals would be able to grow (Silva 2010).

## Psychiatric Hospitals

The primary function of a psychiatric inpatient facility is to provide diagnostic and treatment services for patients who have psychiatric-related illnesses. Specifically, such an institution must have facilities to provide psychiatric, psychological, and social work services. A psychiatric hospital must also have a written agreement with a general hospital for the transfer of patients who may require medical, obstetric, or surgical services (Health Forum 2001).

Historically, state governments have taken the primary responsibility for establishing facilities for the care of the mentally ill. Trends during the 1970s and 1980s resulted in significant deinstitutionalization of the inpatient population who resided in state mental hospitals. As a result, the responsibility for much psychiatric care shifted to psychiatric units in general hospitals, private psychiatric hospitals, other types of residential facilities, and community care programs (Mechanic 1998). However, state mental institutions continue to provide long-term treatment to people with severe and persistent mental illness (Patrick et al. 2006). Between 2000 and 2008, the number of psychiatric hospitals declined from 496 (87,000 beds) to 447 (79,000 beds; US Census Bureau 2011).

## Rehabilitation Hospitals

*Rehabilitation hospitals* specialize in therapeutic services to restore the maximum level of functioning in patients who have suffered recent disability due to an episode of illness or an accident. These hospitals serve patients who generally cannot be cured but whose functioning can be improved. According to Medicare rules, to be classified as a rehabilitation hospital, 75% of a hospital's inpatients must require intensive rehabilitation services for the treatment of stroke, spinal cord injury, major multiple trauma, brain injury, and other specific conditions (Grimaldi 2002). Intensive rehabilitation refers to at least 3 hours of therapy per day. Rehabilitation hospitals also serve amputees, victims of accident or sports injuries, and those needing intensive cardiac rehabilitation. Facilities and staff are available to provide physical therapy, occupational therapy, and speech-language pathology. Most rehabilitation hospitals have special arrangements for psychological, social work, and vocational services and are required to have written arrangements with a general hospital for the transfer of patients who need medical, obstetrical, or surgical care not available at the institution (Health Forum 2001).

In 2006, over 1,200 facilities were Medicare certified. These facilities are referred to as inpatient rehabilitation facilities (IRFs). Medicare accounts for about 70% of the caseload in these hospitals (MedPAC 2008). Medicare has developed a separate IRF prospective payment system that was implemented in 2002. It pays a per discharge prospective rate according to case-mix groups (see Chapter 6).

## Children's Hospitals

Children's hospitals are community hospitals that typically have specialized facilities to deal mainly with complex, severe, or chronic illnesses among children. Nearly all children's hospitals provide neonatal intensive care units, pediatric intensive care units, trauma centers, and transplant services. Thus, these hospitals provide a wide range of high-intensity services for children, such as pediatric surgery, cardiology, orthopedic surgery, cancer treatment, HIV/AIDS treatment, and rehabilitation services (DelliFraine 2006).

There are 45 freestanding children's hospitals in the United States. They have an average capacity of 124 beds. All of these hospitals are nonprofit and are located in major metropolitan areas. Many are affiliated with medical schools and academic medical centers. However, in many large communities, where no specialty children's hospitals exist, general acute care hospitals serve as de facto children's hospitals by providing the same services and treating the same types of patients (DelliFraine 2006).

## Classification by Length of Stay

### Short-Stay Hospitals

A *short-stay hospital* is one in which the average length of stay is 25 days or less. Most hospitals fall in this category. Patients admitted to these hospitals suffer from acute conditions. Hospitals with average stays of more than 25 days are long-stay hospitals. These include state-run, as well as private, psychiatric hospitals; long-term care hospitals (LTCHs) providing subacute care; tuberculosis hospitals; and chronic disease hospitals.

### Long-Term Care Hospitals

The majority of long-stay hospitals in the United States are long-term care hospitals (LTCHs). A long-term care hospital is a special type of long-stay hospital described in section 1886(d)(1)(B)(iv) of the Social Security Act. LTCHs must meet Medicare's conditions of participation for acute (short-stay) hospitals and must have an ALOS greater than 25 days. LTCHs serve patients who have complex medical needs and may suffer from multiple chronic problems requiring long-term hospitalization. Many LTCH patients are admitted directly from short-stay hospital intensive care units with respiratory/ventilator-dependent or other complex medical conditions. The number of LTCHs in the United States grew rapidly from 105 facilities in 1993 to 318 in 2003 (MedPAC 2004). In 2008, there were 386 LTCH facilities, but they were not distributed evenly throughout the nation. Medicare accounted for about 70% of the revenues for these hospitals (MedPAC 2010a).

The Balanced Budget Refinement Act of 1999 (BBRA) mandated a new discharge-based prospective payment system, which was implemented in 2003. The LTCH PPS replaced the previous cost-based system. It uses the Medicare Severity Long-Term Care-Diagnosis Related Groups (MS-LTC-DRGs) as a patient classification system in which each patient stay is grouped into an MS-LTC-DRG based on diagnoses (including secondary diagnoses), procedures performed, age, gender, and discharge status. Each MS-LTC-DRG has a predetermined ALOS, which is updated annually based on the latest available LTCH discharge data. The hospital receives payment for each Medicare patient, based on the MS-LTC-DRG to which that patient's stay is grouped. This grouping reflects the typical resources used for treating such a patient. Cases assigned to an MS-LTC-DRG are paid based on the Federal payment rate, including facility and case-level adjustments. One type of case-level adjustment is an interrupted stay (CMS 2010).

## Other Long-Stay Hospitals

The demand for other types of long-stay hospitals has declined over the years. Tuberculosis hospitals, for example, have practically disappeared, leaving only one in operation as of 2008 (US Census Bureau 2011), mainly because the disease has been largely eradicated or controlled with modern drugs.

## Classification by Location

Based on location, hospitals can be classified as urban or rural. *Urban hospitals* are located in a county that is part of a metropolitan statistical area (MSA). The US Bureau of Census has defined an MSA as a geographic area that includes at least (1) one city with a population of 50,000 or

more or (2) an urbanized area of at least 50,000 inhabitants and a total MSA population of at least 100,000. *Rural hospitals* are located in a county that is not part of an MSA. It is estimated that rural hospitals deliver health care to 54 million Americans, including 9 million Medicare beneficiaries (Slusky 2006).

Compared to rural hospitals, urban hospitals have higher costs because they pay higher salaries in more competitive markets, offer a broader scope of more sophisticated services, and treat patients requiring more complex care. Urban hospitals are located either in inner cities or in the suburbs. Because suburbs of metropolitan areas are more affluent than inner cities or rural areas, both inner city urban hospitals and rural hospitals treat a patient mix that is disproportionately poor and elderly, compared to suburban hospital patients (HCIA, Inc. and Deloitte & Touche 1997). Because of the disproportionate numbers of the elderly and poor in rural areas, rural community hospitals often find themselves in financial trouble. Conversion to a facility that provides nonacute health care services, such as a primary care clinic, a long-term care facility, or a specialty hospital, is sometimes a viable alternative when closure threatens these hospitals. For example, adoption of long-term care strategies has demonstrated to improve profitability of rural hospitals (Stuart et al. 2006).

To save some of the very small rural hospitals, the Balanced Budget Act of 1997 created the Medicare Rural Hospital Flexibility Program (MRHFP). Under this program, certain rural hospitals can be classified as *critical access hospitals* (CAH) if they have no more than 25 acute care and/or swing beds and if they provide 24-hour emergency medical services. An additional

10 beds may be operated for psychiatric and/or rehabilitation services. Although CAH status is not necessarily the best alternative for all small rural hospitals, the number of such hospitals jumped from 850 in 2003 (Mantone 2005) to an estimated 1,300 in 2010. The CMS has authorized few additional CAHs since 2006 (MedPAC 2010b). If a hospital elects CAH status and meets the criteria for CAH designation, it can receive cost-plus reimbursement for inpatient, outpatient, laboratory, therapy, and most postacute services in swing beds. The CAH program has provided the financial stability that many small rural hospitals need.

## Classification by Size

There is no standard way to classify hospitals by size. According to one classification

scheme, hospitals with fewer than 100 beds would be classified as small, those with 100 to 500 beds as medium, and those with 500-plus beds as large. Others may classify by size a little differently. Just over half (51%) of the community hospitals in the United States have 100 beds or more (see Figure 8–6).

Figure 8–12 illustrates expenses per inpatient day by hospital size. Experience in the manufacturing and retail sectors of the economy suggests that large enterprises should realize economies of scale. The reason is that certain overhead costs are fixed or semifixed—they do not increase proportionately as the size of the enterprise increases. Examples are administrative costs and plant maintenance costs. In the hospital industry, economies of scale seem to evaporate when the size exceeds 100 beds. Higher costs in larger hospitals are mainly attributable to

Figure 8–12  Expenses per Inpatient Day by US Hospital Size, Community Hospitals, 2007.

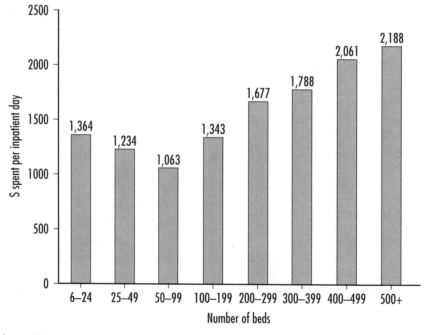

*Source:* Data from *Health, United States, 2009,* p. 415, National Center for Health Statistics.

a more extensive array of specialized and resource-intensive services that these hospitals must be equipped to provide. Such services require sophisticated technology and personnel with advanced training. Large teaching hospitals incur the additional costs of residency training and medical research.

## Other Types of Hospitals

### Teaching Hospitals    *COTH*

To be designated as a *teaching hospital*, a hospital must have one or more graduate residency programs approved by the AMA. The mere presence of nursing programs or training affiliations for other health professionals, such as therapists and dietitians, does not make an institution a teaching hospital.

The term *academic medical center* is commonly used when one or more hospitals, with or without affiliated outpatient clinics, are organized around a medical school. Apart from the training of physicians, research activities and clinical investigations become an important undertaking.

Among the largest and most prestigious teaching hospitals are the members of the Council of Teaching Hospitals and Health Systems (COTH). They usually have substantial teaching and research programs and are affiliated with medical schools of large universities. The approximately 400 COTH member institutions train about three-quarters of the physician residents in the United States (AAMC 2003).

Three main traits separate teaching and nonteaching hospitals:

1. Teaching hospitals provide medical training to physicians, research opportunities to health services researchers, and specialized care to patients. They incur certain costs directly associated with medical education programs, the largest category being the salary and benefits expense for interns and residents. Medicare reimburses the additional costs of graduate medical education in teaching hospitals separately, in addition to the prospective DRG rates (Dalton 1995).

2. Teaching hospitals have a broader and more complex scope of services than nonteaching hospitals. Teaching hospitals often operate several intensive care units, possess the latest medical technologies, and attract a diverse group of physicians representing most specialties and many subspecialties. Major teaching hospitals also offer many unique tertiary care services not generally found in other institutions, such as burn care, trauma care, and organ transplantation. Because services that are more specialized are available, teaching hospitals attract patients who frequently have more complicated diagnoses or need more complex procedures. Because of the greater case-mix complexity of teaching hospitals, greater resources are required for treatment.

3. Many of the major teaching hospitals are located in economically depressed, older inner city areas and are generally owned by state or local governments. Consequently, these hospitals often provide disproportional amounts of uncompensated care to uninsured patients. For example, COTH member institutions provide nearly one-half of all hospital charity care nationwide (AAMC 2011).

## Church-Affiliated Hospitals

Various churches established hospitals mainly during the latter half of the 19th and the early 20th centuries. Various Catholic sisterhoods established the first church-sponsored hospitals in the United States. Later, protestant denominations organized hospitals in accord with their missions of service, and Jewish philanthropic organizations opened hospitals so that Jewish patients could observe their dietary laws more faithfully and Jewish physicians could more easily find sites for training and work opportunities (Raffel 1980).

Church-affiliated hospitals are often community general hospitals. They may be large or small, teaching or nonteaching. Affiliation with a medical school may also vary. They are different only in that they are owned or heavily influenced by the church groups that sponsor them. Church hospitals do not discriminate in rendering care; however, they are generally sensitive to the sponsoring denomination's special spiritual and/or dietary emphasis (Raffel and Raffel 1994).

## Osteopathic Hospitals

Chapter 4 points out the main differences between allopathic and osteopathic medicine. For all practical purposes, osteopathic hospitals are community general hospitals. In 1970, osteopathic hospitals became eligible to apply for registration with the AHA (AHA 1994). For many years after osteopathy was established as a separate branch of medicine in 1874, osteopaths had to develop their own hospitals because of antagonism from the established allopathic medical practitioners. Since then, both groups have inspected each other's medical schools and satisfied themselves that each is

worth associating with and that each could serve on the other's faculties and practice side by side in the same hospitals (Raffel and Raffel 1994). Many osteopathic hospitals today are part of hospital systems and maintain their osteopathic identity within the context of these larger systems. An independent osteopathic hospital is no longer a necessity and seems to be economically out of place in today's market (Hilsenrath 2006). Also, the operation of osteopathic hospitals has been found to be more costly and less productive in comparison to their counterparts (Sinay 2005). Consequently, a number of these hospitals have closed.

# Expectations from Nonprofit Hospitals   *tax-exempt!*

Lay people make a common assumption that nonprofit (sometimes called not-for-profit) health care corporations are driven by the mission to meet the health care needs of patients regardless of their ability to pay. It is further assumed that these corporations do not make a profit. The fact is that every corporation, regardless of whether it is for profit or nonprofit, has to make a profit (surplus of revenues over expenses) to survive over the long term. No business can survive for long if it continually spends more than it takes in. That is true for both the nonprofit and the for-profit sectors (Nudelman and Andrews 1996).

The Internal Revenue Code, Section 501(c)(3), grants tax-exempt status to nonprofit organizations. As such, these institutions are exempt from federal, state, and local taxes, such as income taxes, sales taxes, and property taxes. In general, these organizations must (1) provide some defined public good, such as service, education, or community welfare and (2) not distribute any profits to any individuals. A major goal for a for-profit corporation, on the other hand, is to provide its shareholders with a return on their investment, but it achieves this goal primarily by excelling at its basic mission. For any health services provider, the basic mission is to deliver the highest-quality care at the most reasonable price possible.

Community hospitals owned by various groups, such as local citizens, fraternal orders, churches, and the government, have traditionally been classified as nonprofit and receive substantial tax subsidies. Current rules for tax-exempt hospitals require them to provide charity care, as well as community benefits. The latter broadly refer to services that the government would otherwise have to undertake (Owens 2005). Also, Section 4958 of the IRS code prohibits executive compensation that may be deemed unreasonable for tax-exempt organizations. Nonprofit hospitals have to be prepared to demonstrate not only that they are paying salaries within some reasonable range of industry standards but also that executives are bringing measurable value in key areas of operations, including community benefits (Appleby 2004). Hence, it is recommended that some portion of hospital chief executive officers' salaries directly hinge on their performance in two critical areas: (1) organizational effectiveness (financial performance, market share, quality, daily operations, and achievement of strategic objectives) and (2) community health (charitable care, health promotion and education, and overall state of the community's health; Newman et al. 2001).

The problem is that nonprofit hospitals, in many instances, compete head-on with for-profit hospitals. For example, nonprofit hospitals frequently engage in the same kinds of aggressive marketplace behaviors

that for-profit hospitals pursue. Institutional theory actually predicts such behavior. When for-profit and nonprofit organizations face similar regulatory, legal, and professional constraints, they will imitate each other, according to institutional theory (O'Connell and Brown 2003). In the hospital industry, competition commonly occurs in the same communities for the same patients, with revenues coming from the same public and private third-party sources, and often involving the same physician providers who have admitting privileges at more than one hospital.

The empirical evidence indicates that for-profit and nonprofit hospitals provide similar levels of charity and uncompensated care (Thorpe et al. 2000). Their quality of care and the adoption of new technology are also similar (Sloan 1998). Conversion of nonprofit to for-profit status does not necessarily adversely affect the provision of uncompensated care. However, some reduction in uncompensated care may occur, particularly when public hospitals are acquired by for-profit owners (Thorpe et al. 2000).

Whether nonprofit hospitals are indeed charitable institutions has remained controversial, and both Congress and the states continue to scrutinize nonprofit hospitals. In a 2010 decision by the Illinois Supreme Court, pertaining to *Provena v. Department of Revenue*, the court ruled that the medical center was not entitled to charitable exemption for property taxes because it did not provide sufficient community benefits (Supreme Court of the State of Illinois 2010).

Nonprofit institutions face new demands to deliver charity care under the Patient Protection and Affordable Care Act of 2010. The law requires nonprofit hospitals to (1) assess community health needs and implement plans to meet those needs, (2) provide financial assistance and emergency care, (3) limit certain billing and collection actions, (4) limit charges that the uninsured would have to pay for emergency care, and (5) report on community health needs and provide annual audited financial statements to the Internal Revenue Service (Betbeze 2011).

## Some Management Concepts

From a management standpoint, hospitals are complex organizations. Compared to other business enterprises of similar size, both external and internal environments of hospitals are more complex. A hospital is responsible to numerous stakeholders in its external environment. These stakeholders include the community, the government, insurers, MCOs, and accreditation agencies. Internally, hospital governance involves three major sources of power whose motivations are sometimes at odds. A hospital's organizational structure (see Figure 8–13) also differs substantially from that of other large organizations. The chief executive officer (CEO) receives delegated authority from the board and is responsible for managing the organization with the help of senior managers. In large hospitals, these senior managers often carry the title of senior vice president or vice president for various key service areas, such as nursing services, rehabilitation services, human resources, finance, and so forth.

The medical staff constitute a separate organizational structure parallel to the administrative structure. Such a dual structure is rarely seen in other businesses and presents numerous opportunities for conflict between the CEO and the medical staff. Matters are further complicated when the lines of authority cross between the two structures.

Figure 8–13 Hospitals Governance and Operational Structures.

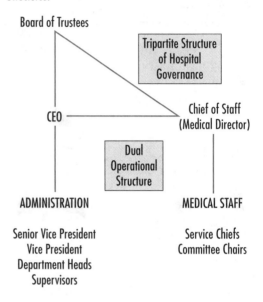

For example, nursing service, pharmacists, diagnostic technicians, and dietitians are administratively accountable to the CEO (via the vertical chain of command) but professionally accountable to the medical staff (Raffel and Raffel 1994). Although most of the medical staff are not paid employees of the hospital, physicians' interest in employment has been growing as they seek ways to stabilize their incomes and achieve a better work-life balance in a changing health care landscape (Shoger 2011). Regardless of whether the physicians are independent practitioners or contracted employees of the hospital, they play a significant role in the hospital's success. It requires special skills on the part of the CEO to manage the dual structure to achieve the organization's overall objectives. On the other hand, boards of trustees are called upon to evaluate, from a strategic standpoint, decisions such as incurring capital expenditures for building and equipment or hiring a new physician (Shoger 2011).

## Sources of authority

## Hospital Governance

Hospital governance has traditionally followed a tripartite structure. The three major sources of authority are the CEO, the board of trustees, and the chief of staff (medical director), as illustrated in Figure 8–13. In earlier periods, when physicians operated their own hospitals, trustees dominated the hospitals. Trustees were often the source of capital investment, and their influence in the community brought prestige to the hospital. Later, as voluntary hospitals increased in number, the balance of power shifted into the hands of physicians because they played a critical role in bringing patients to the hospitals. As changes in the health care environment made the management of hospitals more complex, considerable power shifted from physicians to senior managers.

## Board of Trustees

The *board of trustees* (also referred to as the governing body or board of directors) consists of influential business and community leaders. The board is legally responsible for the operations of the hospital. It is also responsible for defining the hospital's mission and long-term direction and for setting policy guidelines that establish the overall framework for day-to-day operations. It approves long-range plans and annual budgets and monitors performance against plans and budgets (Griffith 1995). The CEO is a member of the board. One or more physicians also sit on the board as voting members. One of the most important responsibilities of the board is to appoint and evaluate the performance of the CEO, who is charged with providing the board timely reports on the institution's progress toward achieving its mission and objectives. The board has the power to remove the CEO. In most hospitals, the board also approves the appointment of physicians and other professionals to the hospital's medical staff.

Boards often function through committees. Standing committees usually include executive, medical staff, human resources, finance, planning, quality improvement, and ethics. Special, or ad hoc, committees are established as needed. The two most important committees, from a governance standpoint, are the executive committee and the medical staff committee. The *executive committee* has continuing monitoring responsibility and authority over the hospital. Usually, it receives reports from other committees, monitors policy implementation, and makes recommendations. The *medical staff committee* is charged with medical staff relations. For example, it reviews admitting privileges and the performance of the medical staff. There is also increased emphasis on the legal and ethical obligations of the hospital regarding patient safety, quality improvement, and patient satisfaction.

## Chief Executive Officer

Formerly, the titles of "superintendent" and later "administrator" were commonly used for a hospital's chief executive. Now, "chief executive officer" and "president" are the common titles used. The CEO's job is to accomplish the organization's mission and objectives through leadership within the organization. He or she has the ultimate responsibility for day-to-day operations.

## Medical Staff

The hospital's medical staff is an organized body of physicians who provide medical services to the hospital's patients and perform related clinical duties. Most physicians are in private practice outside the hospital.

The hospital grants them admitting privileges that enable them to admit and care for their patients in the hospital. Other clinicians, such as dentists and podiatrists, may also be granted admitting privileges. Appointment to the medical staff is a formal process outlined in the hospital's medical staff bylaws. The medical staff use a framework of self-governance, which represents the strong tradition of physician independence. The medical staff are formally accountable to the board. Lines of communication to the CEO and the board of trustees are established through various committee representations.

A medical director, or *chief of staff*, heads the medical staff. In all but the smallest hospitals, the medical staff are organizationally divided by major specialties into departments, such as anesthesiology, internal medicine, obstetrics and gynecology, orthopedic surgery, pathology, cardiology, and radiology. A *chief of service*, such as chief of cardiology, heads each specialty.

The medical staff generally have their own executive committee that sets general policies and is the main decision-making body in medical matters. Other medical staff committees are common to most hospitals. The *credentials committee* grants and reviews admitting privileges for those already credentialed and for new doctors whose skills are yet untested. The *medical records committee* ensures that accurate documentation is maintained on the entire regimen of care given to each patient. This committee also oversees confidentiality issues related to medical records. The *utilization review committee* performs routine checks to ensure that inpatient placements, as well as the length of stay, are clinically appropriate. The *infection control committee* is responsible for reviewing policies and

procedures for minimizing infections in the hospital (Griffith 1995; Rakich et al. 1992). The *quality improvement committee* is responsible for overseeing the program for continual quality improvement.

## Licensure, Certification, and Accreditation

A license to operate a certain number of hospital beds is a basic regulatory requirement. State governments oversee the *licensure* of health care facilities, and each state sets its own standards for licensure. All facilities must be licensed to operate, but they do not have to be certified or accredited. A state's department of health carries out licensure functions. State licensure standards strongly emphasize the physical plant's compliance with building codes, fire safety, climate control, space allocations, and sanitation. Minimum standards are also established for equipment and personnel. State licensure is not directly tied to the quality of care a health care facility actually delivers.

*Certification* gives a hospital the authority to participate in Medicare and Medicaid. Legislation in 1972 mandated federal oversight of hospitals if they wished to admit Medicare and Medicaid patients. The Department of Health and Human Services (DHHS) developed standards called *conditions of participation*. The purpose of the hospital conditions of participation is to protect patient health and safety and help assure that quality care is furnished to all hospital patients. Hospitals must meet the conditions of participation to participate in Medicare or Medicaid. Conditions, as currently revised, are intended to focus primarily on the actual quality of care furnished to patients and the outcomes of that care. Each state's department of health verifies the actual compliance with the standards through periodic inspections.

In contrast with licensure and certification, which are government regulatory mechanisms, *accreditation* is a private mechanism designed to assure that accredited health care facilities meet certain basic standards. Seeking accreditation is voluntary, but the passage of Medicare in 1965 specified that accredited facilities were eligible for purposes of Medicare reimbursement. Accreditation of a hospital by the JCAHO confers *deemed status* on the hospital, meaning the hospital is deemed to have met Medicare and Medicaid certification standards. Thus, an accredited hospital does not need to go through the certification process. Private organizations that have been approved by the CMS to confer deemed status are said to have "deeming authority." In addition to JCAHO, the American Osteopathic Association also has deeming authority to accredit hospitals.

The JCAHO sets standards and accredits most of the nation's hospitals, as well as many of the long-term care facilities, psychiatric hospitals, substance abuse programs, outpatient surgery centers, urgent care clinics, group practices, community health centers, hospices, and home health agencies. Other private organizations also have deeming authority for some of these facilities. Different sets of standards apply to each category of health care organization. Some facilities, such as nursing homes, do not receive deemed status as a result of accreditation and must also be certified by DHHS to receive Medicare and Medicaid reimbursement. Over the years, JCAHO has refined its accreditation standards and process of verifying compliance. Since 2006, JCAHO has moved from scheduled to unannounced inspections, with the objective that hospitals will attempt to comply with all the standards all the time.

# The Magnet Recognition Program®

*Magnet hospital* is a special designation by the American Nurses Credentialing Center, an affiliate of the American Nurses Association, to recognize quality patient care, nursing excellence, and innovations in professional nursing practice in hospitals. The designation was created after a study of 163 hospitals was undertaken in 1983 by the American Academy of Nursing's Task Force on Nursing Practice in Hospitals. The study found that 41 of these hospitals had an environment that attracted and retained well-qualified nurses and promoted quality patient care. These hospitals were labeled as "magnet" hospitals because of their ability to attract and retain professional nurses. The characteristics that seemed to distinguish "magnet" organizations from others became known as the Forces of Magnetism. The Forces of Magnetism have been incorporated into quality indicators and standards of nursing practice as defined in the *ANA Nursing Administration: Scope & Standards of Practice*. The Magnet designation is granted after a thorough and lengthy process that includes data on quality indicators. Studies show that visionary leadership, empowerment, and collaboration have an impact on development and maintenance of healthy work environments and that quality of patient care is related to quality of the nurses' work environment (Kramer et al. 2011).

---

The Magnet Recognition Program® is a registered trademark of the American Nurses Credentialing Center.

# Ethical and Legal Issues in Patient Care

Ethical issues arise in all types of health services organizations, but the most significant occur in acute care hospitals. Increasing levels of technology create situations requiring decision making under complex circumstances. For example, life-sustaining therapies in intensive care and dealing with life and death issues commonly raise ethical concerns. Ethical issues also arise in health care research and in experimental medicine. In management, ethical conduct becomes important when competition is intense or when cost cutting becomes necessary to save an organization from bankruptcy.

## Ethical Principles

Ethics requires judgment. Clear-cut rules are often not available. Hence, medical practitioners and managers have to rely on certain well-established principles as guides to ethical decision making.

Four important principles of ethics are respect for others, beneficence, nonmaleficence, and justice. The principle of respect for others has four elements: autonomy, truth-telling, confidentiality, and fidelity. Autonomy allows people to govern themselves by choosing and pursuing a course of action without external coercion. In health care delivery, it refers to patient empowerment: obtain consent for treatment, explain the various treatment alternatives, allow the patients and their families to participate in decision making and selection of treatment options, and treat the patients with respect and dignity. Constant tension exists between autonomy and paternalism, the view that someone else must direct what the patient must undergo without the patient's involvement. Truth-telling requires a caregiver to be honest. This principle often needs to be balanced with nonmaleficence because a tension is created when truth-telling would result in harm to the patient. The principle of confidentiality sometimes comes into conflict when the legal system requires disclosure of patient information. Fidelity means performing one's duty, keeping one's word, and keeping promises.

The principle of beneficence implies that all individuals have some moral obligation to benefit others. A health services organization is ethically obligated to do all it can to alleviate suffering caused by ill health and injury. This obligation includes providing the needy with certain types of services, such as emergency department services.

The principle of nonmaleficence implies that people have a moral obligation not to harm others, but many health care interventions, including certain preventive measures, such as immunization, often carry risks. Hence, in health care, nonmaleficence requires that the potential benefits from medical treatment sufficiently outweigh the potential harm.

The principle of justice encompasses fairness and equality. It denounces discrimination in the delivery of health care.

## Legal Rights

Ethical concerns are often triggered in decisions related to informed consent and continuation of life support services to terminally ill patients. One of the most critical decisions relates to patient competency and the right to refuse treatment. Although the right of competent patients to refuse medical care is well established, the desires of incompetent or comatose patients present ethical challenges. Unless such patients have expressed their wishes in advance, family members or legal guardians end up making decisions regarding sustained medical treatment, or state laws may govern such decisions. Medical and legal experts and family members may differ, often bitterly, on the controversial issue of withdrawing nutrition and other life support means for dying patients, as the case of Theresa Schiavo, which made national news in 2004, demonstrated in the state of Florida. However, certain legal mechanisms have been established to deal with the issues of patients' rights.

## Bill of Rights and Informed Consent

The Patient Self-Determination Act of 1990 applies to all health care facilities participating in Medicare or Medicaid. The law requires hospitals and other facilities to provide all patients, upon admission, with information on patients' rights. Most hospitals and other inpatient institutions have developed what is referred to as the *patient's bill of rights*. This document reflects the law concerning issues such as confidentiality and consent. Other rights include the right to make decisions regarding medical care, be informed about diagnosis and treatment, refuse treatment, and formulate advance directives.

Based on the principle of autonomy, *informed consent* is a fundamental patient right. It refers to the patient's right to make an informed choice regarding medical treatment. The current climate in medical ethics supports honest and complete disclosure of medical information. In 1972, the Board of Trustees of the AHA affirmed a Patient's Bill of Rights, which states that patients have the right to obtain from their physicians

complete current information concerning their diagnosis, treatment, and prognosis, in terms the patients can be reasonably expected to understand (Rosner 2004). Informed consent is customarily obtained via a signature on preprinted forms and becomes part of the patient's medical record.

Certain principles governing patients' rights are being incorporated into provider mindsets and organizational culture creating what is referred to as *patient-centered care*. Patients' involvement in their own treatment, grounding treatment decisions in patients' preferences, and creating a caregiving environment in which staff solicit patients' inputs and meet their needs for information and education collectively promote patient-centered care (Cross 2004).

## Advance Directives

*Advance directives* refer to the patient's wishes regarding continuation or withdrawal of treatment when the patient lacks decision-making capacity. Advance directives are intended to ensure that the patient's end-of-life wishes are carried out.

Three types of advance directives are in common use: do-not-resuscitate orders, living wills, and durable powers of attorney. A *do-not-resuscitate order* directs medical caregivers not to administer any artificial means to resuscitate the person when his or her heart or breathing stops. It is based on the theory that a patient may prefer to die rather than live when strong odds are against a good quality of life after cardiopulmonary resuscitation because severe disabilities would likely remain. A *living will* communicates a patient's wishes regarding medical treatment when he or she is unable to make decisions due to terminal illness or incapacitation. The main drawback of a living will is that it is general in nature because it cannot possibly cover all possible situations. A *durable power of attorney* for health care is a written legal document in which the patient appoints another individual to act as the patient's agent for purposes of health care decision making in the event that the patient is unable or unwilling to make such decisions. Although a durable power of attorney can cover most circumstances, its main drawback is that the appointed person may not act in the same manner in which the patient would have acted had he or she remained competent.

## Mechanisms for Ethical Decision Making

Many health care organizations, especially large acute care hospitals, have *ethics committees* charged with developing guidelines and standards for ethical decision making in the delivery of health care (Paris 1995). Ethics committees are also responsible for resolving issues related to medical ethics. Such committees are multidisciplinary, including physicians, nurses, clergy, social workers, legal experts, ethicists, and administrators. Although physicians and other caregivers have moral responsibilities on the clinical side, the health care executive who leads the health services organization must also assume the role of a moral agent. As a *moral agent*, the manager morally affects and is morally affected by actions taken. Although executives are entrusted with the fiduciary responsibility to act prudently in managing the affairs of the organization, their responsibilities to patients must take precedence. In governing the affairs of an organization, health care executives must also recognize that ethics is much more than

obeying the law. The law represents only the minimum standard of morality established by society. Similarly, health care professionals must recognize that, even though they are bound by the law, they also have a higher calling, one that includes numerous positive duties to patients, society, and each other (Darr 1991).

## Summary

Hospitals are institutions engaged primarily in the delivery of inpatient acute care services. However, they have increasingly branched out to provide postacute and outpatient services. Hospitals evolved from the almshouses and pesthouses of the 18th and 19th centuries, and early hospitals mainly served a custodial function, providing services that were more akin to social welfare than to medicine. Taking care of the sick did not develop as a main function of hospitals until the late 19th century, when many of the almshouses were replaced by public hospitals to serve the poor. Voluntary hospitals were developed to serve all classes of people. The growth of medical science and technology made it necessary for physicians to use hospitals as the main venue for the practice of medicine and for training residents. Since then, hospitals have moved toward consolidation and diversification aimed at developing a full continuum of health care services.

The growth of hospitals occurred in conjunction with advances in science and medical technology, advances in medical education, the development of professional nursing, and the growth of health insurance. The Hill-Burton Act of 1946 stands as the greatest single factor contributing to the increase in the nation's bed supply. The government played an equally important role in reducing inpatient utilization by means of the prospective payment system, implemented in 1983. The growth of managed care has been significant in reducing inpatient utilization during the 1990s. Some of the key measures of inpatient utilization are discharges, inpatient days, average length of stay, capacity, average daily census, and occupancy rates.

Hospitals can be classified in numerous ways, and the various classification schemes help differentiate one hospital from another. Performance statistics by hospital type can help executives compare their hospital to others in the same category. Although most US hospitals are general community hospitals, various specialty hospitals treat specific types of patients or conditions. Teaching hospitals and academic medical centers play a leading role in graduate medical education. Church-affiliated hospitals are mostly voluntary community hospitals, but they serve a special purpose by emphasizing the sponsoring organization's dietary and spiritual aspects of health care. Osteopathic hospitals are also community general hospitals, for the most part, with an emphasis on holistic medicine. Most public and voluntary hospitals are nonprofit, and, as such, these institutions enjoy some tax advantages. They are expected to provide charity care that is equivalent in value to the tax subsidies received; however, many nonprofit hospitals emulate the behavior of their for-profit counterparts. Court decisions that have denied tax exemption and provisions in the Patient Protection and Affordable Care Act of 2010 emphasize nonprofit hospitals' legal duty to provide community benefits.

Hospitals are among the most complex organizations to manage; they must satisfy numerous external stakeholders and manage a complex internal governance structure. Hospital organization is represented by a triad in which the board of trustees, the CEO, and the medical staff share various aspects of authority. The CEO must possess exceptional skills to manage the day-to-day operations, while satisfying the demands of the board, the medical staff, and the external stakeholders. Hospital administrators have been under growing pressure to handle the issues of resource allocation, cost containment, and uncompensated care.

A hospital cannot legally operate unless licensed by the state in which it is located. To participate in Medicare and Medicaid, a hospital must also be certified by the US Department of Health and Human Services. Certification is maintained by satisfying the conditions of participation. As an alternative to certification, a hospital can voluntarily apply for accreditation by the Joint Commission. Accreditation confers deemed status on a hospital, which exempts the hospital from Medicare and Medicaid certification. Hospitals designated as Magnet hospitals are able to recruit and retain qualified nurses and demonstrate a high level of quality in delivering patient care.

Ethical decision making has been a special area of concern for hospitals. From a medical standpoint, ethical issues often pertain to patient privacy, confidentiality, informed consent, and end-of-life treatment. Bills of rights and advance directives are two of the legal means to address these issues. Active ethics committees must continually address the development of policies and standards for clinicians and administrators. These same multidisciplinary committees also deal with ethical problems as they arise.

## Terminology

academic medical center
accreditation
advance directives
average daily census
average length of stay
board of trustees
certification
chief of service
chief of staff
community hospital
conditions of participation
credentials committee
critical access hospitals
days of care
deemed status
discharge
do-not-resuscitate order

durable power of attorney
ethics committees
executive committee
general hospital
hospital
infection control committee
informed consent
inpatient
inpatient day
investor-owned hospitals
licensure
living will
long-term care hospital
Magnet hospital
medical records committee
moral agent
multihospital system

occupancy rate
patient-centered care
patient's bill of rights
proprietary hospitals
public hospitals
quality improvement
   committee
rehabilitation hospitals
rural hospitals
short-stay hospital
specialty hospitals
swing beds
teaching hospital
urban hospitals
utilization review
   committee
voluntary hospitals

## Review Questions

1. What is the difference between inpatient and outpatient services?

2. As hospitals evolved from rudimentary custodial and quarantine facilities to their current state, how did their purpose and function change?

3. What were the main factors responsible for the growth of hospitals until the latter part of the 20th century?

4. Name the three main forces that have been responsible for hospital downsizing. How have each of these forces been responsible for the decline in inpatient hospital utilization?

5. What is a voluntary hospital? Explain. How did voluntary hospitals evolve in the United States?

6. Discuss the role of government in the growth, as well as the decline, of hospitals in the United States.

7. What are inpatient days? What is the significance of this measure?

8. How does hospital utilization vary according to a person's age, gender, and race?

9. Discuss the different types of public hospitals and the roles they play in the delivery of health care services in the United States.

10. What are some of the differences between private nonprofit and for-profit hospitals?

11. What is a long-term care hospital (LTCH)? What role does it play in health care delivery in the United States?

12. The table below gives some operational statistics for two hospitals located in the same community. Answer the questions following the table.

| Calendar Year 2010 | Nonprofit Community Hospital (A) | Proprietary Community Hospital (B) |
|---|---|---|
| Number of beds in operation | 320 | 240 |
| Total discharges | 12,051 | 9,230 |
| Medicare | 5,130 | 3,876 |
| Medicaid | 3,565 | 2,118 |
| Private insurance | 3,356 | 3,236 |
| Total hospital days | 72,421 | 51,684 |
| Medicare | 36,935 | 26,359 |
| Medicaid | 23,175 | 12,921 |
| Private insurance | 12,311 | 12,404 |
| Total inpatient revenues | $45,755,000 | $35,800,000 |
| Dollar value of charity care | $5,000,000 | $3,500,000 |

(a) Calculate the following measures for each hospital (wherever appropriate, calculate the measure for each pay type). Discuss the meaning and significance of each measure, and point out the differences between the two hospitals.

   (1) Hospital capacity

   (2) ALOS

   (3) Occupancy rate

(b) Operationally, which hospital is performing better? Why?

(c) Do you think the nonprofit hospital is meeting its service obligations to the community in exchange for its tax-exempt status? Explain.

(d) Do you think the hospitals have a problem with excess capacity? If so, what would you recommend?

13. Why have physicians developed their own specialty hospitals? What legal issues can arise when physicians have an ownership interest in a hospital?

14. What criteria does Medicare use to classify a hospital as a rehabilitation hospital?

15. How do you differentiate between a community hospital and a noncommunity hospital?

16. What is a critical access hospital (CAH)? Why was this designation created?

17. What are some of the main differences between teaching and nonteaching hospitals?

18. Can church-affiliated hospitals be classified as voluntary hospitals? Explain.
19. Discuss some of the issues relative to the tax-exempt status of nonprofit hospitals.
20. Why are hospitals among the most complex organizations to manage?
21. Discuss the governance of a modern hospital.
22. In the context of hospitals, what is the difference between licensure, certification, and accreditation?
23. What can a hospital do to address some of the difficult ethical problems relative to end-of-life treatment?

## REFERENCES

American Hospital Association (AHA). 1990. *Hospital statistics 1990–1991 edition.* Chicago: American Hospital Association.

American Hospital Association. 1994. *AHA guide to the health care field 1994 edition.* Chicago: American Hospital Association.

Anderson, K., and B. Wootton. 1991. Changes in hospital staffing patterns. *Monthly Labor Review* 114, no. 3: 3–9.

Appleby, J. 2004. IRS looking closely at what non-profits pay. *USA Today*, September 30. p. 02b.

Arndt, M., and B. Bigelow. 2006. Toward the creation of an institutional logic for the management of hospitals: Efficiency in the early nineteen hundreds. *Medical Care Research and Review* 63, no. 3: 369–394.

Association of American Medical Colleges (AAMC). 2003. Teaching hospitals. Available at: http://www.aamc.org/teachinghospitals.htm. Accessed May 2003.

Association of American Medical Colleges (AAMC). 2011. Teaching hospitals. Available at: https://www.aamc.org/about/112264/teachinghospitals/. Accessed February 2011.

Balotsky, E.R. 2005. Is it resources, habit or both: Interpreting twenty years of hospital strategic response to prospective payment. *Health Care Management Review* 30, no. 4: 337–346.

Betbeze, P. 2011. Reassessing community benefit. *Health Leaders Magazine* 14, no. 1: 50.

Centers for Medicare and Medicaid Services (CMS). 2010. *Long-term care hospital prospective payment system: Interrupted stay fact sheet.* Available at: http://www.cms.gov/MLNProducts/downloads/LTCH-IntStay.pdf. Accessed March 2011.

Clement, J.P., and K.L. Grazier. 2001. HMO penetration: Has it hurt public hospitals? *Journal of Health Care Finance* 28, no. 1: 25–38.

Cross, G.M. 2004. What does patient-centered care mean for the VA? *Forum* (November 2004), Academy Health.

Dalton, M.J. 1995. *Inpatient hospital reimbursement.* In: *Health care administration: Principles, practices, structure, and delivery.* 2nd ed. L.F. Wolper, ed. Gaithersburg, MD: Aspen Publishers, Inc. pp. 166–191.

Darr, K. 1991. *Ethics in health services management.* 2nd ed. Baltimore, MD: Health Professions Press.

DelliFraine, J.L. 2006. Communities with and without children's hospitals: Where do the sickest children receive care? *Hospital Topics* 84, no. 3: 19–26.

Department of Health and Human Services (DHHS). 2002. *Health, United States, 2002.* Hyattsville, MD: National Center for Health Statistics.

Department of Health and Human Services (DHHS). 2006. *Health, United States, 2006.* Hyattsville, MD: National Center for Health Statistics.

Department of Health and Human Services (DHHS). 2011. *Health, United States, 2010.* Hyattsville, MD: National Center for Health Statistics.

Department of Veterans Affairs. 2010. *2010 VHA facility quality and safety report.* Washington, DC: U.S. Department of Veterans Affairs.

Feldstein, M. 1971. *The rising cost of hospital care.* Washington, DC: Information Resource Press.

Feldstein, P.J. 1993. *Health care economics.* 4th ed. Albany, NY: Delmar Publishers.

Griffith, J.R. 1995. *The well-managed health care organization.* Ann Arbor, MI: AUPHA Press/Health Administration Press.

Grimaldi, P.L. 2002. Inpatient rehabilitation facilities are now paid prospective rates. *Journal of Health Care Finance* 28, no. 3: 32–48.

Guterman, S. 2006. Specialty hospitals: A problem or a symptom? *Health Affairs* 25, no. 1: 95–105.

Haglund, C.L., and W.L. Dowling. 1993. The hospital. In: *Introduction to health services.* 4th ed. S.J. Williams and P.R. Torrens, eds. Albany, NY: Delmar Publishers. pp. 135–176.

HCIA, Inc. and Deloitte & Touche. 1997. *The comparative performance of US hospitals: The sourcebook.* Baltimore, MD: HCIA Inc.

Health Forum. 2001. *AHA guide to the health care field. 2001–2002 edition.* Chicago: Health Forum.

Hilsenrath, P.E. 2006. Osteopathic medicine in transition: Postmortem of the osteopathic medical center of Texas. *Journal of the American Osteopathic Association* 106, no. 9: 558–561.

Kahl, A., and D.E. Clark. 1986. Employment in health services: Long-term trends and projections. *Monthly Labor Review* 109, no. 8: 28.

Kramer, M. et al. 2011. Clinical nurses in Magnet hospitals confirm productive, healthy unit work environments. *Journal of Nursing Management* 19, no. 1: 5–17.

Mantone, J. 2005. Critical time at rural hospitals. *Modern Healthcare* 35, no. 10: 22.

Mechanic, D. 1998. Emerging trends in mental health policy and practice. *Health Affairs* 17, no. 6: 82–98.

Medicare Payment Advisory Commission (MedPAC). 2004. *New approaches in Medicare: Report to the Congress.* Washington, DC: Medicare Payment Advisory Commission.

Medicare Payment Advisory Commission (MedPAC). 2006. *Report to the Congress: Physician-owned specialty hospitals revisited.* Washington, DC: Medicare Payment Advisory Commission.

Medicare Payment Advisory Commission (MedPAC). 2010a. *Long-term care hospitals payment system.* Washington, DC: Medicare Payment Advisory Commission.

Medicare Payment Advisory Commission (MedPAC). 2010b. *Critical access hospitals payment system.* Washington, DC: Medicare Payment Advisory Commission.

Muller, R.W. 2003. The changing American hospital in the twenty-first century. *Policy Brief No. 26/2003.* Syracuse, NY: Center for Policy Research, Syracuse University.

Newman, J.F. et al. 2001. CEO performance appraisal: Review and recommendations. *Journal of Healthcare Management* 46, no. 1: 21–37.

Nudelman, P.M., and L.M. Andrews. 1996. The "value added" or not-for-profit health plans. *New England Journal of Medicine* 334, no. 16: 1057–1059.

O'Connell, L., and S.L. Brown. 2003. Do nonprofit HMOs eliminate racial disparities in cardiac care? *Journal of Healthcare Finance* 30, no. 2: 84–94.

Owens, B. 2005. The plight of the not-for-profit. *Journal of Healthcare Management* 50, no. 4: 237–250.

Paris, M. 1995. *The medical staff.* In: *Health care administration: Principles, practices, structure, and delivery.* 2nd ed. L.F. Wolper, ed. Gaithersburg, MD: Aspen Publishers, Inc. pp. 32–46.

Patrick, V. et al. 2006. Facilitating discharge in state psychiatric institutions: A group intervention strategy. *Psychiatric Rehabilitation Journal* 29, no. 3: 183–188.

Raffel, M.W. 1980. *The US health system: Origins and functions.* New York: John Wiley and Sons, Inc.

Raffel, M.W., and N.K. Raffel. 1994. *The US health system: Origins and functions.* 4th ed. Albany, NY: Delmar Publishers.

Rakich, J.S. et al. 1992. *Managing health services organizations.* 3rd ed. Baltimore, MD: Health Professions Press.

Roemer, M.I. 1961. Bed supply and hospital utilization: A natural experiment. *Hospitals* 35, no. 21: 36–42.

Rosner, F. 2004. Informing the patient about a fatal disease: From paternalism to autonomy—The Jewish view. *Cancer Investigation* 22, no. 6: 949–953.

Sanofi-Aventis. 2007. *Managed care digest series, 2007: Hospital/systems digest.* Bridgewater, NJ: Sanofi-Aventis US, LLC.

Sanofi-Aventis. 2010. *Managed care digest series, 2010: Hospital/systems digest.* Bridgewater, NJ: Sanofi-Aventis US, LLC.

Shoger, T.R. 2011. Commonsense contracts. *Trustees* 64, no. 1: 6–7.

Silva, C. 2010. Physician-owned hospitals: Endangered species? *American Medical News,* June 28, 2010. Available at: http://www.ama-assn.org/amednews/2010/06/28/gvsa0628.htm. Accessed February 2011.

Sinay, T. 2005. Cost structure of osteopathic hospitals and their local counterparts in the USA: Are they any different? *Social Science and Medicine* 60, no. 8: 1805–1814.

Sloan, F.A. 1998. Commercialism in nonprofit hospitals. *Journal of Policy Analysis and Management* 17, no. 2: 234–252.

Slusky, R. 2006. An investment in rural hospitals is an investment in healthier communities. *AHA News* 42, no. 5: 4–5.

Snook, I.D. 1981. *Hospitals: What they are and how they work.* Rockville, MD: Aspen Systems Corporation.

Snyder, J. 2003. Specialty hospitals on rise: Facilities source of controversy. *The Arizona Republic,* February 23.

Stewart, D.A. 1973. The history and status of proprietary hospitals. *Blue Cross Reports—Research Series 9.* Chicago: Blue Cross Association.

Stuart, B. et al. 2006. Financial consequences of rural hospital long-term care strategies. *Health Care Management Review* 31, no. 2: 145–155.

Supreme Court of the State of Illinois. 2010. *Provena Covenant Medical Center et al. v. the Department of Revenue et al.* Docket no. 107328. Opinion filed March 18, 2010. Available at: http://www.state.il.us/court/Opinions/SupremeCourt/2010/March/107328.pdf. Accessed February 2011.

Teisberg, E.D. et al. 1991. *The hospital sector in 1992.* Boston: Harvard Business School.

Thorpe, K.E. et al. 2000. Hospital conversions, margins, and the provision of uncompensated care. *Health Affairs* 19, no. 6: 187–194.

US Census Bureau. 2011. *Statistical abstract of the United States, 2011.* Suitland, MD: US Census Bureau.

Vogt, W.B., and R. Town. 2006. *How has hospital consolidation affected the price and quality of hospital care?* Princeton, NJ: The Robert Wood Johnson Foundation.

Weaver, C. 2010. Physician-owned hospitals racing to meet health law deadline. *Kaiser Health News,* October 28, 2010. Available at: http://www.kaiserhealthnews.org/Stories/2010/October/28/physician-owned-hospitals.aspx. Accessed February 2011.

Williams, S.J. 1995. *Essentials of health services.* Albany, NY: Delmar Publishers.

Wolfson, J., and S.L. Hopes. 1994. What makes tax-exempt hospitals special? *Healthcare Financial Management* 4, no. 7: 56–60.

# Chapter 9

# Managed Care and Integrated Organizations

## Learning Objectives

- To review the link between the development of managed care and earlier organizational forms in the US health care delivery system
- To grasp the basic concepts of managed care and how managed care organizations realize cost savings
- To distinguish between the main types of managed care organizations
- To examine the different models under which health maintenance organizations are organized and to understand the advantages and disadvantages of each model
- To understand the concept of integration and the formation of integrated health care delivery systems
- To become familiar with certain provisions of the Patient Protection and Affordable Care Act of 2010 that apply to medical loss ratios, Medicare Advantage plans, and accountable care organizations
- To explore trends and issues in managed care and integration of services

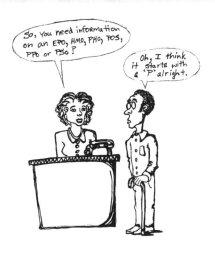

## Introduction

Managed care has been the single most dominant force that has fundamentally transformed the delivery of health care in the United States since the 1990s. At first, some observers had viewed the managed care phenomenon as an aberration, but, as private employers began to realize cost savings and public policy makers and administrators saw the opportunity to slow down the growing expense of providing health care through the Medicare and Medicaid programs, they increasingly turned to managed care. For now, managed care has become firmly entrenched in the US health care system. The health insurance provisions of the Patient Protection and Affordable Care Act (ACA) of 2010 do not go into effect until 2014, and it is unknown exactly how this new law, implemented in its current form, will affect managed care organizations.

Although managed care originated in the United States, its tools have spread internationally. For instance, general practitioners in several European countries regulate access to specialists and have responsibility over a per capital annual budget (Deom et al. 2010).

In the United States, transition to managed care became necessary as employers grappled with the unaffordable excesses of unrestrained delivery of services that led to spiraling health insurance premiums. In the fee-for-service system that prevailed prior to managed care, insurance companies had no incentive to manage the delivery of services and how the providers should be paid. With no controls on delivery and payment, costs got out of hand. The only way to control runaway costs was to integrate delivery and payment with the other two functions of financing and insurance. This integration of functions was accomplished through managed care. Figure 9–1 illustrates the extent

Figure 9–1  Percentage of Enrollment in Managed Care Plans Compared to Traditional Fee-for-Service Plans.

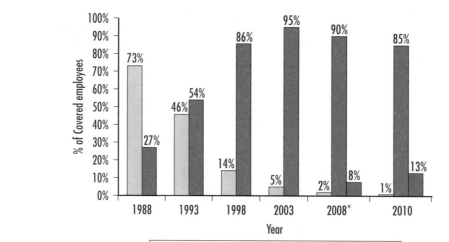

*In 2008, the survey started to include High Deductible Health Plans paired with a savings option (HDHP/SO), [discussed in Chapter 6].
*Source:* Data from *Employer Health Benefits: 2003 Annual Survey; Employer Health Benefits: 2010 Annual Survey;* The Henry J. Kaiser Family Foundation and Health Research and Educational Trust.

to which employer-sponsored health insurance has shifted from traditional fee for service to managed care.

After concerns from physicians and consumers and increased regulation from policy makers in the 1990s, managed care organizations (MCOs) were forced to relax tight controls over cost and utilization. Consequently, managed care evolved as something quite different from what it was intended to be, and it had limited success in controlling health care costs. Managed care faces the challenge of how to further manage cost escalations in hospital care, prescription drugs, and other areas of health care.

Professional dominance in health care delivery had long favored the supply side of the market equation. With the growth of managed care, the balance swung toward the demand side. This occurred in two ways: (1) Employers became active purchasers of health insurance with numerous managed care choices available; and (2) managed care, both directly and indirectly, purchased services from providers and wielded enormous buying power. Market forces have attempted to bring about a better equilibrium between health care providers and MCOs and given rise to new organizational arrangements.

By prompting organizational integration, managed care has literally transformed America's health care delivery landscape. During the 1990s and early 2000s, a wave of hospital mergers and acquisitions, a phenomenon that was national in scope, occurred. Hospital CEOs cited the potential for efficiency gains and strengthening of their financial positions as the main reasons that spurred integration (Williams et al. 2006). This wave of organizational integration occurred simultaneously with the growing power of managed care. True, there can be numerous reasons why health

care organizations have consolidated, such as technology, effects of reimbursement, and growth of services in alternative delivery settings, but the role of managed care cannot be dismissed. For instance, there is some evidence that hospitals gained increased pricing power over managed care organizations subsequent to consolidations (Capps and Dranove 2004). Hence, it can be argued that various types of organizational consolidations were driven, at least in part, by the significant influence of managed care, which had a significant negative impact on the utilization of hospital capacity and, consequently, on the financial performance of hospitals. Ginsburg (2005) reached the same conclusion: "Hospitals correctly perceived that by merging with others in the same community, they would increase their leverage with health plans (managed care plans)" (p. 1514). Conversely, the managed care industry itself has consolidated by absorbing weaker competitors.

Organizational alliances and networks are referred to as integrated delivery systems (IDSs) in this book. These systems are also called "health care systems," "integrated service networks," "integrated health networks," "integrated delivery networks," or "integrated provider networks." Organized networks differ by the degree of integration, but no standard method of classification captures the numerous variations.

## What Is Managed Care?

Managed care can be defined as an organized approach to delivering a comprehensive array of health care services to a group of enrolled members through efficient management of services needed by the members and negotiation of prices or payment arrangements with providers. Managed care is generally discussed in two different contexts. First, and more common, it refers to a mechanism or process of providing health care services and has two main features: Managed care (1) integrates the functions of financing, insurance, delivery, and payment within one organizational setting (Figure 9–2) and (2) exercises formal control over utilization. Second, the term "managed care" can refer to an MCO, which can take a variety of forms subsequently discussed in this chapter. In this context, managed care is an organization that delivers health care services without using an insurance company to manage risk and without using a third-party administrator to make payments.

## Financing

Premiums are based on contract negotiations between employers and the MCO.

Generally, a fixed premium per enrollee includes all health care services provided for in the contract.

## Insurance

The MCO functions like an insurance company by assuming all risk. In other words, it takes the financial responsibility if the total cost of services provided exceeds the revenue from fixed premiums. The percentage of premium revenue spent on medical expenses is called *medical loss ratio* (MLR); the remainder is used for administration, marketing, and profits. Some states have required a minimum MLR, such as 75%. Effective January 1, 2011, the ACA of 2010 required a minimum MLR of 85% in large-group markets, leaving just 15% to cover overhead, including claims administration, customer service, and sales expenses, which also include broker commissions (Wojcik 2011).

Figure 9–2  Integration of Health Care Delivery Functions Through Managed Care.

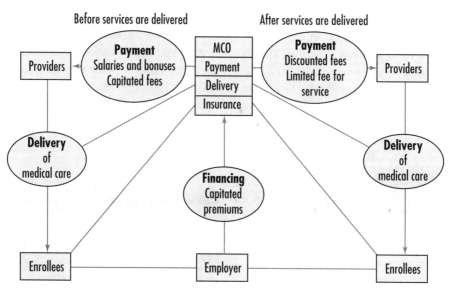

## Delivery

The MCO promises to provide a comprehensive set of services, including preventive services, ambulatory care, inpatient care, surgery, and rehabilitative services. In an ideal scenario, an MCO would operate its own hospitals and outpatient clinics and employ its own physicians. Some large MCOs actually do employ their own physicians on salary. Others have concluded mergers with hospitals and/or group practices. Most MCOs, however, arrange the delivery of medical services through contracts with physicians, clinics, and hospitals operating independently.

## Payment

MCOs use three main types of payment arrangements with providers: capitation, discounted fees, and salaries. The three methods allow risk sharing in varying degrees between the MCO and the providers. Risk sharing puts the burden on the providers to be cost conscious and to curtail unnecessary utilization. Sometimes, a limited amount of fee-for-service is used for specialized services.

① Capitation was discussed in previous chapters. It is a method in which a fixed monthly fee per member is paid to a provider. All health care services are included in the one set fee so that risk shifts from the MCO to the provider.

② The second type of payment arrangement used by MCOs is discounted fees. This arrangement can be regarded as a modified form of fee-for-service. After the delivery of services, the provider can bill the MCO for each service separately but is paid according to a prenegotiated schedule called a *fee schedule*. In this case, risk is borne by the MCO, but the MCO can lower its costs by paying discounted rates. Providers agree to discount their regular fees in exchange for the volume of business the MCO brings them.

③ A third method of payment is salaries, often coupled with bonuses or withholdings. In this case, the provider is an employee of the MCO. The physicians, for instance, are paid fixed salaries. At the end of the year, a pool of money is distributed among the physicians in the form of bonuses based on various performance measures. From an economic perspective, the physicians are paid only partial compensation up front. The remainder is withheld and paid later on condition that the physicians meet certain performance standards. Hence, under this method of payment the risk shifts from the MCO to the physicians.

It is important to note that cost containment is not the only objective managed care seeks to achieve, although the potential for cost containment has been the driving force behind the phenomenal growth of managed care. A survey of physicians and employers reported consensus of the two groups on seven essential features of managed care (Business Word Inc. 1996): cost containment, accountability for quality and cost, measurement of health outcomes and quality of care, health promotion and disease prevention programs, management of resource consumption, consumer education programs, and continuing quality improvement initiatives.

## Evolution of Managed Care

The concept of managed care is not new, even though the widespread adoption of the concept is a more recent phenomenon. The principles on which managed care is based have been around for about a century.

Chapter 3 discusses the prototypes of managed care, and Figure 9–3 summarizes the evolutionary steps.

In retrospect, the first private health insurance arrangement (see Baylor Plan in Chapter 3) was based on capitation, in which a fixed monthly fee was paid to Baylor Hospital for every teacher who enrolled. The idea of managed care evolved from what the medical establishment pejoratively referred to as the corporate practice of medicine, referring to contract practice and prepaid group practice discussed in Chapter 3. Even before private health insurance became widespread, these practices were used sporadically as cost-effective means of providing health care services to certain groups of people. Contract practice takes the idea of capitation a step further by incorporating a defined group of enrollees. Here, an employer is the financier who contracts with one or more providers to furnish health care to a group of enrollees—the employees—at a predetermined fee per enrollee.

Figure 9–3  The Evolution of Managed Care.

Health insurance
  Capitation
  Bearing of risk by providers

Initially, health insurance combined the insurance, delivery, and payment functions of health care, as seen in the Baylor Plan, but further evolution of this initial concept was thwarted by organized medicine. Contract practice moved toward the integration of these functions, bypassing the insurance companies.

Contract practice
  Defined group of enrollees
  Capitation or salary
  Bearing of risk by providers

Prepaid group practice
  Comprehensive services
  Defined group of enrollees
  Capitation
  Bearing of risk by providers

Managed care
  Utilization controls
  Comprehensive services
  Defined group of enrollees
  Capitation, discounted fees, or salary
  Limited fee for service
  Limits on choice of providers
  Sharing of risk with providers
  Financial incentives to providers
  Accountability for plan performance

Prepaid group practice goes another step. First, it preserves the principles of capitation, bearing of risk by the provider, and a defined group of enrollees whose health care contract is financed by their employer. It then adds the provision of comprehensive services.

The subsequent health insurance model loosely retained the insurance and payment functions but abandoned the delivery function. It let those insured decide where they would receive health services. The medical establishment, which strongly preferred the fee-for-service system, strongly influenced this fragmentation. Managed care reemerged in the 1970s with the passage of the Health Maintenance Organization Act (HMO Act) of 1973.

Early MCOs adopted the idea of prepaid group practice. To achieve greater cost efficiency, various utilization control measures were adopted. Management of utilization is, in essence, the "managed" part of managed care. Later, MCOs adopted variations in payment and delivery mechanisms that gave rise to different forms of managed care plans and MCOs.

## The First Prepaid Plans and the HMO Act

Prepaid group practice plans first became popular in some selected large urban markets in the United States. The American Medical Association (AMA) opposed the first plan, the Group Health Association of Washington (started in 1937 in Washington, DC), but the AMA was found guilty of restraint of trade, violating the Sherman Antitrust Act. This verdict may have been crucial in paving the way for the growth of other prepaid group practice plans. Notable among them are the Kaiser-Permanente Medical Care Program, started in 1942; the Group Health Cooperative of Puget Sound, opened in 1947; the

Health Insurance Plan of Greater New York, started in 1947; and the Group Health Plan of Minneapolis, started in 1957 (MacLeod and Prussin 1973). The Health Insurance Plan of Greater New York became one of the most successful health insurance programs, providing comprehensive medical services through organized medical groups of family physicians and specialists, but it provided hospital insurance through Blue Cross. Kaiser-Permanente went a few steps further. It exercised control over hospitals by contracting their services; placing considerable emphasis on preventive medicine; and employing mechanisms, such as penalizing physicians, to curtail excessive use of hospital facilities (Mechanic 1972; Raffel 1980). In due course, Kaiser-Permanente became the model for HMOs.

The HMO Act of 1973 was passed during the Nixon Administration, with the objective of stimulating growth of HMOs by providing federal funds for the establishment and expansion of new HMOs (Wilson and Neuhauser 1985). The underlying reason for supporting the growth of HMOs was the belief that prepaid medical care, as an alternative to traditional fee-for-service practice, would stimulate competition among health plans, enhance efficiency, and slow the rate of increase in health care expenditures. The HMO Act required employers with 25 or more employees to offer an HMO alternative if one was available in their geographic area. The objective was to create 1,700 HMOs to serve 40 million members by 1976 (Iglehart 1994). However, the HMO Act failed to achieve this objective. By 1976, only 174 HMOs had formed, with an enrollment of 6 million (Public Health Service 1995). In 1977, only 4% of those having job-based insurance had enrolled in HMO plans (Gabel 1999).

*HEDIS by NCQA*

By the end of the 1970s, enrollment in HMOs remained below 10 million.

## Alternative Forms of Managed Care

Competition among MCOs gave rise to new forms of managed care arrangements. Various MCO types resulted from the way they differentiated themselves, by offering enrollees greater freedom to choose their providers, adopting variations in the methods of payment to providers, and using creative means of organizing medical care providers. Competition from commercial insurance companies led MCOs to adopt measures that would distinguish them as more cost efficient. Thus, MCOs adopted various methods to control health care costs, active management of utilization being one such method.

## Accreditation of Managed Care Organizations

Since the 1990s, managed care has been the primary vehicle for managing health care for a vast number of Americans. The National Committee for Quality Assurance (NCQA) began accrediting MCOs in 1991. Accreditation began in response to the demand for standardized, objective information about the quality of MCOs. Participation in the accreditation program is voluntary, but about one-half of the plans are accredited. To be accredited, MCOs must comply with NCQA standards. Compliance is determined by a review process and evaluation by physicians and managed care experts. A national oversight committee of physicians supervises the process. Accreditation is combined with a rating system that has five status categories: excellent, commendable, accredited, provisional, and denied (NCQA 2007).

## Quality Assessment in Managed Care

Developed by the NCQA, Healthcare Effectiveness Data and Information Set (HEDIS) performance measures date back to 1989. Originally designed for private employers' needs as purchasers of health insurance, HEDIS has been adapted for use by the general public, public insurers, and regulators. More than 90% of America's health plans use HEDIS measures to measure performance on important dimensions of care and service. These measures have also been used quite extensively to evaluate and compare the quality of care in health plans.

HEDIS 2011 contains 70 measures across seven domains of care: effectiveness of care, access and availability of care, satisfaction with care, use of services, cost of care, health plan descriptive information, and health plan stability (NCQA 2011). The HEDIS program has been criticized because disclosure is voluntary. However, despite this concern, the overall quality of care has consistently improved among all plans reporting to the NCQA (DoBias 2008).

## Growth of Managed Care

As previously mentioned, the main impetus for managed care's growth was rapid cost escalations during the 1970s and 1980s under the dominant fee-for-service system. For example, in the 1980s, health insurance premiums rose on average more than 12% annually. Managed care offered relief from a growing cost burden. Some evidence suggests that, at least initially, managed care was also in a position to take advantage of the weakened economic position of health care providers.

## Flaws in Fee for Service

### Uncontrolled Utilization

Under the former dominant fee-for-service practice of medicine, utilization of medical care and payment to providers were practically unrestricted. In a system dominated by specialists and an absence of primary care gatekeeping, patients were free to go to any provider. Care received from specialists and utilization of sophisticated technology gave patients the impression of high quality. Competition was driven by such impressions rather than by cost. Physicians and hospitals competed for patients by offering the most up-to-date technologies and the most attractive practice settings (Wilkerson et al. 1997). Providers had an incentive to incur high utilization because they could increase their incomes by providing more services than medically necessary (provider-induced demand).

### Uncontrolled Prices and Payment

In traditional health insurance, the insurance company exercised little control over the prices providers charged or patients' utilization of services. Providers set charges at an artificially high level and billed insurance an item-by-item claim. The insurance company was merely a passive payer of claims—it paid what the providers billed, limited only by what the insurer deemed as usual, customary, and reasonable. The insurance company had little incentive to control costs because it could simply increase the premiums the following year based on utilization during the previous year.

### Focus on Illness Rather than Wellness

Conventional insurance paid for services only when a specific medical diagnosis was reported on the insurance claim. Visits for preventive checkups were not covered. The fee-for-service system presented a second and bigger problem. Traditional insurance provided more thorough coverage when a person was hospitalized, and the physician was paid for daily hospital visits when the patient was being treated in the hospital. Thus, costly hospitalization of patients was more lucrative for the physicians.

## Cost Appeal of Managed Care

Mainly due to the flaws in fee-for-service, health care delivery through conventional insurance led to rapid escalation of health care costs. Various methods of cost control were tried during the 1970s and 1980s, but they produced only limited results. At its inception, the concept of managed care was designed to compete against fee-for-service medicine. Up until the 1980s, HMOs were the predominant form of managed care. The price-based competition from HMOs was often referred to as "shadow pricing," in which HMOs would offer more benefits and somewhat lower premiums than fee-for-service plans (Zelman 1996). However, at this stage, managed care plans had limited appeal. Individuals covered by insurance plans that allowed them to choose their own physician or hospital saw little benefit in joining a plan that would restrict these choices. Most providers also saw little benefit in joining an MCO that might restrict their potential income or alter their style of practice (Wilkerson et al. 1997). For the most part, employers remained passive.

Between 1980 and 1990, total cost of private health insurance, on the average, went up at an annual rate of over 12% (Figure 9–4). As premiums escalated unchecked, economic realities forced employers

Figure 9–4   Growth in the Cost of US Health Insurance (Private Employers), 1980–1995.

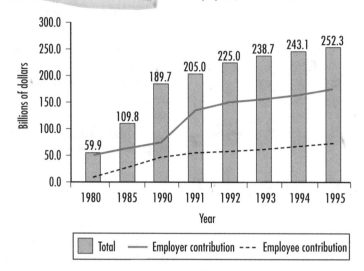

*Source:* Data from *Health, United States, 1998*, p. 348, National Center for Health Statistics.

to make the transition from traditional insurance plans to managed care. Among the US population with employer-sponsored health insurance, the proportion of those enrolled in various managed care plans jumped from 27% in 1988 to 86% in 1998 and to 95% in 2003 (see Figure 9–1).

## Weakened Economic Position of Providers

Indirectly, excess capacity in the health care delivery system may also have contributed to the growth of managed care (McGuire 1994). This was perhaps initially true because the Medicare prospective payment system, introduced in the mid-1980s, had a marked impact on hospital economics. Left with significant unused capacity in the form of empty beds, the bargaining power of hospitals substantially weakened. Physicians initially showed great resistance to managed care, but, as the financing of health care was quickly shifting toward managed care, they

could no longer resist the growing momentum. In most cases, they were left with the choice of participating or being completely left out.

## Efficiencies and Inefficiencies in Managed Care

Managed care achieves efficiencies in several ways. First, by eliminating insurance and payer intermediaries, MCOs can realize some savings. Second, MCOs control costs by sharing risk with providers or by extracting discounts from providers. Risk sharing promotes delivery of health care that is economically prudent. Hence, risk sharing is an indirect method of utilization control. Third, cost savings are achieved by coordinating a broad range of patient services and by monitoring care to determine whether it is appropriate and delivered in the most cost-effective settings (Health Insurance

Association of America 1991). For example, by emphasizing outpatient services, MCOs achieved lower rates of hospital utilization. Some evidence also suggests that HMO plans have lower use of costly procedures, compared to non-HMO plans (Miller and Luft 1997). Last, HMOs provide a substantially higher amount of preventive care than traditional insurance plans (Rizzo 2005). Preventive care keeps people healthy and saves money through prevention, as well as early detection and treatment of more serious illnesses.

Although many of the cost-control measures adopted by managed care have been applauded, other results have not been so commendable. Most providers find the complexity of having to deal with numerous plans overwhelming. A tremendous amount of inefficiency is created for providers, who must deal with differences in each plan's protocols and procedures. Another problem is that many contracts with providers exclude some services. For example, carving out laboratory testing services for outpatients has become a common practice. Many MCOs use one of the large national lab chains, such as Quest Diagnostics or Roche Diagnostics, which may present certain inconveniences for both patients and providers. A third area of inefficiency is the lengthy appeals process that patients and providers must sometimes go through when an MCO denies service. In short, managed care does not always create the well-coordinated, seamless system that patients and providers would like to see (Southwick 1997).

## Cost Control Methods in Managed Care

MCOs use various methods to monitor and control utilization of services. The need for

utilization management emanates from the fact that, in the United States, about 10% of patients—typically those with chronic or complex medical conditions—account for 70% of overall health care spending (Berk and Monheit 2001). Utilization management requires (1) an expert evaluation of which services are medically necessary in a given case, which ensures that unnecessary services are minimized; (2) a determination of how those services can be provided most inexpensively, while maintaining acceptable quality standards; and (3) a review of the process of care and changes in the patient's condition to revise the course of medical treatment if necessary. Utilization management of institutional inpatient services takes priority because such services account for 40% or more of the total expenses in a managed care plan (Kongstvedt 1995a). The methods commonly used for utilization monitoring and control are:

- Choice restriction
- Gatekeeping
- Case management
- Disease management
- Utilization review
- Practice profiling

*For utilization monitoring*

Not all MCOs use all of these mechanisms. Traditionally, HMOs have employed tighter utilization controls than other managed care plans.

### Choice Restriction

As previously discussed, traditional health insurance gave the insured open access to any provider, whether generalist or specialist. Such indiscretion led to overutilization of services. Most managed care plans impose some restrictions on where and from whom the patient can obtain medical care. Patients still have a choice of physicians, but the choice is limited to physicians who are either employees of the MCO or have established contracts with the MCO. A physician who has formal affiliations with an MCO is said to be on the *panel* of the MCO. In a *closed-panel* (or closed-access or in-network) plan, services obtained from providers outside the panel are not covered by the plan. By contrast, an *open-panel* (or open-access or out-of-network option) plan allows access to providers outside the panel, but enrollees almost always have to pay higher out-of-pocket costs.

Because the MCO has greater control over providers who are on its panel, utilization is better managed under closed-panel plans, compared to those that allow access outside the panel. From the enrollees' standpoint,

restricted choice of providers is a trade-off for lower out-of-pocket costs; however, lack of physician choice has been strongly associated with consumers' dissatisfaction with their health plans (Berenson 1997).

## Gatekeeping

Chapter 7 discusses primary care gatekeeping, which requires a primary care physician (PCP) to coordinate all health care services needed by an enrollee and take responsibility for managing utilization. Gatekeeping emphasizes preventive care, routine physical examinations, and other primary care services. Secondary care services, such as diagnostic testing, consultation with specialists, and admission to a hospital, are obtained only on referral from the primary care gatekeeper. Figure 9–5 illustrates the role of primary care gatekeeping.

Figure 9–5  Care Coordination and Utilization Control Through Gatekeeping.

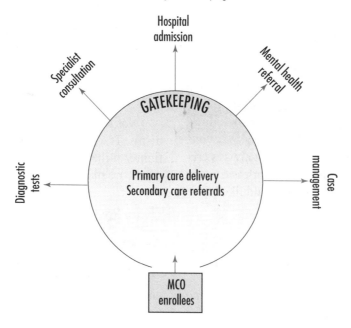

## Case Management

*Case management* is an organized approach to evaluating and coordinating care, particularly for patients who have complex, potentially costly problems that require a variety of services from multiple providers over an extended period. Examples include acquired immune deficiency syndrome (AIDS), spinal cord injury, bone marrow transplant, lupus, cystic fibrosis, and severe workplace injuries. These patients may need secondary and tertiary care services more often, whereas primary care may be needed only occasionally. In such circumstances, a primary care gatekeeper cannot adequately coordinate all of the patient's needs that may also frequently change. In case management, an experienced health care professional, such as a nurse practitioner, with knowledge of available health care resources coordinates an individual's total health care in consultation with primary and secondary care providers. The delivery of services is periodically reviewed to ascertain their appropriateness and efficacy. Case managers are also frequently involved in patient and family support and advocacy. Figure 9–6 illustrates the case management model.

**Figure 9–6** The Case Management Function in Health Services Utilization.

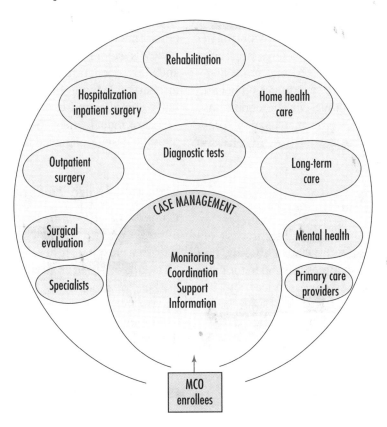

## Disease Management

Whereas case management is typically highly individualized and focuses on coordinating the care of high-risk patients with multiple or complex medical conditions (Short et al. 2003), disease management is a population-oriented strategy for people with chronic conditions, such as diabetes, asthma, depression, and coronary artery disease. Disease management is based on well-established, evidence-based treatment guidelines. After subgroups among all the enrollees in a health plan have been identified according to their specific chronic conditions, disease management focuses on patient education, training in self-management, ongoing monitoring of the disease process, and follow-up to ensure that people are complying with their medical regimens. The goal of disease management is to prevent or delay comorbidities and complications arising from uncontrolled chronic conditions. Cost savings are realized because it is estimated that more than one-half of health care spending is on behalf of people with multiple chronic conditions (Sipkoff 2003). Disease management programs can lower emergency room visits and hospitalizations.

## Utilization Review

*Utilization review* (UR) is the process of evaluating the appropriateness of services provided. It is sometimes misunderstood as a mechanism for denying services, but its main objective is to ensure that appropriate level of services are delivered, care is cost efficient, and subsequent care is planned. Three main types of UR are distinguished by when the review is undertaken: prospective, concurrent, and retrospective.

## Prospective Utilization Review *before*

*Prospective utilization review* determines the appropriateness of utilization before the care is actually delivered. An example of prospective UR is the decision by a primary care gatekeeper to refer or not refer a patient to a specialist. However, not all managed care plans use gatekeepers. Some plans require the enrollee or the provider to call the plan administrators for preauthorization (also called precertification) of services for hospital admissions and surgical procedures. In case of an emergency admission to an inpatient facility, plans generally require notification within 24 hours. Most plans now use preestablished clinical guidelines to determine the appropriateness of services.

One objective of prospective UR is to prevent unnecessary or inappropriate institutionalization; however, it also serves other functions. It notifies the concurrent review system that a case will be occurring and allows concurrent review to prepare for discharge planning. In the event of a potentially complex and expensive case, it notifies case management to evaluate and take over the case (Kongstvedt 1995a).

## Concurrent Utilization Review *during*

*Concurrent utilization review* determines, on a daily basis, the length of stay necessary in a hospital. It also monitors the use of ancillary services and ensures that the medical treatment is appropriate and necessary. When a patient is hospitalized, a certain number of inpatient days are preauthorized. Physicians and nurses then monitor the patient's condition to determine the appropriate length of stay. The UR nurse also coordinates discharge planning.

*Discharge planning* is often part of the overall treatment plan from the outset. It focuses on postdischarge continuity of care. For example, if a patient is admitted with a fractured hip, it is important to estimate whether a rehabilitation hospital or a skilled nursing facility would be more appropriate for convalescent care. If the patient requires care in a skilled nursing facility, discharge planning must find out whether the appropriate level of rehabilitation services would be available and how long the plan will pay for rehabilitation therapies in a long-term care setting. For a patient who will be discharged home, subsequent home health services and the need for durable medical equipment (DME) may be necessary. The objective is "to get all the ducks in a row" to provide seamless services at the lowest cost and in the best interest of the patient.

## Retrospective Utilization Review after

*Retrospective utilization review* refers to a review of utilization after services have been delivered. A close examination of medical records is undertaken to assess the appropriateness of care. Large claims may be reviewed for billing accuracy. Retrospective review may also involve an analysis of utilization data to determine patterns. Such patterns may be provider specific. For example, a particular provider may show patterns of excessive utilization or underutilization compared to his or her peers (Kongstvedt 1995b). Pattern review is often used to furnish feedback to providers. Incentive compensation, such as bonuses, is often tied to pattern reviews in an effort to influence future practice behavior. The analyses may also show planwide variations from previous periods or from established medical

practice norms. Such statistical data can be helpful for taking corrective action and for monitoring subsequent progress.

## Practice Profiling

Also called "profile monitoring," *practice profiling* refers to the development of physician-specific practice patterns and the comparison of individual practice patterns to some norm. Practice profiling may be a byproduct of retrospective UR. Mainly, such profiles are used to decide which providers have the right fit with the plan's managed care philosophy and goals. The profile reports are also used to give feedback to physicians so they can modify their own behavior of medical practice. Other uses include identifying specialists to whom the plan should refer certain types of cases, detecting fraud and abuse, and determining how to focus the UR program (Kongstvedt 1995c).

Physicians become understandably anxious when their practices come under scrutiny. They may think that the standards used to evaluate their work do not consider extenuating circumstances and that their fate may be decided based on sterile reports. For MCOs, the ability to report the behavior of individual physicians provides a powerful tool to discipline nonconforming physicians; however, great care must be exercised when using physician-specific reports. The administrator must look behind the data and investigate reasons for the reported performance. It is necessary to see how the norms for comparisons are established. It is also important to examine provider behavior from the standpoint of total health care resource consumption and outcome and to employ a variety of performance measures (Kongstvedt 1995c). According to one study, about one-half of all physicians affected by practice profiling viewed it positively as a useful tool to improve quality and efficiency, but 40% expressed mixed feelings (Reed et al. 2003).

## Types of Managed Care Organizations

Three main factors led to the development of different types of managed care plans, the first being choice of providers. To compete with HMOs, which employed tight restrictions on the choice of providers, MCO plans offering a greater freedom of choice emerged. Different ways of arranging the delivery of services also led to different forms of MCOs. Payment and risk sharing make up the third major factor. These variables led to the development of different types of managed care plans and various models of HMOs.

## Health Maintenance Organization

Commonly referred to as HMOs, health maintenance organizations were the most common type of MCO until commercial insurance companies developed preferred provider organizations (PPOs) to compete with HMOs. An *HMO* is distinguished from other types of plans by the following main characteristics:

1. In the traditional system, health insurance pays for medical care only when a person is ill. An HMO not only provides medical care during illness but also offers a variety of services to help people maintain their health. Hence, the name "health maintenance" organization. HMOs place considerable emphasis on preventive services and primary care. Compared to other managed care plans, HMOs are also more likely to use disease management as a means for delivering cost-effective health care.

2. The enrollee is generally required to choose a PCP from the panel of physicians. The PCP becomes the first contact to deliver basic care, coordinate all health care services the enrollee may need, and make referrals for secondary care services.

3. The provider receives a capitated fee regardless of whether the enrollee uses health care services and regardless of the quantity of services used.

4. All health care must be obtained from in-network hospitals, physicians, and other health care providers, although some may allow out-of-network use at a higher out-of-pocket cost. Specialty services, such as mental health and substance abuse treatment, are frequently carved out. A *carve out* is a special contract outside regular capitation, which is funded separately by the HMO.

5. The HMO is responsible for ensuring that services comply with certain established standards of quality.

HMO enrollments grew rapidly in the first half of the 1990s (Figure 9–7). Subsequently, other types of managed care plans—notably PPO and point of service (POS) plans—gained in popularity. HMOs fell into disfavor with enrollees because these plans were the most restrictive. The trend since the late 1990s has favored plans offering enrollees greater freedom to select their physicians.

Figure 9–7  Percent of Covered Employees Enrolled in HMO Plans (Selected Years).

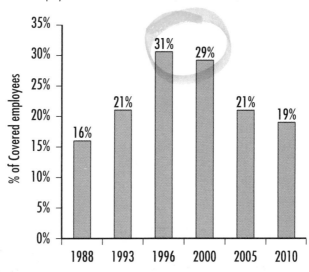

*Source:* Data from *Employer Health Benefits: 2010 Annual Survey*; The Henry J. Kaiser Family Foundation and Health Research and Educational Trust.

There are four common HMO models—staff, group, network, and independent practice association (IPA)—differing primarily in their arrangements with participating physicians. Figure 9–8 depicts the proportionate share of the four models. The IPA model remains dominant, but it continues to lose market share to network and group model HMOs. Figure 9–9 shows enrollment trends. Some HMOs cannot be categorized neatly into any one of the four models because they may use a hybrid arrangement, referred to as a *mixed model.* An example of a mixed model is an HMO that is partially organized as a staff model, employing its own physicians, and partially relies on the group model by contracting with a group practice.

Figure 9–8  Breakdown of HMO Model Types, 2009.

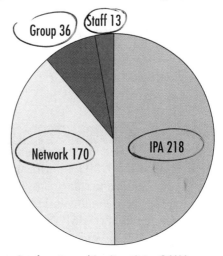

*Source:* Data from *Managed Care Digest Series,* ©2010 Sanofi-Aventis.

Figure 9–9  US Enrollment in HMOs by Model Type, 1993–2009.

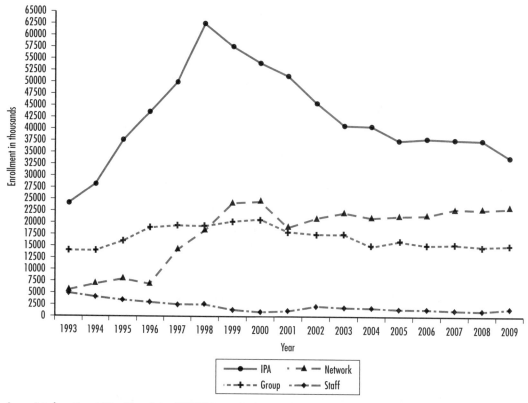

*Source:* Data from *Managed Care Digest Series: HMO-PPO Digest,* © 1996, Hoechst Marion Roussel; *Managed Care Digest Series: HMO-PPO/ Medicare-Medicaid Digest,* © 1999, Hoechst Marion Roussel; *HMO-PPO/Medicare-Medicaid Digest,* © 2003, Aventis Pharmaceuticals; *HMO-PPO Digest,* ©2006, ©2008, and ©2010 Sanofi-Aventis.

## Staff Model

A *staff model* HMO employs its own salaried physicians. Based on the physician's productivity and the HMO's performance, bonuses may be added to salary. Physicians work only for their employer HMO and provide services to that HMO's enrollees (Rakich et al. 1992). Staff model HMOs must employ physicians in all the common specialties to provide for the health care needs of their members. Contracts with selected subspecialties are established for infrequently needed services. The HMO operates one or more ambulatory care facilities that contain physicians' offices; employ support staff; and may have ancillary support facilities, such as laboratory and radiology departments. In most instances, the HMO contracts with area hospitals for inpatient services (Wagner 1995).

Compared to other HMO models, staff model HMOs can exercise a greater degree of control over the practice patterns of their physicians. These HMOs also offer the convenience of "one-stop shopping" for their enrollees because most common services are located in the same clinic (Wagner 1995).

Staff model HMOs also present several disadvantages. The fixed-salary expense can be high, requiring these HMOs to have a large number of enrollees to support operating expenses. Enrollees have a limited choice of physicians. Using the staff model concept, expansion into new markets requires heavy capital outlays (Wagner 1995). Because of such disadvantages, the staff model has been the least popular. Nationwide, the number of staff model HMOs has continued to decline, from 30 (3.3% of all HMOs) in 1998 to 13 (3% of all HMOs) in 2009 (Aventis Pharmaceuticals/SMG Marketing-Verispan LLC 2002; Sanofi-Aventis 2010a).

## Group Model

A *group model* HMO contracts with a single multispecialty group practice and contracts separately with one or more hospitals to provide comprehensive services to its members. The group practice employs the physicians, not the HMO. The HMO pays an all-inclusive capitation fee to the group practice to provide physician services to its members. The group practice may have contracts with other MCOs as well.

Large groups are usually attractive to HMOs because they deliver a large block of physicians with one contract. However, a large group contract can also be a downside for the HMO. If the contract is lost, the HMO will have difficulty meeting its service obligations to the enrollees. As for other advantages, the HMO is able to avoid large expenditures in fixed salaries and facilities.

Affiliation with a reputable multispecialty group practice lends the HMO prestige and creates a perception of quality among its enrollees. Conversely, enrollees may find the choice of physicians limited. In 2009, there were 36 group practice HMOs (8.2% of all HMOs) in the United States (Sanofi-Aventis 2010a).

## Network Model

Under the *network model*, the HMO contracts with more than one medical group practice. This model is especially adaptable to large metropolitan areas and widespread geographic regions where group practices are located. A common arrangement in the network model is to have contracts only with primary care group practices. Enrollees may select PCPs from any of these groups. Each group is paid a capitation fee based on the number of enrollees. The group is responsible for providing all physician services. It can make referrals to specialists but is financially responsible for reimbursing them for any referrals made. In some cases, the HMO may contract with a panel of specialists, in which case referrals can be made only to physicians serving on the panel (Wagner 1995). The network model can offer a wider choice of physicians than the staff or group model. The main disadvantage is the dilution of utilization control. In 2009, there were 170 network model HMOs (38.9% of all HMOs) in the United States (Sanofi-Aventis 2010a).

## Independent Practice Association (IPA) Model

In 1954, a variant of the prepaid group practice plan was established by the San Joaquin

County Foundation for Medical Care in Stockton, California. The plan was a prototype of the *IPA model* and was initiated by the San Joaquin County Medical Society (MacColl 1966). As a result of political pressures from organized medicine, this form of HMO was specifically included in the HMO Act of 1973 (Mackie and Decker 1981).

An *independent practice association* is a legal entity separate from the HMO. The IPA contracts with both independent solo practitioners and group practices. In turn, the HMO contracts with the IPA instead of contracting with individual physicians or group practices (Figure 9–10). Hence, the IPA is an intermediary representing a large number of physicians. The HMO pays a capitation amount to the IPA. The IPA retains administrative control over how it pays its physicians. It may reimburse physicians through capitation or some other means, such as a modified fee for service. The IPA often shares risk with the physicians and assumes the responsibility for utilization management and quality assessment. The IPA also carries stop-loss reinsurance, or the HMO may provide stop-loss coverage to prevent the IPA from going bankrupt (Kongstvedt and Plocher 1995).

Under the IPA model, the HMO is still responsible for providing health care services to its enrollees, but the logistics of arranging physician services shifts to the IPA. The HMO is, thus, relieved of the administrative burden of establishing contracts with numerous providers and controlling utilization. Financial risk also transfers to the IPA. The IPA model provides an expanded choice of providers to enrollees. It also allows small groups and individual physicians the opportunity to participate in managed care and get a slice of the revenues. Community physicians may independently establish IPAs, or the HMO may create an IPA and invite community physicians to participate in it. An IPA may also be hospital based and structured so that only physicians from one or two hospitals are eligible to participate in the IPA (Wagner 1995). One major disadvantage of the IPA model is that, if a contract is lost, the HMO loses a large number of participating physicians.

The IPA acts as a buffer between the HMO and physicians. Hence, the IPA does not have as much leverage in changing physician behavior as a staff or a group model HMO would have. Finally, many IPAs have a surplus of specialists, which creates some pressure to use their services (Kongstvedt and Plocher 1995). Of the four HMO models, the IPA model has been the most successful in terms of the share of all enrollments over time. Perhaps its success can be attributed to the buffer an IPA creates between the HMO and its practicing physicians. This amounts to less direct HMO control over the providers. In 2009, there were 218 IPA model HMOs (49.9% of all HMOs) in the United States (Sanofi-Aventis 2010a).

Figure 9–10  The IPA-HMO Model.

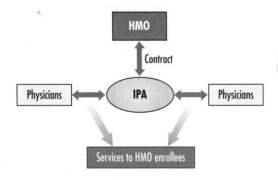

# Preferred Provider Organization

*PPOs* first appeared in the medical marketplace in the late 1970s as a competitive response by insurance companies to HMOs' growing market share. They differentiated the PPO product by offering open-panel options for enrollees and offering noncapitation payment to providers. The enrollees agree to use a selected set of physicians and hospitals with which the PPO has contracts. These providers on the PPO's panel are referred to as "preferred providers." The main appeal of PPOs is that they allow patients the choice of using physicians and hospitals outside the panel, for which the patients must pay higher copayments than if they used in-network providers. The additional out-of-pocket expenses act largely as a deterrent to going outside the panel. If a PPO does not provide an out-of-network option, it is referred to as an *exclusive provider plan*.

Instead of capitation, PPOs make discounted fee arrangements with providers. The discounts can range between 25 and 35% from the provider-established charges. Thus, in paying providers, PPOs substitute discounted fee for service for capitation, which is more commonly used by HMOs—although some HMOs also switched to discounted fee for service to reduce risk for physicians. Negotiated payment arrangements with hospitals can take any of the forms discussed in Chapter 6, such as payments based on diagnosis-related groups (DRGs), bundled charges for certain services, or discounts. Hence, no direct risk sharing with providers is involved.

Insurance companies (including Blue Cross and Blue Shield), independent investors, and hospital alliances own most PPOs. Other PPOs are owned by HMOs, and some are jointly sponsored by a hospital and physicians. Although HMOs have organizational mechanisms to assume corporate responsibility for cost containment and quality assessment, PPOs do not have such intrinsic controls (MacLeod 1995). PPOs also apply fewer restrictions to the care-seeking behavior of enrollees. In most instances, primary care gatekeeping is not employed. Prior authorization (retrospective UR) is generally employed only for hospitalization and high-cost outpatient procedures (Robinson 2002).

As a less stringent choice of managed care for both enrollees and providers, PPOs have enjoyed remarkable success. Figure 9–11 illustrates the growth in enrollments in PPO plans over time.

# Point-of-Service Plan

*Point-of-service plans* combine features of classic HMOs with some of the characteristics of patient choice found in PPOs. Hence, they are sometimes referred to as hybrid plans or open-ended HMOs. When first brought on the market, these plans had a two-pronged objective: (1) retain the benefits of tight utilization management found in HMOs but (2) offer an alternative to their unpopular feature of restricted choice. The features borrowed from HMOs were capitation or other risk-sharing payment arrangements with providers and the gatekeeping method of utilization control. The feature borrowed from PPOs was the patient's ability to choose a nonparticipating provider at the point (time) of receiving services, hence, the name "point of service." Of course, the enrollee had to pay extra for the privilege of using nonparticipating providers because these providers were paid their fee-for-service rates. POS plans grew in popularity soon after they first

Figure 9–11  Percent of Covered Employees Enrolled in PPO Plans (Selected Years).

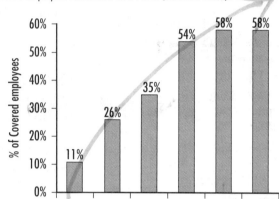

Source: Data from *Employer Health Benefits: 2002 Annual Survey; Employer Health Benefits: 2010 Annual Survey;* The Henry J. Kaiser Family Foundation and Health Research and Educational Trust.

emerged in 1988. Over time, as HMOs relaxed some of their utilization control practices and PPOs already offered a choice of providers, the need for a hybrid plan became less and less important to consumers. After reaching a peak in popularity in 1998 and 1999, enrollment in POS plans has continued to decline (Figure 9–12).

Figure 9–12  Percent of Covered Employees Enrolled in POS Plans (Selected Years).

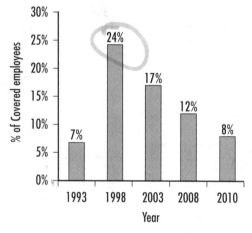

Source: Data from *Employer Health Benefits: 2002 Annual Survey; Employer Health Benefits: 2010 Annual Survey;* The Henry J. Kaiser Family Foundation and Health Research and Educational Trust.

# Trends in Managed Care

## Private Health Insurance Enrollment

Managed care has indeed become a mature industry in the United States. Within a decade, from 1996 to 2006, enrollment in employer-sponsored traditional fee-for-service insurance plans declined from 27 to 3% (Figure 9–13). By 2010, fee-for-service plans

Figure 9–13  Changes in Enrollment in Job-Based Health Plans, 1996 and 2006.

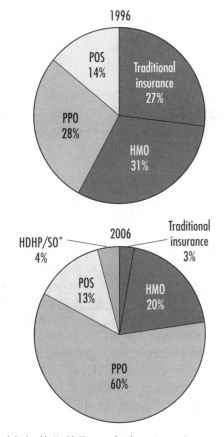

*High Deductible Health Plan paired with a savings options.
*Source:* Data from *Employer Health Benefits: 2002 Annual Survey;*
*Employer Health Benefits: 2006 Annual Survey;* The Henry J. Kaiser
Family Foundation and Health Research and Educational Trust.

were available to only 6% of workers, and only 1% enrolled in these plans (Claxton et al. 2010). Many employers offer their workers a choice of plans with level-dollar employer contribution, meaning workers pay more themselves—in premium contributions, deductibles, and copayments—if they choose a more expensive plan.

For employers, the cost of health insurance remains the biggest economic concern related to employee benefits. Managed care received wide acclaim in the 1990s for slowing the growth rate of health insurance premiums, a burden borne mostly by employers. As employers abandoned traditional insurance plans for managed care, the annual rate of increase in premiums dropped to 0.8% in 1996 (Kaiser/HRET 2002). Since then, the rate of increase did pick up but remained below the rate of general inflation until 1998. The rate of premium increases intensified from 1999 onward but has moderated in recent years (Figure 9–14). Between 2009 and 2010, premiums increased by 5% for single coverage and 3% for family coverage (Claxton et al. 2010). To cope with the rising premiums, employers are requiring increased cost sharing from covered employees. Another emerging strategy is to offer high-deductible health plans in conjunction with health savings accounts (discussed in Chapter 6).

## Medicaid Enrollment

Waivers under the Social Security Act, particularly sections 1115 and 1915(b), allowed states to enroll their Medicaid recipients in managed care plans. The Balanced Budget Act of 1997 gave states the authority to implement mandatory managed care programs without requiring federal waivers (Moscovice et al. 1998). Since then, enrollment of

Figure 9–14   Annual Percent Increase in US Health Insurance Premiums.

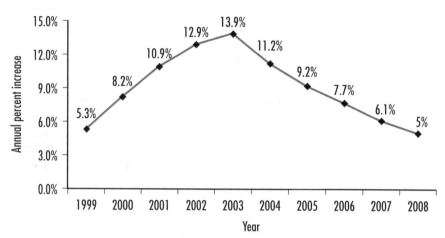

*Source:* Data from *Employer Health Benefits: 2006 Annual Survey*; *Employer Health Benefits: 2007 Annual Survey*; *Employer Health Benefits: 2008 Annual Survey*; The Henry J. Kaiser Family Foundation and Health Research and Educational Trust.

Medicaid beneficiaries into managed care programs has grown rapidly. Enrollment of Medicaid beneficiaries in managed care grew from 56% in 2000 to over 71% in 2009 (CMS 2009).

Some states have developed a different model of managing health care delivery, particularly in rural areas where managed care has not flourished. Medicaid *primary care case management* (PCCM) is a model that requires a Medicaid enrollee to choose a PCP, who is responsible for coordinating the enrollee's care and paid a monthly fee for doing so, on top of payment for providing medical services. In general, all medical services are reimbursed on a fee-for-service basis. Approximately 30 states are using the PCCM model (Cohen 2009).

## Medicare Enrollment

Under the provisions of the Tax Equity and Fiscal Responsibility Act (TEFRA) of 1982, Medicare beneficiaries have the option to enroll in managed care or remain in the traditional fee-for-service program. The legislation introduced a full-risk capitation reimbursement to include all covered services. Another program introduced was the Health Care Prepayment Plan (HCPP) for Part B services only. Under this program, MCOs are paid on a reasonable cost basis for outpatient and other services covered under Part B.

Medicare managed care contracts are commonly referred to as *risk contracts*, in which the MCO is liable for services regardless of their extent, expense, or degree, in exchange for a fixed capitated fee. As an incentive for MCOs to enroll Medicare beneficiaries, generous capitated rates were initially offered. Between 1996 and 2000, Medicare enrollment in managed care had increased from 4.7 million (12% of all beneficiaries) to 6.7 million (17% of all beneficiaries; Hoechst Marion Roussel 1998; Aventis Pharmaceuticals/SMG Marketing-Verispan LLC 2002). Then, in 1997, Congress passed the Balanced Budget Act, which created the Medicare+Choice program to keep managed care as an active player in the delivery of health care services, but the legislation also reduced payments to HMOs. As HMOs withdrew from the Medicare program, 800,000 beneficiaries lost their HMO coverage between 2000 and 2001 (Aventis Pharmaceuticals/SMG Marketing-Verispan LLC 2002). Enrollment in Medicare+Choice fell from 6.3 million in December 1999 to 5 million by February 2002, a decline of 21% (Thorpe and Atherly 2002).

In 2003, Medicare+Choice was renamed Medicare Advantage (MA) with the passage of the Medicare Prescription Drug, Improvement, and Modernization Act of 2003 (MMA 2003). The federal government added generous funding for MA plans as part of the new Part D program, and, once again, enrollment of Medicare beneficiaries in managed care plans was on the rise, albeit at a slow pace. MA plans are luring Medicare beneficiaries by offering richer benefits at lower costs and are moving into new markets (Fine 2005). While most Medicare beneficiaries enroll in the fee-for-service option, enrollment in MA plans increased from 5.3 million (13% of all beneficiaries) in 2003, when the MMA legislation was passed, to 11.1 million (24% of all beneficiaries) in 2010. The ACA of 2010 will gradually phase down payments to MA plans over time, which is expected to ultimately affect enrollment, premiums, and extra benefits (Gold et al. 2010).

## Impact on Cost, Access, and Quality

### Influence on Cost Containment

Managed care has been widely credited with slowing down the rate of growth in health care expenditures during the 1990s.

Between 1990 and 1998, hospitals in high managed care growth areas experienced revenue and cost growth rates 18 percentage points below hospitals in low managed care areas, but this cost containment effect reached a plateau after 1998 (Shen 2005). A backlash from both enrollees and providers prompted MCOs to back away from aggressive cost control measures. Hence, the full cost-containment potential of managed care was never realized. In the absence of other alternatives to deliver cost-effective medical services, both private and public insurance plans have increasingly moved their enrollees away from traditional fee-for-service plans to managed care so that managed care has become the dominant player in the health insurance marketplace. Hence, any further assessments of managed care's ongoing successes in cost containment have not been forthcoming. Future cost reductions may not be realized without tighter restrictions on utilization, particularly on the use of expensive new technology.

A number of HMOs include both conventional and complementary and alternative medicine (CAM) in their range of covered services. In one study, almost 14% of the enrollees reported using CAM therapies, such as acupuncture, naturopathy, massage, and chiropractic (Lafferty et al. 2006). Effective coordination of conventional medical services and CAM has the potential to save money, as well as improve quality. This is because, for some chronic problems, conventional medicine offers few proven benefits. Examples include psychosomatic ailments and cases in which patients have recurring complaints of unexplained painful symptoms or spells of dizziness. Such nagging complaints can rack up high costs and compromise an individual's quality of life. Lower cost therapies, such as stress management and meditation classes, can save numerous trips to physicians and costly diagnostic tests. In the study previously cited, the median expenditures were $39 for CAM care, compared to $74.40 for conventional outpatient care (Lafferty et al. 2006).

## Impact on Access

Managed care enrollees have good access to primary and preventive care. For example, Baker and colleagues (2004) found that timely breast cancer and cervical cancer screening was twice as likely for women receiving services in geographic areas with greater HMO market share, compared to women in areas with low managed care penetration. As people's ability to obtain health care improved between 2001 and 2003, health plan-related barriers that would have led some people to delay care or go without it declined significantly (Strunk and Cunningham 2004). It perhaps reflects relaxed utilization controls adopted by health plans in the years following the bashing of managed care.

On a larger scale, managed care's impact on access is not known. For instance, it is not clear to what extent during the 1990s managed care might have enabled small employers to offer employees health insurance coverage by holding down premium increases. Between 1996 and 2000, the proportion of employers offering health insurance benefits increased from 59 to 67% among firms employing between 3 and 199 workers, and the most notable increase was among the smallest firms employing between 3 and 9 workers (Kaiser/HRET 2002). However, this period also saw unprecedented economic growth that may have enabled more employers to add new benefits.

## Influence on Quality of Care

It is not surprising that quality varies across plans; however, overall quality of care in managed care plans has been found to be at least equivalent to that in traditional fee-for-service plans. Concerns about disparities in quality of care, based on race and socioeconomic status, are also largely unfounded (DeFrancesco 2002). On the other hand, there is evidence that quality of care may be lower in for-profit health plans, compared to nonprofit plans (Himmelstein et al. 1999; Schneider et al. 2005).

During the 1990s, concerns were raised that risk sharing between providers and payers would influence treatment decisions made by physicians, which would result in skimping on necessary services. However, evidence suggests that financial pressures do not lead to significant changes in physician behavior because, under capitation, a physician takes full responsibility for the patient's overall care (Eikel 2002). This is particularly true for life-saving treatment decisions, such as treatment of cancer patients (Bourjolly et al. 2004). On the other hand, there is some evidence that, in MCOs serving Medicaid patients under capitation, the enrollees may not receive certain services for which the PCPs do not get additional compensation, which may have some impact on quality of care (Quast et al. 2008).

Despite anecdotes, individual perceptions, and isolated stories propagated by the news media, no comprehensive research to date has clearly demonstrated that managed care's growth has been at the cost of quality in health care. Actually, available evidence points to the contrary. Quality of health care provided by MCOs has improved over time (Hofmann 2002). Early detection and treatment are more likely in a managed care plan than in a traditional fee-for-service plan (Riley et al. 1999). Higher managed care penetration was associated with increased quality in hospitals when such indicators as inappropriate utilization, wound infections, and iatrogenic complications were used to assess quality (Sari 2002). A more recent national study comparing quality of care in Medicare fee-for-service and MA plans showed that the level of quality, as evaluated by breast cancer screening, quality of diabetes care, and most other HEDIS measures, was significantly higher in MA plans (Brennan and Shepard 2010). There is further confirmation that, in terms of benefits and costs, being white or a member of a minority class makes no difference for Medicare enrollees regardless of whether they are enrolled in Medicare managed care or in the traditional fee-for-service program (Balsa et al. 2007).

A comprehensive review of the literature by Miller and Luft (2002) concluded that HMO and non-HMO plans provided roughly equal quality of care, as measured by a wide range of conditions, diseases, and interventions. At the same time, HMOs lower the use of hospitals and other expensive resources. Hence, managed care plans have been cost effective, while delivering levels of quality that are either comparable to or better than traditional insurance plans.

In the delivery of mental health, earlier reports suggested poorer outcomes in managed care plans (Rogers et al. 1993; Wells et al. 1989). However, more recent investigations conclude otherwise. Examining both qualitative and quantitative aspects of specialty managed outpatient mental health treatment, managed care was found to achieve cost savings but not at the expense of quality of care (Goldman et al. 2003).

# Managed Care Backlash, Regulation, and the Aftermath

The large-scale transition of health care delivery to the managed care system in the 1990s was met with widespread criticism, which turned into a backlash from consumers, physicians, and legislators. There were three main reasons behind the discontent, and widespread media reports further shaped unsympathetic public opinion toward managed care. (1) To restrain the spiraling costs of health insurance premiums, employers around the country switched to managed care by dropping, in many instances, traditional health insurance plans that offered choice of physicians and hospitals. A large number of employees experienced at least some loss of freedom and, to some extent, faced barriers to free access. (2) People did not see a reduction in their own share of the premium costs or a drop in their out-of-pocket expenses when they received health care. (3) In reaction to tight utilization management from MCOs, physicians became openly hostile toward managed care. In national surveys, managed care penetration was found to be negatively correlated with physicians' satisfaction (Landon et al. 2003). Much of this discontent arose from pressures to change the way physicians had traditionally practiced medicine with no accountability for appropriateness of utilization and costs. Physicians' vocal discontent no doubt also helped shape patients' views about managed care. Both physicians and patients perceived that managed care would drive a wedge between the patient–provider relationship. However, as the momentum continued to shift toward enrollment in managed care, physicians had little choice but to contract with managed care or lose patients; employees had little choice but to enroll in managed care plans, or personally bear significantly higher premium costs, or go without health insurance altogether. As this drama unfolded, employers largely remained passive, as their main objective of sharp reductions in premium costs was attained.

## Regulation of Managed Care

In response to widespread complaints and negative publicity against managed care, legislators across states were prompted to take action because the state governments are primarily responsible for overseeing issues pertaining to health insurance. Hence, states passed an extensive array of anti-managed care legislation. Between 1990 and 1999, states adopted more than 1,000 distinct regulatory provisions against managed care (Kronebusch et al. 2009). Congress passed the Newborns' and Mothers' Health Protection Act of 1996, although numerous states already had laws against "drive-through deliveries." The federal law prohibits a health plan to offer less than a 48-hour inpatient maternity coverage for a mother and her child following a normal vaginal delivery and less than a 96-hour coverage following a Caesarean section.

Most states have adopted legislation to limit financial incentives to physicians for curtailing utilization, to expand the rights of health care professionals, to promote continuity of care, and to give patients the right to an expeditious appeals process to review denial of services, including mandatory external reviews. States have also continued to mandate that certain benefits be included in the health plans. Some examples include chiropractic services, women's health screening, diabetic supplies, and obesity care. Increasingly, state legislation also includes provisions for insurer liability, which gives enrollees the right to seek civil remedy in the courts for negligent actions of health plans, including the denial of services (Hurley and Draper 2002). While managed care legislation provides both consumers and providers certain protections, it also has negative implications of increasing costs. Also, as a result of these laws, physicians with a high level of involvement in managed care reported lower levels of clinical autonomy, quality of clinical interactions, and ability to obtain services, compared to physicians with limited involvement in managed care (Kronebusch et al. 2009).

## The Aftermath

The backlash and antimanaged care laws seem to have produced their intended effects. MCOs have relaxed tight controls on utilization and have also taken significant steps to develop better relationships with physicians and other providers. Enthoven (2001) demonstrated that choice restriction was a main cause of the managed care consumer backlash. Satisfaction increases as employers offer more choices among plans. In response, employers have increasingly offered choices among HMO, PPO, POS plans, and, more recent, high-deductible health plans.

Managed care now stands at the crossroads of its past successes and future abilities to control mounting costs. As rising premiums increasingly shift the burden to employees, a greater differentiation among plans will again become necessary, and this differentiation, on a continuum of tight controls to more relaxed management, will have to be reflected in the level of premiums. Employees can then evaluate for themselves each plan's benefits against its costs and make choices that best suit their individual needs.

## Consolidation, Expansion, Diversification, and Integration

Consolidation, diversification, and other forms of organizational integration have occurred in response to cost pressures, development of new alternatives for the delivery of health care, concentration of power on the demand side because of managed care's growth, and the need to more efficiently provide services to populations spread over large geographic areas. Even the Centers for Medicare and Medicaid Services (CMS) recently promoted organizational collaboration for achieving coordinated care (Gregory 2010).

Consolidation, expansion, diversification, and integration are different types of growth strategies used by health services organizations. Although, in previous discussions, these terms have been used rather loosely, they do carry specific meanings. *Consolidation* refers to a concentration of control by a few organizations over other organizations through a consolidation of existing facility assets. Acquisitions, mergers, alliances, and the formation of contractual networks are examples of consolidation. *Expansion* is another growth strategy in which an organization adds new services or services similar to those it has offered before, but there is one difference. Whereas consolidation is achieved through the integration of existing facilities, expansion involves the building of new facilities. Examples include expansion of a nursing home by adding more beds, a multifacility corporation building new facilities to expand into new markets, and a hospital adding a women's health center to its existing services. *Diversification* refers to addition of new services that the organization has not offered before. Diversification can be achieved through consolidation or expansion, but it can also be achieved without the two growth strategies. For example, a hospital may acquire an existing long-term care facility (diversification through consolidation). As a second option, the hospital may diversify into long-term care by converting an unused acute care wing into a long-term care facility (diversification not involving consolidation or expansion but the use of existing idle resources). As a third option, the hospital may build a long-term care facility (diversification through expansion). In each instance, the hospital has realized its strategy of diversification through different means. The term *integration*—more specific, organizational integration—is commonly used as a catch-all expression that may refer to certain consolidations, expansions, or diversifications that involve new products or services. In other words, integration can be achieved via any of these strategies. The ultimate aim of integration is to provide a seamless array of services around a hospital, which functions as the central core. Such an organization would be a veritable health system capable of fulfilling most of a community's health care needs. The highly integrated Kaiser-Permanente model, which has been in use in California since the 1940s, for example, has been known for its cost-effective care with high quality services to its enrollees. This model has started to influence the mindsets and policy development within many European health care systems (Strandberg-Larsen et al. 2007).

# Integrated Delivery Systems

An *integrated delivery system* (IDS) may be defined as a network of organizations that provides or arranges to provide a coordinated continuum of services to a defined population and is willing to be held clinically and fiscally accountable for the outcomes and health status of the population serviced (Shortell et al. 1993). An IDS represents various forms of ownership and other strategic linkages among hospitals, physicians, and insurers. Its objective is to achieve greater integration of health care services along a continuum of care (Shortell and Hull 1996).

Managed care market domination prompted providers to integrate for three main reasons: (1) For MCOs, it is more cost effective to contract with organizations that offer comprehensive services to ensure a full spectrum of services to the MCO's enrollees. Various integrated systems developed so as not to be left out of the expanding managed care market. (2) Managed care also seeks providers who can render services in a cost-efficient manner and who will take responsibility for the quality of those services. Providers seek greater efficiencies by joining with other organizations or by diversifying into providing new services. Large organizations are in a better position to acquire up-to-date management and information systems to monitor their operations and successfully address inefficiencies. (3) Hospitals, physicians, and other providers have been concerned with protecting their autonomy. They found the growing power of managed care invading their turf when they were isolated. By forging linkages, they have strengthened their bargaining power in dealing with MCOs.

Merging with an MCO gives providers the best of both worlds. They can have a say in how the MCO is run and get referrals of patients who are enrollees of the MCO.

Integration adds complexity to an organization's size and management. It can also present obstacles for customers. Many frail and sick people may find it difficult to navigate a large and complicated delivery system. Many of these systems have also failed to live up to their potential to deliver cost-efficient care, and many have experienced significant financial distress (Nader and Walston 2005). For various reasons, the number of IDSs dropped substantially from 574 in 2001 to 453 in 2009. Besides physicians and hospitals, specialized facilities, such as freestanding outpatient surgery centers and diagnostic imaging centers, have been affiliating with IDSs (Sanofi-Aventis 2010b).

# Accountable Care Organizations

In the ongoing pursuit for cost effectiveness and quality, recent emphasis seems to have shifted from IDSs to accountable care organizations. In a general sense, an *accountable care organization* (ACO) describes an integrated group of providers who are willing and able to take responsibility for improving the overall health status, care efficiency, and satisfaction with care for a defined population (DeVore and Champion 2011). The ACO concept evolved from CMS's demonstration projects involving hospitals and physician group practices between 2005 and 2010. In May 2010, an Accountable Care Implementation Collaborative, involving 25 health systems, embarked on a project to develop the key capabilities needed to operate an ACO (DeVore and Champion 2011).

It is conceivable that other collaborative models involving various provider organizations, such as IPAs, multispecialty group practices, and affiliations between hospitals and physicians, could emerge (Goldsmith 2011). The ACA of 2010 authorized the Medicare program to establish care delivery and payment methods involving ACOs, beginning in 2012. However, little is known as to how these arrangements might or might not take shape. For example, many regions of the country have few IDSs, multispecialty group practices, and other clinically integrated entities. Furthermore, the lack of operational experience with ACOs makes the task a particularly complicated one (Lieberman and Bertko 2011). In the longer term, it also remains unclear how such organizations might survive in an environment of increasing government control over both clinical practice and reimbursement.

## Types of Integration

### Integration Based on Major Participants

From the standpoint of integration, the major participants in the health care delivery system have been physicians and hospitals. However, other clinical and nonclinical entities, such as specialized care providers, have joined the integration movement. In the past, several different types of configurations emerged. However, success of these models has been spotty. Lack of experience, misplaced administrative controls, misaligned financial incentives, and unfavorable economic trends have been some of the reasons many of these models failed to gain momentum. A few—namely, management services organizations and physician–hospital

organizations—have survived, but their long-term viability in a rapidly changing health care environment is less than certain.

During the dominant phase of MCOs in the 1980s and early 1990s, physicians recognized that they needed management expertise to survive in the complex health care environment. In recognition of this need, management services organizations (MSOs) emerged to supply management expertise, administrative tools, and information technology to physician group practices. MSO services are still needed, especially by smaller group practices, because they find it uneconomical to employ full-time managers.

A risk-bearing entity that incorporated the insurance function into integrated clinical delivery—referred to as a provider-sponsored organization (PSO)—emerged in the 1990s. PSOs are sponsored by physicians, hospitals, or jointly by physicians and hospitals to compete with regular MCOs by agreeing to provide health care to a defined group of enrollees under capitation. They bypass MCOs by contracting directly with employers and public insurers. When formed jointly by physicians and hospitals, PSOs do not differ much from a physician–hospital organization (PHO). PSOs gained national attention in 1996 when Congress proposed that PSOs could legitimately participate in Medicare risk contracts. Then, the Balanced Budget Act of 1997 opened up the Medicare market to PSOs as an option to HMOs under the Medicare+Choice program. At first, PSOs had been left largely unregulated. Later, the Balanced Budget Act required these entities to carry adequate coverage for risk protection. The initial appeal of PSOs was that they would deal with patients directly rather than through contracted arrangements as an HMO normally would do. However, after they suffered financial losses, PSOs failed in large numbers. In many instances, larger HMOs acquired PSOs. One major reason for PSO failures has been their lack of experience with risk management (the insurance function).

A PHO is a legal entity that forms an alliance between a hospital and local physicians. Apart from contracting with MCOs, if a PHO is large enough, it can also contract its services directly to employers, while engaging a third-party administrator to process claims. The main attraction for physicians to join PHOs was to reap the benefits of integration, while preserving their autonomy. Between 1998 and 2000, the number of hospitals associated with PHOs more than doubled. However, the number of these organizations has steadily declined since. Many failed because of poor management, undercapitalization, and federal antitrust scrutiny. Industry trends, along with rising costs and increased demand for services, continue to affect the manner in which hospitals and physicians compete or align (Sanderson et al. 2008). Hospitals seem to be in the driver's seat as physicians increasingly turn to hospitals for financial support. According to the American Hospital Association (AHA), since 2008, 74% of the hospitals have experienced an increase in physicians seeking hospital employment, and 36% have experienced an increase in the number of physicians seeking to sell their practices (Health Forum 2010).

## Integration Based on Degree of Ownership

Organizational consolidation or expansion can take various forms, as illustrated in Figure 9–15. Ownership involves the purchase of a controlling interest in another company, which can be accomplished through a merger or acquisition. Ownership does not have to be an all-or-nothing deal. Joint ventures allow two or more entities to participate in joint ownership of a new entity. A third approach, which can take various forms, does not involve ownership of another company's assets. In principle, it may simply involve cooperative arrangements and joint responsibilities. There may just be sharing of existing resources among two or more organizations or formation of an organization based on contracts.

## Mergers and Acquisitions

Mergers and acquisitions involve integration of existing assets. *Acquisition* refers to the purchase of one organization by another. The acquired company ceases to exist as a separate entity and is absorbed into the purchasing corporation. A *merger* involves a mutual agreement to unify two or more organizations into a single entity. The separate assets of two organizations combine, typically under a new name. Both entities cease to exist, and a new corporation forms. A merger requires the willingness of all parties, after they have assessed the advantages and disadvantages of merging their organizations.

Small hospitals may merge to gain efficiencies by eliminating duplication of services. A large hospital may acquire smaller hospitals to serve as satellites in a major metropolitan area with sprawling suburbs. A regional health care system may form after a large hospital has acquired smaller hospitals and certain providers of long-term care, outpatient care, and rehabilitation to diversify its services. Multifacility nursing home chains and home health firms often acquire other facilities to enter new geographic markets.

Figure 9–15  Organizational Integration Strategies.

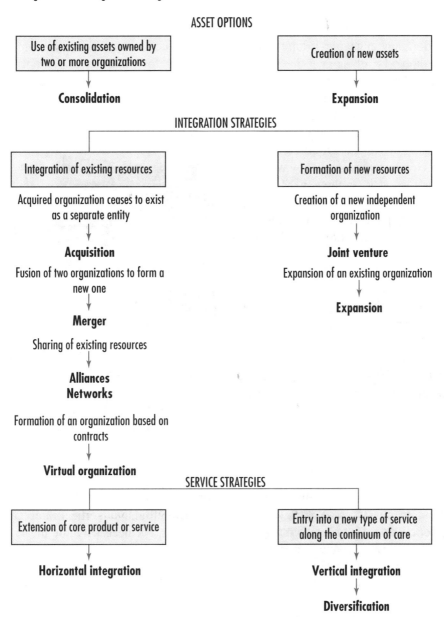

## Joint Ventures

A *joint venture* results when two or more institutions share resources to create a new organization to pursue a common purpose (Pelfrey and Theisen 1989). Each partner in a joint venture continues to conduct business independently. The new company created by the partners also remains independent. Joint ventures are often used to diversify when the new service can benefit all the partners and when competing against each other for that service would be undesirable. Hospitals in a given region may engage in a joint venture to form a home health agency that benefits all partners. An acute care hospital, a multi-specialty physician group practice, a skilled nursing facility, and an insurer may join to offer a managed care plan (Carson et al. 1995). Each participant would continue to operate its own business, and they would all have a common stake in the new MCO.

## Alliances — *Sharing, no joint resources ownership*

In one respect, the health care industry is unique because organizations often develop cooperative arrangements with rival providers. Cooperation instead of competition, in some situations, eliminates duplication of services while ensuring that all the health needs of the community are fulfilled (Carson et al. 1995). An *alliance* is an agreement between two organizations to share their resources without joint ownership of assets. A PHO, for example, can form through a merger, a joint venture, or an alliance. Each type of integration determines the extent to which the hospital controls the assets owned by the physicians.

The main advantages of alliances are (1) They are relatively simple to form. (2) They provide the opportunity to evaluate financial and legal ramifications before a potential "marriage" takes place. Forming an alliance gives organizations the opportunity to evaluate the advantages of an eventual merger. (3) Alliances require little financial commitment and can be easily dissolved, similar to an engagement prior to a marriage.

## Networks

A network is formed through alliances with numerous providers. It is built around a core organization, such as an MCO. Although networks are often sponsored by an MCO, hospitals, physicians, and other organizations, such as an IPA, may form networks. A PHO, for example, may simply be a network, or it may result from a joint venture, a merger, or an acquisition.

## Virtual Organizations

Alliances and networks often involve resource-sharing arrangements between organizations. However, when contractual arrangements between organizations form a new organization, it is referred to as a virtual organization or organization without walls. The formation of networks based on contractual arrangements is called *virtual integration*. IPAs are prime examples of virtual organizations. A PHO may also be a virtual organization. The main advantage of virtual organizations is that they require less capital to enter new geographic or service markets (Gabel 1997). They also help bring together scattered entities under one mutually cooperative arrangement.

## Integration Based on Service Consolidation

Horizontal and/or vertical integration is almost always necessary for the creation of a continuum of integrated services. Of the two strategies, only vertical integration results in diversification (see Figure 9–15).

## Horizontal Integration

*Horizontal integration* is a growth strategy in which a health care delivery organization extends its core product or service. Commonly, the services are similar or may be substitutes for existing services. Horizontal integration may be achieved through internal development, acquisition, or merger. Horizontally linked organizations may be closely coupled through ownership consolidation or loosely coupled through alliances. The main objective of horizontal integration is to control the geographic distribution of a certain type of health care service. Multihospital chains, nursing facility chains, or a chain of drugstores, all under the same management, with member facilities offering the same core services or products, are horizontally integrated. Diversification into new products and/or services is not achieved through horizontal integration.

## Vertical Integration

*Vertical integration* links services at different stages in the production process of health care—for example, organization of preventive services, primary care, acute care, and postacute service delivery around a hospital. The main objective of vertical integration is to increase the comprehensiveness and continuity of care across a continuum of health care services. Hence, vertical integration is a diversification strategy.

Vertical integration may be achieved through ownership consolidation, expansion into new services, joint ventures, or alliances. Formation of networks and virtual organizations can also involve vertical integration. Large hospital systems are particularly attracted to group practices in the interest of vertical integration because group practices can give them a large slice of the patient market. In essence, this kind of integration extends a hospital's control over the delivery of health services to the outpatient setting (Goldfarb 1993). Vertically integrated regional health systems may be the best-positioned organizations to become the providers of choice for managed care or for direct contracting with self-insured employers (Brown 1996).

# Pros and Cons of Integration
## Economies of Scale

In terms of efficiency and the overall effectiveness of the health care delivery system, integration has been a positive development. Fragmentation is often inefficient. Successfully integrated organizations find cost-control opportunities and an increased ability to reach a larger population with their range of services. These organizations are able to transition patients smoothly from their inpatient facilities to less costly outpatient and long-term care settings. Many of these systems also collaborate with independent facilities or other integrated systems to broaden the geographic reach and scope of medical services (Survey identifies top IHNs 2004). Highly integrated systems that include a hospital, a physician component, and at least one systemwide contract with a payer have been on the rise. The number of such highly integrated systems in the United States grew to 329 in 2009 from 325 the year before, the highest such total since 2005 when there were 331 highly integrated systems. The number of hospitals that were part of a highly integrated system increased by almost 7% in 2009. These hospitals enjoy higher occupancy rates and incur lower average length of stay, compared to nonsystem hospitals. The number of medical group practices belonging to systems has grown by 22.4% since 2003 (Sanofi-Aventis 2010b).

## Competition and Antitrust

A side effect of integration is limitation of choice for physicians and patients. Some concern exists that the wave of integration activity may produce a few dominant companies that can squeeze out competition. Erosion of competition can compromise consumer access to affordable quality care (Alpha Center 1997).

Laws have been designed, however, as a check against anticompetitive behavior. If an IDS is formed primarily to stifle competition, it may be found in violation of antitrust legislation (Kongstvedt and Plocher 1995). *Antitrust* policy consists of federal and state laws that make certain types of business practices illegal. The business practices prohibited or regulated by antitrust laws include price fixing, price discrimination, exclusive contracting arrangements, and mergers among competitors. The purpose of antitrust policy is to ensure the competitiveness and, thus, the efficiency of economic markets. Despite antitrust laws, however, large medical systems have come to dominate the health care landscape in some parts of the country, creating virtual monopolies, as smaller players have been bought out because of economic pressures.

### Role of Physicians

Physicians have resented the dominance of managed care and IDSs. Berenson (1997) cogently remarked that physicians are individualistic and strive for personal achievement. They resist management techniques that reduce their authority and autonomy. Physicians and their practice patterns are also the largest single determinant of the level of aggregate national health care expenditures (Sterns 2007). Hence, they must remain active players as new integrated models, such as ACOs, emerge. Physicians possess the knowledge necessary to make the system more efficient in its use of resources and more effective in producing desirable health outcomes (Zwanziger and Melnick 1996). For their part, physicians will have to reexamine their attitudes toward working in

organizational settings. In particular, physicians need to develop greater sensitivity to the cost of providing health care.

### Need for Up-to-Date Information Systems

The need for well-organized information systems (discussed in Chapter 5) presents a critical challenge to MCOs and IDSs. Well-designed information systems strengthen internal planning and quality control to enhance management and clinical functions. Information technology is also critical to providing timely and accurate information for external reporting. Typically, an MCO has to provide periodic reports to multiple external constituencies, which include the NCQA, government agencies, and employers. IDSs face particular challenges in integrating information systems across separate facilities that have become part of an integrated delivery network. Attention and spending in information technology are moving from hardware and software applications toward connectivity, networking, data architecture, and other labor-based services, requiring highly skilled personnel in the application of information technology.

### Summary

Managed care has evolved through an integration of the insurance function with the concepts of contract practice and prepaid group practice of the late 19th and early 20th centuries. Hallmarks of managed care are fixed premiums, risk sharing with providers, comprehensive services, emphasis on primary care, and utilization management. Over time, different managed care plans evolved, particularly to fill consumer desires for a greater choice of providers. Private employers have made almost a complete transition to managed care plans, and the government-sponsored Medicaid and Medicare programs have shown increased enrollments in managed care.

Evidence suggests that managed care has slowed the rate of growth in health care expenditures. Fears of lower quality have been largely unwarranted. Managed care suffered from negative public opinions, only some of which were justified. Legislation enacted to restrain abuses led to lower levels of physician autonomy, quality of clinical interactions, and ability to obtain services. Because of this backlash, managed care lost, at least to some degree, its potential to contain rising health care costs.

Managed care's growth is one force that has led to consolidation and diversification in the health care industry. Various types of integrated organizations emerged but were short lived. Integrated delivery organizations have been successful in realizing economies of scale. However, their widespread development is impractical in many geographic markets. Domination by a few large systems in some markets may also raise concerns about maintaining competition. Conversely, the Kaiser-Permanente model has been highly successful in California.

The Patient Protection and Affordable Care Act of 2010 requires Medicare to start utilizing accountable care organizations by 2012. The development of these organizations is at an experimental stage, and it is unclear how such organizations will evolve and to what extent they would survive in an environment of increasing government control over both clinical practice and reimbursement.

# Test Your Understanding

## Terminology

accountable care
  organization
acquisition
alliance
antitrust
carve out
case management
closed panel
concurrent utilization
  review
consolidation
discharge planning
disease management
diversification
exclusive provider plan
expansion
fee schedule

group model
HMO
horizontal integration
independent practice
  association
integrated delivery system
integration
IPA model
joint venture
medical loss ratio
merger
mixed model
MSO
network model
open panel
panel
PHO

point-of-service plan
PPO
practice profiling
primary care case
  management
prospective utilization
  review
PSO
retrospective utilization
  review
risk contract
staff model
utilization review
vertical integration
virtual integration

## Review Questions

1. What are some of the key differences between traditional health insurance and managed care?

2. Explain how the fee-for-service practice of medicine led to increased health care costs.

3. Despite increasing health care costs, why did the Health Maintenance Organization Act of 1973 fail to achieve its objectives?

4. What are the three main payment mechanisms managed care uses? In each mechanism, who bears the risk?

5. How are cost efficiencies achieved through (a) the integration of financing, insurance, delivery, and payment; (b) risk sharing with providers; and (c) care coordination?

6. What are some of the inefficiencies that have resulted from numerous health plans in the managed care system?

7. Discuss the concept of utilization monitoring and control.

8. What are the various mechanisms used by MCOs to monitor and control utilization? Briefly discuss each mechanism.

9. Describe the three utilization review methods, giving appropriate examples. Discuss the benefits of each type of utilization review.

10. How does case management achieve efficiencies in the delivery of health care?

11. How do case management and disease management differ?

12. What is an HMO? How does it differ from a PPO?

13. Briefly explain the four main models for organizing an HMO. Discuss the advantages and disadvantages of each model.

14. What is a point-of-service plan? Why did it grow in popularity? What caused its subsequent decline?

15. Why has managed care enrollment among Medicare beneficiaries remained relatively low, despite the creation of Medicare Advantage?

16. To what extent has managed care been successful in containing health care costs?

17. Has the quality of health care gone down as a result of managed care? Explain.

18. What is organizational integration? What is the purpose of integration in health care delivery? What are its drawbacks?

19. Explain how managed care has contributed to the development of integrated delivery systems.

20. Why have certain types of integration arrangements been short lived?

21. What is the difference between a merger and an acquisition? What is the purpose of these organizational consolidations? Give examples.

22. When would a joint venture be considered a preferable integration strategy?

23. What is the main advantage of two organizations forming an alliance?

24. State the main strategic objectives of horizontal and vertical integration.

25. What is antitrust policy? Which business practices does antitrust law prohibit? Why do antitrust laws exist?

## REFERENCES

Alpha Center. 1997. Hospital mergers reduce acute care beds but overcapacity remains an issue. *Health Care Financing and Organization Findings Brief,* June, 1.

Aventis Pharmaceuticals/SMG Marketing-Verispan LLC. 2002. *Managed care digest series: HMO-PPO/Medicare-Medicaid digest.* Bridgewater, NJ: Aventis Pharmaceuticals.

Baker, L. et al. 2004. The effect of area HMO market share on cancer screening. *Health Services Research* 39, no. 6: 1751–1772.

Balsa, A. et al. 2007. Does managed health care reduce health care disparities between minorities and Whites? *Journal of Health Economics* 26, no. 1: 101–121.

Berenson, R.A. 1997. Beyond competition. *Health Affairs* 16, no. 2: 171–180.

Berk, M.L., and A.C. Monheit. 2001. The concentration of health expenditures revisited. *Health Affairs* 20, 2: 9–18.

Bourjolly, J.N. et al. 2004. The impact of managed health care in the United States on women with breast cancer and the providers who treat them. *Cancer Nursing* 27, no. 1: 45–54.

Brennan, N., and M. Shepard. 2010. Comparing quality of care in the Medicare program. *American Journal of Managed Care* 16, no. 11: 841–848.

Brown, M. 1996. Mergers, networking, and vertical integration: Managed care and investor-owned hospitals. *Health Care Management Review* 21, no. 1: 29–37.

Business Word Inc. 1996. Physicians and employers identify seven essentials of managed care. *Health Care Strategic Management* 14, no. 12: 4.

Capps, C., and D. Dranove. 2004. Hospital consolidation and negotiated PPO prices. *Health Affairs* 23, no. 2: 175–181.

Carson, K.D. et al. 1995. *Management of healthcare organizations.* Cincinnati, OH: South-Western College Publishing.

Centers for Medicare and Medicaid Services (CMS). 2009. National summary of Medicaid managed care programs and enrollment as of June 30, 2009. Available at: http://www.cms.gov/MedicaidDataSourcesGenInfo/downloads/09Trends.pdf. Accessed February 2011.

Claxton, G. et al. 2010. *Employer health benefits: 2010 Annual Survey.* Menlo Park, CA: Henry J. Kaiser Family Foundation and Chicago, IL: Health Research & Educational Trust.

Cohen, R.K. 2009. Medicaid primary care case management. OLR Research Report, May 26, 2009. Available at: http://www.cga.ct.gov/2009/rpt/2009-R-0216.htm. Accessed February 2011.

DeFrancesco, L.B. 2002. HMO enrollees experience fewer disparities than older insured populations. *Findings Brief: Health Care Financing & Organization* 5, no. 2: 1–2.

Deom, M. et al. 2010. What doctors think about the impact of managed care tools on quality of care, costs, autonomy, and relations with patients. *BMC Health Services Research* 10, no. 331: 2–8.

DeVore, S., and R.W. Champion. 2011. Driving population health through accountable care organizations. *Health Affairs* 30, no. 1: 41–50.

DoBias, M. 2008. Uneven results. *Modern Healthcare* 38, no. 40: 12.

Eikel, C.V. 2002. Fewer patient visits under capitation offset by improved quality of care: Study brings evidence to debate over physician payment methods. *Findings Brief: Health Care Financing & Organization* 5, no. 3: 1–2.

Enthoven, A.C. 2001. Consumer choice and the managed care backlash. *American Journal of Law & Medicine* 27, no. 1: 1–14.

Fine, A. 2005. Medicare managed care plans grow. *Managed Care Quarterly* 13, no. 4: 26–27.

Gabel, J. 1997. Ten ways HMOs have changed during the 1990s. *Health Affairs* 16, no. 3: 134–145.

Gabel, J.R. 1999. Job-based health insurance, 1977–1998: The accidental system under scrutiny. *Health Affairs* 18, no. 6: 62–74.

Ginsburg, P.B. 2005. Competition in health care: Its evolution over the past decade. *Health Affairs* 24, no. 6: 1512–1522.

Gold, M. et al. 2010. *Medicare Advantage 2010 data spotlight: Plan enrollment patterns and trends.* Menlo Park, CA: Henry J. Kaiser Family Foundation.

Goldfarb, B. 1993. Corporate health care mergers. *Medical World News* 34, no. 2: 26–34.

Goldman, W. et al. 2003. A four-year study of enhancing outpatient psychotherapy in managed care. *Psychiatric Services* 54, no. 1: 41–49.

Goldsmith, J. 2011. Accountable care organizations: The case for flexible partnerships between health plans and providers. *Health Affairs* 30, no. 1: 32–40.

Gregory, D.A. 2010. Integrate or disintegrate: Integrated delivery systems, a re-emerging trend. *MGMA Connexion* 10, no. 10: 40–43.

Health Forum. 2010. *AHA hospital statistics, 2009.* Chicago: Health Forum.

Health Insurance Association of America. 1991. *Source book of health insurance data.* Washington, DC: HIAA.

Henry J. Kaiser Family Foundation/Health Research and Educational Trust (Kaiser/HRET). 2002. *Employer health benefits: 2002 annual survey.* Menlo Park, CA: Kaiser Family Foundation.

Himmelstein, D. et al. 1999. Quality of care in investor-owned vs not-for-profit HMOs. *Journal of the American Medical Association* 282, no. 2: 159–163.

Hoechst Marion Roussel. 1998. *Managed care digest series: HMO-PPO/Medicare Medicaid digest.* Kansas City, MO: Hoechst Marion Roussel, Inc.

Hofmann, M.A. 2002. Quality of health care improving. *Business Insurance* 36, no. 38: 1–2.

Hurley, R.E., and D.A. Draper. 2002. Health plan responses to managed care regulation. *Managed Care Quarterly* 10, no. 4: 30–42.

Iglehart, J.K. 1994. The American health care system: Managed care. In: *The nation's health.* 4th ed. P.R. Lee and C.L. Estes, eds. Boston: Jones & Bartlett Publishers. pp. 231–237.

Kongstvedt, P.R. 1995a. Managing hospital utilization. In: *Essentials of managed health care.* P.R. Kongstvedt, ed. Gaithersburg, MD: Aspen Publishers, Inc. pp. 121–135.

Kongstvedt, P.R. 1995b. Managed health care. In: *Health care administration: Principles, practices, structure, and delivery.* 2nd ed. L.F. Wolper, ed. Gaithersburg, MD: Aspen Publishers, Inc. pp. 627–642.

Kongstvedt, P.R. 1995c. Use of data and reports in medical management. In: *Essentials of managed health care.* P.R. Kongstvedt, ed. Gaithersburg, MD: Aspen Publishers, Inc. pp. 173–181.

Kongstvedt, P.R., and D.W. Plocher. 1995. Integrated health care delivery systems. In: *Essentials of managed health care.* P.R. Kongstvedt, ed. Gaithersburg, MD: Aspen Publishers, Inc. pp. 35–49.

Kronebusch, K. et al. 2009. Managed care regulation in the states: The impact on physicians' practices and clinical autonomy. *Journal of Health Politics, Policy, and Law* 34, no. 2: 219–259.

Lafferty, W.E. et al. 2006. Insurance coverage and subsequent utilization of complementary and alternative medicine providers. *The American Journal of Managed Care* 12, no. 7: 397–404.

Landon, B.E. et al. 2003. Changes in career satisfaction among primary care and specialist physicians, 1997–2001. *Journal of the American Medical Association* 289, no. 4: 442–449.

Lieberman, S.M., and J.M. Bertko. 2011. Building regulatory and operational flexibility into accountable care organizations and "shared savings." *Health Affairs* 30, no. 1: 23–31.

MacColl, W.A. 1966. *Group practice and prepayment of medical care.* Washington, DC: Public Affairs Press.

Mackie, D.L., and D.K. Decker. 1981. *Group and IPA HMOs.* Gaithersburg, MD: Aspen Publishers, Inc.

MacLeod, G.K. 1995. An overview of managed health care. In: *Essentials of Managed Health Care.* P.R. Kongstvedt, ed. Gaithersburg, MD: Aspen Publishers, Inc. pp. 1–9.

MacLeod, G.K., and J.A. Prussin. 1973. The continuing evolution of health maintenance organizations. *New England Journal of Medicine* 288, no. 9: 439–443.

McGuire, J.P. 1994. The growth of managed care. *Health Care Financial Management* 48, no. 8: 10.

Mechanic, D. 1972. *Public expectations and health care.* New York: John Wiley & Sons.

Miller, R.H., and H.S. Luft. 1997. Does managed care lead to better or worse quality of care? *Health Affairs* 16, no. 5: 7–26.

Miller, R.H., and H.S. Luft. 2002. HMO plan performance update: An analysis of the literature, 1997–2001. *Health Affairs* 21, no. 4: 63–86.

Moscovice, I. et al. 1998. Expanding rural managed care: Enrollment patterns and prospectives. *Health Affairs* 17, no. 1: 172–179.

Nader, R., and S. Walston. 2005. Transfer pricing and integrated delivery systems: The effects of interdependence and risk. *Managed Care Quarterly* 13, no. 4: 1–8.

National Committee for Quality Assurance (NCQA). 2007. *What accreditation levels can a plan achieve?* Available at: http://web.ncqa.org/tabid/197/Default.aspx. Accessed March 2007.

Pelfrey, S., and B.A. Theisen. 1989. Joint venture in health care. *Journal of Nursing Administration* 19, no. 4: 39–42.

Public Health Service. 1995. *Health United States, 1994.* Washington, DC: Government Printing Office.

Quast, T. et al. 2008. Does the quality of care in Medicaid MCOs vary with the form of physician compensation? *Health Economics* 17, no. 4: 545–550.

Raffel, M.W. 1980. *The US health system: Origins and functions.* New York: John Wiley & Sons.

Rakich, J.S. et al. 1992. *Managing health services organizations.* 3rd ed. Baltimore, MD: Health Professions Press.

Reed, M. et al. 2003. Physicians and care management: More acceptance than you think. *Issue brief* [Center for the Study of Health System Change], January (60): 1–4.

Riley, G.F. et al. 1999. Stage at diagnosis and treatment patterns among older women with breast cancer. *Journal of the American Medical Association* 281: 720–726.

Rizzo, J.A. 2005. Are HMOs bad for health maintenance? *Health Economics* 14, no. 11: 1117–1131.

Robinson, J.C. 2002. Renewed emphasis on consumer cost sharing in health insurance benefit design. *Health Affairs Web Exclusives* 2002: W139–W154.

Rogers, W.H. et al. 1993. Outcomes for adult outpatients with depression under prepaid or fee-for-service care: Results from the Medical Outcomes Study. *Archives of General Psychiatry* 50, no. 7: 517–525.

Sanderson, B. et al. 2008. Physician integration is back—and more important than ever. *Healthcare Financial Management* 62, no. 12: 64–71.

Sanofi-Aventis. 2010a. *Managed care digest series, 2009: HMO-PPO Digest.* Bridgewater, NJ: Sanofi-Aventis US, LLC.

Sanofi-Aventis. 2010b. *Managed care digest series, 2009: Hospitals/Systems Digest.* Bridgewater, NJ: Sanofi-Aventis US, LLC.

Sari, N. 2002. Do competition and managed care improve quality? *Health Economics* 11, no. 7: 571–584.

Schneider, E.C. et al. 2005. Quality of care in for-profit and not-for-profit health plans enrolling Medicare beneficiaries. *American Journal of Medicine* 118, no. 12: 1392–1400.

Shen, Y. 2005. *Is managed care still an effective cost containment device?* The Freeman Spogli Institute for International Studies at Stanford University. Available at http://fsi.stanford.edu /events/is_managed_care_still_an_effective_cost_containment_device. Accessed May 2011.

Short, A.C. et al. 2003. Disease management: A leap of faith to lower-cost, higher-quality health care. *Issue Brief No. 69 (October 2003).* Washington, DC: Center for Studying Health System Change.

Shortell, S.M. et al. 1993. Creating organized delivery systems: The barriers and facilitators. *Hospital and Health Services Administration* 38, no. 4: 447–466.

Shortell, S.M., and K.E. Hull. 1996. The new organization of the health care delivery system. In: *Strategic choices for a changing health care system.* S.H. Altman and U.E. Reinhardt, eds. Chicago: Health Administration Press.

Sipkoff, M. 2003. Health plans begin to address chronic care management. *Managed Care Magazine.* Available at: http://www.managedcaremag.com/archives/0312/0312.kaiserchronic.html. Accessed February 2011.

Southwick, K. 1997. Case study: How United HealthCare and two contracting hospitals address cost and quality in era of hyper-competition. *Strategies for Healthcare Excellence* (COR Healthcare Resources) 10, no. 8 (August): 1–9.

Sterns, J.B. 2007. Quality, efficiency, and organizational structure. *Journal of Health Care Finance* 34, no. 1: 100–107.

Strandberg-Larsen, M. et al. 2007. Kaiser Permanente revisited—Can European health care systems learn? *Eurohealth* 13, no. 4: 24–26.

Strunk, B.C., and P.J. Cunningham. 2004. Trends in Americans' access to needed medical care, 2001–2003. Tracking Report No. 10 (August 2004). Washington, DC: Center for Studying Health System Change.

Survey identifies top IHNs, indicates stabilized growth. 2004. *Healthcare Financial Management* 58, no. 3: 25.

Thorpe, K.E., and A. Atherly. 2002. Medicare+Choice: Current role and near-term prospects. *Health Affairs Web Exclusives 2002:* W242–W252.

Wagner, E.R. 1995. Types of managed care organizations. In: *Essentials of managed health care.* P.R. Kongstvedt, ed. Gaithersburg, MD: Aspen Publishers, Inc. pp. 24–34.

Wells, K.B. et al. 1989. Detection of depressive disorder for patients receiving prepaid or fee-for-service care: Results from the Medical Outcomes Study. *Journal of the American Medical Association* 262, no. 23: 3298–3302.

Wilkerson, J.D. et al. 1997. The emerging competitive managed care marketplace. In: *Competitive managed care: The emerging health care system.* J.D. Wilkerson et al., eds. San Francisco: Jossey-Bass Publishers.

Williams, C.H. et al. 2006. How has hospital consolidation affected the price and quality of hospital care? *Policy Brief No. 9* (February 2006). Princeton, NJ: The Robert Wood Johnson Foundation.

Wilson, F.A., and D. Neuhauser. 1985. *Health services in the United States.* 2nd ed. Cambridge, MA: Ballinger Publishing Co.

Wojcik, J. 2011. Will broker pay change empower group health buyers? *Business Insurance* 45, no. 2: 1, 20.

Zelman, W.A. 1996. *The changing health care marketplace.* San Francisco: Jossey-Bass Publishers.

Zwanziger, J., and G.A. Melnick. 1996. Can managed care plans control health care costs? *Health Affairs* 15, no. 2: 185–199.

# Chapter 10

---

# Long-Term Care

## Learning Objectives

- To comprehend the concept of long-term care and its main features
- To get an overview of the main types of services encompassed in the delivery of long-term care
- To discover who needs long-term care and why
- To become familiar with the large variety of community-based long-term care services and who pays for these services
- To learn about the various types of long-term care institutions and the levels of services they provide
- To get an overview of specialized long-term care facilities
- To get acquainted with the main aspects of the nursing home industry and the patients it serves
- To learn about the main sources of nursing home financing

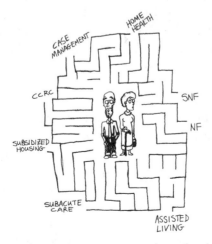

*"Now, honey, where are we supposed to go from here?"*

# Introduction

Long-term care (LTC) is often associated with care provided in nursing homes, but that is a rather narrow view of LTC. Several types of noninstitutional LTC services are provided in a variety of community-based settings. These services include informal care provided by family and surrogates, home health services brought into a person's own home, home-delivered meals, and personal assistance provided in residential settings, such as foster care homes and board-and-care facilities. Older Americans overwhelmingly show a strong desire to remain in their own homes. In one study, 73% of Americans aged 55 and older expected to always live in their current residences (Hoffman 2001). It should also be noted that LTC is not confined to the elderly, but the elderly are the predominant users of these services and most LTC services have been designed with the elderly patient in mind.

This chapter focuses on the elderly as the primary recipients of LTC, but this does not mean that most elderly people are in need of such care. To the contrary, most elderly people are physically and mentally healthy enough to function independently. In 2008, 91% of elderly Americans lived either alone (19%) or with a spouse (72%; Federal Interagency Forum on Aging-Related Statistics 2010). Based on a 3-year average from 2006 to 2008, 77% of adults aged 65 and over assessed their own health status as good to excellent (Figure 10–1), although self-assessed health status for blacks and Hispanics was lower than for whites. Also, health status declines with age because the aging process leads to chronic, degenerative conditions that resist cure. Services that enable people with chronic conditions to live independently for as long as possible are often those that emphasize assistance and care, rather than curing. However, the clients of LTC need a variety of health care services over time. Hence, LTC cannot be an isolated component of the health care delivery system. The LTC system must interface with the rest of the system to provide ease of transition among various types of health care settings and services.

Whereas medical care provided in hospitals is associated with acute episodes, LTC is associated with chronic conditions. Chronic conditions are the leading causes of illness, disability, and death in the United States. In order of their prevalence among the aged population, the most common chronic conditions are hypertension, arthritis, heart disease, cancers, and diabetes for both men and women (Federal Interagency Forum on Aging-Related Statistics 2010). Also common among the elderly are hearing and vision impairments, cognitive loss, and depressive symptoms. Both low cognitive functioning and depressive symptoms are associated with a high risk for functional decline (Mehta et al. 2002). Serious illness or injury can also lead to a rapid decline in a person's health and further limit a person's ability to do things for him- or herself.

It is estimated that one in five Americans has multiple chronic conditions, which increase with age. For example, 62% of Americans over the age of 65 have multiple chronic conditions (Vogeli et al. 2007). Disability and functional limitations rise dramatically among those who have multiple chronic conditions (Figure 10–2). As the elderly population in the United States continues to grow, between 2000 and 2020, the number of Americans with chronic conditions is projected to increase from 125 million (45% of the population) to 157 million (Figure 10–3).

Figure 10–1 Respondent-Assessed Health Status for Adults 65 Years and Over (Age Adjusted), 2005 (Percentage Distribution).

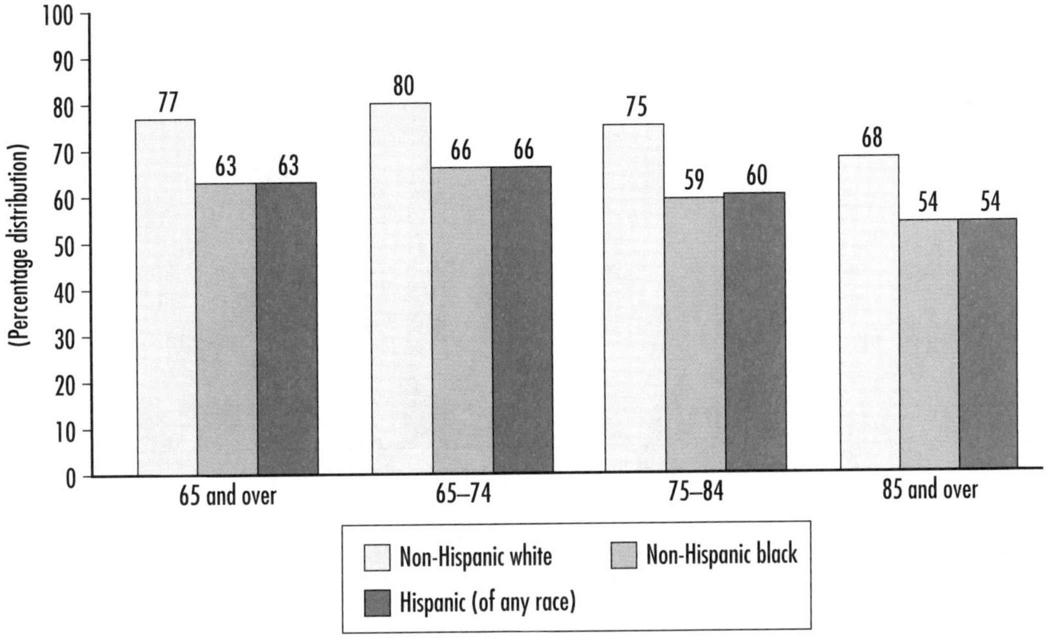

*Source:* Federal Interagency Forum on Aging-Related Statistics. 2010. *Older Americans 2010: Key indicators of well-being.* Washington, DC: US Government Printing Office.

The number of those with multiple chronic conditions will rise to 81 million (25% of the population) by 2020 (Anderson 2003). The number of people 70 years of age and older needing LTC will increase from 10 million in 2000 to 15 million in 2020 and to 21 million in 2030 (National Academy on an Aging Society 2000). However, health and disease trends among the younger population groups will determine the future need for LTC services.

The rest of the developed world also faces aging-related problems and challenges in providing adequate LTC services very similar to those in the United States.

Actually, the elderly population as a proportion of the total population in other developed countries, such as Japan, Germany, France, and Great Britain, is already higher than it is in the United States.

This chapter provides an overview of LTC, its main clients, various types of community-based and institution-based services, and how these services are financed. Both community-based and institution-based services form a continuum of services demanded by the varied needs of a heterogeneous population. Even the elderly, who are the predominant users of LTC services, are not a homogeneous group.

Figure 10–2  People with Multiple Chronic Conditions Are More Likely to Have Activity Limitations.

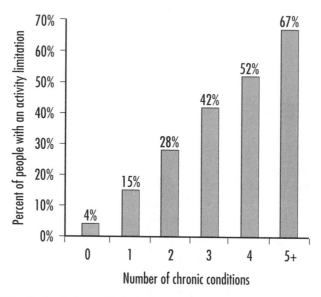

Source: Chronic Conditions: Making the Case for Ongoing Care, Partnership for Solutions, Johns Hopkins University, December 2002, p. 12.

Figure 10–3  The Number of People with Chronic Conditions.

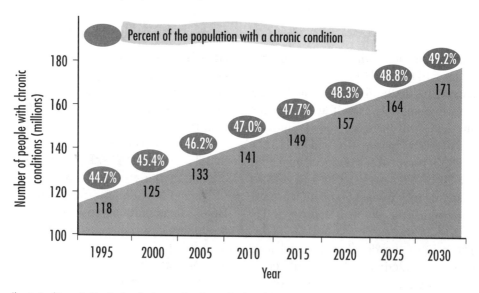

Source: Chronic Conditions: Making the Case for Ongoing Care, Partnership for Solutions, Johns Hopkins University, December 2002.

# The Nature of Long-Term Care

*Long-term care* can be defined as a variety of individualized, well-coordinated services that promote the maximum possible independence for people with functional limitations and are provided over an extended period of time in accordance with a holistic approach, while maximizing their quality of life. To the extent possible, the delivery of LTC should employ appropriate current technology and available evidence-based practices. The main dimensions of LTC delivery apply to both institutional and community-based LTC services.

## Variety of Services

A variety of services is necessary because individual needs, as determined by health status, finances, and other factors, vary greatly among people who require LTC services. Hence, LTC services should (1) fit the needs of different individuals, (2) address the changing needs over time, and (3) suit people's personal preferences.

## Individualized Services

LTC services are tailored to the needs of the individual patient. Those needs are determined by an assessment of the individual's current physical, mental, and emotional condition. Other factors used for this purpose include history of the patient's medical and psychosocial conditions; a social history of family relationships, former occupation, and leisure activities; and cultural factors, such as racial and ethnic background, language, and religious practices. Information obtained from a comprehensive assessment is used to develop an individualized plan of care that addresses each type of need through customized interventions.

## Well-Coordinated Total Care

LTC providers are responsible for managing the total health care needs of an individual client. *Total care* requires that any health care need is recognized, evaluated, and addressed by appropriate clinical professionals (Singh 2010). For example, a patient may need referral to a dentist, optometrist, podiatrist, or mental health professional or transferred to an acute care hospital. Hence, LTC must interface with non-LTC services (Figure 10–4).

Patients needing LTC often require coordination among many services because, as needs change over time, these patients may have to transition among different types of services. For most people, the myriad of LTC services, eligibility requirements, and financing can be overwhelming. Hence, *case management* is regarded as a key coordinating function in the LTC system. It refers to the process of matching client needs with available services that are likely to best address those needs regardless of whether they are obtained within the LTC sector or from the non-LTC sector.

## Promotion of Functional Independence

LTC becomes necessary when there is a remarkable decline in an individual's ability to independently perform certain common tasks of daily living. As a person ages, chronic ailments, comorbidity, disability, and dependency tend to follow each other. Dependency creates the need for LTC.

The goal of LTC is to enable the individual to maintain functional independence to the maximum level possible and practicable. For example, some people can continue to perform certain daily living tasks in spite of their disability by using adaptive devices,

Figure 10–4  Key Characteristics of a Well-Designed Long-Term Care System.

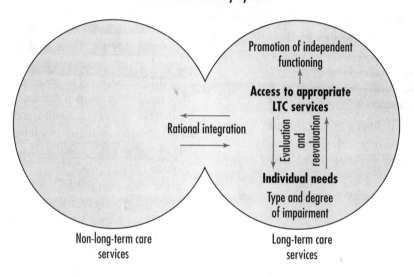

**Health care delivery system**

**KEY CHARACTERISTICS**

1. The LTC system is rationally integrated with the rest of the health care delivery system. This rational integration facilitates easy access to services between the two components of the health care delivery system.
2. Appropriate placement of the patient within the LTC system is based on an assessment of individual needs. For example, individual needs determine whether and when institutionalization may be necessary.
3. The LTC system accommodates changes in individual needs by providing access to appropriate LTC services as determined by a reevaluation of needs.
4. LTC services are designed to compensate for existing impairment and have the objective of promoting independence to the extent possible.

such as walkers and wheelchairs for mobility, adaptive utensils for eating, and portable oxygen devices for breathing. Caregiver assistance becomes necessary when a person is either unable or unwilling to perform daily living tasks. However, caregivers should concentrate on maintaining whatever ability to function a patient still has and on preventing further decline of that ability.

Indicators used to assess functional limitations include the activities of daily living (ADLs) scale and instrumental activities of daily living (IADLs; see Chapter 2 for a description of ADLs and IADLs). Other measures of physical, cognitive, and social functioning can also be included.

## Extended Period of Care

For most LTC clients, the delivery of various services extends over a relatively long period, because most recipients of care will at least require ongoing monitoring to note any deterioration in their health and to address any emerging needs. Certain types of services, such as rehabilitation therapies, postacute convalescence, or stabilization, may be needed for a relatively short duration, generally less than 90 days. The patient subsequently returns to independent living. On the other hand, the need for LTC may necessitate long-range confinement to a nursing care facility. For example, postacute medical complications may occur, leading to a rapid decline in a patient's health, or certain postacute conditions may remain unstable.

## Holistic Care

As discussed in Chapter 2, the holistic model of health proposes that a person's health care needs extend beyond the physical and mental domains; they emphasize well-being in every aspect of what makes a person whole and complete. In holistic care, a patient's physical, mental, social, and spiritual needs and preferences should be incorporated into medical care delivery.

## Quality of Life

A sense of satisfaction, fulfillment, and self-worth are regarded as critical patient outcomes in any health care delivery setting. They take added significance in LTC because (1) a loss of self-worth often accompanies disability and (2) patients remain in LTC settings for relatively long periods, with little hope of full recovery in most instances.

*Quality of life* is a multifaceted concept that recognizes at least five factors: lifestyle pursuits, living environment, clinical palliation, human factors, and personal choices.

- Lifestyle factors are associated with personal enrichment and making one's life meaningful through activities one enjoys. Many older people still enjoy pursuing their former leisure activities, such as woodworking, crocheting, knitting, gardening, and fishing. People also want to engage in spiritual pursuits or spend some time alone. Even those whose functioning has decreased to a vegetative or comatose state must be engaged in something that promotes sensory awakening through visual, auditory, olfactory, and tactile stimulation.

- The living environment must be comfortable, safe, and appealing to the senses. Cleanliness, décor, furnishings, and other aesthetic features are important.

- Clinical *palliation* should be available for relief from unpleasant symptoms, such as pain or nausea, for instance, when a patient is undergoing chemotherapy.

- Human factors refer to caregiver attitudes and practices that emphasize caring, compassion, respect, and preservation of human dignity for the patient. Institutionalized patients find it disconcerting to have lost their autonomy and independence. Quality of life is enhanced when patients residing in a long-term care facility, who are often referred to as residents, have some latitude to govern their own lives. Residents also desire an environment that gives them adequate privacy.

- Being able to make personal choices is important to most people. In nursing facilities, for example, food is often the primary area of discontentment, which can be addressed by offering a selection of menu choices. Also, the ability to set one's own schedule is important to most people. Many elderly resent being awakened early in the morning when caregivers begin their responsibilities to care for patients' hygiene, bathing, and grooming.

## Long-Term Care Services

The large variety of LTC services can include a combination of any of the following services:

- Medical care, nursing, and rehabilitation
- Mental health services
- Social support
- Preventive and therapeutic long-term care
- Informal and formal care
- Community-based and institutional services
- Housing
- End-of-life care

### Medical Care, Nursing, and Rehabilitation

These services focus on three main areas: (1) postacute continuity of care, (2) clinical management of chronic illness and comorbidity, and (3) restoration or maintenance of physical function. LTC generally becomes necessary after the treatment of an acute episode in a hospital. However, patients in LTC settings also encounter acute episodes, such as pneumonia, bone fracture, or stroke, and require admission to a general hospital. For the same medical conditions, the elderly are more prone to hospitalization, compared to younger age groups, who may be treated as outpatients. Hence, the overall utilization of acute care is higher among the elderly.

Nurses, rehabilitation therapists, nutritionists, and other professionals typically provide medical care in LTC settings under the direction of a physician. Preventing complications from chronic conditions (tertiary prevention) is an important aspect of LTC.

### Mental Health Services

It is erroneous to believe that mental disorders are a normal part of aging. Nevertheless, mental disorders affect approximately 20% of the elderly population (Rouse 1995). Hence, LTC patients often suffer from mental conditions, most notably anxiety disorders, depression, delirium, and dementia. Dementias are prevalent among 5% of the elderly population and have an unexplained predominance in women (Ritchie and Lovestone 2002). Psychiatric symptoms and cognitive decline are particularly common among nursing home residents (Scocco et al. 2006). Mental disorders range in severity from problematic to disabling to fatal. Yet, major barriers must be overcome in the delivery of mental health care. In general, assessing psychiatric illness in geriatric patients can be difficult, especially since medical comorbidity may obscure the diagnosis. For example, the patient with multiple chronic illnesses can often have symptoms of either dementia or depression attributed to the primary medical condition rather than to an underlying psychiatric illness (Tune 2001). Hence, elderly people with mental disorders are less likely than younger adults to receive correct diagnosis and needed mental health care.

### Social Support

LTC clients need social and emotional support to help cope with changing life events that may cause stress, frustration, anger, fear, grief, or other emotional imbalances. Adaptation to new surroundings and new people is often necessary. Social support is also needed when problems and issues arise in the interactions among people within social systems. For example, conflicts may arise between what a patient wants for himself or herself and what the family may think is best for the patient. Conflicts also arise between patients and caregivers. Social services are also necessary to facilitate the coordination of total care needs. Examples include transportation services, information, counseling, recreation, and spiritual support. LTC facilities should also establish linkages with the community through a variety of volunteer programs in which community members can participate. Remaining connected with the community and the outside world is an important aspect of social support for many people.

## Preventive and Therapeutic Long-Term Care

One important question pertaining to LTC is how to best prevent and postpone disease and disability and maintain the health, independence, and mobility of an aging population (Satariano 1997). The primary goal is to prevent or delay institutionalization in LTC facilities. Preventive measures call for ensuring that the elderly receive good nutrition and have access to services, such as vaccinations, flu shots, and routine medical care.

Certain community-based social support programs also serve a preventive function. Programs, such as homemaker, chore, and handyman services, can assist with a variety of tasks that older adults may no longer be able to perform. Examples are shopping,

light cleaning, general errands, lawn maintenance, and minor home repairs.

In the initial stages of institutionalization, an emphasis on restorative therapies may be important. For example, after orthopedic surgery or an episode of cardiovascular accident (CVA—stroke), a patient would need rehabilitation therapies. The objective is to curtail the need for long-range institutionalization and to return the patient to the community as soon as possible. Short-term or intermittent LTC services, such as home health care, may still be needed to enable the person to live independently.

## Informal and Formal Care

Contrary to popular belief, most LTC services in the United States are provided informally by family and friends. Informal services are not reimbursed. It is estimated that 92% of community-dwelling residents receive unpaid help, but the extent and nature of these services remains undocumented (Kaye et al. 2010). Family members also play an important role in managing the often critical transitions between settings of care delivery, such as between hospital and nursing home (Levine et al. 2010). Donated care is also the largest source of financing LTC (Holtz-Eakin 2005). Men, minorities, married individuals, and those with less education are more likely to receive care from family and friends and are less likely to receive care in a nursing facility (Alecxih 2001). Adult children and spouses constitute roughly 70% of the caregivers (National Academy on an Aging Society 2000).

Informal care reduces the use of formal home health care and delays nursing home entry (Van Houtven and Norton 2004). Older people who have close access to family or surrogates (neighbors, friends, and church or other community organizations) often continue to live in the community much longer than those who do not have such support. In a population of disabled elderly people, an insufficient informal care level is associated with overall discontinuation of living at home, all-cause mortality, hospitalization, and institutionalization (Kuzuya et al. 2011).

However, the pool of informal caregivers, in relation to the growing elderly population needing LTC, is going to shrink rather dramatically in the future. Various reports suggest that the number of older people who are divorced, unmarried, or without children has been on the rise.

Family caregivers often experience a range of physical, emotional, social, and financial problems. Negative feelings, such as anger, dissatisfaction, guilt, frustration, tension, and family conflict, are some common issues these caregivers face. In general, these caregivers have poorer health and quality of life than noncaregivers (Broe and Jorm 1999; Schofield et al. 1998). Under these circumstances, caregivers experience stress and burnout. *Respite care* is the most frequently suggested intervention to address family caregivers' feelings of stress and burden. The objective is to provide relief or assistance to caregivers for limited periods to allow them some free time without neglecting the patient. Respite care can include any kind of LTC service, such as adult day care (ADC), home health care, or temporary institutionalization.

## Community-Based and Institutional Services

For those who do not have adequate means of informal support, the availability of community-based services provided by formal agencies becomes an important factor in living independently. Services are brought to the patient's home or delivered in a community-based location. Most people have a strong preference for receiving LTC services at home rather than in an institution, which is viewed as an avenue of last resort. Figure 10–5 illustrates various types of community-based services, as well as different types of LTC institutions, which are further discussed in this chapter.

Institutionalization becomes necessary when ADL impairments become high or behavioral problems develop as a result of cognitive impairment (McFall and Miller 1992). Compared to the elderly who can live in the community on their own or with assistance from informal or formal sources of LTC, those in need of institutionalization are more often frail, vulnerable, terminally ill, or functionally and/or cognitively impaired. These individuals are likely to remain in a nursing facility for a long time, perhaps indefinitely. The main objective of LTC in these situations is to manage chronic functional disability in three specific areas. The facility must (1) provide professional help for ADL functions that the patient cannot perform, (2) implement measures to prevent further degeneration of remaining function, and (3) coordinate services with non-LTC providers to address the patient's total care needs.

Most care in LTC institutions is provided by nonphysician staff, such as nurses, nursing assistants, dietitians, social workers, and therapists. Personnel who provide basic ADL services and/or assist licensed and professional staff are technically referred to as *paraprofessionals*. Examples of paraprofessionals are certified nursing assistants and therapy aides.

Figure 10–5 Interlinkages Between Services for Those in Need of Long-Term Care.

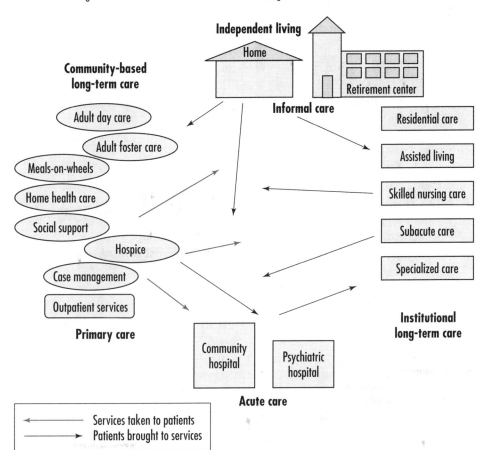

*Source:* Adapted with permission from D.A. Singh, *Nursing Home Administrators: Their Influence on Quality of Care,* p. 15, © 1997, Garland Publishing, Inc.

Residents have the right to be treated by a physician of their choice, who should make regular rounds to visit the patients. Between rounds, the professional nursing staff should communicate with the physician, especially when changes in a patient's condition are noticed or treatment orders are not producing the desired results. A transfer agreement with a local hospital must be in place to facilitate transition between the acute care and LTC facilities. At the onset of an acute episode, such as pneumonia or severe injury from a fall, the patient is hospitalized.

## Housing

Housing is a key social aspect of LTC because health and housing concerns of the elderly and disabled are often interrelated. The physical features of housing affect the ability of frail older people and young disabled individuals to care for themselves and maintain their independence. Congregate housing—multiunit housing with support services—is an option for seniors and disabled adults who do not want to live alone. Congregate housing combines privacy and companionship by offering each resident a private bedroom or apartment and shared living space. Support services may include meals, transportation, housekeeping, building security, and social activities.

Section 202 of the National Affordable Housing Act of 1990 is administered by the Department of Housing and Urban Development (HUD). The program provides federal funds to construct supportive housing designed specifically for the low-income elderly. The program also provides rent subsidies to make such housing affordable.

## End-of-Life Care

Dealing with death and dying is very much a part of LTC. End-of-life care deals with preventing needless pain and distress for terminally ill patients and their families. High emphasis is placed on patient dignity and comfort.

Roughly three-fourths of all deaths occur at 65 years of age or older. Among the elderly, 28% of all deaths are related to heart disease and 22% are related to cancer (Department of Health and Human Services [DHHS] 2010). Other diseases often fatal to the elderly are stroke, chronic lower respiratory disease, Alzheimer's disease, diabetes, pneumonia, and influenza. Care professionals seem to be well-positioned to provide end-of-life care in some LTC settings. In others, terminal patients are referred to a hospice service (see Chapter 7). Regardless of the LTC setting, patients who suffer pain or dyspnea are more likely to be referred to a hospice service (Munn et al. 2006).

## The Clients of Long-Term Care

Almost 13 million Americans need formal LTC services (Kaye et al. 2010). According to the Administration on Aging of the US Department of Health and Human Services, 40% of LTC clients are between the ages of 18 and 64.

LTC clients can be classified into four main categories:

* Older adults
* Children and adolescents
* Young adults
* People with HIV/AIDS

## Older Adults

At the beginning of the 20th century, persons 65 years of age and older constituted just 4% of the population in the United States and numbered 3.1 million. In 2008, the elderly population totaled 39 million, or 12.8% of the population (DHHS 2010). For some time now, the over-85 age group, referred to as the "oldest old," has been the most rapidly growing sector of the US population. Between 2000 and 2008, it grew at an average annual rate of over 3.8%, compared to less than 1% for the entire population. By 2030, when all of the "baby boom generation" will have reached retirement age, the elderly are expected to constitute over 19% of the population, 12% of whom would be 85 years of age and older, according to 2008 projections by the US Census Bureau (Figure 10–6).

Figure 10–7 provides data on activity limitations among the elderly. Although 67% of the elderly had no activity limitations in 2006, with advancing age, chronic ailments, comorbidity, disability, and dependency for

Figure 10–6  Growth of Older Population According to Age Groups.

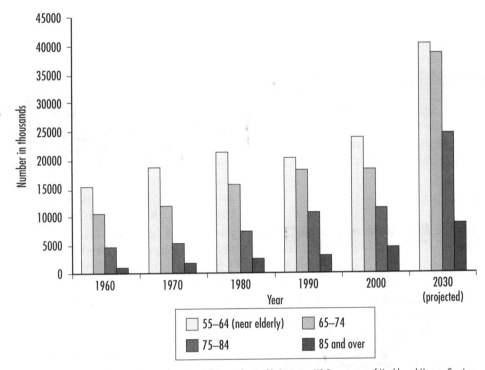

*Source:* Data from *Health, United States, 2002,* p. 79. National Center for Health Statistics, US Department of Health and Human Services. National Population Projections released in 2008 by the US Census Bureau.

Figure 10–7  Activity Limitations Among Medicare Beneficiaries (Percent Distribution), 2006.

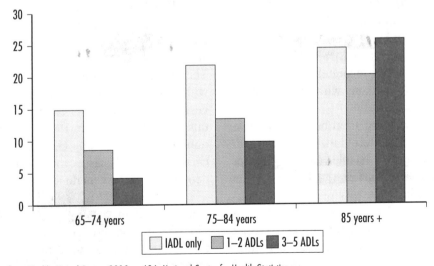

*Source:* Data from *Health, United States, 2010,* p. 406, National Center for Health Statistics.

common daily functions can follow each other, increasing the likelihood that an elderly person would need LTC services. The demographic trends have serious implications for the financing and delivery of LTC services. It is widely believed that a growing elderly population will put severe financial strains on a shrinking cohort of working taxpayers. Elderly in the lowest socioeconomic status are at the greatest risk of need for LTC and are the least able to pay for such services.

## Children and Adolescents

In children, functional impairments are often birth related, such as brain damage, which can occur before or during childbirth. Examples of birth-related disorders include cerebral palsy, autism, spina bifida, and epilepsy. These children grow up with physical disability and need help with ADLs. The term *developmental disability* describes the general physical incapacity such children may face at a very early age. Those who acquire such dysfunctions are referred to as developmentally disabled, or DD for short. *Mental retardation* (MR) or intellectual disability (ID) refers to below-average intellectual functioning, which also leads to DD in most cases. Down syndrome is the most common cause of MR in America. DD and MR can occur separately, but approximately 52% of persons with DD also have MR (Braddock 2001).

The close association between the two is reflected in the terms mentally retarded/developmentally disabled (MR/DD) or intellectually/developmentally disabled. About 6 to 7.5 million mentally retarded individuals live in the United States (Ford-Martin 2003). Most of these people are only mildly retarded, but those with severe retardation and/or DD usually require institutional care in specialized facilities. LTC services for children and adolescents are generally available in special pediatric LTC and MR/DD facilities.

## Young Adults

Permanent disability among young adults commonly stems from neurological malfunctions, degenerative conditions, traumatic injury, or surgical complications. For example, multiple sclerosis is potentially the most common cause of neurological disability in young adults (Compston and Coles 2002). Severe injury to the head, spinal cord, or limbs can occur in victims of vehicle crashes, sports mishaps, or industrial accidents. Other serious diseases, injuries, and respiratory or heart problems following surgery can make it difficult, or even impossible, for a patient to breathe naturally. Such individuals who cannot breathe (or ventilate) on their own require a ventilator. A ventilator is a small machine that takes over the breathing function by automatically moving air into and out of the patient's lungs. Ventilator-dependent patients also require total assistance with their ADLs.

MR/DD is no longer merely a pediatric diagnosis, as was the case in the past. The average life expectancy of those with MR now approaches 66 years (Fisher and Kettl 2005). The aging process begins earlier in people with MR, and 50 years of age has been suggested to demarcate the elderly segment in this population (Altman 1995). This population confronts the same chronic illnesses—cardiovascular disease, cancer, diabetes, and dementia—as the general aging population.

Before the 1970s, MR/DD populations were housed in state-operated institutions. Since then, a serious effort began to move the residents out of state institutions into community-based settings, such as foster care homes. According to the June 1999

US Supreme Court ruling in *Olmstead v. L.C.*, states must provide community-based services for MR/DD patients if treatment professionals determine that such services are appropriate and the affected individuals do not object to such placement, provided the states have the resources to offer such services. Also, states must develop a comprehensive working plan to place qualified MR/DD people in less restrictive settings.

Evidence suggests that MR/DD patients may function better in community-based residential settings than in traditional nursing homes. Studies of patients who had moved out of nursing homes and into community settings demonstrated that these patients had higher levels of adaptive behavior, lifestyle satisfaction, and community integration than residents who remained in nursing homes (Heller et al. 1998; Spreat et al. 1998).

## People with HIV/AIDS

With the increased use of antiretroviral therapy, AIDS has evolved from an end-stage terminal illness into a chronic condition. With reduced mortality, the prevalence of HIV in the population has actually increased, including among the elderly. For example, in 2007, 16.8% of new diagnoses of HIV were in individuals who were older than 50 years (Kearney et al. 2010).

Over a period of time, people with AIDS are subject to a number of debilitating conditions, creating the need for assistance. For instance, nervous system disorders are common in AIDS patients, even though they may survive for several years. Infections of the nervous system, such as cytomegalovirus, can cause blindness and dementia. The accompanying disabilities, despite the availability of advanced treatments, have increased the demand for LTC, and an increasing number of AIDS patients are receiving care in nursing facilities.

Care of HIV/AIDS patients presents special challenges, especially since this population has characteristics that are quite dissimilar to the rest of the LTC population. In LTC facilities, HIV/AIDS patients are likely to be younger than 60 years, male, and black or Hispanic (Shin et al. 2002). They have a significantly higher prevalence of depression, other psychiatric disorders, and dementia associated with AIDS. HIV/AIDS patients also have a significantly higher prevalence of weight loss and incontinence of bladder and bowel (Shin et al. 2002).

## Level of Care Continuum

The importance of providing different levels of services to a heterogeneous population has given rise to a continuum of clinical categories, ranging from basic personal care to subacute care and specialized services.

### Personal Care

*Personal care* refers to light assistance with basic ADLs. Provision of these services is largely the domain of paraprofessionals, such as home health aides, personal care attendants, transportation aides, certified nursing assistants, and therapy aides. Personal care can be provided by informal caregivers, home health agencies, ADC, adult foster care (AFC), and residential and assisted living facilities.

### Custodial Care

*Custodial care* is nonmedical care provided to support and maintain the patient's condition and the essentials of daily living. It requires no active medical or nursing treatments. The focus is on providing routine assistance with ADLs. Services provided are designed to maintain rather than restore functioning, with an emphasis on preventing further deterioration. Examples are personal care with basic ADLs, range-of-motion exercises, bowel and bladder training, and assisted walking. Custodial services are rendered by paraprofessionals, such as aides, rather than licensed nurses or therapists. The settings in which custodial care is provided resemble those for personal care.

## Restorative Care

The goal of *restorative care* or rehabilitation is to help regain or improve function. It is provided immediately after the onset of a disability. Examples of cases requiring short-term restorative therapy include orthopedic surgery, stroke, limb amputation, and prolonged illness. Restorative rehabilitation involves intensive short-term treatments rendered by physical therapists, occupational therapists, and speech–language pathologists. It is based on the philosophy of caregiving in which patients are viewed as participants who can reach their maximum potential in physical and mental functioning. Restorative care can be provided by home health agencies, rehabilitation hospitals, outpatient rehabilitation clinics, ADC centers, and assisted living and skilled nursing facilities (SNFs).

## Skilled Nursing Care

*Skilled nursing care* is medically oriented care provided mainly by a licensed nurse under the overall direction of a physician. Delivery of care includes assessment and reassessment to determine the patient's care needs, monitoring of acute and unstable chronic conditions, and a variety of treatments that may include wound care, tube care management, intravenous therapy, oncology care, HIV/AIDS care, management of neurological conditions, and phlebotomy. Rehabilitation therapies often form an important component of skilled nursing care. Home health agencies and SNFs provide skilled nursing care.

## Subacute Care

The term *subacute care* applies to post-acute services for people who remain critically ill during the postacute phase of illness or injury or who have complex conditions that require ongoing monitoring and treatment or intense rehabilitation. Micheletti and Shlala (1995) suggested four categories of subacute care services: (1) extensive care (parenteral feeding, tracheostomy, etc.), (2) special care (postburn care, pressure sores, intravenous therapy, tube feedings, etc.), (3) clinically complex care (wound care, postsurgical care, etc.), and (4) intensive rehabilitation. These services can be provided in long-term care hospitals (LTCHs—described in Chapter 8), transitional care (or extended care) units in hospitals, or skilled nursing or subacute care facilities that have an adequate number of trained nurses.

## Types of Community-Based Long-Term Care Services

Community-based LTC services have a four-fold objective:

1. To deliver LTC in the most economical and least restrictive setting whenever appropriate for the patient's health care needs,

2. To supplement informal caregiving when more advanced skills are needed than what family members or surrogates can provide,

3. To provide temporary respite to family from caregiving stress, and

4. To delay or prevent institutionalization by meeting the needs of the most vulnerable elderly in community settings.

Financing for formal community-based services comes from a variety of sources: private out-of-pocket payments, private long-term care insurance, Medicaid, Medicare, and other public sources. Title III of the Older Americans Act of 1965 (scheduled for reauthorization in 2011) grants funds to states for a variety of community-based services, such as nutrition programs for the elderly, case management, homemaker services, and ADC services. The services are available to Americans aged 60 years and older, particularly those with social or economic need. Provisions of the act are carried out through an administrative network composed of 56 State Units on Aging (SUA); 655 Area Agencies on Aging (AAA); 243 Indian Tribal Organizations; more than half a million volunteers; and thousands of local community service provider agencies, including more than 5,000 nutrition service providers.

In 1981, the Home and Community Based Services (HCBS) waiver program was enacted under Section 1915(c) of the Social Security Act. The 1915(c) waivers, as they are commonly referred to, allow states to expand community-based LTC services under the Medicaid program. Services are available to those Medicaid beneficiaries who would otherwise require institutional care. Hence, the

main emphasis of the program is to save money on institutional care. Some federal funding available to the states under Title XX Social Services Block Grants from the US Department of Health and Human Services (DHHS) may also be used for community-based LTC services when such services prevent or reduce inappropriate institutionalization. Some states also provide limited assistance with ADLs in a person's home under the Medicaid Personal Care Services program.

## Home Health Care

Chapter 7 discussed home health care and the Medicare rules for eligibility. Chapter 6 covered the prospective payment system (PPS) for home health. The organizational setup commonly requires a community- or hospital-based home health agency that sends health care professionals and paraprofessionals to patients' homes to deliver services approved by a physician.

According to the 2007 Home and Hospice Care Survey, the majority of home health agencies in the United States are private for profit. Of the 14,500 home health and hospice care agencies in 2007, 74.8% provided only home health care; 9.9% were mixed agencies providing both home health and hospice services. Medicare is the single largest payer for home health services (Park-Lee and Decker 2010). Of the total Medicare spending in 2008, 3.5% was paid to home health agencies (1.4% under Part A and 2.1% under Part B; DHHS 2010).

Home health care services are provided mainly to the elderly. Figure 10–8 provides information on ADL and IADL assistance required by home care patients. As Figure 10–9 points out, skilled nursing care is the most common service provided to the patients receiving home health care.

Figure 10–8  The Most Common Types of ADL and IADL Assistance Provided to All Patients Receiving Home Health Care, 2000.

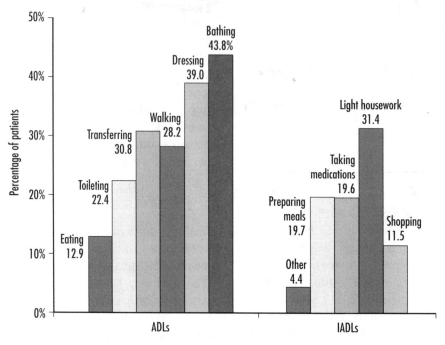

*Source:* Data from *Current Home Health Care Patients* (Table 8, February 2004), National Home and Hospice Care Survey 2000, National Center for Health Statistics.

Figure 10–9   Most Frequently Provided Services to All Home Health Care Patients, 2000.

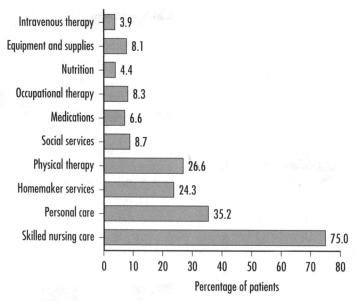

*Source:* Data from *Current Home Health Care Patients* (Table 6, February 2004), National Home and Hospice Care Survey 2000, National Center for Health Statistics.

## Adult Day Care

*Adult day care* (ADC), also referred to as "adult day service," is a daytime group program designed to meet the needs of functionally and/or cognitively impaired adults and provide partial respite to family caregivers. ADC is designed for people who, because of physical or mental conditions, cannot remain alone during the day but who have family members to take care of them. ADC is an important respite program because it enables family caregivers to work during the day or allows informal caregivers to pursue other responsibilities of life.

ADC centers operate programs during normal business hours 5 days a week, although some offer evening and weekend services as well (NADSA 2003). In 2009, there were 4,600 ADC centers across the United States, a 35% increase since 2002 (MetLife Mature Market Institute 2010).

Three models of ADC are commonly recognized: (1) the health-rehabilitative model, (2) the health-maintenance model, and (3) the social-psychological model. All of these programs provide personal care (help with ADLs), midday meals, social services, and transportation. Many programs provide a mix of medical, maintenance, and social–psychological services. Nearly 80% of ADC centers have a nursing professional on staff; nearly 50% have a social work professional; nearly 60% offer case management; and approximately 50% provide physical, occupational, or speech therapy (MetLife Mature Market Institute 2010). Group socialization and therapeutic recreational activities are also important parts of all three models.

① Programs based on the health-rehabilitative model offer more intense medical, nursing, and therapy services, compared to the other two models. Participants in this group may be recovering from various acute episodes, such as stroke or heart attack, or may have late stages of chronic disabling or degenerative conditions, such as arthritis or Parkinson's disease (Kirwin 1991; Tedesco 1996). These programs have formal procedures for evaluating and addressing the participants' medical conditions, rehabilitation goals, and nutritional status. An individualized plan of care is based on this evaluation. The need for ADC is often discontinued once a participant can function independently. This model is the most appropriate for clients who may be candidates for placement in a nursing home.

② Programs using the health-maintenance model focus on participants' physical and psychological needs. The programs are designed to focus on the maintenance of health and function. Hence, they are preventive and generally last longer than the health-rehabilitative programs (Dychtwald et al. 1990).

③ The social-psychological model is best suited for individuals who suffer from dementia, such as Alzheimer's disease. As such, these programs address special concerns in addition to providing basic services similar to those found in the other models.

The primary sources of funding for ADC are Medicaid and private out-of-pocket payments. Medicaid provides some funding under waiver programs that support community-based alternatives to institutional LTC. Medicare does not pay for ADC but may cover rehabilitation services through Part B. In 2009, a bill was introduced in Congress to make ADC a Medicare-covered service, but it failed to pass.

## Adult Foster Care

*Adult foster care* (AFC) is a service characterized by small, family-run homes providing room, board, and varying levels of supervision, oversight, and personal care to nonrelated adults who are unable to care for themselves (AARP Studies Adult Foster Care for the Elderly 1996). Foster care provides services in a community-based dwelling in an environment that promotes the feeling of being part of a family unit (Stahl 1997). Participants in the program are elderly or disabled individuals who have a current medical diagnosis, a psychiatric diagnosis, or a need for assistance with at least one ADL. Typically, the caregiving family resides in part of the home. To maintain the family environment, most states license fewer than 10 beds per family unit; however, many people have made a business of AFC by buying several houses and hiring families to live in them to care for functionally impaired and elderly people (Fein 1994).

The program differs widely from state to state and goes by several names, including adult family care, community residential care, and domiciliary care. Each state has established its own standards for the licensing of foster care homes. Funding for AFCs comes from Medicaid, private insurance, or personal sources. It is estimated that the cost of care averages about one-third of that in nursing homes (Fein 1994), mainly because services in AFC are primarily designed to focus on room and board, supervision, and light assistance with ADLs. Medicare does not pay for AFC but may cover rehabilitation services under Part B.

## Senior Centers

*Senior centers* are local community centers for older adults where seniors can congregate and socialize. Many centers offer one or more meals daily. Others sponsor wellness programs, health education, counseling services, recreational activities, information and referrals, and limited health care services, including health screening, especially for glaucoma and hypertension. Nearly all senior centers receive some public funding. Other common revenue sources are United Way and private donations.

## Home-Delivered and Congregate Meals

The elderly nutrition program (ENP) is the nation's oldest framework for providing community- and home-based preventive nutrition in the United States. The program provides a hot noon meal 5 days a week to Americans 60 years of age and older (and their spouses) who cannot prepare a nutritionally balanced noon meal for themselves. Home-delivered meals for homebound persons are commonly referred to as *meals-on-wheels*. Ambulatory clients are encouraged to get their meals at senior centers or other congregate settings, where they also get the opportunity to socialize.

The ENP program was authorized under the Older Americans Act, which also provides the majority of the funding. Additional funds are provided through Title XX block grants, 1915(c) waivers, and private donations. It is estimated that, in 2009, the program served nearly 7% of the nation's elderly population. Of the 241.6 million meals served, 62% were home delivered (Administration on Aging 2011). Compared with nonparticipants, both ambulatory and homebound ENP clients are better nourished (Millen et al. 2002). However, the demand for services far exceeds the current capacity. The elderly often have to be on waiting lists to participate in the program.

It is a common practice for the Area Agency on Aging to contract out the preparation and delivery of meals to local nursing homes, hospitals, or religious organizations. In the meals-on-wheels program, volunteers carry the meals to homebound participants. Congregate meals may be served on the premises of participating facilities, such as hospitals and nursing homes, or at local senior centers or religious establishments.

## Homemaker Services

Some older adults are relatively healthy but cannot carry out a few simple tasks necessary for independent living. These tasks may be as urgent as repairing a burst pipe or as mundane as cleaning the house. Some tasks, such as grocery shopping, must be performed often, whereas others, such as replacing storm windows, require attention just once or twice a year. Homemaker, chore, and handyman services can assist older adults with a variety of these tasks, including shopping, light cleaning, general errands, and minor home repairs. Homemaker programs may be staffed largely or entirely by volunteers. The Medicaid program may pay for some homemaker services, or these services may be funded through the local seniors programs under Title XX Social Services Block Grants or the Older Americans Act.

## Emergency Response Systems PERS

Many of the frail elderly living alone do not need medical or supportive care, but they may nonetheless be vulnerable in an emergency. Other patients, after returning home from hospitals and nursing homes, are plagued by anxiety about relapses or accidents because people are often unprepared to manage themselves after returning home. Personal emergency response systems (PERS), also referred to as medical emergency response systems, address these needs. A **PERS** provides a cost-effective mechanism that enables at-risk elderly persons to summon help in an emergency. Usually, these people wear or carry a transmitter unit with which they can send a medical alert to a local 24-hour monitoring and response center.

## Case Management

The essential need for case management, which was previously defined, is recognized as a community-based covered service in 1915(c) waiver programs. Case-management services are designed to assess the special needs of older adults, prepare a care plan to address those needs, specify services that are most appropriate, determine eligibility for services, make referrals and coordinate delivery of care, arrange for financing, ensure that clients are receiving services, and reevaluate needs as circumstances change over time.

Three traditional models of case management in LTC have been identified: brokerage model, managed care model, and integrated care model (Scharlach et al. 2001).

### Brokerage Model

In the *brokerage model*, once needs have been independently assessed, case managers arrange services through other providers. The case manager is usually a freestanding agent who is mainly responsible for linking the client with other organizations, agencies, and service providers, with no formal administrative or financial relationship with these entities. Need assessment, development of a service plan, and making referrals are the main functions of case management in this model. There is minimal coordination and monitoring of services. Although private geriatric case managers provide case-management services, in the public domain, most states have implemented *preadmission screening* rules for need assessment and referral for community-based or institutional services. Also, federal regulations mandate a Preadmission Screening and Resident Review (PASRR) process for individuals with serious mental illness or mental retardation who apply to or reside in Medicaid-certified nursing facilities regardless of the source of payment.

## Managed Care Model

This model is offered through a managed care organization (MCO), and it involves capitated financing, which places the MCO at financial risk. Professionally trained nurses and social workers are typically the case managers, who are likely to be more closely involved in the monitoring and coordination of services than is the case in the brokerage model (Scharlach et al. 2001). Delivery of services is arranged through a social health maintenance organization (*S/HMO*), which coordinates acute, chronic, LTC, and social services to address a patient's comprehensive needs. Its primary goal is to prevent or delay placement in a nursing home. Hence, preventive and supportive services are strongly emphasized. There is some evidence that S/HMOs may help at-risk elderly postpone long-term nursing home placement (Fischer 2003). Although most of the emphasis in LTC delivery is on preventing nursing home placement, S/HMOs have also been shown to facilitate successful transition of short-stay residents to the community, thus avoiding the conversion to a long stay in a nursing

home (Thomas et al. 2010). The S/HMO model has so far existed in the form of Medicare demonstration projects in which Medicare beneficiaries have to voluntarily enroll. Once enrolled, the beneficiaries have to obtain all covered services through the MCO. Perhaps for this reason, the model has not gained wide acceptance.

## Integrated Care Model

This model exists within an interdisciplinary organizational structure that strives to provide all necessary services a client may need. Services include medical and social services, such as counseling, advocacy, and ongoing coordination and monitoring. The goal is ongoing prevention of the progression of disability (Scharlach et al. 2001). Similar to the managed care model, capitation is used, for which funding comes from both Medicare and Medicaid programs. Services are delivered through a nonprofit health care organization. At the core of the program is ADC, augmented by home care and meals at home (Gross et al. 2004).

The Program of All-Inclusive Care for the Elderly (PACE) is an example of integrated case management. The PACE program was authorized under the Balanced Budget Act of 1997 after the On Lok project in San Francisco demonstrated that, in many instances, LTC institutionalization could be prevented through appropriate case management. The PACE program focuses on frail elderly who have already been certified for nursing home placement under Medicare and/or Medicaid.

All medical care and social services are coordinated by a PACE team. Providers of PACE services must make all services covered under both Medicare and Medicaid available. PACE has no deductibles and

copayments, which is an incentive for qualified individuals to join the program.

## Institutional Long-Term Care Continuum

Given the variety of LTC services available,
institutional LTC is more appropriate for patients whose needs cannot be adequately met
in a less acute, community-based setting.
The institutional sector of LTC also provides a continuum of services (Figure 10–5)
according to the patient's level of acuity and
dependency for care.

The generic term "nursing home" encompasses a wide spectrum of facilities. All
of these facilities provide room and board,
in addition to varying levels of nursing and
medical care. Various alternative living arrangements now address a variety of care
needs that have gradually filled the gap
between living in one's own home and living in a typical SNF. Retirement living, for
instance, offers the most independence and
provides no nursing or medical services.
Residential care offers some additional services, such as meals, assistance with taking
medications, and basic supervision. Assisted
living goes a step further in providing most
services associated with the ADLs and management of light incontinence. However, the
distinction between some of these alternatives often blurs. Hence, facility labels do
not always clearly define the levels of care.

Unless a resident has a drastic deterioration in health status that necessitates specialized services, such as those offered in an
SNF or an acute care hospital, the changing
health care needs of residents are accommodated in the existing setting, instead of making frequent transfers between facilities.

Institutional LTC may be categorized
in five distinct groups, based on the level
of services: independent or retirement living centers, residential or personal care facilities, assisted living facilities, SNFs, and
subacute care facilities.

## Independent or Retirement Living Centers

As the name suggests, these facilities essentially meet the housing needs of older adults.
They are not LTC institutions in the true sense
because they do not deliver clinical services.
Residents maintain their own independent
lifestyles. The main advantage of special elderly housing, in contrast to ordinary housing,
is found in its physical features and amenities
that are adapted to the needs of the physically
disabled and create a supportive environment
to promote independence. Examples of adaptations are railings in hallways, extra-large
bathrooms that facilitate wheelchair negotiation, grab bars in bathrooms, and pull cords to
summon help in an emergency. In addition,
such facilities often provide transportation
for shopping and outings, and many facilities
organize regular recreational activities and
social events to promote an active lifestyle.
Others provide one or two meals a day in a
congregate setting. Although these facilities
do not provide personal or custodial care, occasional needs for LTC services are met by
obtaining home health care services through
an outside agency.

Depending on the type of housing, independent living arrangements include congregate housing in multiunit rental complexes,
providing self-contained apartments. Up-
scale retirement communities sell individual
apartments and generally require monthly
maintenance fees, all paid through private
funds. More modest housing complexes provide government-assisted, subsidized housing for low-income elderly based on their
incomes.

SNF = skilled nursing facility

## Residential or Personal Care Facilities

These facilities are also known as "domiciliary care facilities" or "board-and-care homes." Sometimes AFC homes (previously discussed) are included in this category. Others have called them "sheltered care facilities." These facilities provide physically supportive dwelling units, monitoring and/ or assistance with medications, oversight, and personal or custodial care. To maintain a residential rather than an institutional environment, many such facilities limit admitting residents who use wheelchairs. Others requiring assistance with ADLs or having cognitive impairments are also generally not admitted because these facilities are not equipped to provide nursing care.

Facilities can range anywhere from spartan to deluxe. The latter are often private pay. For people who have limited incomes, Supplemental Security Income (SSI) can be used along with other types of government assistance funds. Services include meals, housekeeping and laundry services, and social and recreational activities. Transportation is an important support service that allows people to live independently. Minimal staffing is provided 24 hours a day for supervision and assistive purposes. More advanced services can be arranged through an external home health agency when needed.

## Assisted Living Facilities

An *assisted living facility* (ALF) is a residential setting that provides personal care, 24-hour supervision, social services, recreational activities, and some nursing and rehabilitation services. In 2006, the average age of an assisted living resident was 85 years. The typical resident is mobile but needs assistance with two ADLs. The most common areas of ADL assistance are bathing, dressing, and toileting. Also, the majority of residents require help with medications. Approximately one-third of the residents are discharged because they need a higher level of services in a nursing facility; another one-third pass away (National Center for Assisted Living 2006).

Assisted living facilities have burgeoned in popularity as an alternative to the traditional nursing home. The services are specially designed for people who cannot function independently and, therefore, cannot be accommodated in a residential care setting but do not require skilled nursing care. Intermittent skilled nursing care can be arranged through a home health agency if needed. Compared to SNFs, the environment in ALFs is less clinical and more homelike. Hence, people prefer to be in ALFs than in SNFs, provided their needs can be adequately met in ALFs.

Regulation of assisted living facilities is mainly at the state level through the licensing process. These regulations continue to evolve in response to the rising acuity levels of residents. For example, in some states, facilities that serve Alzheimer's or dementia patients face increased oversight. Some states have started to require resident assessment, plan of care, and staff training.

The absence of a common definition for assisted living makes it difficult to pinpoint the number of residences in the United States. According to one source, there were 15,070 ALFs in 2009, up from 14,955 in 2008. Brookdale Senior Living Inc., the largest ALF chain in the nation, with 540 facilities in 35 states, continued to expand, adding 24 new facilities in 2009.

Assisted living is primarily paid for privately. Costs vary widely according to amenities, room size and type (e.g., shared versus private), and the services the resident requires. Most facilities charge a basic monthly rate that covers rent and utilities and then charge separately for services. Many facilities also charge a one-time entrance fee. For people who have limited assets and income, in most states, the Medicaid program for SSI recipients and through Title XX Social Services Block Grants covers assisted living care. However, such funds are limited.

## ④ Skilled Nursing Facilities

Skilled nursing facilities are heavily regulated through licensure and certification requirements. All facilities in a particular state must be licensed and, therefore, must comply with the licensing regulations, which differ considerably from state to state. Most licensing regulations establish minimum qualifications required for administrators and other staff, prescribe minimum staffing levels, establish standards for building construction, and require compliance with the national fire and safety codes. To admit patients covered under the Medicaid and/or Medicare programs, nursing homes must also be certified and must demonstrate compliance with the federal certification standards enforced by the Centers for Medicare & Medicaid Services (CMS).

Until 1989, federal statutes classified nursing homes into two types: SNFs for Medicare and/or Medicaid residents and intermediate care facilities (ICFs) for those covered by Medicaid only. Patients needing a higher level of care were eligible for admission to an SNF, which was required to have a licensed nurse on duty 24 hours a day and a registered nurse (RN) on the day shift. By contrast, ICFs had to have a licensed nurse on duty only on the day shift.

From a clinical standpoint, the Nursing Home Reform Act, passed in 1987, removed the differences between ICFs and SNFs. The reform legislation created two categories for certification purposes. A nursing home certified to admit Medicare patients is called an *SNF*. This facility can be freestanding or a *distinct part*, that is, a section of a nursing home that is distinctly separate and distinguishable from the rest of the facility. When SNF certification applies to a distinct part, Medicare patients can be admitted only to that section. A nursing home certified for Medicaid only (but not for Medicare) is called a nursing facility (*NF*). A facility may be dually certified as an SNF and an NF. Facilities having *dual certification* can admit Medicare and/or Medicaid patients to any part of the facility. The federal certification standards governing SNFs and NFs are essentially the same.

The labels of SNF and NF represent only two types of certifications, often for facilities providing similar levels of care. Thus, the term "skilled nursing facility" has both a regulatory and a clinical meaning. The SNF and NF categories have been created for the two distinct sources of funding. Medicare and Medicaid patients do not receive two different levels of services, although Medicare patients who receive postacute services may have a higher acuity level.

The term "facility" does not necessarily mean a separate physical structure. The term can be used for the facility as a whole, or, within the context of licensure and certification, it may apply more specifically to different sections or units of a building (distinct parts) with different certifications or no certification (see Figure 10-10).

A small proportion of facilities have elected not to participate in the Medicaid and/or Medicare programs. They can admit only patients who have a private funding source for nursing home care. These facilities are *noncertified*; however, they must be licensed under the state licensure regulations. *Private pay patients*—those

Figure 10–10  Distinctly Certified Units in a Nursing Home.

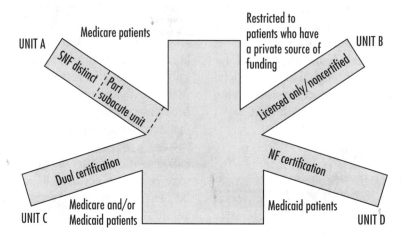

The entire facility must be licensed by the state.

not covered by either Medicare or Medicaid for nursing home care—are not restricted to noncertified facilities. These patients also may be admitted to SNF or NF certified beds. The restriction applies to Medicare and Medicaid patients who cannot be admitted to noncertified facilities.

## Subacute Care Facilities

Subacute care became a prominent service after acute care hospitals were brought under the PPS in the 1980s. The three main institutional locations for subacute care— LTCHs, hospital transitional care units, and SNFs—vary in terms of availability, cost, and quality. Selection of a setting is governed by numerous factors, both clinical and nonclinical. One main nonclinical factor is the availability of subacute care services in a given location (Buntin et al. 2005). Regarding cost, LTCHs are the most expensive. SNFs are often a more cost-effective alternative to LTCHs, and at least some physicians think that the level and intensity of care in the two settings is comparable

(MedPAC 2004). Postacute needs can widely vary among patients, but there is no uniform system of clinical assessment and payment for subacute care. Medicare uses different payment methodologies for the different settings. For example, LTCHs are paid according to severity-based diagnosis-related groups (see MS-LTC-DRGs in Chapter 8), and SNF payments are based on resource utilization groups (see Chapter 6).

## Specialized Facilities

Specialized facilities provide special services for individuals with distinct medical needs.

### Intermediate Care Facility for the Mentally Retarded (ICF/MR)

Federal regulations provide a separate certification category for LTC facilities classified as ICF/MRs since 1971, when Public Law 92–223 authorized Medicaid coverage for the care for MR/DD patients in ICF/MR facilities. Most of these patients have other disabilities, in addition to mental retardation. For example, many of these patients are nonambulatory, have seizure disorders, behavior problems, mental illness, visual or hearing impairments, or have a combination of these conditions. The primary purpose of ICF/MRs is to furnish nursing and rehabilitative services that involve active treatments.

## Alzheimer's Facilities

*Alzheimer's disease* is a progressive degenerative disease of the brain, producing memory loss, confusion, irritability, and severe functional decline. The disease becomes progressively worse and eventually results in death. Alzheimer's facilities provide special programming and have special security features because the residents tend to wander. Carefully designed lighting, color, and signage are employed to help orient the residents (Skaggs and Hawkins 1994).

## Continuing Care Retirement Communities (CCRCs)

A continuing care retirement community (*CCRC*) is specialized in the sense that it integrates and coordinates independent living with some of the other institution-based components of the LTC continuum, such as assisted living and skilled nursing care. Different levels of services are housed in separate buildings, all located on one campus. The range of services is based on the concept of aging in place and yet accommodates the changing needs of older adults. The range of services includes housing, health care, and social services. Residents choose to enter these communities when they are still relatively healthy. The residents' independence is preserved, but assistance and nursing care are provided when needed.

A CCRC commonly has these characteristics (Aaronson 1996):

- Cottages or apartments, in various size options, are available for independent living. Each apartment may have a kitchenette and other facilities to support independence. A congregate dining room provides one or more meals a day. Recreational and social programs promote an active lifestyle.

- Personal care and assisted living are available in an adjoining facility for residents who require some monitoring, assistance with ADLs, and/or basic nursing care. These services represent a midpoint between independent living and nursing care.

- An SNF provides intermittent, as well as permanent, accommodations to residents of the CCRC. SNFs serve the same function for the CCRC that nursing homes serve for the general community.

- A CCRC may require some form of prepayment, such as an entrance fee. In addition, monthly maintenance fees are charged.

- A contract that lasts for more than 1 year and describes the service obligations of the CCRC and the financial obligations of the resident must be signed.

CCRCs, for the most part, require private financing, with the exception of services delivered in a Medicare-certified SNF. Entrance and monthly fees vary considerably, depending on which services are included. The services are directed at middle- and upper-middle-income clientele using a strong customer-oriented marketing approach. The most important reason clients give for joining a CCRC is guaranteed access to institutional LTC services when they are needed (Cohen et al. 1988).

## Nursing Home Industry and Patient Demographics

### Industry Overview

Table 10–1 provides characteristics of the US nursing home industry, based on the 2004 National Nursing Home Survey. Between 1999 and 2004, nationally, the number of nursing homes declined by over 10% and bed capacity declined by almost 8%. This represents a decline from 52 beds to 48 beds per 1,000 elderly persons in the United States. Since 2004, industrywide

Table 10–1  Number and Percentage Distribution of Nursing Homes, Number of Beds and Beds per Home, and Selected Facility Characteristics, 2004

| Facility Characteristic | Nursing Homes Number | % Distribution | Beds Number (1,000) | % Distribution | Beds per Nursing Home | Current Residents Number (1,000) | Occupancy Rate (%) |
|---|---|---|---|---|---|---|---|
| All facilities | 16,100 | | 1,730 | 100 | 107.6 | 1,492 | 86.3 |
| Ownership: | | | | | | | |
| Proprietary | 9,900 | 61.5 | 1,074 | 62.1 | 108.6 | 918 | 85.5 |
| Voluntary nonprofit | 5,000 | 30.8 | 504 | 29.1 | 101.6 | 440 | 87.4 |
| Government and other | 1,200 | 7.7 | 152 | 8.8 | 123.6 | 134 | 88.0 |
| Certification: | | | | | | | |
| Medicare and Medicaid certified (SNF/NF) | 14,100 | 87.6 | 1,600 | 92.5 | 113.5 | 1,380 | 86.3 |
| Medicare only (SNF) | 700 | 4.1 | 33 | 1.9 | 50.6 | 28 | 85.0 |
| Medicaid only (NF) | 1,100 | 6.9 | 76 | 4.4 | 69.0 | 68 | 89.1 |
| Bed size: | | | | | | | |
| Fewer than 50 beds | 2,200 | 13.9 | 76 | 4.4 | 33.8 | 62 | 82.1 |
| 50–99 beds | 6,000 | 37.3 | 455 | 26.3 | 75.7 | 423 | 92.9 |
| 100–199 beds | 6,800 | 42.5 | 903 | 52.2 | 132.0 | 789 | 87.3 |
| 200 beds or more | 1,000 | 6.2 | 296 | 17.1 | 298.2 | 219 | 73.9 |
| Region: | | | | | | | |
| Northeast | 2,800 | 17.4 | 382 | 22.1 | 136.0 | 331 | 86.8 |
| Midwest | 5,300 | 33.0 | 527 | 30.4 | 99.4 | 448 | 85.1 |
| South | 5,400 | 33.6 | 586 | 33.8 | 108.3 | 502 | 85.6 |
| West | 2,600 | 16.0 | 236 | 13.7 | 92.1 | 211 | 89.5 |
| Affiliation: | | | | | | | |
| Chain | 8,700 | 54.2 | 939 | 54.3 | 107.9 | 813 | 86.5 |
| Independent | 7,400 | 45.8 | 791 | 45.7 | 107.2 | 680 | 86.0 |

Source: Data from Nursing Home Facilities (Table 1, December 2006), National Nursing Home Survey 2004, National Center for Health Statistics.

declines have continued so that, by 2009, there were 15,700 nursing homes (1,705,808 beds), with an average of 109 beds per facility. Industry-wide average occupancy rate was 82.2% (DHHS 2010). The decline in the supply of nursing home beds is primarily due to ongoing emphasis on community-based services and assisted living alternatives to nursing home care. Conversely, the number of admissions to nursing homes has risen, spurred by higher short-term Medicare admissions (Sanofi-Aventis 2010).

Between 1999 and 2004, the proportion of dually certified nursing home beds increased from approximately 87 to 93%, and the proportion of beds with NF certification decreased from 9 to 4.4%. This trend has been triggered mainly by low Medicaid reimbursement. In 2008, almost 9% of the national health care expenditures were attributed to nursing homes (DHHS 2010).

Most of the nursing homes in the United States are operated by multifacility chains. The 10 largest chains have at least 90 nursing homes each and, together, operate 14% of the national bed capacity (Table 10–2). Consolidation among nursing home chains has contributed to net income growth in the for-profit sector, even as the nonprofit sector experiences sharp declines (Sanofi-Aventis 2010).

## Services and Patients Served

At least 90% of all nursing home residents are 65 years of age and older. Trends also show a nursing home population that has aged and become more racially diverse. Over 80% of the residents are dependent for their mobility, 66% are incontinent, and 47% require assistance with eating; 37% are dependent in all three areas (DHHS 2006).

Most nursing homes provide a variety of services to fit the varied needs of their patient populations. Restorative care, treatment of skin wounds, and dementia care are the most commonly available services (Table 10–3). The three most common

Table 10–2 Ten Largest Nursing Home Chains in the United States

| Chain/Headquarters | Total Facilities | Total Beds | Avg. Beds/ Facility | # of States |
|---|---|---|---|---|
| 1. Golden Living / Fort Smith, AR | 307 | 31,229 | 102 | 21 |
| 2. Manor Care / Toledo, OH | 282 | 37,520 | 133 | 29 |
| 3. Kindred Healthcare / Louisville, KY | 225 | 27,530 | 122 | 27 |
| 4. Life Care Centers of America / Cleveland, TN | 225 | 29,217 | 130 | 28 |
| 5. Genesis Health Care / Kennett Square, PA | 202 | 25,456 | 126 | 13 |
| 6. Sun Healthcare Group / Irvine, CA | 183 | 20,903 | 114 | 25 |
| 7. Sava Senior Care / Atlanta, GA | 182 | 22,245 | 122 | 19 |
| 8. Evangelical Lutheran Good Samaritan / Sioux Falls, SD | 178 | 13,105 | 74 | 23 |
| 9. Extendicare Health Services / Milwaukee, WI | 176 | 18,288 | 104 | 12 |
| 10. Fundamental Long Term Care Holdings / Sparks, MD | 82 | 9,656 | 118 | 12 |

*Note:* All but No. 8 are for profit.

*Source:* Data from *Managed Care Digest Series: Public Payer Digest, 2010–2011*, p. 43. Bridgewater, NJ: Sanofi-Aventis.

Table 10–3 Percentage of Nursing Homes by Availability of Special Programs, 2004

| | | | | Type of Program | | | | |
|---|---|---|---|---|---|---|---|---|
| | Hospice End of Life | Palliative Care | Dementia Care | Restorative Care | Behavior Problems | Pain Management | Continence Management | Skin Wounds |
| All facilities | 18.8 | 16.7 | 31.5 | 68.9 | 23.8 | 25.6 | 21.7 | 53.5 |
| Ownership | | | | | | | | |
| Proprietary | 16.7 | 14.6 | 28.5 | 71.8 | 23.8 | 23.3 | 22.6 | 54.0 |
| Voluntary nonprofit and other | 22.3 | 20.1 | 36.4 | 64.3 | 23.8 | 29.3 | 20.4 | 52.7 |
| Beds | | | | | | | | |
| Fewer than 50 beds | * | * | * | 45.2 | * | 18.1 | * | 35.6 |
| 50–99 beds | 17.6 | 14.3 | 25.0 | 70.6 | 25.2 | 24.4 | 22.5 | 50.2 |
| 100 beds or more | 21.3 | 19.6 | 41.2 | 74.3 | 25.9 | 28.6 | 23.9 | 61.1 |

*Source:* Data from *Nursing Home Facilities* (Table 18, December 2006), National Nursing Home Survey 2004, National Center for Health Statistics.

Figure 10–11  Percentage of Nursing Home Residents with Various Conditions, 2009.

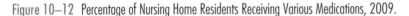

| | |
|---|---|

```
60.0%        56.2%
              █
50.0%        █    52.0%
              █     █    47.3%
40.0%        █     █     █    44.5%
              █     █     █     █
30.0%        █     █     █     █    29.2%
              █     █     █     █     █    24.0%
20.0%        █     █     █     █     █     █
              █     █     █     █     █     █
10.0%        █     █     █     █     █     █    6.5%   6.0%
              █     █     █     █     █     █     █     █
 0.0%
          Bladder  Depression Alzheimer's-type Bowel Behavioral Psychiatric Pressure Skin
       incontinence          dementia incontinence symptoms diagnosis  sores  rashes
```

*Source:* Data from *Managed Care Digest Series: Public Payer Digest, 2010–2011*, p. 45. Bridgewater, NJ: Sanofi-Aventis.

conditions that patients in nursing homes suffer from are bladder incontinence, depression, Alzheimer's-type dementia, and bowel incontinence (Figure 10–11). A relatively large percentage of nursing home residents (over 66%) use psychoactive medications. These are prescription drugs that alter brain function, resulting in temporary changes in perception, mood, consciousness, and behavior. Almost one-half of the residents use antidepressants (Figure 10–12).

## Staffing

Table 10–4 furnishes staffing ratios for nursing staff. For-profit facilities have the lowest per patient day (PPD) staffing ratios. Conclusions of research studies to date are mixed on the quality of care provided in the three categories of facilities by ownership type. If the quality of care is indeed similar, then for-profit facilities gain a cost-effectiveness advantage over the other two ownership types.

Figure 10–12  Percentage of Nursing Home Residents Receiving Various Medications, 2009.

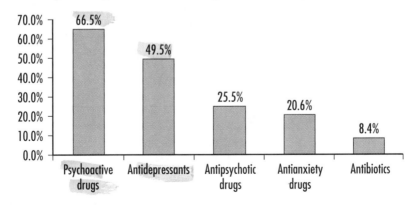

```
70.0%        66.5%
              █
60.0%        █
              █    49.5%
50.0%        █     █
              █     █
40.0%        █     █
              █     █
30.0%        █     █    25.5%
              █     █     █    20.6%
20.0%        █     █     █     █
              █     █     █     █    8.4%
10.0%        █     █     █     █     █
              █     █     █     █     █
 0.0%
        Psychoactive Antidepressants Antipsychotic Antianxiety Antibiotics
          drugs                      drugs         drugs
```

*Source:* Data from *Managed Care Digest Series: Public Payer Digest, 2010–2011*, p. 44. Bridgewater, NJ: Sanofi-Aventis.

Table 10–4  Nursing Home Staffing Ratios per Patient per Day (PPD) by Facility Ownership, 2010

|  | RN | LPN | CNA | Total Nursing |
|---|---|---|---|---|
| **Overall average** | **0.71** | **0.84** | **2.45** | **4.00** |
| For-profit | 0.63 | 0.83 | 2.35 | 3.81 |
| Nonprofit | 0.90 | 0.85 | 2.63 | 4.38 |
| Government | 0.83 | 0.85 | 2.73 | 4.41 |

*Source: CMS Nursing Home Compare,* October 2010.

## Financing

Figure 10–13 provides a comparison of total expenditures for the delivery of hospital care, nursing home care, physician services, prescription drugs, and other personal health care (dental services, home health care, durable medical equipment [DME], vision care, and other professional services). National expenditures for nursing home care have been much lower than those in other sectors of health care delivery. Also, they have not increased as fast as the other

Figure 10–13  Distribution of Personal Health Care Expenditures.

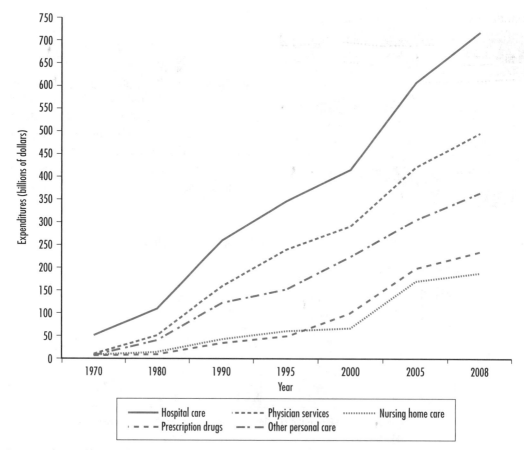

*Source:* Data from *Health, United States, 2002,* pp. 293, 294; *Health, United States, 2009,* pp. 398–399; *Health, United States, 2010,* pp. 371–372; National Center for Health Statistics.

expenditures. For a number of years, expenditures on prescription drugs have exceeded the dollars spent on nursing home care.

Most nursing home care is financed by Medicaid (Figure 10–14), but private sources (mainly, out of pocket and private insurance) also cover a sizable portion of nursing home expenses. Total private financing, however, has been declining for a number of years. In 2008, it paid for 37.8% of nursing home expenses, compared to 43.2% in 2000. One main reason is a rapid rise in Medicare payments, from 10.6% in 2000 to 18.6% in 2008 (DHHS 2010).

## Medicare (for old)

Medicare provides only limited benefits for nursing home care on a postacute basis under Part A. Chapter 6 outlined the criteria for coverage in an SNF. Medicare's share of expenditures has consistently risen, whereas

Medicaid's has declined. Figure 10–15 illustrates the trends in financing from the four main sources.

## Medicaid

Of the 58.2 million Medicaid beneficiaries, only 2.8% received services in nursing facilities and another 0.2% received care in ICF/MRs in 2008 (DHHS 2010). Nursing facilities consumed 16% of total Medicaid expenditures, far more than what Medicaid spent on any other service (Figure 10–16). Medicaid and private pay patients may receive rehabilitation therapies under Medicare Part B, provided those services are certified as medically necessary.

## Private Pay

Private pay refers to out-of-pocket financing for LTC. Many patients are initially

Figure 10–14 Sources of Funding for Nursing Home Care (Nonhospital Affiliated), 2008.

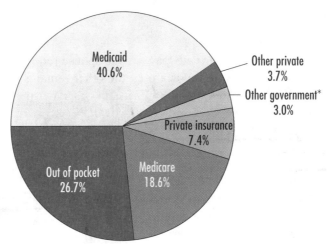

*Other government expenditures include, for example, care funded by the Department of Veterans Affairs.

*Source:* Data from *Health, United States, 2010,* p. 371, National Center for Health Statistics.

Figure 10–15  Main Sources of Financing Nursing Home Care (Nonhospital Affiliated Facilities).

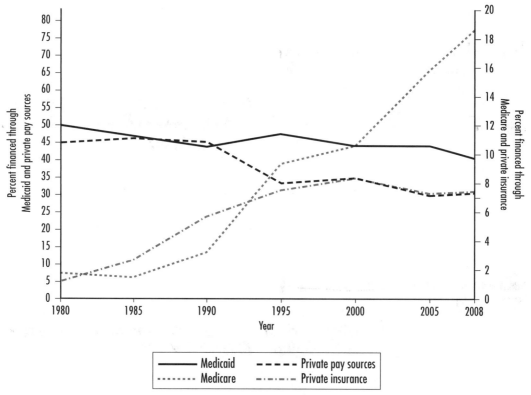

*Source:* Data from *Health, United States, 1999,* p. 289; *Health, United States, 2009,* p. 398; *Health, United States, 2010,* p. 372; National Center for Health Statistics, Department of Health and Human Services.

admitted to a facility with a private pay source of funding. When private funds are exhausted, these patients become eligible for Medicaid assistance. The term *spend-down* refers to exhausting one's assets and one's annual income to the medically needy levels to qualify for Medicaid. If the income and resources of a medically needy individual are above a state-prescribed level, the individual must first incur a certain amount of medical expenses to lower the income and assets to the medically needy level established by the state (Burwell et al. 1996). In the case of married couples, when one spouse requires nursing home care and the other remains in the community, Medicaid rules are intended to prevent the impoverishment of the spouse remaining in the community.

## Private Long-Term Care Insurance

Private LTC insurance is available in a wide range of choices in services covered and prices. In addition to nursing home care, private insurance also covers community-based services, such as home health care or ADC. In 2008, 7.4% of all nursing home

Spend down

Figure 10–16 Trends in the Distribution of Medicaid Expenditures Among Selected Services.

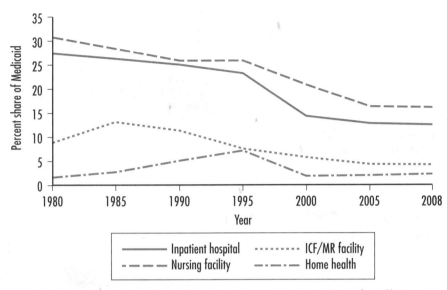

*Source:* Data from *Health, United States, 2002*, p. 328; *Health, United States, 2010*, p. 408. National Center for Health Statistics.

expenditures were paid through private LTC insurance (Figure 10–15).

Private LTC insurance has grown at a slow pace for two main reasons: (1) There is a wide range of policies to choose from, and trying to decide the right coverage can be a daunting task. (2) For most people, the premiums are unaffordable. The costs vary substantially depending on coverage options, such as the daily or monthly benefit amount the insurer would pay, a waiting period (also called elimination period) before benefit payments will begin, the number of years over which benefits will be paid, and inflation protection to cover rising LTC costs in the future. LTC insurance policies are particularly expensive if a plan is purchased in the later years of a person's life. People in younger age groups, for whom the cost of LTC insurance would be more affordable, face other financial priorities, such as saving for retirement, children's college education, life insurance, and buying a home. The need for LTC in the distant future is considered a much lower priority. However, people are learning about the catastrophic financial risks posed by a long stay in a nursing home, and a number of states now offer tax incentives for purchasing LTC policies.

In 2004, 104 companies sold more than 900,000 policies. The market for private LTC insurance grew an average of 18% annually between 1987 and 2002 (America's Health Insurance Plans 2004). However, risk selection is a problem. For example, about 15% of applicants are denied coverage because of their health. Also, recent surveys show that baby boomers have a poor understanding of LTC coverage. Many think that Medicare will pay for LTC services, if and when they need them (Ghose 2007).

## Summary

People of any age may need LTC services, but most of these services are used by the elderly because aging often brings on chronic conditions, multiple illnesses, physical disability, and decreased mental capacity. When such health problems impair the performance of ADL and/or IADL functions, LTC becomes necessary. LTC must be viewed not as an isolated component of the health care delivery system but as a continuum of both community-based and institution-based services that must be rationally linked to the rest of the system. The LTC system can be like a maze. Many people find the various aspects of LTC, such as levels of care, appropriateness of services, and financing, overwhelming. Case management can help clients find an appropriate match of services to address their needs.

LTC includes medical care, social support, and housing alternatives. It encompasses a range of community-based and institutional services to serve a variety of needs. LTC services often complement what people with impaired functioning can do for themselves. Informal caregivers provide the bulk of LTC services in the United States. Respite care can provide family members temporary relief from the burden of caregiving. When the required intensity of care exceeds the capabilities of informal caregivers, available alternatives include professional community-based services to supplement informal care or admission to an LTC facility. Institutional services vary from basic personal assistance to more complex skilled nursing care and subacute care. Some patients may require long-range custodial care without the prognosis of a cure. Others may require short-term postacute convalescence and restorative rehabilitation. Still others may need end-of-life care through a hospice program or dementia care in a specialized facility. A continuing care retirement community offers independent living and institution-based LTC services. Specialized institutions also exist for people with severe mental retardation and/or developmental disability.

LTC facilities can be proprietary, private nonprofit, or government owned. They may be independent or affiliated with a multifacility chain. The average size of a nursing home in the United States is 109 beds with an average occupancy of 82%. Nursing homes require federal SNF certification to admit Medicare patients and NF certification to admit Medicaid patients. Most facility beds in the United States are dually certified as both SNF and NF. Medicaid is the most common source of funding for nursing home care.

---

## Terminology

adult day care
adult foster care
Alzheimer's disease
assisted living facility
brokerage model

case management
CCRC
custodial care
developmental disability
distinct part

## Test Your Understanding

dual certification
long-term care
meals-on-wheels
mental retardation
NF

| | | |
|---|---|---|
| *noncertified* | *preadmission screening* | *S/HMO* |
| *PACE* | *private pay patients* | *skilled nursing care* |
| *palliation* | *quality of life* | *SNF* |
| *paraprofessionals* | *respite care* | *spend-down* |
| *PERS* | *restorative care* | *subacute care* |
| *personal care* | *senior centers* | *total care* |

## Review Questions

1. Long-term care services must be individualized, integrated, and coordinated. Elaborate on this statement, pointing out why these elements are essential in the delivery of LTC.

2. Age is not the primary determinant for long-term care. Comment on this statement, explaining why this is or is not true.

3. What is meant by "quality of life?" Briefly discuss the five main features of this multifaceted concept.

4. What are some of the challenges in the delivery of mental health services for the elderly?

5. Discuss the preventive and therapeutic aspects of long-term care.

6. How do formal and informal long-term care differ? What is the importance of informal care in LTC delivery?

7. What are the main goals of community-based and institution-based long-term care services?

8. What implications does an aging population have for long-term care services?

9. Why is it that some children and adolescents may need long-term care?

10. Why has long-term care become an important service for people with HIV/AIDS?

11. Discuss the three different models of adult day care. Which services are common to all three models?

12. Enumerate the main functions of long-term care case management.

13. Briefly discuss the three main models of case management in the delivery of long-term care.

14. What are the similarities and differences between the S/HMO and PACE models?

15. Briefly discuss the continuum of institutional long-term care services.

16. What is the difference between licensure and certification? What are the two types of certifications? What purpose does each serve from (1) a clinical standpoint and (2) a financial standpoint?

17. What are the main institutional settings for the delivery of subacute care?

18. Which services does a continuing care retirement community provide?

19. Even though the elderly are the primary users of nursing homes and, generally speaking, Medicare is the primary source of payment for health care services provided to the elderly, why does Medicare pay only a small fraction of the cost of nursing home care?

20. Why has private long-term care insurance not gained popularity with consumers?

## REFERENCES

Aaronson, W. 1996. Financing the continuum of care: A disintegrating past and an integrating future. In: *The continuum of long-term care: An integrated systems approach.* C.J. Evashwick, ed. Albany, NY: Delmar Publishers. pp. 223–252.

AARP Studies Adult Foster Care for the Elderly. 1996. *Public Health Reports* 111, no. 4: 295.

Administration on Aging. 2011. *Nutrition services (OAA Title IIIC).* Available at: http://www.aoa .gov/aoaroot/aoa_programs/hcltc/nutrition_services/index.aspx. Accessed March 2011.

Alecxih, L. 2001. The impact of sociodemographic change on the future of long-term care. *Generations* 25, no. 1: 7–11.

Altman, B.M. 1995. *Elderly persons with developmental disabilities in long-term care facilities.* AHCPR Pub. No. 95–0084. Rockville, MD: Agency for Health Care Policy and Research.

America's Health Insurance Plans. 2004. *Long term care insurance in 2002: Research findings.* Washington, DC: AHIP.

Anderson, G.F. 2003. Physician, public, and policymaker perspectives on chronic conditions. *Archives of Internal Medicine* 163, no. 4: 437–442.

Braddock, D. 2001. Expert witness report of David Braddock, Ph.D. for the United States District Court Northern District of Illinois in *Boudreau v. Ryan*, Case Number 00 C 5392. Available at: http://www.iacdd.org/braddock.html. Accessed February 2011.

Broe, G., and A. Jorm. 1999. Carer distress in the general population: Results from the Sydney Older Persons Study. *Age and Ageing* 28, no. 3: 307–311.

Buntin, M.B. et al. 2005. How much is postacute care use affected by its availability? *Health Services Research* 40, no. 2: 413–434.

Burwell, B. et al. 1996. Financing long-term care. In: *The continuum of long-term care: An integrated systems approach.* C.J. Evashwick, ed. Albany, NY: Delmar Publishers. pp. 193–221.

Cohen, M.A. et al. 1988. Attitudes toward joining continuing care retirement communities. *The Gerontologist* 28, no. 5: 637–643.

Compston, A., and A. Coles. 2002. Multiple sclerosis. *Lancet* 359, no. 9313: 1221–1231.

Department of Health and Human Services (DHHS). 2006. *Health, United States, 2006.* Hyattsville, MD: Department of Health and Human Services.

Department of Health and Human Services (DHHS). 2010. *Health, United States, 2010.* Hyattsville, MD: Department of Health and Human Services.

Dychtwald, K. et al. 1990. *Implementing eldercare services: Strategies that work.* New York: McGraw-Hill.

Federal Interagency Forum on Aging-Related Statistics. 2010. *Older Americans 2010: Key indicators of well-being.* Washington, DC: US Government Printing Office.

Fein, E.B. 1994. Foster care for elderly: Like a new home. *New York Times.* March 8, A1.

Fischer, L.R. 2003. Community-based care and risk of nursing home placement. *Medical Care* 41, no. 12: 1407–1416.

Fisher, K., and P. Kettl. 2005. Aging with mental retardation. *Geriatrics* 60, no. 4: 26–29.

Ford-Martin, P.A. 2003. *Mental retardation.* Available at: http://www.healthatoz.com/healthatoz /Atoz/common/standard/transform.jsp?requestURI=/healthatoz/Atoz/ency/mental_retardation .jsp. Accessed March 2003.

Ghose, M. 2007. Press release by the American Health Insurance Plans, November 5, 2007. Available at: http://www.ahip.org/content/pressrelease.aspx?docid=21354. Accessed March 2011.

Gross, D.L. et al. 2004. The growing pains of integrated health care for the elderly: Lessons from the expansion of PACE. *The Milbank Quarterly* 82, no. 2: 257–282.

Heller, T. et al. 1998. Impact of age and transitions out of nursing homes for adults with developmental disabilities. *American Journal of Mental Retardation* 103, no. 3: 236–248.

Hoffman, E. 2001. When the old age home is your own. *Business Week* December 10: 94–96.

Holtz-Eakin, D. 2005. *CBO testimony: The cost of financing of long-term care services.* Before the Subcommittee on Health Committee on Energy and Commerce. US House of Representatives. April 27, 2005.

Kaye, H.S. et al. 2010. Long-term care: Who gets it, who provides it, who pays, and how much? *Health Affairs* 29, no. 1: 11–21.

Kearney, F. et al. 2010. The ageing of HIV: Implications for geriatric medicine. *Age and Ageing* 39, no. 5: 536–541.

Kirwin, P.M. 1991. *Adult day care: The relationship of formal and informal systems of care.* New York: Garland Publishing.

Kuzuya, M. et al. 2011. Impact of informal care levels on discontinuation of living at home in community-dwelling dependent elderly using various community-based services. *Archives of Gerontology & Geriatrics* 52, no. 2: 127–132.

Levine, C. et al. 2010. Bridging troubled waters: Family caregivers, transitions, and long-term care. *Health Affairs* 29, no. 1: 116–124.

Luckasson, R.A. et al. 1992. *Mental retardation: Definition, classification, and systems of support.* 9th ed. Washington, DC: American Association on Mental Retardation.

Medicare Payment Advisory Commission (MedPAC). 2004. *New approaches in Medicare: Report to the Congress.* Washington, DC: Medicare Payment Advisory Commission.

Mehta, K.M. et al. 2002. Cognitive impairment, depressive symptoms, and functional decline in older people. *Journal of the American Geriatric Society* 50, no. 6: 1045–1050.

MetLife Mature Market Institute. 2010. *The MetLife national study of adult day services.* Westport, CT: Metropolitan Life Insurance Company.

Micheletti, J.A., and T.J. Shlala. 1995. Understanding and operationalizing subacute services. *Nursing Management* 26, no. 6: 49–56.

Millen, B.E. et al. 2002. The elderly nutrition program: An effective national framework for preventive nutrition interventions. *Journal of the American Dietetic Association* 102, no. 2: 234–240.

Munn, J.C. et al. 2006. Is hospice associated with improved end-of-life care in nursing homes and assisted living facilities? *Journal of the American Geriatrics Society* 54, no. 3: 490–495.

National Academy on an Aging Society. 2000. *Caregiving: Helping the elderly with activity limitations.* Washington, DC: National Academy on an Aging Society.

National Adult Day Services Association (NADSA). 2003. Available at: http://www.nadsa.org. Accessed March 2003.

National Center for Assisted Living. 2006. Assisted living resident profile. Available at: http://www.ncal.org. Accessed January 2007.

Park-Lee, E.Y., and F.H. Decker. 2010. *Comparison of home health and hospice care agencies by organizational characteristics and services provided: United States, 2007.* Hyattsville, MD: National Center for Health Statistics.

Ritchie, K., and S. Lovestone. 2002. The dementias. *Lancet* 360, no. 9347: 1759–1766.

Rouse, B.A. 1995. *Substance abuse and mental health statistics sourcebook.* DHHS Publication No. (SMA) 953064. Washington, DC: Government Printing Office.

Sanofi-Aventis. 2010. *Managed care digest series, 2010–2011: Public Payer Digest.* Bridgewater, NJ: Sanofi-Aventis US, LLC.

Satariano, W.A. 1997. Editorial: The disabilities of aging—Looking to the physical environment. *American Journal of Public Health* 87, no. 3: 331–332.

Scharlach, A.E. et al. 2001. *Case management in long-term care integration: An overview of current programs and evaluations.* Center for the Advanced Study of Aging Services, University of California, Berkeley, November 2001.

Schofield H. et al. 1998. *Family caregivers: Disability, illness and ageing.* Sydney: Allen & Unwin.

Scocco, P. et al. 2006. Nursing home institutionalization: A source of eustress or distress for the elderly. *International Journal of Geriatric Psychiatry* 21, no. 3: 281–287.

Shin, J.K. et al. 2002. Quality of care measurement in nursing home AIDS care: A pilot study. *Journal of the Association of Nurses in AIDS Care* 13, no. 2: 70–76.

Singh, D.A. 2010. *Effective management of long-term care facilities.* 2nd ed. Boston: Jones and Bartlett Publishers.

Skaggs, R.L., and H.R. Hawkins. 1994. Architecture for long-term care facilities. In: *Essentials of long-term care administration.* S.B. Goldsmith, ed. Gaithersburg, MD: Aspen Publishers, Inc. pp. 254–284.

Spreat, S. et al. 1998. Improve quality in nursing homes or institute community placement? Implementation of OBRA for individuals with mental retardation. *Research in Developmental Disabilities* 19, no. 6: 507–518.

Stahl, C. 1997. Adult foster care: An alternative to SNFs? *ADVANCE for Occupational Therapists* September 29: 18.

Tedesco, J. 1996. Adult day care. In: *The continuum of long-term care: An integrated systems approach.* C.J. Evashwick, ed. Albany, NY: Delmar Publishers.

Thomas, K.E. et al. 2010. Conversion diversion: Participation in a social HMO reduces the likelihood of converting from short-stay to long-stay nursing facility placement. *Journal of the American Medical Directors Association* 11, no. 5: 333–337.

Tune, L. 2001. Assessing psychiatric illness in geriatric patients. *Clinical Cornerstone* 3, no. 3: 23–36.

Van Houtven, C.H., and E. Norton. 2004. Informal care and health care use of older adults. *Journal of Health Economics* 23, no. 6: 1159–1180.

Vogeli, C. et al. 2007. Multiple chronic conditions: Prevalence, health consequences, and implications for quality, care management, and costs. *Journal of General Internal Medicine* 22, Suppl. 3: 391–395.

# Chapter 11

## Health Services for Special Populations

### Learning Objectives

- To learn about population groups facing greater challenges and barriers in accessing health care services
- To understand the racial and ethnic disparities in health status
- To get acquainted with the health concerns of America's children and the health services available to them
- To learn about the health concerns of America's women and health services available to them
- To appreciate the challenges faced in rural health and to learn about measures taken to improve access to care
- To learn about the characteristics and health concerns of the homeless population
- To understand the nation's mental health system
- To understand the AIDS epidemic in America, the population groups affected by it, and the services available to HIV/AIDS patients

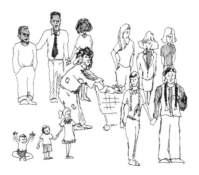

*They all have something in common.*

## Introduction

Certain population groups in the United States face greater challenges than the general population in accessing timely and needed health care services (Lurie 1997; Shortell et al. 1996). They are at greater risk of poor physical, psychological, and/or social health (Aday 1994). Various terms are used to describe these populations, such as "underserved populations," "medically underserved," "medically disadvantaged," "underprivileged," and "American underclasses." The causes of their vulnerability are largely attributable to unequal social, economic, health, and geographic conditions. These population groups consist of racial and ethnic minorities, uninsured children, women, those living in rural areas, the homeless, the mentally ill, the chronically

ill and disabled, and those with human immunodeficiency virus (HIV)/acquired immune deficiency syndrome (AIDS). These population groups are more vulnerable than the general population and experience greater barriers in access to care, financing of care, and racial or cultural acceptance. After presenting a conceptual framework to study vulnerable populations, this chapter defines these population groups, describes their health needs, and summarizes the major challenges they face.

## Framework to Study Vulnerable Populations

The vulnerability framework (see Exhibit 11–1) is an integrated approach to studying

Exhibit 11–1  The Vulnerability Framework

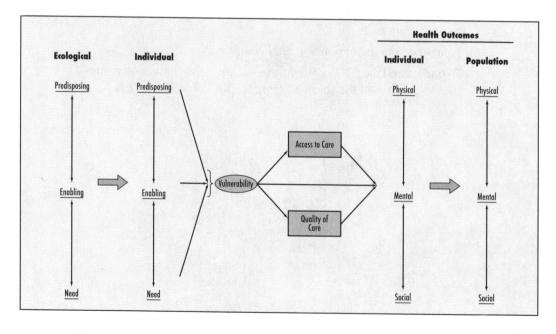

vulnerability (Shi and Stevens 2010). From a health perspective, vulnerability refers to the likelihood of experiencing poor health or illness. Poor health can be manifested physically, psychologically, and/or socially. Because poor health along one dimension is likely to be compounded by poor health along others, the health needs are greater for those with problems along multiple dimensions than those with problems along a single dimension.

According to the framework, vulnerability is determined by a convergence of (1) predisposing, (2) enabling, and (3) need characteristics at both individual and ecological (contextual) levels (see Exhibit 11–2). Not only do these predisposing, enabling, and need characteristics converge and determine individuals' access to health care, they also ultimately influence individuals' risk of contracting illness or, for those already sick, recovering from illness. Individuals with multiple risks (i.e., a combination of two or more vulnerability traits) typically experience worse access to care, care of lesser quality, and inferior health status than do those with fewer vulnerability traits.

Understanding vulnerability as a combination or convergence of disparate factors is preferred over studying individual factors separately because vulnerability, when defined as a convergence of risks, best captures reality. This approach not only reflects the co-occurrence of risk factors, but underscores the belief that it is difficult to address disparities in one risk factor without addressing others.

The vulnerability model previously presented has a number of distinctive characteristics. First, it is a comprehensive model, including both individual and ecological attributes of risk. Second, this is a general model, focusing on the attributes of vulnerability for the total population rather than focusing on vulnerable traits of subpopulations. Although we recognize individual differences in exposure to risks, we also think there are common, crosscutting traits affecting all vulnerable populations. Third, a major distinction of our model is the emphasis on the convergence of vulnerability. The effects of experiencing multiple vulnerable traits may lead to cumulative vulnerability that is additive or even multiplicative. Examining vulnerability as a multidimensional construct can also demonstrate gradient relationships between vulnerability status and outcomes of interest and, thus, improve our understanding of the patterns and factors related to the outcomes of interest.

Exhibit 11–2 Predisposing, Enabling, and Need Characteristics of Vulnerability

**Predisposing Characteristics**
- Racial/ethnic characteristics
- Gender and age (women and children)
- Geographic location (rural health)

**Enabling characteristics**
- Insurance status (uninsured)
- Homelessness

**Need characteristics**
- Mental health
- Chronic illness/disability
- HIV/AIDS

# Racial/Ethnic Minorities

The 2010 census questionnaire lists 15 racial categories, as well as places to write in specific races not listed on the form (US Census Bureau 2009). These are White, Black, American Indian or Alaska Native, Asian Indian, Chinese, Filipino, Japanese, Korean, Vietnamese, Other Asian, Native Hawaii, Guamanian or Chamorro, Samoan, Other Pacific Islander, or some other race. The 2010 Census continues the option first introduced in the 2000 Census for respondents to choose more than one race.

The US Census Bureau estimated that, in 2008, over 34% of the US population was made up of minorities: Black or African Americans (12.2%), Hispanics or Latinos (15.4%), Asians (4.4%), Native Hawaiian and Other Pacific Islanders

(0.1%), and American Indian and Alaska Natives (0.8%). In addition, 1.5% identified as two or more races (US Census Bureau 2010).

Significant differences exist across the various racial/ethnic groups on health-related lifestyles and health status. For example, in 2006, the percentage of live births weighing less than 2,500 grams (low birth weight) was greatest among Blacks, followed by Asians or Pacific Islanders, American Indians or Native Americans, Whites, and Hispanics (Figure 11–1). Asians and Pacific Islanders were most likely to begin prenatal care during their first trimester, followed by Whites, Hispanics, Blacks, and American Indians or Alaska Natives (Table 11–1). Mothers of Asian and Pacific Islander origin are least likely to smoke cigarettes during pregnancy, followed by Hispanics, Blacks,

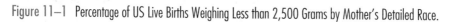

Figure 11–1   Percentage of US Live Births Weighing Less than 2,500 Grams by Mother's Detailed Race.

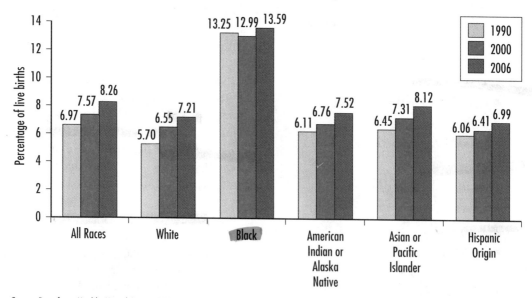

*Source:* Data from *Health, United States, 2009*, p. 163.

Table 11–1  Characteristics of US Mothers by Race/Ethnicity

| Item | 1970 | 1980 | 1990 | 2000 | 2006 |
|---|---|---|---|---|---|
| **Prenatal care began during 1st trimester** | | | | | |
| All mothers | 68.0 | 76.3 | 75.8 | 83.2 | 83.2 |
| White | 72.3 | 79.2 | 79.2 | 85.0 | 84.7 |
| Black | 44.2 | 62.4 | 60.6 | 74.3 | 76.0 |
| American Indian or Alaskan Native | 38.2 | 55.8 | 57.9 | 69.3 | 69.5 |
| Asian or Pacific Islander | — | 73.7 | 75.1 | 84.0 | 84.8 |
| Hispanic origin | — | 60.2 | 60.2 | 74.4 | 77.3 |
| **Education of mother 16 years or more** | | | | | |
| All mothers | 8.6 | 14.0 | 17.5 | 24.7 | 26.6* |
| White | 9.6 | 15.5 | 19.3 | 26.3 | 27.9* |
| Black | 2.8 | 6.2 | 7.2 | 11.7 | 13.4* |
| American Indian or Alaska Native | 2.7 | 3.5 | 4.4 | 7.8 | 8.5* |
| Asian or Pacific Islander | — | 30.8 | 31.0 | 42.8 | 47.1* |
| Hispanic origin | — | 4.2 | 5.1 | 7.6 | 8.7* |
| **Low birth weight (less than 2,500 grams)** | | | | | |
| All mothers | 7.93 | 6.84 | 6.97 | 7.57 | 8.26 |
| White | 6.85 | 5.72 | 5.70 | 6.55 | 7.21 |
| Black | 13.90 | 12.69 | 13.25 | 12.99 | 13.59 |
| American Indian or Alaska Native | 7.97 | 6.44 | 6.11 | 6.76 | 7.52 |
| Asian or Pacific Islander | — | 6.68 | 6.45 | 7.31 | 8.12 |
| Hispanic origin (selected states) | — | 6.12 | 6.06 | 6.41 | 6.99 |

*Source:* Data from *Health, United States, 2007*, p. 144; *Health, United States, 2009*, pp. 159, 163.
*Data from 2003.

and Whites (Figure 11–2). The White adult population is more likely to consume alcohol than other races (Figure 11–3). Among women 40 years of age and older, utilization of mammography is the highest among Whites and lowest among Hispanics (Figure 11–4).

## Black Americans

Black Americans are more likely to be economically disadvantaged than Whites. Likewise, they fall behind in health status, despite progress made during the past few decades. Blacks have shorter life expectancies than

Figure 11–2  Percentage of US Mothers Who Smoked Cigarettes During Pregnancy According to Mother's Race.

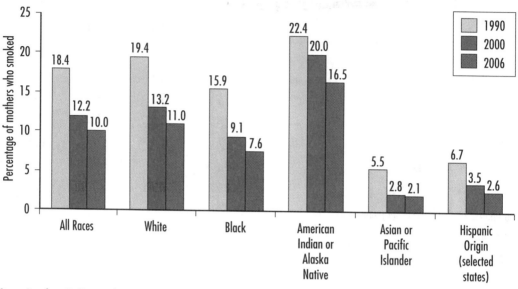

Source: Data from Health, United States, 2009, p. 162.

Figure 11–3  Alcohol Consumption by Persons 18 Years of Age and Over.

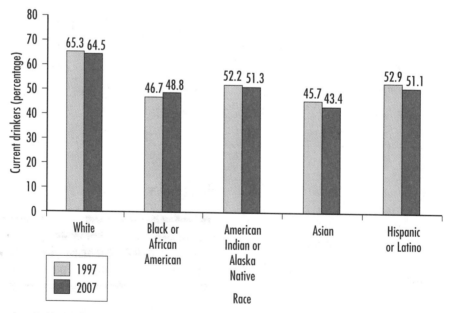

Source: Data from Health, United States, 2009, p. 286.

Figure 11–4 Use of Mammography by Women 40 Years of Age and Over, 2008.

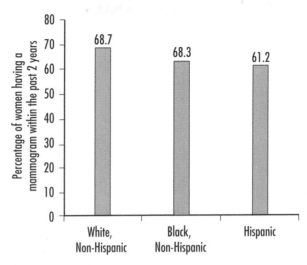

*Source:* Data from *Health, United States, 2009,* p. 329.

Whites (Figure 11–5); higher age-adjusted death rates for leading causes of death (Table 11–2); higher age-adjusted maternal mortality rates (Figure 11–6); and higher infant, neonatal, and postneonatal mortality rates (Table 11–3). On self-reported measures of health status, Blacks are more likely to report fair or poor health status

Figure 11–5 US Life Expectancy at Birth, 1970–2006.

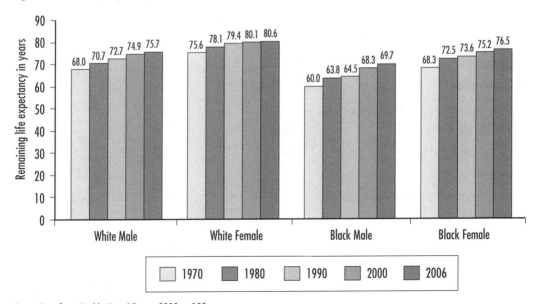

*Source:* Data from *Health, United States, 2009,* p. 123.

Table 11–2  Age-Adjusted Death Rates for Selected Causes of Death (1970–2006)

| Race and Cause of Death | 1970 | 1980 | 1990 | 2000 | 2006 |
|---|---|---|---|---|---|
| **All persons** | Deaths per 100,000 standard population | | | | |
| All causes | 1,222.6 | 1,039.1 | 938.7 | 869.0 | 776.5 |
| Diseases of the heart | 492.7 | 412.1 | 321.8 | 257.6 | 200.2 |
| Ischemic heart disease | — | 345.2 | 249.6 | 186.8 | 134.9 |
| Cerebrovascular diseases | 147.7 | 96.2 | 65.3 | 60.9 | 43.6 |
| Malignant neoplasms | 198.6 | 207.9 | 216.0 | 199.6 | 180.7 |
| Chronic lower respiratory diseases | 21.3 | 28.3 | 37.2 | 44.2 | 40.5 |
| Influenza and pneumonia | 41.7 | 31.4 | 36.8 | 23.7 | 17.8 |
| Chronic liver disease and cirrhosis | 17.8 | 15.1 | 11.1 | 9.5 | 8.8 |
| Diabetes mellitus | 24.3 | 18.1 | 20.7 | 25.0 | 23.3 |
| Human immunodeficiency virus (HIV) disease | — | — | 10.2 | 5.2 | 4.0 |
| Unintentional injuries | 60.1 | 46.4 | 36.3 | 34.9 | 39.8 |
| Motor vehicle-related injuries | 27.6 | 22.3 | 18.5 | 15.4 | 15.0 |
| Suicide | 13.1 | 12.2 | 12.5 | 10.4 | 10.9 |
| Homicide | 8.8 | 10.4 | 9.4 | 5.9 | 6.2 |
| **White** | | | | | |
| All causes | 1,193.3 | 1,012.7 | 909.8 | 849.8 | 764.4 |
| Diseases of the heart | 492.2 | 409.4 | 317.0 | 253.4 | 197.0 |
| Ischemic heart disease | — | 347.6 | 249.7 | 185.6 | 134.2 |
| Cerebrovascular diseases | 143.5 | 93.2 | 62.8 | 58.8 | 41.7 |
| Malignant neoplasms | 196.7 | 204.2 | 211.6 | 197.2 | 179.9 |
| Chronic lower respiratory diseases | 21.8 | 29.3 | 38.3 | 46.0 | 42.6 |
| Influenza and pneumonia | 39.8 | 30.9 | 36.4 | 23.5 | 17.7 |
| Chronic liver disease and cirrhosis | 16.6 | 13.9 | 10.5 | 9.6 | 9.1 |
| Diabetes mellitus | 22.9 | 16.7 | 18.8 | 22.8 | 21.2 |
| Human immunodeficiency virus (HIV) disease | — | — | 8.3 | 2.8 | 2.1 |
| Unintentional injuries | 57.8 | 45.3 | 35.5 | 35.1 | 41.0 |
| Motor vehicle-related injuries | 27.1 | 22.6 | 18.5 | 15.6 | 15.4 |
| Suicide | 13.8 | 13.0 | 13.4 | 11.3 | 12.1 |
| Homicide | 4.7 | 6.7 | 5.5 | 3.6 | 3.7 |

**Black**

| | | | | | |
|---|---|---|---|---|---|
| All causes | 1,518.1 | 1,314.8 | 1,250.3 | 1,121.4 | 982.0 |
| Diseases of the heart | 512.0 | 455.3 | 391.5 | 324.8 | 257.7 |
| Ischemic heart disease | — | 334.5 | 267.0 | 218.3 | 161.6 |
| Cerebrovascular diseases | 197.1 | 129.1 | 91.6 | 81.9 | 61.6 |
| Malignant neoplasms | 225.3 | 256.4 | 279.5 | 248.5 | 217.4 |
| Chronic lower respiratory diseases | 16.2 | 19.2 | 28.1 | 31.6 | 28.1 |
| Influenza and pneumonia | 57.2 | 34.4 | 39.4 | 25.6 | 19.6 |
| Chronic liver disease and cirrhosis | 28.1 | 25.0 | 16.5 | 9.4 | 7.0 |
| Diabetes mellitus | 38.8 | 32.7 | 40.5 | 49.5 | 45.1 |
| Human immunodeficiency virus (HIV) disease | — | — | 26.7 | 23.3 | 18.6 |
| Unintentional injuries | 78.3 | 57.6 | 43.8 | 37.7 | 38.3 |
| Motor vehicle-related injuries | 31.1 | 20.2 | 18.8 | 15.7 | 14.6 |
| Suicide | 6.2 | 6.5 | 7.1 | 5.5 | 5.1 |
| Homicide | 44.0 | 39.0 | 36.3 | 20.5 | 21.6 |

*Source:* Data from *Health, United States, 2009*, pp. 190–191, Centers for Disease Control and Prevention, National Center for Health Statistics.

Figure 11–6  Age-Adjusted Maternal Mortality Rates.

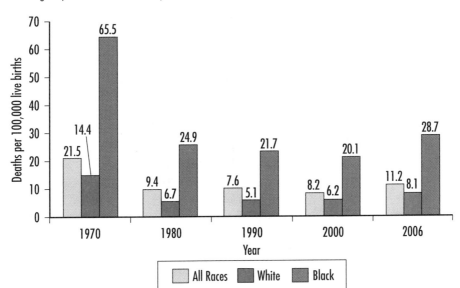

*Source:* Data from *Health, United States, 2009*, p. 231.

Table 11–3  Infant, Neonatal, and Postneonatal Mortality Rates by Mother's Race (per 1,000 live births)

| Race of Mother | Infant Deaths | | | | Neonatal Deaths | | | | Postneonatal Deaths | | | |
|---|---|---|---|---|---|---|---|---|---|---|---|---|
| | 1983 | 1990 | 2000 | 2005 | 1983 | 1990 | 2000 | 2005 | 1983 | 1990 | 2000 | 2005 |
| All mothers | 10.9 | 8.9 | 6.9 | 6.9 | 7.1 | 5.7 | 4.6 | 4.5 | 3.8 | 3.2 | 2.3 | 2.3 |
| White | 9.3 | 7.3 | 5.7 | 5.7 | 6.1 | 4.6 | 3.8 | 3.8 | 3.2 | 2.7 | 1.9 | 2.0 |
| Black | 19.2 | 16.9 | 13.5 | 13.3 | 12.5 | 11.1 | 9.1 | 8.9 | 6.7 | 5.9 | 4.3 | 4.3 |
| American Indian or Alaska Native | 15.2 | 13.1 | 8.3 | 8.1 | 7.5 | 6.1 | 4.4 | 4.0 | 7.7 | 7.0 | 3.9 | 4.0 |
| Asian or Pacific Islander | 8.3 | 6.6 | 4.9 | 4.9 | 5.2 | 3.9 | 3.4 | 3.4 | 3.1 | 2.7 | 1.4 | 1.5 |
| Hispanic origin (selected states) | 9.5 | 7.5 | 5.6 | 5.6 | 6.2 | 4.8 | 3.8 | 3.9 | 3.3 | 2.9 | 1.8 | 1.8 |

Source: Data from *Health, United States, 2009*, p. 176.

Figure 11–7  Respondent-Assessed Health Status.

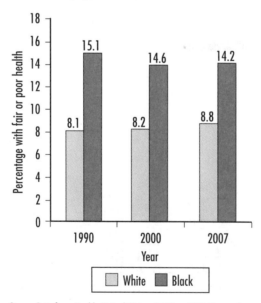

Source: Data from *Health, United States, 1995*, p. 172, Centers for Disease Control and Prevention, National Center for Health Statistics, 1996, and *Health, United States, 2009*, p. 270.

Figure 11–8   Current Cigarette Smoking by Persons 18 Years of Age and Over, Age Adjusted, 2007.

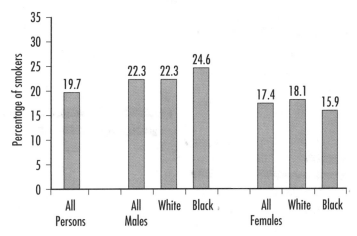

Source: Data from *Health, United States, 2009*, p. 276, Centers for Disease Control and Prevention, National Center for Health Statistics, 2010.

than Whites (Figure 11–7). In terms of behavioral risks, Black males are slightly more likely to smoke cigarettes than White males (24.6 versus 22.3%), but White females are more likely to smoke than Black females (18.1 versus 15.9%) (Figure 11–8), although smoking among Black females has increased. Conversely, Blacks have lower levels of serum cholesterol than Whites (Table 11–4).

Table 11–4   Serum Cholesterol Levels Among Persons 20 Years and Older, 2003–2006

| Sex and Race* | Percentage of Persons 20 Years of Age and Over with Hypertension | Mean Serum Cholesterol Level (mg/dl) of Persons 20 Years of Age and Over | Percentage of Overweight Persons 20 Years of Age and Over |
|---|---|---|---|
| Both sexes | 31.3 | 200 | 66.7 |
| White | | | |
| Male | 31.2 | 198 | 71.8 |
| Female | 28.3 | 203 | 57.9 |
| Black | | | |
| Male | 40.6 | 193 | 71.6 |
| Female | 44.1 | 195 | 79.8 |

*20–74 years, age adjusted.

*Source:* Data from *Health, United States, 2009*, pp. 293, 296, 301, Centers for Disease Control and Prevention, National Center for Health Statistics, Division of Health Examination Statistics, 2010.

## Hispanic Americans

The Hispanic segment of the US population is growing at a significantly higher rate than other population segments. Between 2000 and 2008, the Hispanic segment increased by 33%, compared to the 8% increase in the total population (US Census Bureau 2010). In 2008, the Hispanic population numbered nearly 47 million and is projected to reach 57 million by the year 2015. Hispanic Americans are also one of the youngest groups among Americans. In 2008, the median age among Hispanic Americans was 27.7, compared to 41.1 years for non-Hispanic Whites, and 11.3% are below age 5, compared to 5.6% of non-Hispanic Whites (US Census Bureau 2010). As of 2005, 58.5% of Hispanic Americans 25 years of age and older had completed high school, compared to 87.5% of Whites, and 12% of Hispanic Americans 25 years of age and older had completed college, compared to 28% of Whites (US Census Bureau 2007). In 2007, 20.7% of Hispanic persons lived below the federal poverty level (FPL), compared to 9.0% of non-Hispanic White persons (US Census Bureau 2010).

Many Hispanic Americans experience significant barriers in accessing medical care. Many Hispanic families who immigrated to the United States may not qualify for Medicaid (Rosenbaum and Darnell 1997). This represents a greater problem for those from Central America (79% foreign born) and South America (75% foreign born) than those from Spain (17% foreign born) or Mexico (28% foreign born). Place of birth is also related to Hispanic people's inability to speak English, which is another factor associated with reduced access to medical services (Solis et al. 1990). Low education is related to employment and occupational status. Hispanic Americans have higher unemployment rates than non-Hispanic Whites (12.8 versus 8.8% in 2010; BLS 2010) and are more likely to be employed in semiskilled, nonprofessional occupations (US Census Bureau 2007). Due to the close association between employment status and health insurance, Hispanic Americans are more likely to be uninsured or underinsured than non-Hispanic Whites. In 2007, 31.8% of Hispanic persons were uninsured, compared to 16.3% of non-Hispanic Whites and 17% of non-Hispanic Blacks or African Americans (National Center for Health Statistics 2010). Among Hispanics, 34.7% of Mexican Americans were uninsured, followed by 20.7% of Cubans, 12.8% of Puerto Ricans, and 32.7% of other Hispanics (National Center for Health Statistics 2010).

Homicide was the sixth leading cause of death for Hispanic males in 2006. They have the highest ranking, along with Blacks, for this cause of death (National Center for Health Statistics 2010).

Hispanic Americans are less likely to take advantage of preventive care than non-Hispanic Whites and certain other races. Hispanic women 40 years of age or older were least likely to use mammography (61.2 versus 68.9% for non-Hispanic Whites and 68.3% for non-Hispanic Blacks; see Figure 11–4). In 2006, fewer Hispanic mothers began their prenatal care during the first trimester than mothers of other ethnic groups (76.7% for Hispanic mothers versus 85.4% for White mothers and 84.8% for Asian and Pacific Islander mothers; see Table 11–1). In 2007, 78% of Hispanic children aged 19–35 months had received the combined series vaccines (4:3:1:3:3:1), compared to 78% of White children, 79% of Asian children, 75% of Black children, and 83% of American Indian and Alaska

Native children (National Center for Health Statistics 2010). Among Hispanics 2 years of age and older in 2007, 55.8% had at least one dental visit during a year, compared to 68.7% for non-Hispanic Whites (National Center for Health Statistics 2010). Among Hispanics 2 years of age and older in 2007, 55.8% had at least one dental visit during a year, compared to 68.7% for non-Hispanic Whites (National Center for Health Statistics 2010).

People of Hispanic origin also experience greater behavioral risks than Whites and certain other racial/ethnic groups. For example, among individuals 18 years of age or older in 2007, a higher proportion of Hispanics were current drinkers than people of other ethnic origins (51.1% for Hispanics versus 48.8% for Blacks and 43.3% for Asians; see Figure 11–3). However, fewer Hispanics smoked, compared to people from other ethnic groups. In 2007, 18.7% of Hispanic males 18 years of age and older identified themselves as "current smokers," compared to 24.1% of non-Hispanic White males and 25.5% of non-Hispanic Black males (National Center for Health Statistics 2010). Among female adults, 9.7% of Hispanics smoked in 2007, compared to 20.7% of non-Hispanic Whites and 17.1% of non-Hispanic Blacks (National Center for Health Statistics 2010).

## Asian Americans

Minority health epidemiology has typically focused on Blacks, Hispanics, and American Indians or Alaska Natives because Asian Americans (AAs) have relatively small numbers. To include the diversity of AAs, the National Center for Health Statistics has expanded the race codes into nine categories: White, Black, Native American, Chinese, Japanese, Hawaiian, Filipino, Other Asian/Pacific Islanders, and other races. But even the category of "Other Asian/Pacific Islander" is extremely heterogeneous, encompassing 21 subgroups with different health profiles. In 2008, Asians accounted for 4.5% of the US population and numbered 13.5 million (US Census Bureau 2010).

AAs constitute one of the fastest-growing population segments in the United States. The percent change in the Asian population was 28% between 2000 and 2008, compared to 5.3% for the population as a whole (US Census Bureau 2010). The US Census Bureau (2010) projects that the AA population will reach 16.5 million by 2015.

In education, income, and health, Asian Americans and Pacific Islanders (AA/PI) are very diverse. In 2008, 88.7% AA/PIs 25 years of age or older had at least 4 years of high school education, compared with 87.1% of non-Hispanic Whites; in addition, the percentage of AA/PIs with a bachelor's degree or higher was 52.6%, compared to 29.8% for non-Hispanic Whites (US Census Bureau 2010). Educational attainment varies greatly among the subgroups. For example, in 1990, 88% of the adults of Japanese descent had graduated from high school, whereas among Vietnamese it was 61% and only 31% among Hmong adults (Kuo and Porter 1998). In 2007, the median income for Asian males (aged 15 years and older) was $37,193, compared to $35,141 for non-Hispanic White males (US Census Bureau 2010). In addition, in 2007, a smaller percentage of Asians (10.2%) lived below the FPL, compared to Whites (10.5%), Blacks (24.5%), and Hispanics (21.5%; US Census Bureau 2010).

The heterogeneity of the AA/PI population is reflected in the various indicators of health status. For instance, a greater percentage of Vietnamese and Korean (17.2 and 12.8%, respectively) people assess their own health status as fair or poor, compared to people of Chinese, Filipino, and Japanese descent (6.1 to 7.4%) (Kuo and Porter 1998). The incidence of low-birth-weight babies varies greatly, from 4.5% among Chinese to 7% among Filipinos. Cambodian refugees have extremely high rates of posttraumatic stress disorder, dissociation, depression, and anxiety. Although US smoking rates are reported to be lowest among AA/PIs, 92% of Laotians, 71% of Cambodians, and 65% of Vietnamese are smokers (Yoon and Chien 1996). Compared with Whites, Korean-American men have a five-fold incidence of stomach cancer and an eight-fold incidence of liver cancer. Cultural practices and attitudes may prevent AA/PI women from receiving adequate breast cancer screening and prenatal care. A study analyzing National Health Interview Survey data from 1997 to 2000 found that Chinese, Asian Indian, Filipino, and other AA/PI children were more likely to be without contact with a health professional within the past 12 months, compared to non-Hispanic White children. Citizenship/nativity status, maternal education attainment, and poverty status were all significant independent risk factors for health care access and utilization (Yu et al. 2004). Ignorance of this bipolar distribution contributes to the myth of a minority population that is both healthy and economically successful. For example, the 1985 Department of Health and Human Services (DHHS) Task Force Report on Black and Minority Health stated that, as a group, the AA/PI population in the United States is at lower risk of early death than the White population. Such a misunderstanding demonstrates an essential need for more in-depth, ethnic-specific health research.

## American Indians and Alaska Natives

In 2008, 3.1 million people identified their race as American Indian or Alaska Native alone, and nearly 4.9 million people identified themselves American Indian or Alaska Native in combination with other races (US Census Bureau 2010). More than one-half live in urban areas (IHS 2010a). According to the Census Bureau, this subpopulation is growing at a rate of 1.7% per year (IHS 2010a). Concomitantly, demand for expanded health care has been on the rise for several decades and is becoming more acute. The incidence and prevalence of certain diseases and conditions, such as diabetes, hypertension, infant mortality and morbidity, chemical dependency, and AIDS- and HIV-related morbidity, are all high enough to be matters of prime concern. Compared to the general US population, Native Americans also have much higher death rates from alcoholism, tuberculosis, diabetes, injuries, suicide, and homicide (IHS 2010b).

It is also no secret that Native Americans continue to occupy the bottom of the socioeconomic strata. American Indians/Alaska Natives are approximately twice as likely to be poor, unemployed, and not to have a college degree, compared to the general populations of the areas in which they live (Castor et al. 2006). A strong positive association exists between socioeconomic status and health status. For example, poverty, not cultural factors, has been found to be associated with the high injury-related mortality rate among Indian children. The effects of Indian poverty are exacerbated by an acute political disempowerment.

The health status of American Indian people appears to be improving, yet it significantly lags behind the health status of the population at large. In the years 1972 to 1974,

poverty = low health

the mortality rate among Native American expectant mothers was 27.7 per 100,000 live births (Pleasant 2003). By 1996, the occurrence rate was only 6.1%—a 78% drop. Infant mortality also declined from 22.2 per 1,000 births in 1972 to 8.1 per 1,000 births in 2005. Still, Native Americans experience significant health disparities when compared to the general US population. The life expectancy of Native Americans is 4.6 years fewer than the US population as a whole (IHS 2010b). Native Americans die at higher rates than other Americans from alcohol (519% higher), tuberculosis (500% higher), diabetes (195% higher), unintentional injuries (149% higher), homicide (92% higher), and suicide (72% higher; IHS 2010b).

The provision of health services to American Indians by the federal government was first negotiated in 1832, as partial compensation for land cessions. Subsequent laws have expanded the scope of services and allowed American Indians greater autonomy in planning, developing, and administering their own health care programs. These laws explicitly permit the practice of traditional, as well as Western, medicine.

## Indian Health Care Improvement Act

The Indian Health Care Improvement Act was enacted in 1976. This law, and later amendments in 1980, outlined a 7-year effort to help bring American Indian health to a level of parity with the general population. Although appropriations were significantly increased to improve or develop sanitation services, health care programs, and medical facilities, limited fiscal support undermined the Act's goal of achieving health parity for American Indians. Other features of the Act provided for specific funding for programs to improve access to health care for urban Indians and educational scholarships to increase the number of Indian health care professionals. Thus, the Act has at least been successful in minimizing prejudice, building trust, and putting responsibility back into the hands of American Indians.

## Indian Health Service   IHS

Chapter 6 introduced the federal program administered by the Indian Health Service (IHS). The goal of the IHS is to ensure that Native Americans and Alaska Natives are provided with comprehensive and culturally acceptable health services (Pleasant 2003). The IHS serves the members and descendants of more than 560 federally recognized American Indian and Alaska Native tribes (IHS 2010c). However, the health care needs of a rapidly expanding American Indian population have grown faster than medical care resources, and most American Indian communities continue to be medically underserved.

IHS is divided into 12 area offices, each responsible for program operations in a particular geographic area. Each area office is composed of branches dealing with various administrative and health-related services. Delivery of health services is the responsibility of 161 tribally managed service units operating at the local level (IHS 2010c). The IHS mandate has been made particularly difficult because the locations of Indian reservation communities are among the least geographically accessible (Burks 1992; Kozoll 1986). Relative isolation and impassable roads continue to present unique challenges.

Over the years, the IHS system has evolved to include not only primary care services but also preventive strategies (Rhodes 1987). Within these environmental, educational, and outreach preventive strategies are special initiatives that focus on areas such as injury control, alcoholism, diabetes, mental health, maternal and child health, Indian youth and children, and elder care (IHS 1999b). Programs have also been established for AIDS, otitis media, and health care database management. Additional proposals include a focus on traditional medicine, domestic violence and child abuse, oral health, sanitation, and new initiatives to improve advocacy for Indian health interests (IHS 1999a). However, despite limitations in the IHS's scope of service, many American Indians do not avail themselves of the system's services.

## The Uninsured

Chapter 6 discussed the number of uninsured and the reasons why so many Americans have been without health insurance. Although uninsurance among adults has increased, lack of health insurance coverage among children declined from 13.2 to 8.2% in the first 9 months of 2009 (CDC 2009), mainly because of the success of the CHIP program (see Chapter 6). Nevertheless, 11% of children under the age of 18 remained uninsured (US Census Bureau 2010).

Ethnic minorities are more likely than Whites to lack health insurance. The US Census Bureau (2010) estimated that, in 2007, 32.1% of Hispanic residents were uninsured, compared with 19.5% of Blacks, 16.8% of AAs, and 14.3% of Whites. About 1 in 10 uninsured persons lacks insurance by personal choice (Bennefield 1995). Most of them are young workers in low-paying jobs. Lack of coverage is also more prevalent in the South and the West of the United

States, among individuals who lack a high school diploma and the unemployed.

For the most part, the uninsured tend to be poor, less educated, working in part-time jobs, and/or employed by small firms. Many of the poor do not qualify for Medicaid because of stringent means-test criteria. The uninsured also tend to be younger (25–40 years of age) because most of the elderly (65 years of age or older) are covered by Medicare.

Generally, the uninsured are in poorer health than the general population (Donelan et al. 1996). Numerous studies have also shown that the uninsured use fewer health services than the insured (Freeman and Corey 1993). In 2009, 26% of uninsured people reported having no regular source of health care (Kaiser Commission on Medicaid and the Uninsured 2010). Decreased utilization of lower cost preventive services can ultimately result in an increased need for more expensive emergency health care. Even when the uninsured can access health care, they often have serious problems paying medical bills. It used to be a common practice for teaching hospitals, private physicians, and community clinics to provide discounted or even free medical care to the uninsured, but managed care practices have seriously reduced the ability of this social safety net to provide care for the uninsured (Donelan et al. 1996). In 2003, 47% of uninsured people postponed seeking medical care because of cost, compared to 15% of insured people (Kaiser Commission on Medicaid and the Uninsured 2006).

The plight of the uninsured affects those who have insurance. Medical expenditures for uncompensated care to the uninsured was estimated to be $41 million in 2004 (Kaiser Commission on Medicaid and the Uninsured 2006). Much of this cost is absorbed by Medicaid, federal grants to nonprofit hospitals, and charitable organizations.

# Children

In 2007, 29.8% of children under the age of 18 were covered under Medicaid and 59.8% under private insurance (National Center for Health Statistics 2010). Vaccinations of children for selected diseases differ by race, poverty status, and area of residence (Table 11–5). White children have greater vaccination rates for diphtheria-tetanus-pertussis (DTP), polio, measles, *Haemophilus influenzae* serotype b (Hib), and combined series than Blacks. Children who come from families with incomes below the federal poverty line or who live in central city areas have lower vaccination rates than those at or above poverty or who live in non-inner city areas.

When children have inadequate access to health care, their ability to learn is compromised. Some children stay home and miss school for long periods when they do not receive needed medical care. Some sick children go to school because of unavailability of child care or inability of working parents to get leave. Once in school, children may also expose other children to contagious illnesses (Wenzel 1996).

In 2007, the United Nations published *The State of the World's Children*, which

*[handwritten margin note: Health + Education]*

Table 11–5  Vaccinations of Children 19–35 Months of Age for Selected Diseases According to Race, Poverty Status, and Residence in a Metropolitan Statistical Area, 2007 (%)

| Vaccination | Race | | | Poverty Status | | Inside MSA | |
|---|---|---|---|---|---|---|---|
| | Total | White | Black | Below Poverty | At or Above Poverty | Central City | Remaining Areas |
| DTP[1] | 85 | 85 | 82 | 81 | 86 | 85 | 85 |
| Polio[2] | 93 | 93 | 91 | 92 | 93 | 92 | 93 |
| Measles containing (MMR)[3] | 92 | 92 | 92 | 91 | 93 | 92 | 93 |
| HIB[4] | 93 | 93 | 91 | 91 | 93 | 92 | 94 |
| Combined series[5] | 77 | 78 | 75 | 73 | 76 | 75 | 77 |

[1]Diphtheria-tetanus-pertussis, four doses or more.

[2]Three doses or more.

[3]Respondents were asked about measles-containing or MMR (measles-mumps-rubella) vaccines.

[4]Haemophilus B, three doses or more.

[5]The combined series consists of four doses of DTP vaccine, three doses of polio vaccine, and one dose of measles-containing vaccine (4:3:1:3:3:1).

*Source:* Data from *Health, United States, 2009*, p. 321.

ties children's health and rights to women's health and rights. This report suggests that greater gender equality will lead to profound and positive impact on children's well-being and development (UN 2007).

Children's health has certain unique aspects in the delivery of health care. Among these are children's developmental vulnerability, dependency, and differential patterns of morbidity and mortality. *Developmental vulnerability* refers to the rapid and cumulative physical and emotional changes that characterize childhood and the potential impact that illness, injury, or disruptive family and social circumstances can have on a child's life-course trajectory. *Dependency* refers to children's special circumstances that require adults—parents, school officials, caregivers, and sometimes neighbors—to recognize and respond to their health needs, seek health care services on their behalf, authorize treatment, and comply with recommended treatment regimens. These dependency relationships can be complex, change over time, and affect utilization of health services by children.

Children increasingly are affected by a broad and complex array of conditions, collectively referred to as "new morbidities." *New morbidities* include drug and alcohol abuse, family and neighborhood violence, emotional disorders, and learning problems from which older generations do not suffer. These dysfunctions originate in complex family or socioeconomic conditions rather than exclusively biological causes. Hence, they cannot be adequately addressed by traditional medical services alone. Instead, these conditions require a continuum of comprehensive services that include multidisciplinary assessment, treatment, and rehabilitation, as well as community-based prevention strategies.

Serious chronic medical conditions, leading to disabling conditions, are less prevalent in children. Estimates of the total number of young people with disabilities range from 5 to 20% of the child population. By the most conservative estimates, at least 3 million children 18 years of age and under are disabled, and 1 million children in the United States have a severe chronic illness. Medical problems in children are usually related to birth or congenital conditions rather than degenerative conditions that affect adults. These differences call for an approach to the delivery of health care that is uniquely designed to address the needs of children.

## Children and the US Health Care System

The various programs that serve children have distinct eligibility, administrative, and funding criteria that can present barriers to access. The patchwork of disconnected programs also makes it difficult to obtain health care in an integrated and coordinated fashion. These programs can be categorized into three broad sectors: the personal medical and preventive services sector, the population-based community health services sector, and the health-related support services sector.

Personal medical and preventive health services include primary and specialty medical services, which are delivered in private and public medical offices, health centers, and hospitals. Personal medical services are principally funded by private health plans, Medicaid, and by families' out-of-pocket payments.

The population-based community health services include communitywide health promotion and disease prevention services. Examples are immunization delivery and monitoring programs, lead screening and abatement programs, and child abuse and neglect prevention. Other health services include special child abuse treatment programs and rehabilitative services for children with complex congenital conditions or other chronic and debilitating diseases. Community-based programs also provide assurance and coordination functions, such as case management and referral programs, for children with chronic diseases and early interventions and monitoring for infants at risk for developmental disabilities. Funding for this sector comes from federal programs, such as Medicaid's Early Periodic Screening, Diagnosis, and Treatment (EPSDT) program; Title V (Maternal and Child Health) of the Social Security Act; and other categorical programs.

The health-related support services sector includes such services as nutrition education, early intervention, rehabilitation, and family support programs. An example of a rehabilitation service is education and psychotherapy for children with HIV. Family support services include parent education and skill building in families with infants at risk for developmental delay because of physiological or social conditions, such as low birth weight or very low income. Funding for these services comes from diverse agencies, such as the Department of Agriculture, which funds the Supplemental Food Program for Women, Infants, and Children (WIC), and the Department of Education, which funds the Individuals with Disabilities Education Act (IDEA).

## Women

Women are playing an increasingly important role in the delivery of health care. Not only do women remain the leading providers of care in the nursing profession, but they are also well represented in various other health professions, including allopathic and osteopathic medicine, dentistry, podiatry, and optometry (Figure 11–9).

Figure 11–9  Percentage of Female Students of Total Enrollment in Schools for Selected Health Occupations, 2006–2007.

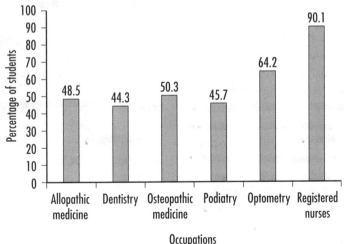

Source: Data from *Health, United States, 2009*, p. 383.

Women in the United States can now expect to live almost 8 years longer than men, but they suffer greater morbidity and poorer health outcomes. Morbidity is greater among women than among men, even after childbearing-related conditions are factored out. For instance, nearly 38% of women report having chronic conditions that require ongoing medical treatment, compared to 30% of men (Salganicoff et al. 2005). Women also have a higher prevalence of certain health problems than men do over the course of their lifetimes (Sechzer et al. 1996). Heart disease and stroke account for a higher percentage of deaths among women than men at all stages of life. In contrast to 24% of men, 42% of women who have heart attacks die within a year (Misra 2001). Research has also demonstrated that health problems restrict women's activities by 25% more days each year than they do for men, even when reproductive conditions are statistically controlled. Women are bedridden 35% more days than men are each year because of infectious or parasitic diseases, respiratory diseases, digestive system conditions, injuries, and other acute conditions (Regier et al. 1988).

According to the 2004 Kaiser Women's Health Survey, 87% of women had at least one visit to a health care provider in the previous year, compared to 74% of men (Salganicoff et al. 2005). Compared to men, women have only a slightly higher mean number of specialty care visits and emergency department visits. However, women have higher annual charges than men do for all types of care, including primary, specialty, emergency, and diagnostic services, indicating that women receive more intensive services (Bertakis et al. 2000).

The differences between men and women are equally pronounced for mental illness. For example, anxiety disorders and major depression affect two to three times as many women as men (Kaiser Family Foundation 2005; Misra 2001). Clinical depression is a major mental health problem for both men and women; however, 6.6% women, compared to 4.4% men, had depression during 2005–2006 (National Center for Health Statistics 2010). An estimated 12% of women in the United States, compared with 7% of men, will suffer from major depression during their lifetime (Misra 2001). Certain other mental disorders also affect more women at different stages of life.

Eating disorders are among the illnesses predominantly affecting women and have been the subject of relatively little rigorous study to date. Up to 3% of women are affected by eating disorders (i.e., anorexia nervosa and bulimia), although between 29 and 38% report dieting at any given time (Misra 2001). At least 90% of all eating disorder cases occur in young women, and eating disorders account for the highest mortality rates among all mental disorders (Misra 2001; Weissman and Klerman 1977).

Some disorders once thought to primarily affect men are now affecting women in increasing numbers. For example, death rates among women who abuse alcohol are 50–100% higher than rates for men who abuse alcohol (Misra 2001). Compared to older men, older women are at substantially greater risk of Alzheimer's disease, a disease responsible for 60–70% of all cases of dementia and one of the leading causes of nursing home placement for older adults (Herzog and Copeland 1985).

## Office on Women's Health    OWH

The Public Health Service's Office on Women's Health (OWH) is dedicated to the achievement of a series of specific goals that span the spectrum of disease and disability. These goals range across the life cycle and address cultural and ethnic differences among women. The OWH stimulates, coordinates, and implements a comprehensive women's health agenda on research, service delivery, and education across the agencies of the Public Health Service (PHS) that include the National Institutes of Health (NIH), the Centers for Disease Control and Prevention (CDC), the Food and Drug Administration (FDA), and others.

The OWH was responsible for implementing the National Action Plan on Breast Cancer (NAPBC), a major public–private partnership, dedicated to improving the diagnosis, treatment, and prevention of breast cancer through research, service delivery, and education. The OWH also worked to implement measures to prevent physical and sexual abuse against women, as delineated in the Violence Against Women Act of 1994. The OWH is also active in projects promoting breastfeeding, women's health education and research, girl and adolescent health, and heart health.

Within the Substance Abuse and Mental Health Services Administration (SAMHSA), the Office for Women's Services has targeted six areas for special attention: physical and sexual abuse of women; women as caregivers; women with mental and addictive disorders; women with HIV infection or AIDS, sexually transmitted diseases, and/or tuberculosis; older women; and women detained in the criminal justice system. The Women's Health Initiative, supported by the NIH, took place in more than 50 centers across the country. It was the largest clinical trial conducted in US history, involving over 161,000 women (NIH 2002). It focused on diseases that are the major causes of death and disability among women—heart disease, cancer, and osteoporosis. In 2002, the Women's Health Initiative published a groundbreaking study, finding detrimental effects of postmenopausal hormone therapy on women's development of invasive breast cancer, coronary heart disease, stroke, and pulmonary embolism (NIH 2002). Within the NIH, the National Institute of Mental Health has issued a specific program announcement to broaden the full spectrum of research on issues pertinent to women's health. Both the National Institute on Drug Abuse (NIDA) and the National Institute of Alcohol Abuse and Alcoholism (NIAAA), also within the NIH, support research related to women's health.

## Women and the US Health Care System

Women face a distinct disadvantage in employer-based health insurance coverage because they are more likely than men to work part time, receive lower wages, and have interruptions in their work histories. Hence, women are more likely to be covered as dependents under their husbands' plans and are at a higher risk of being uninsured. Women must also place greater reliance on Medicaid for their health care coverage.

Even among women who have health insurance, gaps in benefit coverage discourage them from seeking medical and preventive services. Women are more likely than men to use contraceptives (Figure 11–10), but contraceptives are among the most poorly covered reproductive health care service in the United States. As of September 2004, 21 states required private health insurance plans to cover prescription contraceptives if they covered other prescription drugs (Kaiser Family Foundation 2004). Many nonsurgical contraceptors, such as

Figure 11-10  Contraceptive Use in the Past Month Among Women 15–44 Years Old, 2002.

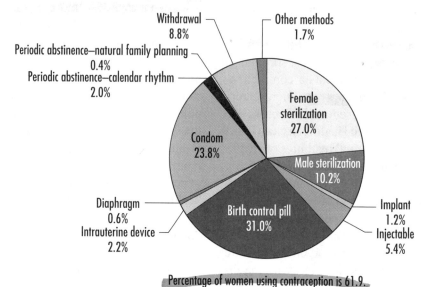

Withdrawal
8.8%

Other methods
1.7%

Periodic abstinence—natural family planning
0.4%

Periodic abstinence—calendar rhythm
2.0%

Female sterilization
27.0%

Condom
23.8%

Male sterilization
10.2%

Diaphragm
0.6%

Intrauterine device
2.2%

Birth control pill
31.0%

Implant
1.2%

Injectable
5.4%

Percentage of women using contraception is 61.9.

*Source:* Data from *Health, United States, 2009*, pp. 171–172.

diaphragms, Norplant implants, intrauterine devices (IUDs), and oral contraceptives, are either not covered or inadequately covered.

# Rural Health

Poor economic conditions are often reflected in diminished access to health care and poor health of rural citizens (Cohen et al. 1994). Access to health care is affected by poverty, long distances, rural topography, weather conditions, and limited availability of personal transportation.

Geographic maldistribution that creates a shortage of health care professionals in rural settings results in barriers in access to care. Reasons for the maldistribution are discussed in Chapter 4. About 20% of the US population resides in areas where primary care health professionals are in short supply (HRSA Bureau of Health Professions 2002). An estimated 22 million-plus rural Americans live in a federally designated area of primary health care provider shortages (HHS Rural Task Force 2002). The scarcity of health care providers encompasses a broad spectrum of professionals, including pediatricians, obstetricians, internists, dentists, nurses, and allied health professionals (Patton and Puskin 1990). Additionally, rural hospitals tend to be smaller and provide fewer services than urban hospitals. Rural hospitals also face financial hardships because they serve a disproportionately higher number of poor, uninsured, and underinsured patients. Closing of rural hospitals further diminishes access to health care. Rural residents, especially poor residents, seek health care services less frequently throughout their lives than do urban residents (Stratton et al. 1993).

Various measures have been taken to improve access in rural America, including the promotion of the National Health Service Corps (NHSC), the designation of Health Professional Shortage Areas (HPSAs) and Medically Underserved Areas (MUAs), the development of Community and Migrant Health Centers (C/MHCs), and the enactment of the Rural Health Clinics Act. In addition, the Office of Rural Health Policy, within the Health Resources and Services Administration of the US Department of Health and Human Services, was established in 1987 to promote better health care in rural America (HRSA Office of Rural Health Policy 2007).

## The National Health Service Corps

The NHSC was created in 1970, under the Emergency Health Personnel Act, to recruit and retain physicians to provide needed services in physician shortage areas. A 1972 amendment created a scholarship program targeting HPSAs. The scholarship and loan repayment program applies to doctors, dentists, nurse practitioners, midwives, and mental health professionals who serve a minimum of 2 years in underserved areas. Since 1972, over 27,000 health professionals have been placed in medically underserved communities in hospitals and clinics (HRSA Bureau of Health Professions 2003). In 2005, the NHSC awarded a record 1,223 loan repayment contracts to health professionals (HRSA Bureau of Health Professions 2007a).

## Health Professional Shortage Areas

The Health Professions Educational Assistance Act of 1976 provided the designation criteria for Health Manpower Shortage Areas, later renamed Health Professional Shortage Areas (Fitzwilliams 1977; HRSA Bureau of Health Professions 2007b). The act provided that three different types of HPSAs could be designated: geographic areas, population groups, and medical facilities. A geographic area must meet the following three criteria for designation as a primary care HPSA: (1) The geographic area involved must be rational for the delivery of health services. (2) One of the following conditions must prevail in the area: a) the area has a population to full-time equivalent primary care physician (PCP) ratio of at least 3,500:1, or b) the area has a population to full-time equivalent PCP ratio of less than 3,500:1 but greater than 3,000:1 and has unusually high needs for primary care services or insufficient capacity of existing primary care providers. (3) Primary care professionals in contiguous areas are overutilized, excessively distant, or inaccessible to the population of the area under consideration (HRSA Bureau of Health Professions 2007c).

A population group can be designated as an HPSA for primary care if it can be demonstrated that access barriers prevent members of the group from using local providers. Medium- and maximum-security federal and state correctional institutions and public or nonprofit private residential facilities can be designated as facility-based HPSAs. HPSAs are classified on a scale from one to four, with one or two signifying areas of greatest need.

## Medically Underserved Areas

The primary purpose of the MUA designation, in the HMO Act of 1973, was to target the community health center and rural health clinic programs. The statute required that several factors be considered in designating MUAs, such as available health resources in relation to area size and population, health indices, and care and demographic factors affecting the need for care. To meet this mandate, the Index of Medical Underservice was developed, comprising four variables: (1) percentage of population below poverty income levels, (2) percentage of population 65 years of age and older, (3) infant mortality rate, and (4) PCP per 1,000 population. The index yields a single numerical value on a scale from 0 to 100; any area with a value less than 62 (the median of all counties) is designated an MUA. Only one-half of the MUA population lives in a physician shortage area.

## Community and Migrant Health Centers

These centers provide services to low-income populations on a sliding-fee scale, thereby addressing both geographic and financial barriers to access. For more than 4 decades, C/MHCs have provided primary care and preventive health services to populations in designated MUAs. These designated areas receive national priority in meeting their health care needs and are targeted for special federal health initiative programs. Traditionally, these areas have had trouble attracting private physicians, particularly in primary care specialties. As a result, C/MHCs heavily rely on nonphysician providers (NPPs) for the delivery of services. The migrant program supports 134 grantees, who run approximately 400 clinics in 40 states and Puerto Rico (HRSA Bureau of Primary Health Care 2007a). They serve approximately 727,000 migrants and seasonal farm workers (HRSA Bureau of Primary Health Care 2007b). Although community health centers must

be located in areas designated as MUAs, migrant centers must be located in "high-impact" areas, defined as areas that serve at least 4,000 migrant and/or seasonal farm workers for at least 2 months per year.

## The Rural Health Clinics Act

The Rural Health Clinics Act was developed to respond to the concern that isolated rural communities could not generate sufficient revenue to support the services of a physician. In many cases, the only source of primary care or emergency services was NPPs, who were ineligible at that time for Medicare or Medicaid reimbursement. The Act is a reimbursement mechanism that strengthens the financial viability of eligible entities by increasing the opportunities for Medicare and Medicaid reimbursement. The Act permitted physician assistants (PAs), nurse practitioners (NPs), and certified nurse midwives (CNMs) associated with rural clinics to practice without the direct supervision of a physician; enabled rural health clinics (but not NPPs directly) to be reimbursed by Medicare and Medicaid for their services; and tied the level of Medicaid payment to the level established by Medicare. To be designated as a rural health clinic, a public or private sector physician practice, clinic, or hospital must meet several criteria, including location in an MUA, geographic HPSA, or a population-based HPSA. Over 3,000 rural health clinics provide primary care services to over 7 million people in 47 states (NARHC 2007).

## Rural Managed Care

Rural managed care faces demographic, geographic, and infrastructure challenges. The demographic and geographic characteristics of rural communities pose important barriers to managed care. Some rural communities do not have large enough populations to support the array of practitioners and services necessary to provide cost-efficient health care. At the same time, health care needs in rural areas are as great as or greater than those in urban areas because of high rates of chronic disease and other unmet needs. Moreover, rural incomes remain low, making it difficult for managed care plans to generate the revenues that comparable resources might generate in an urban area.

Apart from shortages of physicians and hospitals in rural areas, some rural physicians cannot meet board certification or eligibility requirements imposed by managed care plans. Many physicians practicing in rural areas may find the corporate culture of managed care plans alien. The isolation of rural practice can attract individualistic practitioners who are used to making independent decisions and who are unwilling to be held accountable to a managed care organization (MCO).

## The Homeless

Although an exact number is unknown, an estimated 3.5 million people (1.35 million of them children) are likely to experience homelessness in a given year (National Coalition for the Homeless 2006a). Nationally, approximately 26 million people (14% of the US population) are homeless at some point in their lives. Although most homeless persons live in major urban areas, a surprising 19% live in rural areas.

The homeless population includes 43% single men, 17% single women, and 39% children under the age of 18 (National Coalition for the Homeless 2006b). About 33% of the homeless population are families with children (National Coalition for the Homeless 2006b). About 40% of all homeless men are veterans of war (National Coalition for the Homeless 2006b).

Homeless women in particular face major difficulties: economic and housing needs and special gender-related issues that include pregnancy, child care responsibilities, family violence, fragmented family support, job discrimination, and wage discrepancies. Homeless women, regardless of parenting status, should be linked with social services, family support, self-help, and housing resources. Mentally ill women caring for children need additional consideration, with an emphasis on parenting skills and special services for children. Thus, homelessness is a multifaceted problem related to personal, social, and economic factors.

The economic picture of homeless persons is dismal, as would be expected, and suggests that they are severely lacking in the financial and educational resources necessary to access health care. Further, almost one-half of homeless people have not graduated from high school and have been unemployed for 4 years on average. Despite these figures, only 20% receive income maintenance and only 26% have health insurance. These numbers remain low because of federal restrictions that prohibit federal help to those without a physical street address.

The shortage of adequate low-income housing is the major precipitating factor for homelessness. Unemployment, personal or family life crises, rent increases that are out of proportion to inflation, and reduction in public benefits can also directly result in the loss of a home. Illness, on the other hand, tends to result in the loss of a home in a more indirect way. Other indirect causes of homelessness include deinstitutionalization from public mental hospitals, substance abuse programs, and overcrowded prisons and jails.

Community-based residential alternatives for mentally ill individuals vary from independent apartments to group homes staffed by paid caregivers. Independent living may involve either separate apartments or single-room occupancy units (SROs) in large hotels, whereas group homes are staffed during at least a portion of the day and traditionally provide some on-site mental health services (Schutt and Goldfinger 1996).

The homeless, adults and children, have a high prevalence of untreated acute and chronic medical, mental health, and substance abuse problems. The reasons are debatable. Some argue that people may become homeless because of a physical or mental illness. Others argue that homelessness itself may lead to the development of physical and mental disability because homelessness produces risk factors, which include excessive use of alcohol, illegal drugs, and cigarettes; sleeping in an upright position, which results in venous stasis and its consequences; extensive walking in poorly fitting shoes; and grossly inadequate nutrition.

Homeless persons are also at a greater risk of assault and victimization regardless of whether they live in a shelter or outdoors. They are also subject to exposure to extreme heat, cold, and other weather conditions. The homeless are also exposed to illness because of overcrowding in shelters and overexposure to weather.

## Barriers to Health Care

The homeless face barriers to ambulatory services but incur high rates of hospitalization. A high use of inpatient services in this manner amounts to the substitution of inpatient care for outpatient services.

Both individual factors (competing needs, substance dependence, and mental illness) and system factors (availability, cost, convenience, and appropriateness of care) account for the barriers to adequate ambulatory services.

Other barriers include accessible transportation to medical care providers and competing needs for basic food, shelter, and income than obtaining health services or following through with a prescribed treatment plan. Homeless individuals who experience psychological distress and disabling mental illness may be in the greatest need of health services and yet may be the least able to obtain them. This inability to obtain health care may be attributable to such individual traits of mental illness as paranoia, disorientation, unconventional health beliefs, lack of social support, lack of organizational skills to gain access to needed services, or fear of authority figures and institutions resulting from previous institutionalization. The social conditions of street life also affect compliance with medical care because of a lack of proper sanitation and a stable place to store medications. They also lack resources to obtain proper food for a medically indicated diet necessary for conditions like diabetes or hypertension.

Federal efforts to provide medical services to the homeless population are primarily through the Health Care for the Homeless (HCH) program. Community health centers supported by the 1985 Robert Wood Johnson Foundation/Pew Memorial Trust HCH program (subsequently covered by the 1987 McKinney Homeless Assistance Act) have addressed many of the access and quality-of-care issues faced by the homeless. In 2004, community health centers served approximately 703,000 homeless patients (HRSA Bureau of Primary Health Care 2007b).

A critical aspect of these programs is outreach, in which teams of health care professionals bring a wide range of services to homeless persons in shelters, hotels, soup lines, beaches and parks, train and bus stations, religious facilities, and other places where homeless people may gather. Such programs help overcome some of the barriers to care. Outreach teams are typically based in health care centers, to which clinicians can refer homeless patients who need additional medical attention. In addition, a walk-in appointment system reduces access barriers at these medical facilities. Medical care, routine laboratory tests, substance abuse counseling, and some medications are provided free of charge to eliminate financial barriers.

The Mental Health Services for the Homeless Block Grant program sets aside funds for states to implement services for homeless persons with mental illness. These services include outreach services; community mental health services; rehabilitation; referrals to inpatient treatment, primary care, and substance abuse services; case management services; and supportive services in residential settings.

Services for homeless veterans are provided through the Department of Veterans Affairs (VA). The Homeless Chronically Mentally Ill Veterans Program provides outreach, case management services, and psychiatric residential treatment for homeless mentally ill veterans in community-based facilities in 45 US cities. The Domiciliary Care for Homeless Veterans Program addresses the health needs of veterans who have psychiatric illnesses or alcohol or drug abuse problems, operating 1,800 beds at 31 sites across the country (US Dept of Veterans Affairs 2006).

The Salvation Army also provides a variety of social, rehabilitation, and support services for homeless persons. Its centers include adult rehabilitation and food programs and permanent and transitional housing.

# Mental Health

Mental disorders are common psychiatric illnesses affecting adults and present a serious public health problem in the United States (Barker et al. 1989; Klerman and Weisman 1989; Myers et al. 1984; Regier et al. 1988; Romanoski et al. 1992). Mental disorders are the leading cause of disability for people aged 15–44 (NIMH 2007). Mental illness is a risk factor for death from suicide, cardiovascular disease, and cancer. Suicide is currently the 10th leading cause of death in the United States and the 4th leading cause of death among persons aged 18–65. Non-Hispanic White men 85 years of age or older have one of the highest rates of suicide, with 47 suicide deaths per 100,000. American Indian and Alaska Natives are at higher risk for suicides as well, with 14.3 suicide deaths per 100,000 (CDC 2011).

Mental health disorders can be either psychological or biological in nature. Many mental health diseases, including mental retardation (MR), developmental disabilities (DD), and schizophrenia, are now known to be biological in origin. Other behaviors, including those related to personality disorders and neurotic behaviors, are still subject to interpretation and professional judgment. Defining what is and is not normal in a population is difficult and often raises far-reaching moral and ethical issues (Williams 1995).

National studies have concluded that the most common mental disorders include phobias; substance abuse, including alcohol and drug dependence; and affective disorders, including depression. Schizophrenia is considerably less common, affecting an estimated 1.1% of the population (NIMH 2006a).

About one in four adults suffers from a diagnosable mental disorder every year (NIMH 2007). In 2009, 45.1 million adults (18 years of age or older) had a mental illness, including 11 million with severe mental illness (SMI). Among this population, only a small percentage sought care. Prevalence of SMI was higher among women and individuals in the 18–25 age group (NIMH 2008; Substance Abuse and Mental Health Services Administration 2010).

Most mental health services are provided in the general medical sector—a concept first described by Regier and colleagues (1988) as the de facto mental health service system—rather than through formal mental health specialist services. The de facto system combines specialty mental health services with general counseling services, such as those provided in primary care settings, nursing homes, and community health centers by ministers, counselors, self-help groups, families, and friends. Specifically, mental health services are provided through public and private resources in both inpatient and outpatient facilities. These facilities include state and county mental hospitals, private psychiatric hospitals, nonfederal general hospital psychiatric services, VA psychiatric services, residential treatment centers, and freestanding psychiatric outpatient clinics (Table 11–6). Total expenditures for mental disorders have increased since 1996, from $35.2 billion to $57.5 billion in 2006 (NIMH 2006a). Per person, the cost was $1,591, including $1,931 per child (NIMH 2006b). Despite the cost of mental health care for individuals with any

Table 11–6   Mental Health Organizations (Numbers in Thousands), 2004

| Service and Organization | Number of MH Organizations |
|---|---|
| All organizations | 2,891 |
| State and county mental hospitals | 237 |
| Private psychiatric hospitals | 264 |
| Nonfederal general hospital psychiatric services | 1,230 |
| Residential treatment centers for emotionally disturbed children | 458 |
| All other | 702 |

Source: Data from Health, United States, 2009, p. 385.

mental illness, only 37.9% received mental health services and only 60.2% of individuals covered under Medicare Part B received care (Substance Abuse and Mental Health Services Administration 2010). The nation's mental health system is composed of two subsystems: one primarily for individuals with insurance coverage or private funds and the other for those without private coverage.

## The Uninsured and Mental Health

Patients without insurance coverage or personal financial resources are treated in state and county mental health hospitals and in community mental health clinics. Care is also provided in short-term, acute care hospitals and emergency departments. Local governments are the providers of last resort, with the ultimate responsibility to provide somatic and mental health services for all citizens regardless of ability to pay.

## The Insured and Mental Health

For patients who have insurance coverage or personal ability to pay, availability of both inpatient and ambulatory mental health care has expanded tremendously. Inpatient mental health services for patients with insurance are usually provided through private psychiatric hospitals. These hospitals can be operated on either a nonprofit or a for-profit basis. There has been substantial growth in national chains of for-profit mental health hospitals. Patients with insurance coverage are also more likely to receive care through the offices of private psychiatrists, clinical psychologists, and licensed social workers. Mental health services are also provided by the VA and by the military health care system; however, access to these services is limited by eligibility.

## Managed Care and Mental Health

Managed care has expanded its services into mental health delivery. State and local governments are also contracting with MCOs to manage a full health care benefit package that includes mental health and substance-abuse services for their Medicaid enrollees.

Many health maintenance organizations (HMOs) contract with specialized companies that provide managed behavioral health care, an arrangement called a carve-out. This is mainly because HMOs lack the in-house capacity to provide treatment. Using case managers and reviewers, most of whom are psychiatric nurses, social workers, and psychologists, these specialized companies oversee and authorize the use of mental health and substance abuse services. The case reviewers, using clinical protocols to guide them, assign patients to the least expensive appropriate treatment, emphasizing outpatient alternatives over inpatient care.

Working with computerized databases, a reviewer studies a patient's particular problem and then authorizes an appointment with an appropriate provider in the company's selective network. On average, psychiatrists constitute about 20% of any given provider network, psychologists constitute 40%, and psychiatric social workers constitute another 40%.

## Mental Health Professionals

A variety of professionals provide mental health services (Table 11–7), including but not limited to psychiatrists, psychologists, social workers, nurses, counselors, and therapists.

*Psychiatrists* are specialist physicians who specialize in the diagnosis and treatment of mental disorders. Psychiatrists receive postgraduate specialty training in mental health after completing medical school. Psychiatric residencies cover medical, as well as behavioral, diagnosis and treatments. A relatively small proportion of the total mental health workforce consists of psychiatrists, but they exercise disproportionate influence in the system by virtue of their authority to prescribe drugs and admit patients to hospitals.

*Psychologists* usually hold a doctoral degree, although some hold master's degrees. They are trained in interpreting and changing the behavior of people. Psychologists cannot prescribe drugs; however, they provide a wide range of services to patients with neurotic and behavioral problems. Psychologists use such techniques as psychotherapy and counseling, which psychiatrists

Table 11–7  Full-Time Equivalent Patient Care Staff in Mental Health Organizations, 1998

| Staff Discipline | Number | Percentage |
|---|---|---|
| All patient care staff | 531,532 | 78.1 |
| Professional patient care staff | 304,449 | 44.8 |
| Psychiatrists | 28,374 | 4.2 |
| Other physicians | 3,561 | 0.5 |
| Psychologists | 28,729 | 4.2 |
| Social workers | 72,367 | 10.6 |
| Registered nurses | 78,562 | 11.5 |
| Other mental health professionals | 78,854 | 11.6 |
| Physical health professionals and assistants | 14,002 | 2.1 |
| Other mental health workers | 130,551 | 33.4 |

Source: Section VI, Chapter 18, Table 7, Mental Health, United States, 2002. Ronald W. Manderscheid, Marilyn J. Henderson, eds. Rockville, MD: US Department of Health and Human Services, Substance Abuse and Mental Health Services Administration, Center for Mental Health Services.

typically do not engage in. Psychoanalysis is a subspecialty in mental health that involves the use of intensive treatment by both psychiatrists and psychologists.

Social workers receive training in various aspects of mental health services, particularly counseling. Social workers are trained at the master's degree level. They also compete with psychologists for patients.

Nurses are involved in mental health through the subspecialty of psychiatric nursing. Specialty training for nurses had its origins in the latter part of the 1800s. Nurses provide a wide range of mental health services.

Many other health care professionals contribute to the array of available services, including marriage and family counselors, recreational therapists, and vocational counselors. Numerous people work in related areas, such as adult day care (ADC), alcohol and drug abuse counseling, and as psychiatric aides in institutional settings.

# The Chronically Ill and Disabled

Chronic diseases are now the leading cause of death in the United States—heart disease, cancer, and stroke account for more than 50% of deaths each year. Seven out of 10 deaths each year are from chronic diseases (CDC 2010a). Heart disease is the number one cause of death in the United States, at 204.3 per 100,000 persons (National Center for Health Statistics 2007). The prevalence of heart disease in 2009 was 12%, which is equal to 26.8 million Americans (National Center for Health Statistics 2009). In 2005, almost 1 in 2 adults had at least one chronic illness, roughly 133 million Americans. This large prevalence of disease results in adverse consequences such as limitations on daily living activities.

The loss in human potential and work days notwithstanding, chronic disease is expensive, incurring more than 75% of the total medical expenditure ($1.4 trillion annually; National Center for Chronic Disease Prevention and Health Promotion 2005). Chronic disease places a huge economic demand on the nation. The estimated annual direct medical expenditures for the most common chronic diseases are $313.8 billion in 2009 for cardiovascular disease and stroke, $89.0 billion for cancer in 2007, and $116 billion for diabetes in 2007 (CDC 2009).

*Four modifiable behaviors*
1- Physical Activity
2- Nutrition
3- Smoking
4- Alcohol

Much of the burden of chronic diseases is the result of four modifiable risk behaviors: physical activity, nutrition, smoking, and alcohol (CDC 2010a). There is a lack of physical activity among the US population, with 23% reporting no leisure-time physical activity at all in the preceding month of the 2008 Physical Activity Guidelines for Americans survey. There has also been a decline in participation of physical education classes among high school students, from 42% in 1991 to 30% in 2007, showing that all age groups do not partake in regular physical activity. The nation also suffers from poor nutrition. Less than 25% of adults and children eat the required five or more servings of fruit and vegetables, although the majority consumes more than the recommended amount of saturated fat (CDC 2009).

Chronic illness can often lead to disability. The chronic conditions most responsible for disabilities are arthritis, heart disease, back problems, asthma, and diabetes (Kraus et al. 1996). The disabled also tend to be covered by public sources (30% by Medicare and 10% by Medicaid), compared to those who have no disabilities, who are more likely to pay for care with private coverage (Kraus et al. 1996).

Disability can be categorized as mental, physical, or social; tests of disability tend to be more sensitive to some categories than others. Physical disability usually addresses a person's mobility and other basic activities performed in daily life, mental disability involves both the cognitive and emotional states, and social disability is considered the most severe disability because management of social roles requires both physical and mental well-being (Ostir et al. 1999). About 19.4% of the noninstitutionalized US population, or 48.9 million Americans, have a disability (Kraus et al. 1996).

The two commonly used measures of disability, activities of daily living (ADLs) and instrumental activities of daily living (IADLs), were covered in Chapter 2. Another tool for assessing disability is the Survey of Income and Program Participation (SIPP), which measures disability by asking participants about functional limitations (difficulty in performing activities such as seeing, hearing, walking, having one's speech understood, etc.), but ADL and IADL scales are more widely used.

Despite the availability of community-based and institutional long-term care services for people with functional limitations, many people are not getting the help they need with the basic tasks of personal care. It is estimated that more than one-third of people with chronic conditions do not receive assistance with ADLs. Consequently, these people do not bathe or shower because of a fear of falling, are unable to follow a dietary regimen, and sustain falls. Ultimately, unmet needs lead to exacerbated health problems, costly treatments, and unnecessary pain and suffering (The Robert Wood Johnson Foundation 1996).

## HIV/AIDS

In July 1982, acquired immune deficiency syndrome (AIDS) was officially named a disease. Figure 11–11 illustrates trends in AIDS reporting. The number of AIDS cases reported increased between 1987 and 1993, decreased between 1994 and 1999, increased between 2000 and 2004, and decreased from 2005 through 2007 (US Census Bureau 2010).

Deaths from AIDS have declined since 1998 and decreased 11.3% between 2003 and 2006, from 13,658 to 12,113 (US

Figure 11–11  US AIDS Cases Reported, 1987–2007.

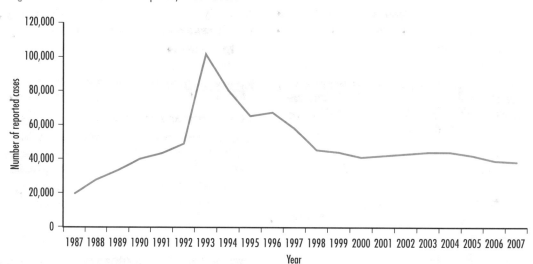

*Source:* Reprinted from US Centers for Disease Control and Prevention, *Statistical Abstracts of the United States, 2001,* p. 119; and *Statistical Abstracts of the United States, 2007,* p. 120; *Statistical Abstracts of the United States, 2008,* p. 121; *Statistical Abstracts of the United States, 2009,* p. 120; *Statistical Abstracts of the United States, 2010,* p. 122.

Census Bureau 2010). Declines in reported AIDS cases between 1994 and 1999 were ascribed to new treatments; decreasing death rates may reflect the fact that benefits from new treatments are being fully realized. Meanwhile, the number of people living with AIDS continues to increase. In 2006, 446,098 people were living with AIDS; in 2001, the figure was 341,332 (CDC 2010b).

AIDS is believed to be caused by the human immunodeficiency virus (HIV). HIV is an unusual type of virus, called a retrovirus, which causes the immune system suppression leading to AIDS. Individuals infected with HIV develop antibodies within a short period but may exhibit no symptoms for many years. Typically, the immune system weakens gradually and the blood level of CD4 cells (a type of white

blood cell known as a T-helper/inducer lymphocyte) drops below the normal level of between 1,200 and 1,400/mm. Persons with few CD4 cells are prone to *opportunistic infections*. Symptoms, such as persistent fever, night sweats, and weight loss, begin to occur more often when the CD4 count drops below 500/mm. The development of AIDS is estimated to occur at 11 years on average from the time of HIV infection.

Certain widely recognized risk factors promote the transmission of HIV, including male-to-male sexual contact; male-to-female sexual contact; injection drug use (IDU); blood product exposure; and perinatal transmission from mother to infant during pregnancy, delivery, or possibly during breastfeeding (Table 11–8).

Most individuals infected with HIV produce antibodies within 6 to 9 months of

Table 11–8  Reports of All AIDS Cases: All Years Through 2007

| Sex and Diagnosis | Percentage Distribution | Number of Reported Cases |
|---|---|---|
| All races | 100% | 1,021,242 |
| Men who have sex with men | 43.6% | 445,645 |
| Injecting drug use | 23.1% | 235,842 |
| Men who have sex with men and injecting drug use | 6.6% | 67,797 |
| Hemophilia/coagulation disorder | 0.5% | 5,567 |
| Heterosexual sex with injecting drug user | 3.8% | 38,766 |
| Other heterosexual contact | 10.2% | 104,086 |
| Transfusion | 0.9% | 9,315 |
| Undetermined | 11.2% | 114,224 |

*Source:* Data from *Statistical Abstract of the United States, 2010*, p. 122.

exposure, although some people do not form antibodies until 2 to 3 years after exposure to HIV. Consequently, an individual can be exposed to HIV and not develop the antibodies for several years. Further, people may transmit HIV before they know they have been exposed, making transmission unsuspecting. HIV infection was the sixth leading cause of death among persons 25 to 34 years of age in 2006 (US Census Bureau 2010).

For Blacks, Hispanics, and minority women, AIDS/HIV is still a major public health concern. In 2004, males and Blacks continued to have significantly higher rates of HIV/AIDS than females and Whites (Table 11–9). Also, only among Black males is HIV infection a leading cause of death (CDC 2010b). In 2007, rates of AIDS cases per 100,000 people were 47.3 in the Black population, 15.2 in the Hispanic population, 6.9 in the American Indian/Alaska Native population, 5.2 in the White population,

3.6 in the Asian population, and 18.3 in the Native Hawaiian/Other Pacific Islander population (CDC 2007). Blacks accounted for 51% of all HIV/AIDS cases diagnosed in 2007 (CDC 2007). Racial differences in HIV/AIDS infection probably reflect social, economic, behavioral, and other factors associated with HIV transmission risks.

New York and Maryland lead the states in the proportion of individuals afflicted with AIDS, at 24.8 cases per 100,000 population (Table 11–10). Vermont has the lowest AIDS rate, at 1.0 per 100,000 population. California has more reported AIDS cases than any other state, followed by New York, Florida, Texas, and Georgia. Vermont has the smallest number of reported AIDS cases, followed by North Dakota and Wyoming (US Census Bureau 2010).

HIV infection has risen to the level of a global pandemic and has become the world's modern-day plague. In 2009,

Table 11–9  US AIDS Cases Reported Through 2007

| Characteristic | All Years | | 2007 | |
| --- | --- | --- | --- | --- |
| | Number | Percentage | Number | Percentage |
| Total | 1,018,429 | 100.0 | 35,962 | 100.0 |
| Sex | | | | |
| Male (13 and over) | 810,676 | 79.6 | 26,355 | 73.3 |
| Female (13 and over) | 198,544 | 19.5 | 9,599 | 26.6 |
| Children under 13 years | 9,209 | 0.9 | 28 | 0.1 |
| Race/ethnic group | | | | |
| White | 404,465 | 40.0 | 10,467 | 29.3 |
| Black | 426,002 | 42.1 | 17,507 | 49.3 |
| Hispanic | 169,138 | 16.7 | 6,920 | 19.5 |
| Asian | 7,512 | 0.7 | 474 | .02 |
| Native Hawaiian or other Pacific Islander | 720 | 0.1 | 76 | .04 |
| American Indian/Alaska Native | 3,492 | 0.3 | 158 | .04 |

Source: Data from Health, United States, 2009, p. 252.

Table 11–10  Top and Bottom 10 States for AIDS, According to Cases per 100,000 Population, 2007

| Top States | Reported Cases | Cases per 100,000 Population | Bottom States | Reported Cases | Cases per 100,000 Population |
| --- | --- | --- | --- | --- | --- |
| California | 4,952 | 13.6 | Rhode Island | 66 | 6.3 |
| New York | 4,810 | 24.8 | New Hampshire | 51 | 3.9 |
| Florida | 3,961 | 21.8 | Maine | 46 | 3.5 |
| Texas | 2,964 | 12.4 | Alaska | 32 | 4.7 |
| Georgia | 1,877 | 19.7 | Montana | 25 | 2.6 |
| Pennsylvania | 1,750 | 14.1 | Idaho | 23 | 1.5 |
| Maryland | 1,394 | 24.8 | South Dakota | 15 | 1.9 |
| Illinois | 1,348 | 10.5 | Wyoming | 13 | 2.5 |
| New Jersey | 1,164 | 13.5 | North Dakota | 8 | 1.3 |
| North Carolina | 1,024 | 11.3 | Vermont | 6 | 1.0 |

Source: Data from Statistical Abstract of the United States, 2010.

33.3 million people were estimated to be living with HIV worldwide (UNAIDS 2010). An estimated 2.6 million people acquired HIV in 2009, including 370,000 children younger than 15 years of age (UN-AIDS 2010). AIDS caused the deaths of an estimated 1.8 million people, including 260,000 children younger than 15 years of age (UNAIDS 2010). These figures represent a decrease over previous years, but the global HIV/AIDS epidemic is far from under control, particularly in sub-Saharan Africa, where 22.5 million of the world's 33.3 million cases of people living with HIV reside (UNAIDS 2010).

Many public health experts believe that cases of AIDS still remain underreported. The reasons for such underreporting include poor reporting standards in health departments (Selike et al. 1993), physicians desiring to protect the confidentiality of their patients because of the stigma of HIV/AIDS (AIDS Forecasting 1989), lack of physician knowledge about the diagnosis of AIDS (Anonymous 1988), patients' denial of the risk behaviors that are likely to transmit HIV, and the absence of or decreased access to health care (Robertson et al. 1974), which prevents the diagnosis of HIV. With the advent of combination antiretroviral therapy, AIDS surveillance data no longer reflect trends in HIV transmission because this therapy has effectively delayed the progression of HIV to AIDS (CDC 1999a).

HIV testing is anonymous or confidential. In anonymous HIV testing, patient-identifying information or other locating information is not linked to the HIV test, whereas, in confidential HIV testing, the test result is linked (CDC 1999c). In September 2006, CDC released new recommendations for HIV testing, which called for routine HIV screening of adults, adolescents, and pregnant women in health care settings in the United States (Branson et al. 2006).

The implementation of rapid HIV testing—versus the previous method, ELISA (enzyme-linked immunosorbent assay)—makes it possible to get early results, permitting the initiation of combined antiretroviral therapy earlier in the disease process. Furthermore, the rapid HIV test may improve the outreach at clinics where testing and counseling are offered together.

Both the rapid HIV test and ELISA require a second testing, using a Western blot or an immunofluorescence assay (IFA) to confirm positive test results. The ELISA test (also known as enzyme immunoassays or EIAs) required special equipment. Blood samples had to be sent to laboratories and test results were not available for 1 or 2 weeks, requiring the clients to make a second visit to the testing site. Many people did not return for their results. The CDC estimated that, in 2000, 31% of patients who tested positive for HIV at public-sector testing points did not return to get their results (Greenwald 2006). With rapid HIV testing, results are available in 5 to 30 minutes, and the test is as accurate as the ELISA. Thus, testing and counseling can be available during the same visit.

Current treatment for HIV/AIDS centers on therapies for slowing the progress of HIV and preventing opportunistic infections (OI), reducing the number of people with HIV who develop and die from AIDS. For example, medications, such as oral antibiotics, are often used to prevent a common pneumonia (pneumocystis carinii or PCP), an OI that often develops in persons with AIDS. Other OIs include tuberculosis, toxoplasmosis, and mycobacterium avium complex (MAC). OIs occur when organisms naturally present in the body get out of control and cause health problems due to a weakened immune system. Protease inhibitors, a combination of new, more effective drugs, are now taken in conjunction with antiretrovirals, the initial drugs used in AIDS/HIV therapy. Combination drug therapy—known as highly active antiretroviral therapy (HAART) or "drug cocktail"—has been more effective because it can reduce the viral load (level of HIV particles circulating in the blood) to extremely low levels; however, the long-term effectiveness of HAART is unknown, and it is extremely expensive. The high cost of HAART makes the treatment unavailable to many patients in the United States and keeps it out of reach in developing countries, where more than 90% of the new HIV infections occur. Also, the complicated drug regimen requires coordination of many pills and doses, which makes it easier to skip medications or doses so that some patients temporarily stop treatment. This lack of regimen adherence not only makes the treatment less effective but also increases the chance of developing a drug-resistant strain of HIV. It is suspected that HIV will eventually develop multidrug resistance. After experiencing improvements in one's condition, complacency may lead to relaxed preventive behavior, which would risk spreading a potential drug-resistant strain of HIV (CDC 1998, 1999b).

## HIV Infection in Rural Communities

Spread of HIV into rural communities in the United States has grown. CDC reported 23,615 new cases of AIDS in nonmetropolitan areas of the United States between March 1994 and February 1995 (CDC 1995b). In 1999, 7% of cumulative adult/adolescent AIDS cases were reported from nonmetropolitan areas (CDC 2001).

Rural persons with HIV and AIDS are more likely to be young, non-White, and female and to have acquired their infection through heterosexual contact. Additionally, a growing number of these HIV-infected persons live in the rural South, a region historically characterized by a disproportionate number of poor and minority persons, strong religious beliefs and sanctions, and decreased access to comprehensive health services (CDC 1995a, 1995b; DHHS, Office of Minority Health 2003; Morrison 1993). Trends in new cases of HIV and AIDS in rural areas indicate that poor and non-White residents are disproportionately affected (Aday 1993; Lam and Liu 1994; Rumby et al. 1991).

## HIV in Children

In the absence of specific therapy to interrupt transmission of HIV, an infected woman has a 25% chance of having a child born with HIV. Therefore, in 1994 and 1995, the US Public Health Service (PHS) began recommending that pregnant women be counseled and voluntarily tested for HIV and that zidovudine (AZT) be given to infected women during pregnancy and delivery, as well as to the infant after delivery. The drop in perinatal transmission rates has been attributed to this strategy, and, in one study, perinatal transmission rates dropped from 21 to 11% after use of AZT, according to PHS guidelines. The number of children with a diagnosis of AIDS who had been perinatally exposed to HIV declined from 122 in 2000 to 47 in 2004 (CDC 2005). The importance of preventing perinatal transmission is underscored by the fact that 91% of all AIDS cases among US children are caused by mother-to-child transmission in pregnancy, labor, delivery, or breastfeeding

(CDC 1999d, 1999f). The earliest and most common symptom in HIV-positive children is enlarged lymph nodes, which are often associated with an enlarged spleen (Johnson and Vink 1992). HIV-infected children also have severe and persistent skin infections. Children who are born with AIDS suffer from failure to thrive, the inability to grow and develop as healthy children. Without intervention, this failure to thrive may lead to developmental delays that can have negative lifetime consequences for the child and his or her family.

HIV infection causes morbidity in two different but equally destructive ways. First, viruses like HIV cause illness by direct infection of cells; HIV can infect every organ system in the body and has a particular affinity for cells of the nervous system. Second, as HIV infects and destroys CD4 cells and weakens the immune system, the child becomes increasingly susceptible to various illnesses (O'Hara and D'Orlando 1996).

Family-centered care provides care and support to all immediate family members of children with HIV. It allows health care providers to develop and implement an interdisciplinary treatment plan to manage HIV infection for all children regardless of how they acquired the infection. For example, as the child becomes symptomatic, health care providers may add new therapies to the already prescribed medication regimen. Providers may also perform numerous diagnostic procedures to rule out potential problems or to diagnose a particular disease process to reduce pain and suffering.

## HIV in Women

Women are a rapidly growing proportion of the population with HIV/AIDS. In 2004, women made up approximately one-half of

HIV/AIDS cases worldwide (WHO 2004). For US women 25 to 44 years of age, HIV/AIDS is a leading cause of death. Between 2001 and 2005, the estimated number of AIDS cases increased 17% for women and 16% for men (CDC 2006a). For women, heterosexual exposure to HIV, followed by IDU, is the greatest cause for exposure. Aside from the inherent risks in IDU, drug use overall contributes to a higher risk of contracting HIV if heterosexual sex with an IDU user occurs or when sex is traded for drugs or money (CDC 2002). Black and Hispanic minority women are at particular risk. Despite representing less than one-fourth of the total US female population, Black and Hispanic women represent more than three-fourths (79%) of all AIDS cases in women (National Institute of Allergy and Infectious Diseases 2006).

Because of women's position in society, HIV-positive women face many problems not confronted by men with HIV. For instance, the social expectation is that women are the caregivers for those who are ill in the family. As a result, women with HIV often care for their partner or children when they are ill themselves. Domestic violence has been increasingly identified among women living with HIV.

## HIV/AIDS-Related Issues

### Need for Research

HIV-related research seeks to develop a vaccine to prevent HIV-negative people from acquiring HIV. Researchers are also seeking to develop a therapeutic vaccine to prevent HIV-positive people from developing symptoms of AIDS.

People with HIV/AIDS often belong to groups that differ from each other. For example, women with AIDS may have different concerns than adolescents with AIDS. People with HIV/AIDS represent a broad spectrum of social classes, races, ethnicities, sexual orientations, and genders. Behavioral intervention research, therefore, should focus particularly on populations that are most vulnerable to HIV infection and are in urgent need of preventive interventions. These populations include gay youth and young adults, especially Black and Hispanic; disenfranchised and impoverished women; heterosexual men, again, Black and Hispanic in particular; inner city youth; and out-of-treatment substance abusers and their sexual partners. Research should be aimed not only at the individual but also at the impact of broader interventions (e.g., among drug users or those involved in sexual networks or communitywide groups) that change behavioral norms and, consequently, affect individual behavior (Merson 1996).

## Public Health Concerns

AIDS underscores the synergy between poverty and intravenous drug use. The despair commonly caused by poverty is often mitigated only by addictions, such as drug use. Further, control of the HIV epidemic among the poor is hampered by their preoccupation with other problems related to survival, such as homelessness, crime, and lack of access to adequate health care.

Additionally, a relationship exists between the current tuberculosis epidemic and HIV. Indeed, tuberculosis, an opportunistic infection, is the worldwide leading cause of death among HIV-infected people. Tuberculosis in HIV-infected persons is also a particular public health concern because HIV persons are at greater risk of developing

multidrug-resistant tuberculosis. Multidrug-resistant tuberculosis is understandably difficult to treat and can be fatal (CDC 1999e, 1999g).

Reducing the spread of AIDS requires the understanding and acceptance of a variety of sexual issues, ranging from the likelihood that even heterosexual men may engage in anonymous homosexual intercourse to the difficulty that adolescents may have controlling their sexual urges. Prejudice against gays and lesbians is manifested as *homophobia*, a fear and/or hatred of these individuals. Homophobia explains the initial slow policy-related response to the HIV epidemic.

A variety of traditional public health measures have been used during the HIV crisis to reduce the spread of HIV, from mass testing for HIV to subjecting the exposed to lifelong quarantine—although quarantine has rarely been used. For several reasons, these traditional measures are much less effective when applied to HIV/AIDS, as opposed to sexually transmitted diseases (STDs), such as gonorrhea or syphilis. The primary purpose for testing for STDs is to limit their spread. This goal is easily accomplished because the symptoms of STDs appear early and are generally treatable and curable. Testing for the presence of HIV, however, may not limit its spread because many people who learn their HIV status do not change the behaviors that contribute to its spread. Further, HIV has no cure. Current treatments do not affect the transmissibility of HIV, and some treatments are of questionable use for treatment of the symptoms of AIDS. Quarantine has generally not been used to contain the spread of HIV. Because HIV-positive people can transmit HIV throughout their lives, lifetime quarantine is not only legally impossible but also economically unfeasible.

Criminal law has also been used to contain the spread of HIV and to protect public health. For example, several laws nationwide require that those convicted of sex offenses be tested for HIV. Most of these laws, however, are disproportionately enforced against prostitutes. These laws suggest that those who test HIV-positive may receive greater prison sentences; however, it is questionable whether this type of punishment actually reduces the spread of HIV.

Health promotion efforts, including those used to reduce the transmission of HIV, are often hamstrung by many psychosocial and other systematic factors. Some of the psychosocial factors include the fact that humans have a hard time changing their behavior. People have a tendency to justify it. Further, much human behavior is associated with functional needs (e.g., unsafe sex might fulfill a need for intimacy). Because of the strength of these psychosocial factors, knowledge about how HIV is actually transmitted may be too weakly correlated with behavior change. The social learning theory explains that behavior change, first, requires knowledge, followed by a change of attitude or perspective.

## Discrimination

HIV-positive people may experience discrimination in access to health care, which could range from refusal of treatment to breach of confidentiality. Even though HIV is difficult to transmit through casual contact, some health care workers often refuse to treat HIV-positive people. Some providers fear losing other patients. A physician who becomes HIV-positive would almost certainly lose patients in his or her practice. Many health care workers simply do not like homosexuals and IV drug users because they do not accept their behavior.

The policies of various government agencies intended to help have also had a discriminatory impact on people with HIV/AIDS. For example, the Social Security Administration has not historically considered many of the HIV-related symptoms of women and IV drug users in adjudicating disability claims. Although the Department of Defense provides adequate medical care to individuals who acquire HIV in the military, recruits who test HIV-positive cannot join the military.

## Provider Training

In a study of the HIV-related training needs of health care providers, medical information was identified as the primary training need. Patients with HIV, on the other hand, emphasized that their health care providers needed psychosocial skills, cultural competency, and sensitivity, in addition to medical proficiency. According to HIV patients, the criteria for appropriate care should include providers' attitudes toward patients (e.g., body language denoting respect, treating the consumer as an equal partner in decision making about care) and providers' concern about nonmedical aspects of consumer quality of life (e.g., child care, transportation, and emotional well-being).

Increased knowledge about HIV and personal contact with people who have HIV have improved the attitudes of health care providers toward individuals with HIV and contributed to their willingness to care for people with HIV. Training should encompass not only medical and treatment-related information but also a range of competencies related to interpersonal interaction.

In the area of psychosocial skills, the following characteristics are essential for an effectively trained provider: good communication skills (ability to establish rapport, ask questions, and listen), positive attitudes (respect, empowerment, trust), and an approach that incorporates principles of holistic care. In the area of cultural competence, essential elements include understanding of and respect for the person's specific culture; understanding that racial and ethnic minorities have important and multiple subdivisions or functional units; acknowledging the issues of gender and sexual orientation within the context of cultural competence; and respecting the customs, including modes of communication, of the person's culture. In the area of substance abuse, the following key elements are essential for primary care providers: understanding the complex medical picture presented by a person who suffers both from HIV and addiction; understanding the complicated psychosocial, ethical, and legal issues related to care of addicted persons; and being aware of the personal attitudes about addiction that may impair the providers' ability to give care objectively and nonjudgmentally (e.g., in the administration of pain medication; Gross and Larkin 1996).

The risk of transmission of HIV from an infected health care worker to a patient lies somewhere between 1 in 4,000 and 1 in 40,000 (Pell et al. 1996). Guidelines adopted in the United Kingdom on the management of HIV-infected health care workers encompass three main principles: a duty to protect patients, a duty of confidentiality toward infected health care workers, and the concept that the risk of HIV transmission is restricted to certain exposure-prone procedures from which infected staff should refrain (Pell et al. 1996):

- Infected health care workers should stop performing exposure-prone procedures immediately after diagnosis.

- Patients who have undergone an exposure-prone procedure, when the infected health care worker was the sole or main operator, should be notified of this situation, offered reassurance and counseling, and administered an HIV test if requested.

- If possible, letters to patients should be sent so that they arrive before or on the day of the planned press statement.

- A dedicated local telephone helpline should be established as soon as possible.

- Health care workers have a right to confidentiality, which can be breached only in exceptional circumstances when required in the public interest.

## Cost of HIV/AIDS

Medical care for an HIV/AIDS patient is extremely expensive. Pharmaceutical companies claim that the high prices they charge for AIDS drugs are related to their extensive investment in research and development of drugs. At least for HIV/AIDS-related drugs, the government must pay these prices without question. Medicaid covers an estimated 200,000 to 240,000 people with HIV (Kaiser Family Foundation 2008). In fiscal year (FY) 2008, combined federal and state Medicaid spending on HIV totaled $7.5 billion, making it the largest source of public financing for HIV/AIDS care in the United

States. Of this, the federal share was $4.1 billion in FY 2008, or 35% of federal HIV care spending (Kaiser Family Foundation 2008). Lack of insurance and underinsurance represent formidable financial barriers to HIV/AIDS care.

The US government also invests substantial amounts of money in research and development through research supported at NIH and CDC. Government programs spend money in several areas for HIV (Figure 11–12).

Much of the cost of medical care for a person infected with HIV is concentrated in the relatively brief period after a diagnosis of full-blown AIDS. From the time of entering HIV care, per person projected life expectancy is 24.2 years, discounted lifetime cost is $385,200, and undiscounted cost is $618,900 for adults who initiate HAART when the CD4 cell count is 350/L. Seventy-three percent of the cost is antiretroviral medications, 13% inpatient care, 9% outpatient care, and 5% other HIV-related medications and laboratory costs. For patients who initiate HAART when the CD4 cell count is 200/L, projected life expectancy is 22.5 years, discounted lifetime cost is $354,100 and undiscounted cost is $567,000. Results are sensitive to drug manufacturers' discounts, HAART efficacy, and use of enfuvirtide for salvage. If costs are discounted to the time of infection, the discounted lifetime cost is $303,100. Indirect costs include lost productivity, largely because of worker morbidity and mortality. However, other factors affect cost projections associated with the HIV epidemic, including the level of employment of HIV-positive people; regional differences in the cost of care, which

Figure 11–12  US Federal Spending for HIV/AIDS by Category, FY 2011 Budget Request.

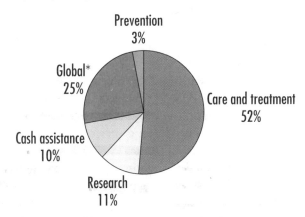

Prevention
3%

Global*
25%

Cash assistance
10%

Research
11%

Care and treatment
52%

*Categories may include funding across multiple agencies/programs; global category includes international HIV research at NIH.

*Source:* Adapted from Kaiser Family Foundation. US Federal Funding for HIV/AIDS: The President's FY 2011 Budget Request. HIV/AIDS Policy Fact Sheet, February 2010.

is often associated with the lack of subacute care in many parts of the country; and the rate at which HIV spreads.

Containment of escalating medical costs, including the coordination of medical care, is the objective of two HIV-specific efforts: the *Medicaid waiver program* and the Ryan White Comprehensive AIDS Resources Emergency (CARE) Act. Through the Medicaid waiver program, states may design packages of services to specific populations, such as the elderly, the disabled, and those who test HIV positive. At this time, it is unknown whether the program is cost effective.

The passage of the Ryan White CARE Act in 1990 by Congress provided much-needed federal money to develop treatment and care options for persons with HIV and AIDS (Summer 1991). This legislation's main purpose was to provide emergency assistance to cities significantly affected by HIV/AIDS, allowing them to provide an array of testing, counseling, and other services, including case management, to people with HIV/AIDS. Title II of this legislation is administered by states and has been used to establish HIV clinics and related services in areas lacking the resources needed to offer this specialty care. Some public health systems have used Ryan White money to provide HIV and AIDS services in rural communities in which poor or medically underserved persons lack access to adequate care. Through the allocation of Ryan White funds, persons with HIV infection have been provided medical care, medicines, and care coordination within the public health system. The Act focuses on the development of cost-effective service schemes by funding innovative and existing services. Federal spending for Ryan White was estimated to total $2.1 billion in 2007 (Kaiser Family Foundation 2007).

## AIDS and the US Health Care System

The course of AIDS is characterized by a gradual decline in a patient's physical, cognitive, and emotional function and well-being. Such a comprehensive decline requires a continuum of care, including emergency care, primary care, housing and supervised living, mental health and social support, nonmedical services, and hospice care. The continuum can encompass elements like outreach and case finding, preventive services, outpatient and inpatient care, and coordination of private and public insurance benefits.

As HIV disease progresses, many persons become disabled or lose their jobs and rely on public entitlement or private disability programs for income and health care benefits. These programs include Social Security Disability Income and Supplemental Security Income, administered by the Social Security Administration. Medicare and Medicaid become primary payers for health care because of the onset of disability and depletion of personal funds.

## Summary

This chapter examines the major characteristics of certain US population groups that face challenges and barriers in accessing health care services. These population groups are racial/ethnic minorities, children and women, those living in rural areas, the homeless, the mentally ill, and those with HIV/AIDS. The health needs of these population groups are summarized, and services available to them are described. The gaps that currently exist between these population groups and the rest of the population indicate that the nation must make significant efforts to address the unique health concerns of US subpopulations.

## Test Your Understanding

### Terminology

| | | |
|---|---|---|
| *AIDS* | *disability* | *new morbidities* |
| *chronic* | *HIV* | *opportunistic infections* |
| *dependency* | *homophobia* | *psychiatrists* |
| *developmental* | *Medicaid waiver program* | *psychologists* |
|    *vulnerability* | *mental health system* | |

### Review Questions

1. How can the framework of vulnerability be used to study vulnerable populations in the United States?
2. What are the racial/ethnic minority categories in the United States?
3. Compared with White Americans, what health challenges do minorities face?
4. Who are the AA/PIs?
5. What is the Indian Health Service?
6. What are the health concerns of children?
7. Which childhood characteristics have important implications for health system design?
8. Which health services are currently available for children?
9. What are the health concerns of women?
10. What are the roles of the Office on Women's Health?
11. What are the challenges faced in rural health?
12. What measures are taken to improve access to care in rural areas?
13. What are the characteristics and health concerns of the homeless population?
14. How is mental health provided in the United States?
15. Who are the major mental health professionals?
16. How does AIDS affect different population groups in the United States?
17. Which services and policies currently combat AIDS in America?

## REFERENCES

Aday, L.A. 1993. *At risk in America: The health and health care needs of vulnerable populations in the United States*. San Francisco, CA: Jossey-Bass Publishers.

Aday, L.A. 1994. Health status of vulnerable populations. *Annual Review Public Health* 15: 487–509.

Barker, P.R. et al. 1989. *Serious mental illness and disability in the adult household population: United States, 1989*. Hyattsville, MD: National Center for Health Statistics.

Bennefield, R. 1995. Current population reports: Health insurance coverage 1995. Bureau of the Census. [Online]. Available at: http://www.census.gov/prod/99pubs/p60–208.pdf. Accessed October 1999.

Bertakis, K.D. et al. 2000. Gender differences in the utilization of health services. *Journal of Family Practice* 49: 147–152.

Branson, B.M. et al. 2006. Revised recommendations for HIV testing of adults, adolescents, and pregnant women in health care settings. *MMWR* 55, no. RR14: 1–17.

Bureau of Labor Statistics (BLS). 2010. Bureau of Labor Statistics news release dated 11-5-10. Available at: http://www.bls.gov/news.release/empsit.nr0.htm. Accessed November 2010.

Burks, L.J. 1992. Community health representatives: The vital link in Native American health care. *The IHS Primary Care Provider* 16, no. 12: 186–190.

Castor, M.L. et al. 2006. A nationwide population-based study identifying health disparities between American Indians/Alaska Natives and the general populations living in select urban counties. *American Journal of Public Health* 96, no. 8: 1478–1484.

Centers for Disease Control and Prevention (CDC). 1995a. *Facts about women and HIV/AIDS*. Atlanta, GA: CDC.

Centers for Disease Control and Prevention (CDC). 1995b. *HIV/AIDS surveillance report, February*. Atlanta, GA: CDC.

Centers for Disease Control and Prevention (CDC). 1998. Update: HIV counseling and testing using rapid tests—United States, 1995. *Morbidity and Mortality Weekly Report* 47, no. 11: 211–215.

Centers for Disease Control and Prevention (CDC). 1999a. Guidelines for national human immunodeficiency virus case surveillance, including monitoring for human immunodeficiency virus infection and acquired immunodeficiency syndrome. *Morbidity and Mortality Weekly Report* 48, no. RR-13: 2–7.

Centers for Disease Control and Prevention (CDC). 1999b. *Rapid HIV tests: Questions/answers*. Available at: http://www.cdc.gov/nchstp/hiv_aids/pubs/rt/rapidqas.htm. Accessed December 2010.

Centers for Disease Control and Prevention (CDC). 1999c. Anonymous or confidential HIV counseling and voluntary testing in federally funded testing sites—United States, 1995–1997. *Morbidity and Mortality Weekly Report* 48, no. 24: 509–513.

Centers for Disease Control and Prevention (CDC). 1999d. *CDC fact sheet: HIV/AIDS among US women: Minority and young women at continuing risk*. Available at: http://www.cdc.gov/nchstp/hiv_aids/pubs/facts.htm. Accessed December 2010.

Centers for Disease Control and Prevention (CDC). 1999e. *CDC fact sheet: Recent HIV/AIDS treatment advances and the implications for prevention*. Available at: http://www.cdc.gov/nchstp/hiv_aids/pubs/facts.htm. Accessed December 2010.

Centers for Disease Control and Prevention (CDC). 1999f. *CDC fact sheet: Status of perinatal HIV prevention: US declines continue*. Available at: http://www.cdc.gov/nchstp/hiv_aids/pubs/facts.htm. Accessed December 2010.

Centers for Disease Control and Prevention (CDC). 1999g. *CDC fact sheet: The deadly intersection between TB and HIV*. Available at: http://www.cdc.gov/nchstp/hiv_aids/pubs/facts.htm. Accessed December 2010.

Centers for Disease Control and Prevention (CDC). 2001. *National Center for HIV, STD, and TB Prevention. Commentary*. Available at: http://www.cdc.gov/hiv/stats/hasrsupp62/commentary.htm. Accessed December 2010.

Centers for Disease Control and Prevention (CDC). 2002. *CDC fact sheet: HIV/AIDS among African-Americans, key facts*. Available at: http://www.cdc.gov/hiv/pubs/facts/afam.pdf. Accessed April 2003.

Centers for Disease Control and Prevention (CDC). 2005. *HIV/AIDS surveillance report, 2004*. Vol. 16. Atlanta: US Department of Health and Human Services.

Centers for Disease Control and Prevention (CDC). 2006. *HIV/AIDS surveillance report, 2005*. Vol. 17. Atlanta: US Department of Health and Human Services.

Centers for Disease Control and Prevention (CDC). 2007. *HIV/AIDS surveillance report*. Available at: http://www.cdc.gov/hiv/surveillance/resources /reports/2007report/table6b.htm. Accessed December 2010.

Centers for Disease Control and Prevention (CDC). 2009. *The power of prevention*. Available at: http://www.cdc.gov/chronicdisease/overview/index.htm. Accessed January 2011.

Centers for Disease Control and Prevention (CDC). 2010a. *Chronic disease and health promotion*. Available at: http://www.cdc.gov/chronicdisease/pdf/2009-Power-of-Prevention.pdf. Accessed January 2011.

Centers for Disease Control and Prevention (CDC). 2010b. Deaths among persons with AIDS through December 2006. *HIV/AIDS surveillance report*, volume 14, no. 3. Available at: http://www.cdc.gof/hiv/surveillance/resources/reports/2009supp_vol14no3/ pdf/table1.pdf. Accessed December 2010.

Centers for Disease Control and Prevention (CDC), National Center for Injury Prevention and Control. 2011. *Web-based injury statistics query and reporting system (WISQARS)*. Available at: www.cdc.gov/ncipc/wisqars. Accessed January 2011.

Cohen, S.E. et al. 1994. The geography of AIDS: Patterns of urban and rural migration. *Southern Medical Journal* 85, no. 6: 599.

Department of Health and Human Services (DHHS), Office of Minority Health. 2003. *HIV impact, AIDS in rural America*. Washington, DC: Government Printing Office. pp. 10–11.

Donelan, K. et al. 1996. Whatever happened to the health insurance crisis in the United States? *Journal of the American Medical Association* 276, no. 16: 1346–1350.

Fitzwilliams, J. 1977. Critical health manpower shortage areas: Their impact on rural health planning. *Agricultural Economic Report* No. 361. Washington, DC: Economic Research Service, Department of Agriculture.

Freeman, H.E., and C.R. Corey. 1993. Insurance status and access to health services among poor persons. *Health Services Research* 28: 531–541.

Greenwald, J.L. et al. 2006. A rapid review of rapid HIV antibody tests. *Current Infectious Disease Reports* 8: 125–131.

Gross, E.J., and M.H. Larkin. 1996. The child with HIV in day care and school. *Nursing Clinics of North America* 31, no. 1: 231–241.

Health Resources and Services Administration (HRSA), Bureau of Health Professions. 2003. National Health Service Corps. Available at: http://nhsc.bhpr.hrsa.gov/about/. Accessed December 2008.

Health Resources and Services Administration (HRSA), Bureau of Health Professions. 2007a. About NHSC. Available at: http://nhsc.bhpr.hrsa.gov/about/history.asp. Accessed December 2008.

Health Resources and Services Administration (HRSA), Bureau of Health Professions. 2007b. Shortage designation. Available at: http://bhpr.hrsa.gov/shortage/. Accessed December 2008.

Health Resources and Services Administration (HRSA), Bureau of Health Professions. 2007c. Health professional shortage area primary medical care designation criteria. Available at: http://bhpr.hrsa.gov/shortage/hpsacritpcm.htm. Accessed December 2008.

Health Resources and Services Administration (HRSA), Bureau of Primary Health Care. 2007a. Migrant health centers. Available at: http://bphc.hrsa.gov/migrant/. Accessed December 2008.

Health Resources and Services Administration (HRSA), Bureau of Primary Health Care. 2007b. America's health centers. Available at: http://bphc.hrsa.gov/chc/charts/healthcenters.htm. Accessed December 2008.

Health Resources and Services Administration (HRSA), Office of Rural Health Policy. 2007. Strategic plan 2005–2010. Available at: http://ruralhealth.hrsa.gov/policy/StrategicPlan.asp. Accessed December 2008.

Herzog, D.B., and P.N. Copeland. 1985. Medical progress: Eating disorders. *New England Journal of Medicine* 313, no. 5: 295–303.

HHS Rural Task Force. 2002. Report to the Secretary: One department serving rural America. Available at: http://ruralhealth.hrsa.gov/PublicReport.htm#2001. Accessed December 2008.

Indian Health Service (IHS). 1999a. *A quick look*. Washington, DC: Public Health Service, September: 1.

Indian Health Service (IHS). 1999b. *Fact sheet: Comprehensive health care program for American Indians and Alaskan Natives*. Washington, DC: Public Health Service, October: 1.

Indian Health Service (IHS). 2010a. *Indian population. IHS fact sheet*. Washington, DC: Public Health Service. January 2010.

Indian Health Service (IHS). 2010b. *Indian health disparities. IHS fact sheet*. Washington, DC: Public Health Service. January 2010.

Indian Health Service (IHS). 2010c. *IHS year 2010 profile. IHS fact sheet*. Washington, DC: Public Health Service. January 2010.

Johnson, J.P., and P.E. Vink. 1992. Diagnosis and classification of HIV infection in children. In: *Management of HIV infection in infants and children*. R. Yogev and E. Connor, eds. St. Louis, MO: Mosby–Year Book. pp. 117–128.

Kaiser Commission on Medicaid and the Uninsured. 2006. *The uninsured: A primer*. Available at: http://www.kff.org/uninsured/upload/7451-021.pdf. Accessed December 2008.

Kaiser Commission on Medicaid and the Uninsured. 2010. *The uninsured and the difference health insurance makes*. Washington DC: Kaiser Commission on Medicaid and the Uninsured. September 2010.

Kaiser Family Foundation. 2004. *Health care and the 2004 elections: Women's health policy.* Available at: http://www.kff.org/womenshealth/7184.cfm#repro. Accessed December 2008.

Kaiser Family Foundation. 2005. *Women and health care: A national profile.* Available at: http://www.kff.org/womenshealth/7336.cfm. Accessed December 2008.

Kaiser Family Foundation. 2007. *Fact sheet: The Ryan White Program.* Available at: http://www.kff.org/hivaids/upload/7582_03.pdf. Accessed December 2008.

Kaiser Family Foundation. 2008. *Medicaid and HIV/AIDS. HIV/AIDS policy fact sheet.* Washington, DC: Kaiser Family Foundation. February 2009.

Klerman, G.L., and M.M. Weissman. 1989. Increasing rate of depression. *Journal of the American Medical Association* 261, no. 24: 2229–2235.

Kozoll, R. 1986. Indian health care. In: *New dimensions in rural policy: Building upon our heritage.* Washington, DC: Government Printing Office. pp. 447–480.

Kraus, L.E. et al. 1996. *Chartbook on disability in the United States, 1996. An InfoUse Report.* Washington, DC: US National Institute on Disability and Rehabilitation Research.

Kuo, J., and K. Porter. 1998. *Health status of Asian Americans: United States, 1992–94.* Advance data from vital and health statistics. Hyattsville, MD: National Center for Health Statistics. no. 298: 1–3.

Lam, N., and K. Liu. 1994. Spread of AIDS in rural America, 1982–1990. *Journal of Acquired Immune Deficiency Syndrome* 7, no. 5: 485–490.

Lurie, N. 1997. Studying access to care in managed care environment. *Health Services Research* 32: 691–701.

Merson, M.H. 1996. Returning home: Reflections on the USA's response to the HIV/AIDS epidemic. *Lancet* 347, no. 9016: 1673–1676.

Misra, D. ed. 2001. *Women's health data book: A profile of women's health in the United States,* 3rd ed. Washington, DC: Jacobs Institute of Women's Health and the Henry J. Kaiser Family Foundation.

Morrison, C. 1993. Delivery systems for the care of persons with HIV infection and AIDS. *Nursing Clinics of North America* 28, no. 2: 317–333.

Myers, J.K. et al. 1984. Six-month prevalence of psychiatric disorders in three communities. *Archives of General Psychiatry* 41, no. 10: 959–967.

National Association of Rural Health Clinics (NARHC). 2007. Available at: http://www.narhc.org/about_us/about_us.php. Accessed December 2008.

National Center for Chronic Disease Prevention and Health Promotion. 2005. *Chronic disease: Overview.* Available at: http://www.cdc.gov/nccdphp/overview.htm. Accessed December 2008.

National Center for Health Statistics. 2007. *Deaths: Final data for 2007, table B, national vital statistics report.* Hyattsville, MD: Department of Health and Human Services.

National Center for Health Statistics. 2009. *Summary health statistics for U.S. adults: National health interview survey, 2009, tables 1, 2.* Hyattsville, MD: Department of Health and Human Services.

National Center for Health Statistics. 2010. *Health, United states, 2009.* Hyattsville, MD: Department of Health and Human Services.

National Coalition for the Homeless. 2006a. *NCH fact sheet #2: How many people experience homelessness?* Available at: http://www.nationalhomeless.org/publications/facts/How_Many .pdf. Accessed December 2008.

National Coalition for the Homeless. 2006b. *NCH fact sheet #3: Who is homeless?* Available at: http://www.nationalhomeless.org/publications/facts/Whois.pdf. Accessed December 2008.

National Institute of Allergy and Infectious Diseases. 2006. *Fact sheet: HIV infection in women.* Available at: http://www.niaid.nih.gov/factsheets/womenhiv.htm. Accessed December 2008.

National Institute of Health (NIH). July 9, 2002. *News release: NHLBI stops trial of estrogen plus progestin due to increased breast cancer risk, lack of overall benefit.* Available at: http://www. nhlbi.nih.gov/new/press/02-07-09.htm. Accessed December 2006.

National Institute of Mental Health (NIMH). 2006a. *The numbers count.* Available at: http://www .nimh.nih.gov/publicat/numbers.cfm#Schizophrenia. Accessed December 2008.

National Institute of Mental Health (NIMH). 2006b. *Total expenditures for the five most costly health conditions (1996, 2006).* Available at: http://www.nimh.nih.gov/statistics/4TOT_ MC9606.shtml. Accessed January 2011.

National Institute of Mental Health (NIMH). 2007. *Statistics.* Available at: http://www.nimh.nih .gov/healthinformation/statisticsmenu.cfm. Accessed December 2008.

National Institute of Mental Health (NIMH). 2008. *Prevalence of serious mental illness among U.S. adults by sex, age, race in 2008.* Available at: http://www.nimh.nih.gov/statistics/SMI_AASR .shtml. Accessed January 2011.

O'Hara, M.J., and D. D'Orlando. 1996. Ambulatory care of the HIV-infected child. *Nursing Clinics of America* 31, no. 1: 179–205.

Ostir, G.V. et al. 1999. Disability in older adults 1: Prevalence, causes, and consequences. *Behavioral Medicine* 24: 147–154.

Patton, L., and D. Puskin. 1990. *Ensuring access to health care services in rural areas: A half century of federal policy.* Essential Health Care Services Conference Center at Georgetown University Conference Center. Washington, DC.

Pell, J. et al. 1996. Management of HIV infected health care workers: Lessons from three cases. *British Medical Journal* 312, no. 7039: 1150–1152, discussion 1152–1153.

Pleasant, R. 2003. Minority health. In: *The Department of Health and Human Services: 50 years of service.* DHHS. pp. 92–95.

Regier, D.A. et al. 1988. One month prevalence of mental disorders in the United States: Based on five epidemiologic catchment area sites. *Archives of General Psychiatry* 45, no. 11: 977–986.

Rhodes, E.R. 1987. The organization of health services for Indian people. *Public Health Reports* 102, no. 4: 361–365.

Robertson, L.S. et al. 1974. *Changing the medical care system: A controlled experiment in comprehensive care.* New York: Praeger Publishers.

Romanoski, A.J. et al. 1992. The epidemiology of psychiatrist-ascertained depression and DSM-III depressive disorders: Results from the Eastern Baltimore Mental Health Survey Clinical Reappraisal. *Psychological Medicine* 22, no. 3: 629–655.

Rosenbaum, S., and J. Darnell. 1997. *An analysis of the Medicaid and health-related provisions of the Personal Responsibility and Work Opportunity Reconciliation Act of 1996 (P.L. 104–193).* Washington, DC: The Kaiser Commission on the Future of Medicaid.

Rumby, R.L. et al. 1991. AIDS in rural Eastern North Carolina. Patient migration: A rural AIDS burden. *AIDS* 5, no. 11: 1373–1378.

Salganicoff, A. et al. 2005. *Women and health care: A national profile.* Menlo Park, CA: The Henry J. Kaiser Family Foundation.

Schutt, R.K., and S.M. Goldfinger. 1996. Housing preferences and perceptions of health and functioning among homeless mentally ill persons. *Psychiatric Services* 47, no. 4: 381–386.

Sechzer, J.A. et al. 1996. Women and mental health. New York: *Academy of Sciences.*

Selike, R.M. et al. 1993. HIV infection as leading cause of death among young adults in US cities and states. *Journal of the American Medical Association* 269, no. 23: 2991–2994.

Shi, L., and G. Stevens. 2010. *Vulnerable Populations in the United States.* 2nd ed. San Farncisco, CA: Jossey-Bass Publishers, Inc.

Shortell, S.M. et al. 1996. *Remaking health care in America.* San Francisco, CA: Jossey-Bass Publishers.

Solis, J.M. et al. 1990. Acculturation, access to care, and use of preventive services by Hispanics: Findings from HHANES 1982–84. *American Journal of Public Health* 80 (Suppl): 11–19.

Stratton, T. et al. 1993. *A demographic analysis of nurse shortage counties: Implications for rural nursing policy.* Grand Forks, ND: University of North Dakota Rural Health Research Center.

Substance Abuse and Mental Health Services Administration. 2010. Results from the 2009 National Survey on Drug Use and Health: Mental Health Findings. Rockville, MD: Office of Applied Studies, NSDUH Series H-39, HHS Publication No. SMA 10-4609.

Summer, L. 1991. *Limited access: Health care for the rural poor.* Washington, DC: Center on Budget and Policy Priorities.

The Robert Wood Johnson Foundation. 1996. *Chronic care in America: A 21st century challenge.* Available at: http://www.rwjf.org/files/publications/other/ChronicCareinAmerica.pdf?gsa=1. [O1] Accessed December 2000.

United Nations (UN). 2007. *The state of the world's children 2007.* Available at: http://www.unicef.org/sowc07/docs/sowc07.pdf[O2]. Accessed December 2008.

UNAIDS. 2010. UNAIDS report on the global AIDS epidemic 2010. Available at: http://www.unaids.org/globalreport/Global_report.htm. Accessed December 2010).

US Census Bureau. 2007. *Statistical abstract of the United States, 2007: The National Data Book.* Washington, DC: Government Printing Office.

US Census Bureau. 2009. *The 2010 census questionnaire: Informational copy.* Available at: http://2010.census.gov/2010census/pdf/2010_Questionnaire_Info_Copy.pdf. Accessed April 2009.

US Census Bureau. 2010. *Statistical abstract of the United States, 2010.* Washington, DC: Government Printing Office.

US Department of Veteran Affairs. 2006. *Fact sheet: VA programs for homeless veterans.* Available at: http://www1.va.gov/opa/fact/hmlssfs.asp. Accessed December 2008.

Weissman, M.M., and G.L. Klerman. 1977. Sex differences and the epidemiology of depression. *Archives of General Psychiatry* 34, no. 1: 98–111.

Wenzel, M. 1996. A school-based clinic for elementary school in Phoenix, Arizona. *Journal of School Health* 66, no. 4: 125–127.

Williams, S.J. 1995. *Essentials of health services.* Albany, NY: Delmar Publishers.

World Health Organization (WHO). 2004. *Women and AIDS: Have you heard us today?* Available at: http://www.who.int/features/2004/aids/en/. Accessed December 2008.

Yoon, E., and F. Chien. 1996. Asian American and Pacific Islander health: A paradigm for minority health. *Journal of the American Medical Association* 275, no. 9: 736–737.

Yu, S.M. et al. 2004. Health status and health services utilization among US Chinese, Asian Indian, Filipino, and other Asian/Pacific Islander children. *Pediatrics* 113, no. 1 part 1: 101–107.

# PART IV

---

# System Outcomes

# Chapter 12

# Cost, Access, and Quality

## Learning Objectives

- To understand the meaning of health care costs and review recent trends
- To examine the factors that have led to cost escalations in the past
- To become familiar with both regulatory and market-oriented approaches to contain costs
- To understand why some regulatory cost-containment approaches were unsuccessful
- To appreciate the framework and various dimensions of access to care
- To learn about access indicators and measurement
- To understand the nature, scope, and dimensions of quality
- To understand the difference between quality assurance and quality assessment

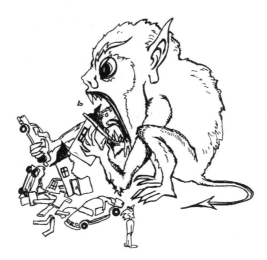

*The health care sector of the economy is like a monster with a voracious appetite that needs to be controlled.*

## Introduction

Cost, access, and quality are three major cornerstones of health care delivery (Al-Assaf 1993a). For many years, employers and third-party payers in the United States have been preoccupied with controlling the growth of health care expenditures. Cost and access go hand in hand, meaning expansion of access will increase health care expenditures. This is one main reason that attempts to implement universal coverage in the United States have failed in the past. Although cost and access have remained the primary concerns within the US health care delivery system, quality of health care has taken center stage.

Cost, access, and quality have some interdependencies. From a macro perspective, costs of health care are commonly viewed in terms of national health expenditures (NHE). As pointed out in Chapter 6, a widely used measure of NHE is the proportion of the gross domestic product (GDP) a country spends on the delivery of health care services. From a micro perspective, health care expenditures refer to costs incurred by employers to purchase health insurance and out-of-pocket costs incurred by individuals when they receive health care services. Improving access to health care and equal access to quality health care are contingent on expenditures at both the macro and micro levels. High-quality care is also the most cost-effective care. Hence, cost is an important factor in the evaluation of quality. On the other hand, quality is achieved by having up-to-date capabilities, using evidence-based processes, and measuring outcomes. Quality goals are accomplished when the system capabilities and practices employed in the delivery of health care

achieve desirable outcomes for individuals and populations.

This chapter discusses the major reasons for the dramatic rise in health care expenditures. Costs are compared with those in other countries, and the impact of cost-containment measures is examined. Dimensions of access are presented. Finally, quality of care and its measurement are discussed.

## Cost of Health Care

The term "cost" can carry different meanings in the delivery of health care, depending on whose perspective is considered. (1) When consumers and financiers speak of the "cost" of health care, they usually mean the "price" of health care. This could refer to the physician's bill, the price of a prescription, or the premiums employers pay to purchase health insurance for their employees. (2) From a national perspective, health care costs refer to how much a nation spends on health care, that is, NHE or health care spending (see Chapter 6). Since expenditures (E) equal price (P) times quantity (Q), growth in health care spending can be accounted for by growth in prices charged by the providers of health services and by increases in the utilization of services (see Figure 6–1). (3) A third perspective is that of the providers, for whom the notion of cost refers to the cost of producing health care services. Such things as staff salaries, capital costs for buildings and equipment, rental of space, and purchase of supplies are included in the cost of production.

### Trends in National Health Expenditures

Chapter 6 gave an overview of national and personal health expenditures, their composition, and the proportional share between the private and public sectors. Health care spending spiraled upward at double digit rates during the 1970s, right after the Medicare and Medicaid programs created a massive growth in access in 1965. By 1970, government expenditures for health care services and supplies had grown by 140%, from $7.9 to $18.9 billion (DHHS 1996). During much of the 1980s, average annual growth in national health spending continued in the double digits, but the rate of increase slowed considerably (Figure 12–1). In the 1990s, medical inflation was finally brought under control, down to a single digit rate of growth, mainly due to control over payment and utilization through managed care. The rate of growth has again started

to accelerate, but at a relatively slow pace (Table 12–1).

Trends in NHE are commonly evaluated in three ways. One is to compare medical inflation to general inflation in the economy, which is measured by annual changes in the consumer price index (CPI). Except for a brief period between 1978 and 1981, when the US economy was experiencing hyperinflation, the rates of change in medical inflation have remained consistently above the rates of change in the CPI (Figure 12–2). The second method compares changes in NHE to those in the GDP. With only isolated exceptions (in 1983 to 1984, after the implementation of diagnosis-related group [DRG]-based payments to hospitals, and in 1995 to 1998, after significant managed

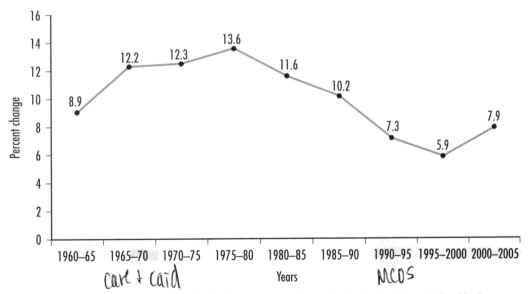

Figure 12–1  Average Annual Percentage Growth in US National Health Care Spending During Five-Year Periods, 1960–2005.

*Source:* Data from *Health, United States, 1995*, p. 244; *Health, United States, 2002*, p. 291; *Health, United States, 2009*, p. 396, Department of Health and Human Services.

Table 12–1　Average Annual Percentage Increase in US National Health Care Spending, 1975–2007

| Periods | % Increase | Periods | % Increase |
|---|---|---|---|
| 1975–1980 | 13.6 | 1990–1995 | 7.3 |
| 1975–1976 | 14.7 | 1990–1991 | 9.2 |
| 1976–1977 | 13.7 | 1991–1992 | 9.5 |
| 1977–1978 | 11.9 | 1992–1993 | 6.9 |
| 1978–1979 | 12.9 | 1993–1994 | 5.1 |
| 1979–1980 | 14.8 | 1994–1995 | 4.9 |
| 1980–1985 | 11.6 | 1995–2000 | 5.9 |
| 1980–1981 | 16.1 | 1995–1996 | 4.6 |
| 1981–1982 | 12.5 | 1996–1997 | 4.7 |
| 1982–1983 | 10.0 | 1997–1998 | 5.4 |
| 1983–1984 | 9.7 | 1998–1999 | 5.7 |
| 1984–1985 | 9.9 | 1999–2000 | 6.9 |
| 1985–1990 | 10.2 | 2000–2005 | 7.9 |
| 1985–1986 | 7.6 | 2000–2001 | 8.7 |
| 1986–1987 | 8.5 | 2001–2002 | 9.3 |
| 1987–1988 | 11.9 | 2002–2003 | 8.2 |
| 1988–1989 | 11.2 | 2003–2004 | 5.9 |
| 1989–1990 | 12.1 | 2004–2005 | 6.5 |
| | | 2005–2010 | |
| | | 2005–2006 | 6.7 |
| | | 2006–2007 | 6.1 |

Source: Data from Health, United States, 1995, p. 243; Health, United States, 1996–97, p. 249; Health, United States, 1999, p. 284; Health, United States, 2000, p. 322; Health, United States, 2002, p. 288; Health, United States, 2005, p. 363; Health, United States, 2006, p. 377; Health, United States, 2008, p. 415; Health, United States, 2009, p. 396; K. Levit et al. Trends in US health care spending, 2003. Health Affairs Vol. 22, no. 1: 154–164.

care penetration), health care spending growth rates have consistently surpassed growth rates in the general economy (Figure 12–3). When spending on health care grows at a faster rate than GDP, it means that health care consumes a larger share of the total economic output. Put another way, a growing share of total economic resources is devoted to the delivery of health care.

International comparison is the third method. Compared to other nations, the United States uses a larger share of its economic resources for health care (Table 12–2). In addition, the United States has outpaced

Consumer Price Index

Figure 12–2  Annual Percentage Change in CPI and Medical Inflation, 1975–2008.

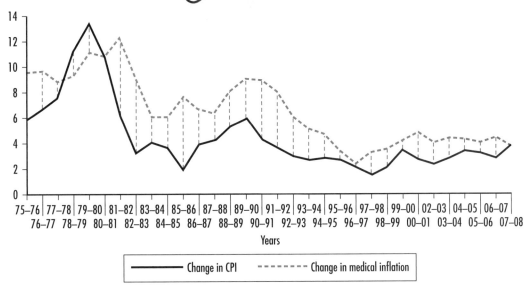

*Source:* Data from *Health, United States, 1995*, p. 241; *Health, United States, 1996–97*, p. 251; *Health, United States, 2002*, p. 289; *Health, United States, 2006*, p. 375; *Health, United States, 2008*, p. 413; *Health, United States, 2009*, p. 394.

Figure 12–3  Annual Percentage Change in US National Health Care Expenditures and GDP, 1980–2007.

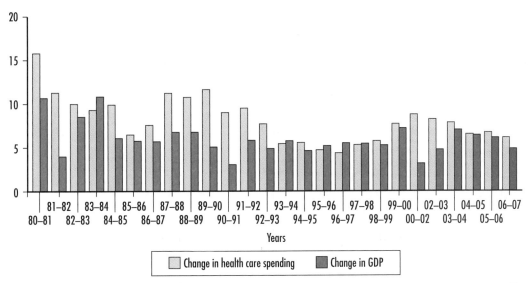

*Source:* Data from *Health, United States, 1996–97*, p. 249; *Health, United States, 2002*, p. 288; *Health, United States, 2006*, p. 374; *Health, United States, 2008*, p. 412; *Health, United States, 2009*, p. 393.

Table 12—2  Total US Health Care Expenditures as a Proportion of GDP and Per Capita Health Care Expenditures (Selected Years, Selected OECD Countries; Per Capita Expenditures in US Dollars)

|  | 1990 | 1995 | 2000 | 2005 |
|---|---|---|---|---|
| Australia | 7.8 | 8.2 | 9.0 | 8.8 |
|  | $1,307 | $1,745 | $2,220 | $2,999 |
| Austria | 7.0 | 8.0 | 7.6 | 10.3 |
|  | $1,338 | $1,870 | $2,184 | $3,507 |
| Belgium | 7.4 | 8.4 | 8.7 | 10.6 |
|  | $1,345 | $1,820 | $2,279 | $3,385 |
| Canada | 9.0 | 9.2 | 8.9 | 9.9 |
|  | $1,737 | $2,051 | $2,503 | $3,460 |
| Denmark | 8.5 | 8.2 | 8.4 | 9.5 |
|  | $1,567 | $1,848 | $2,382 | $3,179 |
| Finland | 7.8 | 7.5 | 6.7 | 8.3 |
|  | $1,422 | $1,433 | $1,718 | $2,523 |
| France | 8.6 | 9.5 | 9.3 | 11.1 |
|  | $1,568 | $2,033 | $2,456 | $3,306 |
| Germany | 8.5 | 10.6 | 10.6 | 10.7 |
|  | $1,748 | $2,276 | $2,761 | $3,251 |
| Italy | 7.9 | 7.3 | 8.1 | 8.9 |
|  | $1,391 | $1,535 | $2,049 | $2,496 |
| Japan | 5.9 | 6.8 | 7.6 | 8.2 |
|  | $1,115 | $1,538 | $1,971 | $2,474 |
| Netherlands | 8.0 | 8.4 | 8.3 | 9.5* |
|  | $1,438 | $1,826 | $2,259 | $3,156* |
| Sweden | 8.4 | 8.1 | 8.4 | 9.2 |
|  | $1,579 | $1,738 | $2,273 | $3,012 |
| United Kingdom | 6.0 | 7.0 | 7.3 | 8.2 |
|  | $986 | $1,374 | $1,833 | $2,580 |
| United States | 11.9 | 13.3 | 13.1 | 15.2 |
|  | $2,738 | $3,654 | $4,539 | $6,347 |

*Data from 2004

[1]Proportion of GDP.

[2]Per capita expenditures adjusted to US dollars using GDP purchasing power parities.

Source: Data from Health, United States, 2009, p. 392.

the growth in health care spending in other countries (Figure 12–4). Numerous reasons have been given for the growth of health care expenditures, and several initiatives have been employed over the years to prevent out-of-control spending. These topics are subsequently discussed in this chapter.

The rate of growth in health spending came down to its lowest level in 4 decades (5.7% average annual growth) between 1993 and 2000 as managed care proliferated (Levit et al. 2003), but the good news ended as the year 2002 recorded the fastest annual growth (9.3%) since 1992. However, the rate of growth has been slowing down each year (see Table 12–1). In 2008, the rate of growth slowed down to 4.4% over 2007. This was the slowest rate of growth in health care spending over the previous 48 years. This decrease is largely attributed to the most severe recession the nation had

experienced since 1933. As a result, personal health care expenditures that are paid mostly by private sources increased just 2.8%, the lowest rate since the 1990s, when managed care implemented tight cost control measures (Hartman et al. 2011). Future growth of health care expenditures will depend on two main factors: (1) the impact of the Patient Protection and Affordable Care Act (ACA) of 2010 and (2) GDP growth in the general economy. Higher utilization of health care services will no doubt lead to medical care cost inflation unless measures are employed to slow down the rise in P and Q.

In 2008, the United States spent $2.34 trillion on health care. This amounted to a per capita spending of $7,681 and 16.2% of GDP (DHHS 2011). According to the Congressional Budget Office, if present trends continue, health care spending will amount to 25% of GDP by 2025, 37% by 2050, and

Figure 12–4 US Health Care Spending as a Percentage of GDP for Selected OECD Countries, 1985 and 2005.

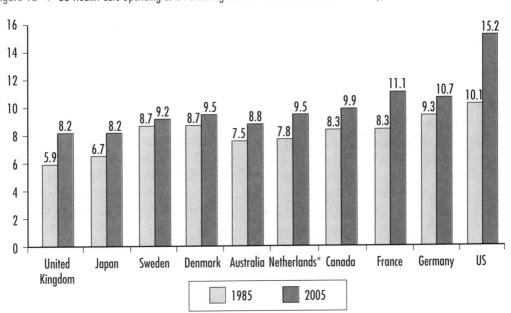

\*Netherlands data from 2004.

*Source:* Data from *Health, United States, 2002,* p. 287; *Health, United States, 2009,* p. 392.

49% by 2082 (CBO 2007). These forecasts portend that the health care sector will remain one of the fastest-growing components of the US economy. Increased demand for services will expand job opportunities for various types of health professionals and administrators. On the other hand, we can expect to see policy debates and new initiatives to keep costs from getting out of control.

## Should Health Care Costs Be Contained?

Americans view growth in expenditures in other sectors of the economy, such as manufacturing, much more favorably than expenditures on medical care. Increased medical expenditures create new health care jobs, do not pollute the air, save rather than destroy lives, and alleviate pain and suffering. Why shouldn't society be pleased that more resources are flowing into a sector that cares for the aged and the sick? It would seem to be a more appropriate use of a society's resources than spending those same funds on faster cars, fancy clothes, or other consumable items. Yet, increased expenditures for these other consumable items do not cause the concern that arises when medical expenditures increase (Feldstein 1994).

Unlike other goods and services in the economy, health care is not delivered under free market conditions (see Chapter 1). For the consumption of various other goods and services, the free market determines how much people and the nation should spend, depending on their economic capabilities. In the United States, the private sector and the government share roughly equally in the financing of health care. In a quasi-market, such as health care in the United States, it would be almost impossible to determine how much the nation should spend. Hence,

in the United States, we depend on three main sources to assess whether we spend too much:

1. The first source is international comparisons (Table 12–2), which is actually not an unbiased tool because, in these other nations, the government decides how much should be spent on health care and various rationing measures—such as supply-side controls, comparatively little spending on developing new technology, and price controls (for pharmaceuticals, for example)—are used to maintain certain levels of predetermined spending.

2. The second source is the rise in health insurance premiums in the private sector. This is what triggered private employers to abandon traditional fee-for-service insurance plans, sometime in the 1980s, and to seek employee coverage through HMO plans. In the United States, employer-based health insurance covers almost 160 million people, which is about 90% of the nonelderly, privately insured population (Kaiser Family Foundation 2010).

3. How much the government has to spend on health care for beneficiaries who receive health care through various public insurance programs is the third source. Concerns about the short- and long-term sustainability of the Medicare trust funds were discussed in Chapter 6.

Experts generally agree that the United States spends too much on health care, and, therefore, expenditures must be controlled. The main reasons are as follows:

1. Rising health care costs consume greater portions of the total economic output. Because economic resources are limited, rising health care costs mean that Americans have to forgo other goods and services when more is spent on health care.

2. Limited economic resources should be directed to their highest valued uses. In a free market, consumers make purchasing decisions based on their perception of value, knowing that an expenditure on one good means forgoing other goods and services (Feldstein 1994). In health care delivery, comprehensive health insurance creates moral hazard and provider-induced demand (as discussed in Chapter 1), both of which fuel inefficiencies in the consumption of resources.

3. American businesses argue that rising insurance premium costs have to be passed on to consumers in the form of higher prices, which may interfere with the ability of businesses to stay globally competitive. For example, health insurance premiums have consistently increased faster than inflation in the general economy or workers' wages in recent years. Between 1999 and 2008, the cumulative growth in health insurance premiums was 119%, whereas cumulative inflation was 29% and cumulative wage growth 34% (Kaiser Family Foundation 2009).

4. Rising premium costs limit the ability of many employers, especially small businesses, to offer health benefits, and, when those benefits are offered, they limit the ability of some employees to contribute toward the purchase of employer-sponsored insurance coverage (Kaiser Family Foundation 2010).

5. Rising health care costs take a toll on average- and low-income Americans. The 2010 Commonwealth Fund International Health Policy Survey pointed out that affordability of health care was one of the biggest economic problems for many Americans (Health Council of Canada 2010). Only 25% of Americans were very confident in their ability to afford care in case of serious illness. Twenty-two percent of Americans (compared to an average of 8% in other countries) had a medical problem but did not visit a doctor because of cost.

6. The government has only a limited ability to raise people's taxes, given that most American tax payers believe that they already pay more than their fair share of taxes. Paradoxically, as has been widely reported, half of Americans, many of whom use tax-financed health care, pay no federal income taxes (USA Today 2010).

## Reasons for Cost Escalation

Numerous factors have been attributed to rising health care expenditures. They interact in complex ways. Hence, one cannot just point to one or two main causes. General inflation in the economy is a more visible cause of health care spending because it affects the cost of producing health care services through such things as higher wages and cost of supplies. Some of the other factors mentioned subsequently were also discussed in earlier chapters. They are included here, along with additional pertinent details, to provide a comprehensive picture of the reasons behind medical cost inflation:

- third-party payment
- imperfect market
- growth of technology
- increase in elderly population
- medical model of health care delivery
- multipayer system and administrative costs
- defensive medicine
- waste and abuse
- practice variations

## Third-Party Payment

Health care is among the few services for which a third party, not the consumer, pays for most services used. Whether payment is made by the government or by a private insurance company, individual out-of-pocket expenses are far lower than the actual cost of the service (Altman and Wallack 1996). Hence, patients are generally insensitive to the cost of care. Introduction of prospective payment methods and capitation has, to a large extent, minimized provider-induced demand. However, the backlash against managed care (see Chapter 9) from consumers and providers alike has, in a sense, kept the door open to overuse of high-cost technologies and other services. Also, fee-for-service reimbursement and its discounted fee variation are still widely used in the outpatient sector of health care delivery. Hence, provider-induced demand has not been expunged from the system.

## Imperfect Market

Prices charged by providers for health care services are likely to be much closer to the cost of producing the services in a highly regulated or highly competitive market (Altman and Wallack 1996). Because the US health care delivery system follows neither the highly regulated single-payer model nor a free market model, utilization remains largely unchecked; prices charged for health care services remain higher than the true economic costs of production (Altman and Wallack 1996). A quasi-market results in increased health care expenditures because both Q and P remain unchecked. *quantity + price*

## Growth of Technology

The United States has been characterized as following an early-start-fast-growth pattern in the adoption and diffusion of intensive procedures (TECH Research Network 2001). Factors that drive technology innovation, diffusion, and utilization and their impact on cost escalation were discussed in Chapter 5. According to the Centers for Disease Control and Prevention (CDC), the use of advanced imaging scanning during visits to physician offices and outpatient departments more than tripled from 1996 to 2007 (National Center for Health Statistics 2010a). Medicare Part B spending for imaging services under the physician fee schedule more than doubled between 2000 and 2006, from $6.9 billion to $14.1 billion (US GAO 2008).

New technology is expensive to develop, and costs incurred in research and development (R&D) are included in total health care expenditures. One reason Canada and European nations, compared to the United States, have incurred lower costs is because they have proportionally invested far less in R&D. Hence, compared to other nations, the overall diffusion and utilization of technology is greater in the United States (Reinhardt et al. 2002).

## Increase in Elderly Population

Since the early part of the 20th century, life expectancy in the United States has consistently risen (see Figure 12–5). Life expectancy at birth increased by over 30 years, from 47.3 years in 1900 to 77.4 years in 2005 (National Center for Health Statistics 2010b). Consequently, the United States— and other industrialized nations as well— is experiencing an aging boom. Growth

in the US elderly population has outpaced growth in the nonelderly population since 1900. Figure 12–6 shows changes in the makeup of the US population from 1970 to 2007. Most remarkable is the growth in the age group 85 years and older, whereas the youngest age group is shrinking. Growth of the elderly population is projected to continue through the middle of the 21st century. Between 2000 and 2030, the proportion of the US population that is 65 years of age and older is expected to rise from 12.4 to 20%, or 1 in 5. The number in the 85-and-older category is projected to more than double. The swelling of the elderly population will result from the aging of the baby boom

Figure 12–5  Life Expectancy of Americans at Birth, Age 65, and Age 75, Selected Years 1900–2005.

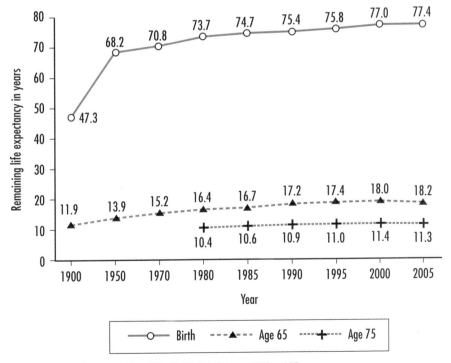

Figure 12–6  Change in US Population Mix Between 1970 and 2007, and Projections for 2030.

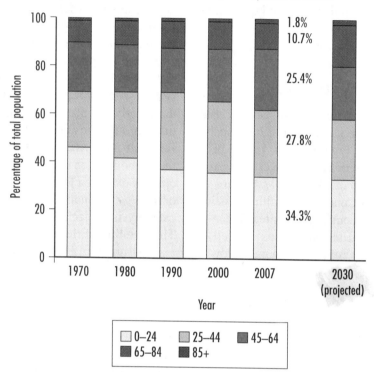

*Source:* Data from *Health, United States, 2009,* p. 147, National Center for Health Statistics; *Census 2000,* US Census Bureau; *Projections of the Total Resident Population by 5-Year Age Groups, and Sex with Special Age Categories: Middle Series, 2025 to 2045,* US Census Bureau.

generation of roughly 77 million Americans born between 1946 and 1964. The youngest of the baby boomers will be 66 years old in 2030.

Elderly people consume more health care than younger people. In 2004, the average medical expenses for people 65 years of age and older was $17,619 per person, compared to $4,754 per person for those under the age of 65 (National Center for Health Statistics 2010b). In other words, health care costs for the elderly are 3.7 times more than those for the nonelderly. Hence, health care expenditures are sure to rise unless drastic steps are taken to curtail spending. Total Medicare expenditures are projected to increase from

2.7% of GDP in 2005 to 9% of GDP in 2050 (Van de Water and Lavery 2006).

## Medical Model of Health Care Delivery

As discussed in Chapter 2, the medical model emphasizes medical interventions after a person has become sick. It does not put an equal emphasis on prevention and lifestyle behavior changes to promote health. Although health promotion and disease prevention are not the answer to every health problem, these principles have not been accorded their rightful place in the US health care delivery system. Consequently, more costly health care resources must be deployed to treat health problems that could have been prevented. For example, smoking-related illnesses are estimated to cost the United States $75.5 billion annually for direct medical care and an additional $167 billion in lost productivity (CDC 2005). Evidence suggests that smoking cessation programs have the potential for significant cost savings without imposing an undue cost burden on insurers and employers (Levy 2006). Although the prevalence of cigarette smoking has been slowly declining, in 2007, 22.3% of American adult males and 17.4% of women still smoked (National Center for Health Statistics 2010b).

Overweight conditions and obesity have reached alarming rates in the United States and in many other developed nations. In 2006, 66.7% of Americans 20 years of age and over were overweight, of which 33.4% were obese (National Center for Health Statistics 2010b). Overweight and obesity substantially elevate the risk of heart disease, diabetes, some types of cancers, musculo-skeletal disorders, and gallbladder problems. Recent estimates suggest that, of the total medical spending in the United States, 10% ($147 billion) could be attributed to overweight and obesity, rivaling that attributed to smoking (Finkelstein et al. 2009). Both Medicare and Medicaid spend a disproportionate share to treat overweight- and obesity-related health problems. On average, obese Medicare beneficiaries incur $600 per beneficiary per year in extra costs, compared to beneficiaries with normal weight (Finkelstein et al. 2009).

## Multipayer System and Administrative Costs

*Administrative costs* are associated with the management of the financing, insurance, delivery, and payment functions. They include

management of the enrollment process, setting up contracts with providers, claims processing, utilization monitoring, denials and appeals, and marketing and promotional expenses. The enrollment process in private, employer-financed health plans and in publicly financed Medicaid and Medicare programs includes determination of eligibility, enrollment, and disenrollment. Each activity has associated costs. Private insurers also incur enrollment and disenrollment costs, in addition to marketing costs to promote and sell their plans. Providers have to deal with numerous plans in which the extent of benefits and reimbursement is not standardized. It is difficult and costly to remain current with the numerous and frequently changing rules and regulations. Denials of payment result in appeals and follow-up. Denial of services also results in appeals and incurs costs for the insurer to review the appeals and for the provider to furnish justifications for the delivery of services. Utilization review and authorization of care incur additional costs for both payers and providers. According to the Center for Medicare and Medicaid Services (CMS), the administrative costs, taxes, profits, and other nonbenefit expenses of private health plans have averaged about 12% of premiums over the last 40 years (Lemieux 2005). The ACA of 2010 requires health plans to standardize electronic data exchange to reduce administrative costs, although there is no specific guidelines as to how information must be transferred (Blanchfield et al. 2010).

## Defensive Medicine

The US health care delivery system is characterized by legal risks for providers, which promote defensive medicine (see Chapter 1). The practice of defensive medicine leads to tests and services that are not medically justified but are performed by physicians to protect themselves against potential malpractice lawsuits. Induction of labor and cesarean sections are commonly overused procedures in the United States. Fear of legal liability is one of the main reasons for carrying out unnecessary cesarean sections because it makes it easier to defend a potential birth injury case. Unrestrained malpractice awards by the courts and increased malpractice insurance premiums for physicians add significantly to the cost of health care.

## Fraud and Abuse

Fraud and (system) abuse are another type of waste in health care, which were introduced in Chapter 6. Fraud has been identified as a major problem in the Medicare and Medicaid programs.

*Fraud* involves a knowing disregard of the truth. Fraudulent activities are both illegal and immoral. Fraud occurs when billing claims or cost reports are intentionally falsified. A mere oversight or an inadvertent error will not rise to the level of fraud; however, a pattern of oversights or errors may be tantamount to fraud (Lovitky 1997). Fraud may also occur when more services are provided than are medically necessary or when services not provided are billed. *Upcoding* is another fraudulent practice in which a higher-priced service is billed when a lower-priced service is actually delivered. These practices are illegal under the False Claims Act.

Under the Anti-Kickback statute (Medicare and Medicaid Patient Protection Act of 1987), it is illegal to provide any remuneration to any individual or entity in exchange for a referral for services to be paid by the Medicare or Medicaid program.

Knowingly providing such financial inducements amounts to a federal crime punishable by imprisonment. The Stark Law prohibits physician self-referral for laboratory or other designated health services. This law prevents physicians from referring a patient to laboratories in which they or members of their immediate families have a financial interest (Lovitky 1997).

## Practice Variations

The work of John Wennberg and others brought to the fore a disturbing aspect of physician behavior, accounting for wide variations in treatment patterns for similar patients. Numerous studies in the United States and abroad have documented notable differences in utilization rates for hospital admissions and surgical procedures among different communities, as well as for the same specialties (Feldstein 1993). These practice variations are referred to as *small area variations* (SAV) because the differences in practice patterns have only been associated with geographic areas of the country. For example, in earlier studies, variations in the rate of tonsillectomies in New England counties could not be explained by differences in the demographics or other characteristics of the populations studied (Wennberg and Gittelsohn 1973); the overall inpatient hospital utilization by an aged population in East Boston was higher than that by an equivalent population in New Haven, after controlling for several variables (Wennberg et al. 1987). More recent investigations on regional differences in Medicare spending demonstrated that higher rates of inpatient-based care and specialist services were associated with higher costs but not with improved quality of care, health outcomes, access to services, or satisfaction with care (Fisher et al. 2003a, 2003b). This variation, which can be as great as two-fold, cannot be explained by age, gender, race, pricing variations, or health status (Baucus and Fowler 2002). Geographic variations, as discussed here, signal gross inefficiencies in the US health care delivery system because they increase costs without yielding appreciably better outcomes. This variation is also unfair because workers and Medicare beneficiaries in low-cost, more efficient regions subsidize the care of those in high-cost regions (Wennberg 2002). SAVs cannot be explained by demand inducement. For example, no incentives exist for physicians to induce demand in Canada or Britain, yet variations similar to those in the United States also exist in those countries. SAVs indicate that patients in some parts of the country are receiving too much treatment, whereas others may be receiving too little. Medical opinions often differ on the appropriateness of clinical interventions because physicians use different criteria for hospital admissions and surgical interventions (Gittelsohn and Powe 1995).

## Cost Containment — Regulatory Approaches

Many attempts to control health care spending have been undertaken in the United States; however, most of these attempts have met with only limited success, mainly because the United States has never been able to implement a systemwide cost-control initiative. Cost-containment measures have been piecemeal, affecting only certain targeted sectors of the health care delivery system at a time. So, for instance, when prices have been regulated, utilization has been left untouched; or when capital expenditures have required preapprovals, operating costs of production have been exempted. In a fragmented system, it is impossible to implement cost-control measures in a systematic and global manner.

A *single-payer system* in which centralized controls would allow cost-containment efforts to sweep through the entire health care delivery system has never been tried in the United States because that would require a major overhaul of the system. Other industrialized nations have created national regulatory mechanisms to keep their health care spending in line with their national income. Many of these countries follow what is referred to as *top-down control* over total expenditures. They establish budgets for entire sectors of the health care delivery system. Funds are distributed to providers in accordance with these global budgets. Thus, total spending remains within established budget limits. The downside to this approach is that, under fixed budgets, providers are not as responsive to patient needs and the system provides little incentive to be efficient in the delivery of services. Once budgets are expended, providers are forced to cut back services, particularly for illnesses that are not life threatening or do not represent an emergency. This top-down approach is in sharp contrast to the "bottom-up" approach used in the United States, where each provider and managed care organization (MCO) establishes its own fees or premiums (Altman and Wallack 1996). Competition, created by employers shopping for the best premium rates and by MCOs contracting with providers who agree to favorable fee arrangements, determines what the total expenditures will be. To some extent, the United States also uses regulatory cost control, although it is not as comprehensive as it is in countries with national health care programs.

Cost-control efforts in the United States are characterized by a combination of government regulation and market-based competition. A fragmented approach to cost control allows providers to shift costs (see Cost Shifting in Chapter 6), mainly from low payers to higher payers or from one delivery sector to another. For example, when regulatory controls are employed to squeeze costs out of the inpatient sector, providers experience reduced revenues from inpatient services. To make up for the lost revenues, they increase utilization of outpatient services if that sector is free of controls. In another scenario, when the government implements cost-control measures, providers may start charging higher prices to private payers. This practice is very common in the nursing home industry, in which reimbursement is restricted under Medicaid rate-setting criteria. In this case, nursing home administrators make a conscious attempt to make up for lost revenues by admitting more private-pay residents and by establishing higher private-pay charges.

Regulatory approaches to cost containment typically control the capacity of the supply side, prices, and utilization (Exhibit 12–1). Supply-side constraints are accomplished through "health planning," also called supply-side rationing. Planning enables policy makers to limit the number of hospital beds and diffusion of costly technology, but regulatory limits on the health care system's capacity inevitably create monopolies on the supply side. To make sure that these artificially created monopolies do not exploit their economic power, health planning is always coupled with stiff price and budgetary controls (Reinhardt 1994).

## Health Planning

*Health planning* refers to a government undertaking to align and distribute health care resources so that, at least in the eyes of the government, the system will achieve desired health outcomes for all people. The planning function becomes critical in a centrally controlled national health care program so that the basic health care needs of the population are met and expenditures are maintained at predetermined levels.

The central planning function does not fit well in a system in which more than one-half of health care financing is in private hands and there is no central administrative agency to monitor the system. Instead, the types of health care services, their geographic distribution, access to these services, and the prices charged by providers develop independently of any preformulated plans. Levels of expenditures cannot be predetermined, and such a system is not conducive to achieving broad social objectives. Nevertheless, the United States has tried some forms of health planning on voluntary or mandated bases, but these efforts have met limited success.

## Health Planning Experiments in the United States

Some of the early efforts to control health care costs in the United States took the form of voluntary health planning. The goal was to minimize duplication of services. Early forms of health planning in the 1930s and 1940s were primarily the result of communitywide voluntary organizations, called hospital councils, which were established by hospitals in some of the largest cities. Hospitals agreed to share or consolidate services, or they traded the closing of a service in one hospital for the expansion of

Exhibit 12–1  Regulation-Based and Competition-Based Cost-Containment Strategies

| Regulation-Based Cost-Containment Strategies | |
|---|---|
| Supply-side controls | Restrictions on capital expenditures (new construction, renovations, and technology diffusion) |
| | Example: Certificate of need |
| | Restrictions on supply of physicians |
| | Example: Entry barriers for foreign medical graduates |
| Price controls | Artificially determined prices |
| | Examples:  Reimbursement formulas |
| | Prospective payment systems |
| | Diagnosis-related groups |
| | Resource utilization groups |
| | Global budgets |
| Utilization controls | Peer review organizations |
| **Competition-Based Cost-Containment Strategies** | |
| Demand-side incentives | Cost sharing |
| | Sharing of premium costs |
| | Deductibles and copayments |
| Supply-side regulation | Antitrust regulation |
| Payer-driven competition | Competition among insurers |
| | Competition among providers |
| Utilization controls | Managed care |

another service (Williams 1995). Voluntary planning worked only on a limited basis and only in instances where participating hospitals could gain an advantage through cooperative planning. Consequently, voluntary planning contributed little to overall efficiency (Gottlieb 1974).

The federal government got involved in health planning after the passage of Medicare and Medicaid in the 1960s. These programs were designed to achieve broad social objectives by extending health care access to the underprivileged, but the passage of these programs generated an explosion in health care spending. Recognizing the increasing dollars the federal government was putting into health care, Congress believed that it had the right to control escalating costs (Williams 1995). The comprehensive health planning legislation of the mid-1960s mandated the establishment of local and state health planning agencies. These agencies assessed local health care needs and advocated better coordination and distribution of resources. However, the agencies had little or no actual regulatory power and were largely ineffective (Williams 1995). When these agencies were evaluated, planned and unplanned areas had the same amount of duplication of facilities and services and the rate of increase in hospital costs was the same (May 1974).

## Certificate-of-Need Statutes

The federal Health Planning and Resource Development Act of 1974 was enacted to provide incentives and penalties that would encourage states to adopt *certificate-of-need* (CON) legislation (Feldstein 1993) in an attempt to implement an enhanced regulatory approach.

As discussed in Chapter 5, CON statutes were state-enacted legislation whose primary purpose was to control capital expenditures by health facilities. The CON process required prior approval from a state government agency for construction of new facilities, such as hospitals and nursing homes. Similar approvals were required for the expansion of existing facilities or the acquisition of expensive equipment. Approvals were based on the demonstration of a community need for additional services. Although the reasons given for the CON legislation were better planning of resources and control of increasing expenditures, in reality, the adoption of CON was easier in states having greater competition among hospitals (Wendling and Werner 1980), indicating

that hospitals supported CON legislation when it was to their own benefit. These hospitals did not want additional capital spending on new construction and equipment by their competitors.

CON laws did not seem to lower hospital expenditures on a per patient day basis. CON also represented a conservative approach to containing the rise in hospital costs because it did not address reimbursement and provided no incentives to change utilization behavior in patients or physicians (Feldstein 1993). In the case of nursing homes, however, CON regulations have been used to contain Medicaid costs. In the face of a growing demand for nursing home beds, the CON regulations have restricted the supply of nursing home beds that otherwise would have been utilized. More recent, however, the Home and Community Based Services (HCBS) waiver program— also referred to as 1915(c) waivers (see Chapter 10)—has been used to curtail nursing home utilization and costs.

In the early 1980s, the US government moved away from its commitment to health planning. The federal Health Planning and Resource Development Act was repealed in 1986, and it was left strictly up to the states to decide whether to have or not have CON regulations.

## Price Controls

In 1971, under pressure from Congress, President Nixon imposed the Economic Stabilization Program (ESP) as an economywide measure to contain general inflation through wage and price controls. The ESP limited the amount by which hospitals could raise their prices from year to year (Williams and Torrens 1993). The ESP

ESP

also imposed controls on physicians' fees. Although controls on most of the economy were dropped by the end of 1971, the special problems of health care inflation led the administration to keep tight controls on the health care sector through 1974 (Altman and Wallack 1996). The ESP controls did generate a moderating influence on price increases for most medical services; however, the program had placed no limits on the quantity of services (Altman and Eichenholz 1976). For example, the quantity of services delivered to Medicare patients increased by about 10% during the first year of the ESP and between 8 and 15%, depending on physician specialty, during the second year (Gabel and Rice 1985). Also, the costs of production remained relatively unchanged. Therefore, once controls were lifted, inflation returned to its precontrol levels (Altman and Eichenholz 1976). ESP demonstrated that, although price increases can be limited for a short period, effective controls on total spending require much more extensive limits on the costs of production, as well as on the quantity of services utilized (Altman and Wallack 1996).

During 1984 and 1986, Medicare froze physician fees; however, during each year fees were frozen, per-enrollee physician expenditures increased by at least 10% (Mitchell et al. 1988) because physicians could induce demand and, thus, increase the quantity of services provided. Similar results from price controls have been demonstrated in other countries.

## Price Control Through Prospective Payment Methods

Perhaps the most important effort to control prices of inpatient hospital care was the conversion of hospital Medicare reimbursement from cost-plus to a prospective payment system (PPS) based on DRGs authorized under the Social Security Amendments of 1983 (see Chapter 6). The DRG-based reimbursement significantly reduced growth in inpatient hospital spending but had little impact on total per capita Medicare cost inflation because costs were shifted from the inpatient to the outpatient sector (Figure 12–7). Use of per capita spending data in Figure 12–7 controls for the growth in Medicare population; hence, changes in spending are mainly attributable to utilization of services. As explained in Chapter 6, Medicare has implemented other price control measures through various reimbursement methods that apply to physicians, home health care, and various inpatient service providers. These programs seem to have been successful. For example, before the implementation of the resource-based relative value scale (RBRVS) for physician payments, the per capita Medicare spending for physician services had increased at an average annual rate of 11.7% between 1980 and 1990 (much higher than the CPI). After RBRVS, per capita Medicare spending for physician services increased by only 5% annually between 1995 and 2005, based on data from the CMS.

Most states have also employed price-control measures to control their Medicaid expenditures. Both retrospective and prospective methods have been used to define payment rates for hospitals and nursing homes. Often, complex formulas are used, which, in essence, produce arbitrary reimbursement rates and rate ceilings. For example, two neighboring states can have sizable differences in Medicaid reimbursement for practically the same level of services.

Figure 12–7  Increase in US Per Capita Medicare Spending, Selected Years: 1970–2008.

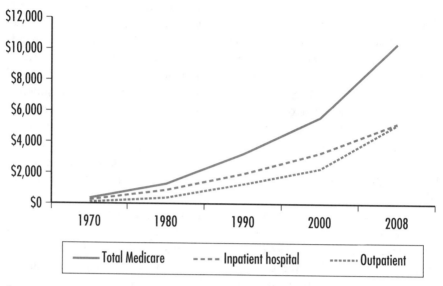

*Source:* Data from *Health, United States, 2010*, p. 402; National Center for Health Statistics.

## Pay-for-Performance

A recent development in Medicare reimbursement is the move toward pay-for-performance (P4P), introduced in Chapter 6. P4P, which is receiving attention in both the private and public sectors, aims to align provider payments with the quality of care provided. In 2003, as part of the Medicare Prescription Drug, Improvement, and Modernization Act, the US Congress asked the Institute of Medicine (IOM) to assess the potential for implementing P4P in the Medicare program (IOM 2004). Specifically, the IOM studied the performance measure set that could be used, the payment policy that could be used, and the key implementation issues involved, such as data and information technology requirements. The IOM found mixed evidence regarding the effectiveness of P4P payments, and it noted that unintended adverse consequences of P4P could include decreased access to care, increased disparities in care, and impediments to innovation. However, the IOM concluded that careful monitoring of P4P could minimize these adverse consequences. Further, the IOM argued that, if Medicare payment structures were left unchanged, they would pose a barrier to improved quality of care. However, to date, there is little evidence that hospitals respond to P4P incentives as expected (Nicholas et al. 2011). Alternative incentive structures need to be developed to motivate greater response.

The Medicare program is not alone in considering P4P strategies. At least 12 states have instituted P4P in their Medicaid programs (CMS 2007). While these programs are in the early stages of development, CMS is offering technical assistance to states for implementing and evaluating P4P.

## Peer Review

The term *peer review* refers to the general process of medical review of utilization and quality when it is carried out directly by or under the supervision of physicians (Wilson and Neuhauser 1985). Based on this concept, the Social Security Amendments of 1972 required the establishment of professional standards review organizations (PSROs). These associations of physicians reviewed professional and institutional services provided under Medicare and Medicaid. The stated purpose was monitoring and control of both cost and quality. When Congress evaluated the performance of PSROs for their cost-control effectiveness, the program had not produced any net savings. Because of their questionable effectiveness, the PSROs were replaced in 1984 by a new system of peer review organizations (PROs), now called quality improvement organizations (QIOs). QIOs are private organizations composed of practicing physicians and other health care professionals in each state who are paid by the CMS under contract to review the care provided to Medicare beneficiaries. To control utilization, QIOs determine whether care is reasonable, necessary, and provided in the most appropriate setting. CMS is required to publish a report to Congress every fiscal year that outlines the administration, cost, and impact of the QIO program.

## Cost Containment — Competitive Approaches

*Competition* refers to rivalry among sellers for customers (Dranove 1993). In health care delivery, it means that providers of health care services will try to attract patients who can choose among several different providers. Although competition more commonly refers to price competition, it may also be based on technical quality, amenities, access, or other factors (Dranove 1993). Because competition is an essential element for the operation of free markets, competitive approaches are also referred to as market-oriented approaches.

During the Reagan presidency in the 1980s, competitive reforms were given preference because of growing interest in market-oriented approaches in many sectors of the economy. These reforms were accompanied by waning interest in comprehensive health care reform at the national level. Market-oriented reforms were accompanied by mounting cost-containment efforts in the private sector and the growth of managed care. Competitive reforms have been diverse and have often entailed simultaneous reforms in the regulation of health care markets (Arnould et al. 1993). Competitive strategies fall into four broad categories: demand-side incentives, supply-side regulation, payer-driven price competition, and utilization controls (Exhibit 12–1).

## Demand-Side Incentives

The underlying notion of cost sharing (discussed in Chapter 6) is that, if consumers pay more of the insurance cost, they will be more cost conscious in selecting the insurance plan that best serves their needs. They will not automatically opt for the most comprehensive plan. Also, when consumers pay out of pocket a larger share of the cost of health care services they use, they will consume services more judiciously. In essence, cost sharing encourages consumers to ration their own health care. For example, cost sharing leads people to forgo professional services for minor ailments, not for serious problems (Wong et al. 2001).

Cost sharing (now a common feature of almost all health plans) became popular after the Rand Health Insurance Experiment empirically demonstrated the effects of cost sharing. The most comprehensive study of its type, the experiment ran from 1974 through 1981. It enrolled more than 7,000 people into 1 of 14 different health plans. They included a free plan carrying no deductible or copayments. The other plans involved varying degrees of cost sharing. It was found that cost sharing resulted in lower costs, compared to the free plan. Coinsurance rates of 25% resulted in a 19% decline in expenditures because out-of-pocket costs reduced health care utilization. Increased coinsurance rates resulted in further declines in utilization and expenditures. Another important finding of the Rand Experiment was that lower utilization due to cost sharing did not affect most measures of health status. People enrolled in the free plan did better in three areas: vision, blood pressure, and dental health, but the average appraised mortality risk for people on the free plan was close to the risk for those with cost sharing (Feldstein 1993).

## Supply-Side Regulation

As pointed out in Chapter 9, US antitrust laws prohibit business practices that stifle competition among providers. These practices include price fixing, price discrimination, exclusive contracting arrangements, and mergers the Department of Justice deems anticompetitive. The purpose of antitrust policy is to ensure the competitiveness and, thus, the efficiency of economic markets. In a competitive environment, MCOs, hospitals, and other health care organizations have to be cost efficient to survive.

## Payer-Driven Price Competition

Generally speaking, consumers drive competition. However, because health care markets are imperfect, patients are not typical consumers in the marketplace because insured patients lack the incentive to be good shoppers and because patients face information barriers that prevent them from being efficient shoppers. Despite the information boom, it is extremely difficult for individual patients or their surrogates to obtain needed information on cost and quality. Payer-driven competition in the form of managed care has overcome the drawbacks of patient-driven competition (Dranove 1993). Payer-driven competition occurs at two different points. First, employers shop for the best value, in terms of the cost of premiums and the benefits package (competition among insurers). Second, MCOs shop for the best value from providers of health services (competition among providers).

## Utilization Controls

Managed care also helps overcome some of the other inefficiencies of an imperfect health care market. The utilization controls in managed care (discussed in Chapter 9) have cut through some of the unnecessary or inappropriate services provided to consumers. Managed care is designed to intervene in the decisions made by care providers to ensure that they give only appropriate and necessary services and that they provide the services efficiently. MCOs base this intervention on information that is not generally available to consumers. MCOs, thus, act on the consumer's behalf (Dranove 1993).

# Access to Care

Fundamentally, *access* refers to the ability of a person to obtain health care services when needed. More broadly, access to care is the ability to obtain needed, affordable, convenient, acceptable, and effective personal health services in a timely manner. It may also refer to whether an individual has a usual source of care (such as a primary care physician), indicate the ability to use health care services (based on availability, convenience, referral, etc.), or reflect the acceptability of particular services (according to an individual's preferences and values). Access has several key implications for health and health care delivery.

- Access to medical care is one of the key determinants of health, along with environment, lifestyle, and heredity factors (see Chapter 2).

- Access is a significant benchmark in assessing the effectiveness of the medical care delivery system. For example, access can be used to evaluate national trends against specific goals, such as those proposed in Healthy People 2010 and 2020 (see Chapter 2).

- Measures of access reflect whether or not the delivery of health care is equitable.

- Access is also linked to quality of care and the efficient use of needed services.

## Framework of Access

The conceptualization of access to care (see Figure 12–8) can be traced to Andersen (1968) and was later refined by Aday and Andersen (1975) and Aday and colleagues (1980). Andersen (1968) believed that, in addition to need, predisposing and enabling conditions also prompt some people to use more medical services than others. Predisposing conditions include an individual's sociodemographic characteristics, such as age, sex, education, marital status, family size, race and ethnicity, and religious preference. These factors indicate a person's propensity to use medical care. For example, holding everything else constant, elderly people are more likely to use medical care than young people. The enabling conditions are income, socioeconomic status, price of medical services, financing of medical services, and occupation. They focus on the individual's means, enabling that person to use medical care. For example, holding everything else constant, those with high incomes are more likely to use medical care than those with low incomes, particularly in countries that do not provide national health insurance.

The distinction between predisposing and enabling conditions can be applied to assess the equity of a health care system (Aday et al. 1993). To the extent that significant differences in medical care utilization can be explained by need and certain predisposing characteristics (e.g., age, gender), the delivery of medical care is considered equitable. When enabling characteristics create significant differences in medical care utilization, the delivery of medical care is considered inequitable.

This access to care model has been expanded to include characteristics of health policy and the health care delivery system (Aday et al. 1980). Examples of health policy include major health care financing initiatives (Medicare, Medicaid, and CHIP) and organization of health services delivery (Medicaid managed care, community health centers). Characteristics of the health care

Figure 12–8  The Expanded Behavioral Model.

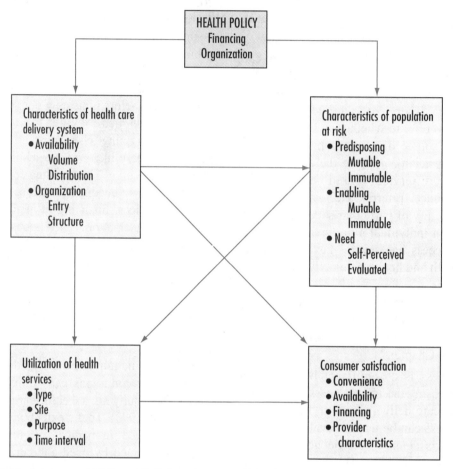

Source: L.A. Aday, R. Andersen, and G.V. Fleming, *Health Care in the US: Equitable for Whom?*, p. 49, Copyright © 1980 by Sage Publications, Inc. Reprinted by permission of Sage Publications, Inc.

delivery system include availability (volume and distribution of services) and organization (mechanisms of entry into and movement within the system). Both health policy and the health care delivery system are aggregate components in contrast to the individual components of predisposing, enabling, and need characteristics. The expanded model recognizes the importance of systemic and structural barriers to access

and is useful in comparing access to care among countries with different health policies and health care delivery systems.

Managed care's growth and the ensuing integration of the health care delivery functions represent a fundamental change in health care delivery. Accordingly, the access framework must be updated to reflect the new paradigm under managed care. Gold contributed a revised framework for access in the context of managed care (Docteur et al. 1996; see Figure 12–9). According to this framework, access to care is a two-stage process in a managed care environment. In the first stage, individuals select among the health plans available to them, constrained by structural, financial, and personal characteristics. In the second stage, individuals seek medical care, constrained by both plan-specific and nonplan factors. The framework accounts for people enrolling and staying with the plan or disenrolling. It also links actual utilization with clinical and policy outcomes. Although comprehensive models are useful in conceptualizing access to care, they are difficult to test because of the range of variables and the differing levels of analysis they require.

Figure 12–9   Framework for Access in the Managed Care Context.

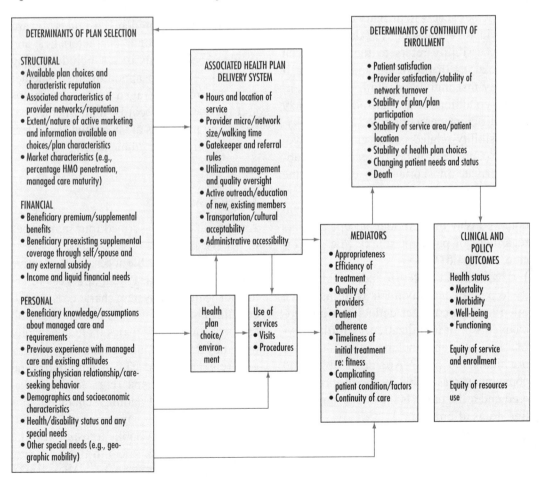

*Source:* Reprinted from E.R. Docteur, D.C. Colby, and M. Gold, "Shifting the Paradigm," *Health Care Financing Review* 17, no. 4 (1996): p. 12.

## Dimensions of Access

Penchansky and Thomas (1981) described access to care as consisting of five dimensions: availability, accessibility, accommodation, affordability, and acceptability.

(1)  Availability refers to the fit between service capacity and individuals' requirements. Availability-related issues include whether primary and preventive services are available to patients; whether enabling services, such as transportation, language, and social services, are made available by the provider; whether the health plan has sufficient specialists to care for patients' needs; and whether access to primary care services is provided 24 hours a day, 7 days a week.

(2)  Accessibility refers to the fit between the locations of providers and patients. It is likely that individuals with different enabling conditions (e.g., transportation) may have different perceptions of accessibility. Accessibility-related issues include convenience (Can the provider be reached by public or private transportation?), design (Is the provider site designed for convenient use by disabled or elderly patients?), and payment options (Will the provider accept patients regardless of payment source [e.g., Medicare, Medicaid]?).

(3)  Affordability refers to individuals' ability to pay. Even individuals with insurance often have to consider deductibles and co-payments prior to utilization. Affordability-related questions include Are insurance premiums too high? Are deductibles and copayments reasonable for the services covered under the plan? Is the cost of prescription drugs affordable?

(4)  Accommodation refers to the fit between how resources are organized to provide services and the individual's ability to use the arrangement. Accommodation-related questions include Can a patient schedule an appointment? Are scheduled office hours compatible with most patients' work and way of life? Can most of the urgent cases be seen within one hour? Can most patients with acute, but nonurgent, problems be seen within one day? Can most appropriate requests for routine appointments, such as preventive exams, be met within one week? Does the plan permit walk-in services?

(5)  Acceptability is based on the attitudes of patients and providers and refers to the compatibility between patients' attitudes about providers' personal and practice characteristics and providers' attitudes toward their clients' personal characteristics and values. Acceptability issues include waiting time for scheduled appointments; whether patients are encouraged to ask questions and review their records; and whether patients and providers are accepted regardless of race, religion, or ethnic origin.

## Types of Access

Andersen (1997) described four main types of access: potential access, realized access, equitable or inequitable access, and effective and efficient access. Potential access refers to both health care system characteristics and enabling characteristics. Examples of health care system characteristics include capacity (e.g., physician–population ratio), organization (e.g., managed care penetration), and financing mechanisms (e.g., health insurance coverage). Enabling characteristics include personal (e.g., income) and community resources (e.g., public transportation).

Realized access refers to the type, site, and purpose of health services (Aday 1993).

The type of utilization refers to the category of services rendered: physician, dentist, or other practitioners; hospital or long-term care admission; prescriptions; medical equipment; and so on. The site of utilization refers to the place where services are received (e.g., inpatient setting, such as short-stay hospital, mental institution, or nursing home; or ambulatory setting, such as hospital outpatient department, emergency department, physician's office, staff-model HMO, public health clinic, community health center, freestanding emergency center, or patient's home). The purpose of utilization refers to the reason medical care was sought: for health maintenance in the absence of symptoms (primary prevention), for the diagnosis or treatment of illness to return to well-being (secondary prevention or illness related), or for rehabilitation or maintenance in the case of a chronic health problem (tertiary prevention or custodial care).

Equitable access refers to the distribution of health care services according to the patient's self-perceived need (e.g., symptoms, pain, physical and functional status) or evaluated need as determined by a health professional (e.g., medical history, test results). Inequitable access refers to services distributed according to enabling characteristics (e.g., income, insurance status).

Effective and efficient care links realized access to health outcomes (Institute of Medicine 1993). For example, does adequate prenatal care lead to successful birth outcomes as measured by birth weight? Is immunization related to reduction of vaccine-preventable childhood diseases, such as diphtheria, measles, mumps, pertussis, polio, rubella, and tetanus? Are preventive services related to the early detection and diagnosis of treatable diseases? The concepts of effectiveness and efficiency link access to quality of care.

## Measurement of Access

Using the conceptual models, access can be measured at three different levels: individual, health plan, and the delivery system. Access indicators at the individual level include (1) measures of medical services utilization relative to enabling and predisposing factors, while controlling for need for care (Aday and Andersen 1975) and (2) the patient's assessment of the interaction with the provider. Examples include differences in physician visits by race/ethnicity, gender, age, income, and insurance. Patients' perceived level of access is closely related to patient satisfaction with care and is part of the access framework (Aday et al. 1984).

At the health plan level, indicators include (1) plan characteristics that affect enrollment, such as cost of premium, deductibles, copayments, coverage for preventive care, authorization of new and expensive procedures, physician referral incentives, and out-of-plan use; (2) plan practices that affect access, such as travel time to a usual source of care and waiting time to see a physician (accessibility), whether an appointment is necessary, hours of operation, language and other enabling services (accommodation), the content of provider–patient encounters, including tests ordered and done, and referral to specialists (contact); and (3) plan quality as measured by the Health Plan Employer Data and Information Set (HEDIS) (see Chapter 9) and patient satisfaction surveys.

Indicators of access at the level of the health care delivery system comprise ecological measures that affect populations rather than individuals. System indicators help study access in an environmental context, that is, how context affects the access of persons and groups. Examples of system access indicators include health policies or programs related to access, physician–population ratio, hospital beds per 1,000 population, percentage of population with insurance coverage, median household income, state per capita spending on welfare and preventive care, and percentage of population without access to primary care physicians.

Population-based surveys supported by federal statistical agencies are the major sources of data for conducting access-to-care analyses. Large national surveys, such as the National Health Interview Survey, the Medical Expenditure Panel Survey (MEPS), and the Community Tracking Survey are the leading data sources used to monitor access trends and other issues of interest. Other well-known national surveys include the Current Population Survey, the National Hospital Discharge Survey, the Ambulatory Medical Care Survey, the National Nursing Home Survey, and the Home and Hospice Care Survey (HHCS). In addition, the federal government may periodically collect data on special topics, such as human immunodeficiency virus (HIV) and acquired immune deficiency syndrome (AIDS); mental health; health care utilization by veterans, military staff, and their dependents; patient satisfaction; and community health centers.

In addition to the federal government, states, associations, and research institutions also regularly collect data on topics of interest to them. Examples of state-based initiatives include state health services utilization data (all-payer hospital discharge data systems), state managed care data (managed care encounter data), and state

Medicaid enrollee satisfaction data (Medicaid enrollee satisfaction surveys). Examples of association-based initiatives include data on physicians (American Medical Association's Physician Masterfile and the Periodic Survey of Physicians 1969 to present) and hospitals (American Hospital Association's Annual Survey of Hospitals 1946 to present). Examples of research institution-based initiatives include collecting data on the health care delivery system (Center for Evaluative Clinical Sciences: Dartmouth Atlas of Health Care in the US), women's health (Kaiser Family Foundation: Women's Health Survey 2004), minority health (Commonwealth Fund: Minority Health Survey 1997), family health (Urban Institute National Survey of America's Families 1997, 1999, and 2002), health insurance (Commonwealth Fund Bienniel Health Insurance Survey 2005), and access to care (Robert Wood Johnson Foundation National Access Surveys).

Access to care data for vulnerable populations is systematically collected by the Sentinel Centers Network (SCN) initiative, currently composed of 37 participants located in the majority of states in the United States. Approximately 650 health care practitioners provide services to 1 million registered users within the SCN. The SCN data system is the first primary care administrative database that focuses exclusively on care delivery and outcomes for medically underserved populations.

## Current Status of Access

In the United States, barriers to access still exist at both the individual and the system level. Many of these barriers are experienced by vulnerable population groups (discussed in Chapter 11). Access is best predicted by face, income, and occupation. These three factors are interrelated. People belonging to minority groups tend to be poor, not well educated, and more likely to work in jobs that pose greater health risks. For example, rural Americans face barriers because they are more likely to be low-income, suffer from chronic impairment and diseases, and be elderly than their urban counterparts (Hutchison et al. 2005). A national survey places access to quality health services as the top-ranking priority among rural health care stakeholders and leaders (Hutchison et al. 2005). It has been suggested that the United States has an overall surplus of resources, such as hospital beds and physicians, in urban areas. The problem is that these surpluses are not shifted to respond to areas of biggest need (Brown 1992).

Tables 12–3 and 12–4 summarize physician contacts by categories of age, sex, race, income, and geographic location. Table 12–5 summarizes dental visits. These results are not adjusted for health need,

however, and, therefore, are not true indicators of access. Rather, they provide utilization measures as a proxy for access.

## Quality of Care

One reason the pursuit of quality in health care has trailed behind the emphasis on cost and access is the difficulty of defining and measuring quality. Since the 1990s, when cost containment became a major priority, emphasis on quality has taken center stage in the delivery of health care because of intuitive concerns that cost control may negatively impact quality. In spite of the progress made, however, there is still a long road ahead to specify what constitutes good quality in medical care, how to ensure it for patients, and how to reward providers and health plans whose outcomes indicate successes in quality improvement. One challenge in achieving such a goal is that patients, providers, and payers each define

Table 12–3 Visits to Office-Based Physicians, 2007

| Characteristic | Number of Visits (million) | Percentage Distribution | Visits per 100 Persons/Year |
|---|---|---|---|
| All visits | 994.3 | 100.0 | 335.6 |
| Age | | | |
| Under 15 years old | 167.5 | 16.8 | 275.3 |
| 15–44 years old | 284.3 | 28.6 | 445.4 |
| 45–64 years old | 283.9 | 28.6 | 373.3 |
| 65–74 years old | 127.8 | 12.9 | 668.9 |
| 75 years old and over | 130.4 | 13.1 | 761.0 |

*Source:* Data from US Bureau of the Census. *Statistical Abstracts of the United States, 2010,* Washington, DC, p. 113.

Table 12–4　Number of Health Care Visits According to Selected Patient Characteristics, 2007

| Characteristic | None | 1–3 Visits | 4–9 Visits | 10+ Visits |
|---|---|---|---|---|
| Total | 164% | 47.2% | 23.6% | 12.8% |
| Sex | | | | |
| Male | 21.3% | 47.3% | 20.9% | 10.5% |
| Female | 11.5% | 47.1% | 26.3% | 15.1% |
| Race and age | | | | |
| White | 16.2% | 46.8% | 24.0% | 13.0% |
| Black | 15.2% | 48.4% | 23.4% | 12.7% |
| % Poverty level | | | | |
| Below 100% | 19.3% | 39.5% | 23.3% | 18.0% |
| 100–200% | 20.5% | 42.1% | 23.3% | 14.0% |
| 200% + | 14.6% | 50.0% | 23.7% | 11.7% |
| Geographic region | | | | |
| Northeast | 13.0% | 47.7% | 26.2% | 13.2% |
| Midwest | 15.5% | 48.8% | 22.4% | 13.3% |
| South | 16.9% | 45.3% | 24.8% | 13.0% |
| West | 19.1% | 48.2% | 21.1% | 11.7% |
| Location of residence | | | | |
| Within MSA | 16.5% | 47.7% | 23.5% | 12.4% |
| Outside MSA | 15.9% | 44.4% | 24.4% | 15.0% |

*Source:* Data from *Health, United States, 2009,* pp. 317–319, National Center for Health Statistics, Division of Health Interview Statistics, 2010.

quality differently, which translates into different expectations of the health care delivery system and, thus, differing evaluations of its quality (McGlynn 1997).

The IOM has defined *quality* as "the degree to which health services for individuals and populations increase the likelihood of desired health outcomes and are consistent with current professional knowledge" (McGlynn 1997). The definition has several implications: (1) Quality performance occurs on a continuum, theoretically ranging from unacceptable to excellent. (2) The focus is on services provided by the health care delivery system as opposed to individual behaviors. (3) Quality may be evaluated from the perspective of individuals and populations or communities. (4) The emphasis is on desired health outcomes, and scientific research must identify the services that improve health outcomes. (5) In the absence of scientific evidence regarding

Table 12–5 Dental Visits in the Past Year Among Persons 18–64 Years of Age, 2007

| Characteristic | Percentage of Persons |
|---|---|
| All persons | 62.7 |
| Poverty status | |
| Poor | 46.7 |
| Near poor | 47.0 |
| Nonpoor | 69.3 |
| Race and Hispanic origin | |
| White, non-Hispanic | 67.3 |
| Black, non-Hispanic | 55.1 |
| Hispanic | 48.9 |
| Sex | |
| Male | 58.8 |
| Female | 66.5 |

*Source:* Data from *Health, United States, 2009*, p. 345, National Center for Health Statistics.

appropriateness of care, professional consensus can be used to develop criteria for the definition and measurement of quality (McGlynn 1997).

Although complete in many respects, the IOM definition leaves out the role of cost in the evaluation of quality. Even though the United States spends more of its national income on health care than other nations, Americans are not the healthiest people in the world. For example, based on comparative data on 37 countries, 27 nations had better outcomes than the United States on infant mortality rates in 2006, and 20 countries had better outcomes on life expectancy at birth for both males and females in 2007 (National Center for Health Statistics 2010a). On the other hand, even though these two comparative measures are widely used as proxies for medical quality, such national comparisons are debatable as to whether the US medical system should be faulted for the disparities. For example, Blum's model of health and wellness (presented in Chapter 2) clearly points to a more significant role that numerous factors other than medical care play in determining health and well-being of individuals and populations. Nevertheless, more health care expenditures do not produce better health, and high quality care must also be cost effective. The delivery of most medical care at the flat of the curve (see Chapter 5) clearly points to a greater need to incorporate cost of care in the assessment of quality.

## Dimensions of Quality

Quality needs to be viewed from both micro and macro perspectives. The micro view focuses on services at the point of delivery and their subsequent effects. It is associated with the performance of individual caregivers and health care organizations. The macro view looks at quality from the standpoint of populations. It reflects the performance of the entire health care delivery system.

### The Micro View

The micro dimension of health care quality encompasses the clinical aspects of care delivery, the interpersonal aspects of care delivery, and quality of life.

#### Clinical Aspects

Clinical aspects of care deal with technical quality, which evaluates the appropriateness of care according to several criteria. Some of the key criteria evaluated to determine clinical appropriateness of care are the facilities where care is delivered, the qualifications and skills of caregivers, the processes and interventions used, cost efficiency of care, and the results or effects on patients' health. Small area variations, previously discussed in this chapter, compromise clinical quality. Geographic variations also indicate widespread inefficiencies. Hence, addressing the problem of clinical variations would result in improved cost, as well as improved quality. Although standardized clinical practice guidelines are intended to address clinical variability, the delivery of medical care will always leave room for physicians' judgment and competence.

Incidents of medical errors in hospitals have been widely reported. For example, the IOM reported that 44,000 to 98,000 patients die in American hospitals each year because of medical errors, making "adverse events" the eighth leading cause of death in the United States (IOM 2000). The Agency for Healthcare Research and Quality (AHRQ) identifies four types of medical errors. Medication errors, or adverse drug events (ADEs), are errors in prescribing and administering medicines to patients. Surgical errors are errors in performing surgical operations. Diagnostic inaccuracies may lead to incorrect treatment or unnecessary testing. Systemic factors, such as organization of health care delivery and distribution of resources, may also contribute to preventable adverse events (AHRQ 2000).

## Interpersonal Aspects

When quality is viewed from the patient's perspective, clinical quality remains important, but interpersonal aspects of care take on added significance. Patients lack technical expertise and often judge the quality of technical care indirectly by their perceptions of the practitioner's interest, concern, and demeanor during clinical encounters (Donabedian 1985). Interpersonal relations and satisfaction become even more important when placed within the holistic context of health care delivery. Positive interactions between patients and practitioners are major contributors to treatment success through greater patient compliance and return for care (Svarstad 1986). Expressions of love, hope, and compassion can enhance the healing effects of medical treatments. Without these elements, the quality of health care remains incomplete.

Interpersonal aspects of quality are also important from the standpoint of organizational management. Consumers—that is, patients and their surrogates—gain lasting impressions of organizational quality from the way they are treated by an organization's employees. Such employee–customer interactions include not just the direct caregivers but a variety of other employees associated with the health care organization, such as receptionists, cafeteria workers, housekeeping employees, and billing clerks.

To measure interpersonal aspects of quality, patient satisfaction surveys have been widely used by various types of health care organizations. Ratings by consumers provide the most appropriate method for evaluating interpersonal quality (McGlynn and Brook 1996). Satisfaction surveys have been used to give physicians feedback on important dimensions of interpersonal communication and service quality. Evidence suggests that such feedback has achieved widespread acceptance by physicians, with more than three-fourths of the physicians affected by such surveys reacting positively to their use (Reed et al. 2003).

## Quality of Life  HRQL

The concept of quality of life has received a great deal of attention in recent years because patients with chronic and/or debilitating diseases are living longer but in a declining state of health. Chronic problems often impose serious limitations on patients' functional status (physical, social, and mental functioning), access to community resources and opportunities, and sense of well-being (Lehman 1995). In a composite sense, during or subsequent to disease, a person's own perception of health, ability to function, role limitations stemming from physical or emotional problems, and personal happiness are referred to as health-related quality of life (*HRQL*).

General HRQL refers to the essential or common components of overall well-being that are more broadly applicable to almost everyone. Other elements of quality of life are relevant only to a particular patient or to patients suffering from a specific disease. Hence, disease-specific HRQL focuses entirely on impairments that are caused by a specific disorder and the effects and side effects of treatments for that disorder. For example, arthritis quality of life is concerned with joint pain and mobility and the side effects of anti-inflammatory agents; depression quality of life deals with the symptoms of depression, such as suicidal thoughts, and such medication side effects as blurred vision, dry mouth, constipation, and impotence (Bergner 1989); and cancer-specific HRQL may include anxiety about cancer recurrence (Ganz and Litwin 1996) and pain management.

*Institution-related quality of life* is also an important attribute of quality in addition to the clinical and interpersonal aspects. It refers to a patient's quality of life while confined in an institution as an inpatient. Factors contributing to institutional quality of life can be classified into three main groups: environmental comfort, self-governance, and human factors. Cleanliness, safety, noise levels, odors, lighting, air circulation, environmental temperature, and furnishings are some of the key comfort factors that are particularly relevant to the physical aspects of institutional living. Self-governance means autonomy to make decisions, freedom to air grievances without fear of reprisal, and reasonable accommodation of personal likes and dislikes. Human factors are associated with caregiver attitudes and practices. Human factors include privacy and confidentiality, treatment from staff in a manner that maintains respect and dignity, and freedom from physical and/or emotional abuse.

## The Macro View

The macro view encompasses systemwide efficiencies and outcomes, which include cost, access, and population health. Some of the other indicators of macro level quality are life expectancy, mortality rates, cause-specific mortality, low-birth-weight deliveries, and incidence and prevalence of specific diseases or chronic conditions. Individual lifestyle and behaviors, along with adequate access to preventive and primary care services, play a major role in determining both individual and population health.

## Quality Assurance

The terms "quality assessment" and "quality assurance" are often encountered in literature on health care quality. Yet, these terms are not always well defined or differentiated. *Quality assessment* refers to the measurement of quality against an established standard. It includes the process of defining how quality is to be determined, identification of specific variables or indicators to be measured, collection of appropriate data to make the measurement possible, statistical analysis, and interpretation of the results of the assessment (Williams and Brook 1978). *Quality assurance* is synonymous with quality improvement. It is the process of institutionalizing quality through ongoing assessment and using the results of assessment for continuous quality improvement (CQI; Williams and Torrens 1993). Quality assurance, then, is a step beyond quality assessment. It is a systemwide or organizationwide commitment to engage in the improvement of quality on an ongoing basis. Although the two activities—quality assessment and quality assurance—are related, quality assurance cannot occur without quality assessment. Quality assessment becomes an integral part of the process of quality assurance. Conversely, it is possible to conduct quality assessment without engaging in quality assurance.

In the past, quality assurance focused on observing deviations from established standards by means of inspection techniques and was used in conjunction with punitive actions for noncompliance. The nursing home industry presents a typical case. Standards of patient care in nursing homes and the system for evaluating performance were developed mainly in conjunction with the certification of facilities for Medicare and Medicaid. Federal regulations developed by CMS are viewed as minimum standards or baseline criteria for defining quality of resident care in certified facilities. Compliance with the standards is monitored through periodic inspections of the facilities, and serious noncompliance is punishable by monetary fines and threats of expulsion from Medicare and Medicaid. Although such external monitoring of quality is necessary (Lohr 1997), it is not quality assurance in the true sense. Rather, it is a rudimentary form of quality assessment that would be more appropriately referred to as "periodic monitoring of quality." Quality assurance is based on the principles of total quality management (*TQM*), also referred to as CQI. The philosophy of TQM was developed and used in other industries before it was adapted for health care delivery. The adoption of TQM by many hospitals and health systems has streamlined administration, reduced lengths of stay, improved clinical outcomes, and produced higher levels of patient satisfaction (HCIA Inc. and Deloitte & Touche 1997).

TQM is an integrative management concept of continually improving the quality of delivered goods and services through the participation of all levels and functions of the organization (Evans 1993) to meet the needs and expectations of the customer. TQM encompasses five main elements:

1. Quality is an integrative concept. It must permeate everything that a health care organization does. In other words, it is not simply confined to the delivery of health services to patients but applies equally to activities that support clinical care. Examples of supportive services include business office, housekeeping, and building and equipment maintenance functions. Hence, everyone working in the organization plays a part in quality improvement.

2. TQM must have the support and commitment of the top management and managers at all levels. Management must allocate the necessary resources, such as staff training for measuring quality; organizing staff functions and work flows so that CQI becomes a part of what people do on a daily basis; and implementing a reward program for achieving quality goals.

3. The organization is committed to ongoing improvement. This means that the standards against which quality is assessed do not remain static. As soon as the current standards of performance are achieved, higher standards are set. The ultimate goal is to achieve a zero error rate or a 100% success rate. Even though such a state of perfection may never be attained, goals must nevertheless be set toward its achievement.

4. TQM emphasizes striving to exceed prevailing standards. This can be accomplished by studying the processes throughout the organization by which health care is produced and provided (Laffel and Blumenthal 1993). Defects, delays, duplications, and waste in processes of health care delivery are identified and improved.

5. TQM is customer driven. The efforts of TQM are directed toward customer satisfaction. In a general sense, customers are the recipients, not necessarily the purchasers, of a service or product. From the organizational perspective, there are both internal and external customers. The organization's internal customers are the users of products or services that ultimately influence the quality of patient care. For example, nursing units are customers of the pharmacy, which must furnish the right medications as ordered by the physicians. The pharmacy is the customer of the physicians, who must prescribe legibly and correctly. Patients and communities are the external customers who ultimately benefit from the results of TQM.

## Quality Assessment

Quality assessment is particularly difficult because it requires the measurement of phenomena that are often subjective or qualitative. They must be quantified to be measured and compared. When quality is defined by qualitative concepts, measurement scales are developed to assess quality. Before these scales are used, their validity and reliability must be established. The *validity* of a scale is the extent to which it actually assesses what it purports to measure. If a measure is supposed to reflect the quality of care, one would expect improvements in quality to affect the measure positively. In other words, the measurement scale would show a higher score for improved quality and vice versa. *Reliability* reflects the extent to which the same results occur from repeated applications of a measure. The subsequent sections survey some of the main criteria and mechanisms used to evaluate quality.

## The Donabedian Model

In his well-known model to help define and measure quality in health care organizations,

Donabedian proposed three domains in which health care quality should be examined: structure, process, and outcomes. Donabedian noted that all three domains are equally important. He also emphasized that these three approaches are complementary and should be used collectively to monitor care quality (Al-Assaf 1993b).

Structure, process, and outcomes are closely linked (Figure 12–10). The three domains are also hierarchical. Structure is the foundation of the quality of health care. Good processes require a good structure. In other words, deficiencies in structure have a negative effect on the processes of health care delivery. Structure and processes together influence quality outcomes. Structure primarily influences process and has only a secondary direct influence on outcome. For improvement of quality, outcomes must be measured and compared against pre-established benchmarks. When desired outcomes are not achieved, one must examine the processes and structures to identify and correct deficiencies.

The model views quality strictly from the perspective of health care delivery. It does not account for social and individual lifestyle or behavior factors that also have a significant influence on health status.

## Structure

Structure has been defined as "the relatively stable characteristics of the providers of care, of the tools and resources they have at their disposal, and of the physical and organizational settings in which they work" (Donabedian 1980). Structural criteria refer to the resource inputs, such as facilities, equipment, staffing levels, staff qualifications, programs, and the administrative organization (Guralnik et al. 1991; McElroy

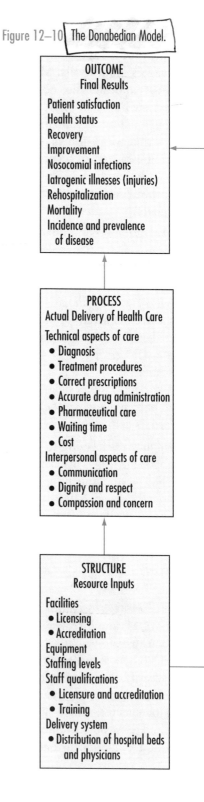

Figure 12–10  The Donabedian Model.

OUTCOME
Final Results

Patient satisfaction
Health status
Recovery
Improvement
Nosocomial infections
Iatrogenic illnesses (injuries)
Rehospitalization
Mortality
Incidence and prevalence
 of disease

PROCESS
Actual Delivery of Health Care

Technical aspects of care
• Diagnosis
• Treatment procedures
• Correct prescriptions
• Accurate drug administration
• Pharmaceutical care
• Waiting time
• Cost
Interpersonal aspects of care
• Communication
• Dignity and respect
• Compassion and concern

STRUCTURE
Resource Inputs

Facilities
• Licensing
• Accreditation
Equipment
Staffing levels
Staff qualifications
• Licensure and accreditation
• Training
Delivery system
• Distribution of hospital beds
 and physicians

and Herbelin 1989). Structural measures indicate the extent to which health care organizations have the capability to provide adequate levels of care (Williams and Torrens 1993). Hence, structure provides an indirect measure of quality under the assumption that a good structure enables health delivery professionals to employ good processes that would lead to good outcomes.

In the past, it was common to rely mostly on the evaluation of structural measures for quality assessment. As such, they were designed to ensure that certain minimum standards were met. Examples are licensing of facilities, accreditation of facilities by the Joint Commission on Accreditation of Healthcare Organizations (JCAHO), and licensing and certification of health care professionals to ensure they meet the required minimum qualifications. Training of personnel is designed to improve the structural elements of quality. From a systemwide macro perspective, structural elements include the number of physicians and hospital beds available per 1,000 population; the geographic distribution of physicians, hospitals, and nursing home beds; and the mix between primary care and specialist physicians.

## Process

Process refers to the specific way in which care is provided. Examples of process are correct diagnostic tests, correct prescriptions, accurate drug administration, waiting time to see a physician, and interpersonal aspects of care delivery. Peer review, previously discussed in this chapter, was designed to serve a dual purpose: control costs and ensure that quality does not suffer. The activities of QIOs rely mainly on process indicators in evaluating the quality of care provided to Medicare patients (Al-Assaf 1993a).

Quality of structures and processes determines quality of outcomes. Some significant initiatives toward process improvement have been undertaken. Some main developments are clinical practice guidelines, cost efficiency, critical pathways, and risk management.

### Clinical Practice Guidelines

*Clinical practice guidelines* (also called medical practice guidelines) are explicit descriptions representing preferred clinical processes for specified conditions. Hence, clinical practice guidelines are scientifically based protocols to guide clinical decisions. A clinical practice guideline constitutes a plan to manage a clinical problem based on evidence whenever possible and on consensus in the absence of evidence (Larsen 1996). Proponents believe that these guidelines simultaneously promote lower costs and better outcomes. Critics view guidelines as an administrative mechanism to reduce utilization.

Congress established the Agency for Health Care Policy and Research in 1989, now called the Agency for Healthcare Research and Quality (AHRQ). Although the agency has a broad research agenda, one of its primary mandates is to build the scientific base of which health care practices work and which do not work. AHRQ has established a National Guideline Clearinghouse (NGC) in partnership with the American Medical Association (AMA) and America's Health Insurance Plans. The NGC is a comprehensive database of evidence-based clinical practice guidelines and related documents. It facilitates access to information produced by different organizations by making it all available at one site.

The NGC is an Internet-based resource that enables health care professionals to compare clinical recommendations. As of November 2010, the NGC contains 7,236 clinical practice guidelines, submitted by 282 health care organizations, associations, medical societies, and federal agencies, (AHRQ 2010a). Guidelines have been catalogued in the areas of diseases; chemicals and drugs; analytical, diagnostic and therapeutic techniques and equipment, and behavioral disciplines and activities.

After some initial reluctance by physicians, there is evidence that clinical practice guidelines are being viewed positively. According to one report, among physicians affected by this care management tool, 66% expressed a positive view (only 8% were negative) on its overall effect on quality and efficiency of medical practice (Reed et al. 2003).

## Cost Efficiency

Also referred to as cost effectiveness, cost efficiency (discussed in Chapter 5 in conjunction with technology assessment) is an important concept in quality assessment. A service is cost efficient when the benefit received is greater than the cost incurred to provide the service. Cost efficiency uses the health production function to evaluate the relationship between increasing medical expenditures (or health risks) and improvements in health levels. As medical interventions and expenditures are increased, there is a curvilinear, rather than a constant, effect on improved health (Feldstein 1994). At the start of medical treatment, each unit is likely to deliver benefits exceeding its costs or benefits exceeding the potential risks. The marginal (i.e., additional) health benefits become smaller and risks become bigger as more care is delivered and greater costs are incurred (see Figure 5–2). An optimum point

is reached when additional health benefits approximately equal the additional costs (or risks). Beyond this point, additional interventions result in fewer benefits in relation to the additional costs, or the risks are greater than the benefits. In economic terms, additional services beyond the optimum point produce diminishing marginal returns. This point also represents optimal quality, which serves as a point of demarcation between underutilization and overutilization.

*Underutilization* (underuse) occurs when the benefits of an intervention outweigh its risks or costs, and yet it is not used (Chassin 1991). Potential adverse health outcomes related to underutilization include hospitalizations that could be avoided by providing better medical access and timely care, low birth weight due to lack of prenatal care, infant mortality due to lack of early pediatric care, and low cancer survival rates due to lack of early detection and treatment. Conversely, *overutilization* (overuse) occurs when the costs or risks of treatment outweigh its benefits, and yet additional care is delivered. When health care is overused, precious resources are wasted. Hence, inefficiency can be regarded as unethical because it deprives someone else of the potential benefits of health care.

The principles of cost efficiency indicate that health care costs can be reduced without lowering quality of care. Conversely, quality can be improved without increasing costs. A trade-off does not have to occur between cost and quality. Introduction of PPS by Medicare is an example. The resulting discharge of patients "quicker and sicker" triggered by PPS initially raised some alarm concerning decreased quality, but it was found that processes of care in hospitals actually improved and mortality rates were unchanged or lower (Rogers et al. 1990). Other potential negative health outcomes that can be avoided by curtailing overuse include life-threatening drug interactions, nosocomial infections, and iatrogenic illnesses.

## Critical Pathways

*Critical pathways* are outcome-based and patient-centered case management tools that are interdisciplinary, facilitating coordination of care among multiple clinical departments and caregivers. A critical pathway is a timeline that identifies planned medical interventions, along with expected patient outcomes, for a specific diagnosis or class of cases, often defined by a DRG. The outcomes and interventions included in the critical pathway are broadly defined. In addition to technical outcomes, pathways may measure such factors as patient satisfaction, self-reported health status, mental health, and activities of daily living (ADLs). Interventions include treatments, medications, diagnostic tests, diet, activity regimens, consultations, discharge planning, and patient education. A critical pathway serves as a plan of action for all disciplines caring for a patient and incorporates a system for documenting and evaluating variances from the critical path plan. Critical pathways are unique to the institutions that develop them because they are based on the particular practices of that facility and its caregivers. A pathway also is customized to the patient population being served and the available patient care resources. Finally, critical pathways are meant to promote interdisciplinary collaboration within the environment of the hospital and its market. The latter occurs by making patients and families active participants in the process. For these reasons, critical pathways are difficult to replicate from one organization to another. Use of critical pathways reduces costs and improves quality by reducing errors, improving coordination among interdisciplinary players, streamlining case management functions, providing systematic data to assess care, and reducing variation in practice patterns (Giffin and Giffin 1994).

## Risk Management

*Risk management* consists of proactive efforts to prevent adverse events related to clinical care and facilities operations and is especially focused on avoiding medical malpractice (Orlikoff 1988). In response to the threat of lawsuits, initiatives undertaken by a health care organization to review clinical processes and establish protocols for the specific purpose of reducing malpractice litigation can actually enhance quality. Because malpractice concerns also result in defensive medicine, risk management approaches should employ the principles of cost efficiency along with standardized practice guidelines and critical pathways.

Threat of malpractice litigation also has a downside. Fear of litigation actually leads to a reluctance by hospitals and physicians to disclose preventable harm and actual medical errors. In this respect, it is believed that fear of litigation may actually conceal problems that may compromise patient safety (Lamb et al. 2003).

## Outcomes

*Outcomes* refer to the effects or results obtained from utilizing the structure and processes of health care delivery. Many view outcomes as the bottom-line measure of the effectiveness of the health care delivery system (McGlynn and Brook 1996). Positive outcomes suggest recovery from disease and improvement in health. They also suggest an overall improvement in health status through health promotion and disease prevention and adequate access to health care services. Outcomes are often gauged through a comparative assessment—between two time intervals—of the measures of morbidity, mortality, and health status presented in Chapter 2. Other outcome measures include postoperative infection rates, nosocomial infections, iatrogenic illnesses, and rates of rehospitalization. Malpractice litigation is sometimes used as an outcome indicator because litigation seeks damages for negative outcomes. Another indicator of positive outcome is patient satisfaction, which is assessed through questionnaires completed by patients and/or surrogates.

Quality outcomes are also evaluated using interview techniques and self-administered questionnaires to report on functional status, neuropsychiatric function, social function, and emotional and spiritual health. Determination of HRQL is an example. Typically, HRQL data are collected with self-report questionnaires, called "instruments," using survey research techniques. These instruments contain questions or items organized into scales. Each scale measures a different aspect or domain of HRQL. Some scales comprise dozens of items, whereas others may include only one or two items (Ganz and Litwin 1996). HRQL domains can be general, disease-specific, or institution-related.

None of the outcome measures provides a perfect assessment. Each measure focuses on a particular aspect of quality. Hence, using a combination of measures is likely to produce more objective results, but there is a cost and benefit trade-off. The greater the number of measures used for evaluating

quality, the more costly the assessment process.

## Public Reporting of Quality

Public reporting on macro levels of quality expanded in the early 2000s. This section summarizes the major public reporting initiatives.

### CMS Programs on Quality *Transparency*

CMS began developing a large public reporting program known as Hospital Compare, which initially measured and reported process-based measures of high-quality care for acute myocardial infarction, heart failure, pneumonia, and general surgery (Ross 2010). That effort was followed by Nursing Home Quality Initiative, Home Health Quality Initiative, and End Stage Renal Disease (ESRD) Quality Initiative (CMS 2010). Hospital Compare has been further expanded to include hospital 30-day risk standardized mortality and readmission rates for acut myocardial infarction, heart failure, and pneumonia, as well as patient satisfaction and medical imaging usage (Ross 2010). CMS and AHRQ, together, developed the Hospital Consumer Assessment of Healthcare Providers and Systems (CAHPS) survey, which collects uniform measures of patient perspectives on various aspects of their inpatient care (CMS 2005). Results are publicly reported on the CMS Hospital Compare website. Results are used by health care organizations, public and private purchasers, consumers, and researchers to inform their purchasing or contracting decisions and to improve the quality of health care services (AHRQ 2010b). CMS collects and reports performance data by home health agencies with the Outcome and Assessment Information Set (OASIS; CMS 2010).

## AHRQ Quality Indicators

Since 2003, AHRQ has published National Healthcare Quality Report and National Healthcare Disparities Report annually (AHRQ 2010c). In identifying key measures for these reports, Interagency Workgroup focused on priority areas established in Healthy People 2010 (AHRQ 2005). AHRQ has a set of quality indicators (QIs) that measure quality of process of care in an outpatient or an inpatient setting (AHRQ 2006). Prevention QIs identify hospital admissions that could have been avoided. Inpatient QIs and patient safety indicators both reflect quality of care inside hospitals, with the former focusing on inpatient mortality and the latter on potentially avoidable complications and iatrogenic events. Pediatric quality indicators reflect quality of care received by children inside hospitals and identify potentially avoidable hospitalizations.

## State Public Reporting of Hospital Quality

A study published in 2010 found that 25 states have state public reporting programs (Ross 2010). The vast majority of these programs provide data on hospital outcomes of care with focus on acquired infection, readmission rates, and mortality rates following hospitalization for the same clinical conditions currently reported by CMS (acute myocardial infarction, heart failure, and pneumonia), although most states use AHRQ's Inpatient Quality Indicators (Ross 2010). One of the advantages of state public reporting programs is that their reporting is not limited to Medicare fee-for-service beneficiaries but also includes younger adults and older adults insured through private plans and Medicaid-affiliated HMOs (Ross 2010).

---

# Summary

Increasing costs, lack of access, and concerns about quality pose the greatest challenges to health care delivery in the United States. To some extent, the three issues are interrelated. Increasing costs limit the system's ability to expand access. A lack of universal coverage negatively affects the health status of uninsured groups. Despite spending the most resources on health care, the United States continues to rank in the bottom quartile among developed countries on outcome indicators such as life expectancy and infant mortality.

Nations that have national health insurance can control systemwide costs through top-down controls, mainly in the form of global budgets. This approach is not possible in the United States because it has a multipayer system. In the United States, regulatory approaches have been used to try to constrain the supply side, but the major emphasis has been on constricting reimbursement to providers. Several competitive approaches have been used, mainly through the expansion of managed care. A move toward prospective payments and the growth of managed care can be largely credited with the brakes put on rising health care spending during the 1990s.

Access to medical care is one of the key determinants of health status, along with environment, lifestyle, and hereditary factors. Access is also regarded as a significant benchmark in assessing the effectiveness of the medical care delivery system. Access is explained in terms of enabling and predisposing factors, as well as factors related to health policy and health care delivery. Access has five dimensions: availability, accessibility, accommodation, affordability, and acceptability. Measures of access can relate to individuals, health care plans, and the health care delivery system.

Quality in health care has been difficult to define and measure, although it has received increasing emphasis. At the micro level, health care quality encompasses the clinical aspects of care delivery, the interpersonal aspects of care delivery, and quality of life. Indicators of quality at the macro level are commonly associated with life expectancy, mortality, and morbidity. Quality assessment is the measurement of quality against an established standard. Quality assurance emphasizes improvement of quality using the principles of continual quality improvement. Donabedian proposed that quality should be assessed along three dimensions: structure, process, and outcomes. These three dimensions are complementary and should be used collectively to monitor quality of care. Reliability and validity are important concepts in the measurement of quality. Since 2000, several federal and state initiatives have been implemented to report on certain macro levels of quality.

---

## Terminology

## Test Your Understanding

| | | |
|---|---|---|
| access | HRQL | reliability |
| administrative costs | institution-related quality | risk management |
| certificate-of-need | of life | single-payer system |
| clinical practice guidelines | outcomes | small area variations |
| competition | overutilization | top-down control |
| cost efficiency | peer review | TQM |
| critical pathways | QIO | underutilization |
| defensive medicine | quality | upcoding |
| fraud | quality assessment | validity |
| health planning | quality assurance | |

---

## Review Questions

1. What is meant by the term "health care costs"? Describe the three meanings of the term "cost."

2. Why should the United States control the rising costs of health care?

3. How do findings of the Rand Health Insurance Experiment reinforce the relationship between growth in third-party reimbursement and increase in health care costs? Explain.

4. Explain how, under imperfect market conditions, both prices and quantity of health care are higher than they would be in a highly competitive market.

5. What are some of the reasons for increased health care costs that are attributed to the providers of medical care?

6. What are some of the main differences between broad cost-containment approaches used in the United States and those used in countries with national health insurance?

7. Discuss the effectiveness of certificate-of-need (CON) regulation in controlling health care expenditures.

8. Discuss price controls and their effectiveness in controlling health care expenditures.

9. Discuss the role of quality improvement organizations (QIOs) in cost containment.

10. What are the four competition-based cost-containment strategies?

11. What are the implications of access for health and health care delivery?

12. What is the role of enabling and predisposing factors in access to care?

13. Briefly describe the five dimensions of access.

14. What are the four main types of access described by Andersen?

15. Describe the measurement of access at the individual, health plan, and delivery system levels.

16. What are some of the implications of the definition of quality proposed by the Institute of Medicine (IOM)? In what way is the definition incomplete?

17. Discuss the dimensions of quality from the micro and macro perspectives.

18. Discuss the two types of health-related quality of life (HRQL).

19. Distinguish between quality assessment and quality assurance.

20. What are the basic principles of total quality management (TQM; or continual quality improvement [CQI])?

21. Give a brief description of the Donabedian model of quality.

22. Discuss the main developments in process improvement that have occurred in recent years.

## REFERENCES

Aday, L.A. 1993. Indicators and predictors of health services utilization. In: *Introduction to health services*. 4th ed. S.J. Williams and P.R. Torrens, eds. Albany, NY: Delmar Publishers. pp. 46–70.

Aday, L.A., and R. Andersen. 1975. *Development of indices of access to medical care*. Ann Arbor, MI: Health Administration Press.

Aday, L.A. et al. 1980. *Health care in the US: Equitable for whom?* Newbury Park, CA: Sage.

Aday, L.A. et al. 1984. *Access to medical care in the US: Who has it, who doesn't?* Research Series No. 32. Chicago, IL: Center for Health Administration Studies, University of Chicago, Pluribus Press Inc.

Aday, L.A. et al. 1993. *Evaluating the medical care system: Effectiveness, efficiency, and equity.* Ann Arbor, MI: Health Administration Press.

Agency for Healthcare Research and Quality (AHRQ). 2000. *Reducing errors in health care: Translating research into practice.* AHRQ Publication No. 00-PO58, April 2000. Available at: http://www.ahrq.gov/qual/errors.htm. Accessed January 2011.

Agency for Healthcare Research and Quality (AHRQ). 2005. *National healthcare quality report: Background on the measures development process.* Available at: www.ahrq.gov/qual/nhqrmeasures/nhqrprelim.htm. Accessed January 2011.

Agency for Healthcare Research and Quality (AHRQ). 2006. *What are the AHRQ QIs?* Available at: www.qualityindicators.ahrq.gov/general_faq.htm#1. Accessed January 2011.

Agency for Healthcare Research and Quality (AHRQ). 2010a. The National Guideline Clearinghouse. Available at: www.guideline.gov/browse/bytopic.aspx. Accessed December 2010.

Agency for Healthcare Research and Quality (AHRQ). 2010b. *Consumer Assessment of Healthcare Providers and Systems (CAHPS).* Available at: www.cahps.ahrq.gov. Accessed January 2011.

Agency for Healthcare Research and Quality (AHRQ). 2010c. *Measuring healthcare quality.* Available at: www.ahrq.gov/qual/measurix.htm. Accessed January 2011.

Al-Assaf, A.F. 1993a. Introduction and historical background. In: *The textbook of total quality management.* A.F. Al-Assaf and J.A. Schmele, eds. Delray Beach, FL: St. Lucie Press. pp. 3–12.

Al-Assaf, A.F. 1993b. Outcome management and TQ. In: *The textbook of total quality management.* A.F. Al-Assaf and J.A. Schmele, eds. Delray Beach, FL: St. Lucie Press. pp. 221–237.

Altman, S.H., and J. Eichenholz. 1976. Inflation in the health industry: Causes and cures. In: *Health: A victim or cause of inflation?* M. Zubkoff, ed. New York: Milbank Memorial Fund. pp. 1–32.

Altman, S.H., and S.S. Wallack. 1996. Health care spending: Can the United States control it? In: *Strategic choices for a changing health care system.* S.H. Altman and U.E. Reinhardt, eds. Chicago: Health Administration Press.

Andersen, R. 1968. *A behavioral model of families' use of health services.* Research Series No. 25. Chicago, IL: Center for Health Administration Studies, University of Chicago.

Andersen, R. 1997. *Too big, too small, too flat, too tall: Search for "just right" measures of access in the age of managed care.* Chicago, IL: Paper presented at the Association for Health Services Research Annual Meeting.

Arnould, R.J. et al. 1993. Competitive reforms: Context and scope. In: *Competitive approaches to health care reform.* R.J. Arnould, R.F. Rich, and W.D. White, eds. Washington, DC: The Urban Institute Press. pp. 3–18.

Baucus, M., and E.J. Fowler. 2002. Geographic variation in Medicare spending and the real focus of Medicare reform. *Health Affairs Jul–Dec, Suppl Web Exclusives*: W115–W117.

Bergner, M. 1989. Quality of life, health status, and clinical research. *Medical Care* 27, no. 3 (Suppl): S148–S156.

Blanchfield, B.B. et al. 2010. Saving billions of dollars and physicians' time by streamlining billing practices. *Health Affairs*, 29, no. 6: 1248–1254.

Brown, K. 1992. Death and access: Ethics in cross-cultural health care. In: *Choices and conflict: Explorations in health care ethics.* E. Friedman, ed. Chicago, IL: American Hospital Publishing.

Centers for Disease Control and Prevention (CDC). 2005. Annual smoking-attributable mortality, years of potential life lost, and productivity losses—United States, 1997–2001. *Morbidity and Mortality Weekly Report* 54, no. 25: 625–628.

Centers for Medicare & Medicaid Services (CMS). 2005. *Costs and benefits of HCAHPS.* Available at: www.cms.gov/HospitalQualityInits/downloads/HCAHPSCostsBenefits200512.pdf. Accessed January 2011.

Centers for Medicare & Medicaid Services (CMS). 2007. *Pay for performance.* Available at: http://www.cms.hhs.gov/MedicaidSCHIPQualPrac/04_P4P.asp. Accessed January 2011.

Chassin, M.R. 1991. Quality of care—Time to act. *Journal of the American Medical Association* 266, no. 24: 3472–3473.

Congressional Budget Office (CBO). 2007. *The long-term outlook for health care spending.* November 2007. Available at: www.cbo.gov/ftpdocs/87xx/doc8758/11-13-LT-Health.pdf. Accessed January 2011.

Department of Health and Human Services (DHHS). 1996. *Health, United States, 1995.* Hyattsville, MD: National Center for Health Statistics.

Department of Health and Human Services (DHHS). 2011. *Health, United States, 2010.* Hyattsville, MD: National Center for Health Statistics.

Docteur, E.R. et al. 1996. Shifting the paradigm: Monitoring access in Medicare managed care. *Health Care Financing Review* 17, no. 4: 5–21.

Donabedian, A. 1980. *Explorations in quality assessment and monitoring: The definition of quality and approaches to its assessment.* Vol. 1. Ann Arbor, MI: Health Administration Press.

Donabedian, A. 1985. *Explorations in quality assessment and monitoring: The methods and findings of quality assessment and monitoring.* Vol. 3. Ann Arbor, MI: Health Administration Press.

Dranove, D. 1993. The case for competitive reform in health care. In: *Competitive approaches to health care reform.* R.J. Arnould, R.F. Rich, and W.D. White, eds. Washington, DC: The Urban Institute Press. pp. 67–82.

Evans, J.R. 1993. *Applied production and operations management.* 4th ed. Minneapolis/St. Paul, MN: West Publishing Co.

Feldstein, P. 1994. *Health policy issues: An economic perspective on health reform.* Ann Arbor, MI: AUPHA Press/Health Administration Press.

Feldstein, P.J. 1993. *Health care economics.* 4th ed. Albany, NY: Delmar Publishers.

Finkelstein, E.A. et al. 2009. Annual medical spending attributable to obesity: Payer- and service-specific estimates. *Health Affairs* 28, no. 5: W822–W831.

Fisher, E.S. et al. 2003a. The implications of regional variations in Medicare spending. Part 1: The content, quality, and accessibility of care. *Annals of Internal Medicine* 138, no. 4: 273–287.

Fisher, E.S. et al. 2003b. The implications of regional variations in Medicare spending. Part 2: Health outcomes and satisfaction with care. *Annals of Internal Medicine* 138, no. 4: 288–298.

Gabel, J., and T. Rice. 1985. Reducing public expenditures for physician services: The price of paying less. *Journal of Health Politics, Policy and Law* 9, no. 4: 595–609.

Ganz, P.A., and M.S. Litwin. 1996. Measuring outcomes and health-related quality of life. In: *Changing the US health care system: Key issues in health services, policy, and management.* R.M. Andersen et al., eds. San Francisco, CA: Jossey-Bass Publishers.

Giffin, M., and R.B. Giffin. 1994. Market memo: Critical pathways produce tangible results. *Health Care Strategic Management* 12, no. 7: 1–6.

Gittelsohn, A., and N.R. Powe. 1995. Small area variation in health care delivery in Maryland. *Health Services Research* 30, no. 2: 295–317.

Gottlieb, S.R. 1974. A brief history of health planning in the United States. In: *Regulating health facilities construction.* C.C. Havighurst, ed. Washington, DC: American Enterprise Institute for Public Policy Research.

Guralnik, J.M. et al. 1991. Morbidity and disability in older persons in the years prior to death. *American Journal of Public Health* 81, no. 4: 443–447.

Hartman, M. et al. 2011. Health spending growth at a historic low in 2008. *Health Affairs* 29, no. 1: 147–155.

HCIA Inc. and Deloitte & Touche. 1997. *The comparative performance of US hospitals: The sourcebook.* Baltimore, MD: HCIA Inc.

Health Council of Canada. (2010). *How Do Canadians rate the health care system?* Results from the 2010 Commonwealth Fund International Health Policy Survey. Canadian Health Care Matters, Bulletin 4. Toronto: Health Council of Canada.

Hutchison, L. et al. 2005. *Access to quality health services in rural areas—long-term care: A literature review.* Available at: http://www.srphtamhsc.edu/centers/rhp2010/Volume_3/Vol3Ch1LR .pdf. Accessed January 2011.

Institute of Medicine (IOM). 1993. *Access to health care in America.* M. Millman, ed. Washington, DC: National Academy Press.

Institute of Medicine (IOM). 2000. *To err is human: Building a safer health system.* L.T. Kohn, J.M. Corrigan, and M.S. Donaldson, eds. Washington, DC: National Academy Press.

Institute of Medicine (IOM). 2004. *Rewarding provider performance: Aligning incentives in Medicare.* Washington, DC: National Academy Press.

Kaiser Family Foundation. 2009. *Trends in health care costs and spending, March 2009.* Available at: http://www.kff.org/insurance/upload/7692_02.pdf. Accessed January 2010.

Kaiser Family Foundation, Health Research and Education Trust. 2010. *Employer health benefits 2010 annual survey.* Available at: http://ehbs.kff.org. Accessed January 2011.

Laffel, G., and D. Blumenthal. 1993. The case for using industrial quality management science in health care organizations. In: *The textbook of total quality management.* A.F. Al-Assaf and J.A. Schmele, eds. Delray Beach, FL: St. Lucie Press. pp. 40–50.

Lamb, R.M. et al. 2003. Hospital disclosure practices: Results of a national survey. *Health Affairs* 22, no. 2: 73–83.

Larsen, R.R. 1996. Narrowing the gray zone: How clinical practice guidelines can improve the decision-making process. *Postgraduate Medicine* 100, no. 2: 17–24.

Lehman, A.F. 1995. Measuring quality of life in a reformed health system. *Health Affairs* 14, no. 3: 90–101.

Lemieux, J. 2005. *Perspective: Administrative costs of private health insurance plans*. Available at: http://www.ahipresearch.org/pdfs/Administrative_Costs_030705.pdf. Accessed March 2011.

Levit, K. et al. 2003. Trends in US health care spending, 2001. *Health Affairs* 22, no. 1: 154–164.

Levy, D.E. 2006. Employer-sponsored insurance coverage of smoking cessation treatments. *American Journal of Managed Care* 12, no. 9: 553–562.

Lohr, K.N. 1997. How do we measure quality? *Health Affairs* 16, no. 3: 22–25.

Lovitky, J.A. 1997. Health care fraud: A growing problem. *Nursing Management* 28, no. 11: 42, 44–45.

May, J. 1974. The planning and licensing agencies. In: *Regulating health facilities constructions*. C.C. Havighurst, ed. Washington, DC: American Enterprise Institute for Public Policy Research.

McElroy, D., and K. Herbelin. 1989. Assuring quality of care in long-term care facilities. *Journal of Gerontological Nursing* 15, no. 7: 8–10.

McGlynn, E.A. 1997. Six challenges in measuring the quality of health care. *Health Affairs* 16, no. 3: 7–21.

McGlynn, E.A., and R.H. Brook. 1996. Ensuring quality of care. In: *Changing the US health care system: Key issues in health services, policy, and management*. R.M. Andersen, T.H. Rice, and G.F. Kominski, eds. San Francisco, CA: Jossey-Bass Publishers.

Mitchell, J. et al. 1988. *Impact of the Medicare fee freeze on physician expenditures and volume: Final report*. Baltimore, MD: Health Care Financing Administration.

National Center for Health Statistics. 2002. *National vital statistics reports* 49, no. 12. Atlanta, GA: Centers for Disease Control and Prevention.

National Center for Health Statistics. 2010a. *Health, United States, 2009: With special feature on medical technology*. Hyattsville, MD: US Department of Health and Human Services.

National Center for Health Statistics. 2010b. *Health, United States, 2009*. Hyattsville, MD: US Department of Health and Human Services.

Nicholas L.H. et al. 2011. Do hospitals alter patient care effort allocations under pay-for-performance? *Health Services Research* 46, no. 1: 61–81.

Orlikoff, J.E. 1988. *Malpractice prevention and liability control for hospitals*. 2nd ed. Chicago, IL: American Hospital Publishing.

Penchansky, R., and J.W. Thomas. 1981. The concept of access: Definition and relationship to consumer satisfaction. *Medical Care* 19: 127–140.

Reed, M. et al. 2003. Physicians and care management: More acceptance than you think. Issue brief. *Center for the Study of Health System Change*, January, no. 60: 1–4.

Reinhardt, U.E. 1994. Providing access to health care and controlling costs: The universal dilemma. In: *The nation's health*. 4th ed. P.R. Lee and C.L. Estes, eds. Boston: Jones & Bartlett Publishers. pp. 263–278.

Reinhardt, U.E. et al. 2002. Cross-national comparisons of health systems using OECD data, 1999. *Health Affairs* 21, no. 3: 169–181.

Rogers, W.H. et al. 1990. Quality of care before and after implementation of the DRG-based prospective payment system: A summary of effects. *Journal of the American Medical Association* 264, no. 15: 1989–1994.

Ross, J.S., Sheth, S., and H. M. Krumholz. 2010. State-sponsored public reporting of hospital quality: Results are hard to find and lack uniformity. *Health Affairs* 29, no. 12: 2317–2322.

Svarstad, B.L. 1986. Patient-practitioner relationships and compliance with prescribed medical regimens. In: *Applications of social sciences to clinical medicine and health policy*. L.H. Aiken and D. Mechanic, eds. New Brunswick, NJ: Rutgers University Press.

TECH Research Network. 2001. Technology change around the world: Evidence from heart attack care. *Health Affairs* 20, no. 3: 25–42.

USA Today. 2010. Our view on financing government: When 47% don't pay income tax, it's not healthy for USA. *USA Today*, updated 4/15/2010. Available at: http://www.usatoday.com /news/opinion/editorials/2010-04-16-editorial16_ST_N.htm. Accessed March 2011.

U.S. Government Accountability Office (GAO). 2008. *Medicare Part B imaging services: Rapid spending growth and shift to physician offices indicate need for CMS to consider additional management practices*. Available at: http://www.gao.gov/products/GAO-08-452. Accessed January 2011.

Van de Water, P.N., and J. Lavery. 2006. Medicare finances: Findings of the 2006 trustees report. *Medicare Brief* 13: 1–8.

Wendling, W., and J. Werner. 1980. Nonprofit firms and the economic theory of regulation. *Quarterly Review of Economics and Business* 20, no. 3: 6–18.

Wennberg, J.E. 2002.Unwarranted variations in healthcare delivery: Implications for academic medical centres. *British Medical Journal* 325, no. 7370: 961–964.

Wennberg, J.E., and A. Gittelsohn. 1973. Small area variations in health care delivery. *Science* 183: 1102–1108.

Wennberg, J.E. et al. 1987. Are hospital services rationed in New Haven or over-utilized in Boston? *Lancet* 1, no. 8543: 1185–1189.

Williams, K.N., and R.H. Brook. 1978. Quality measurement and assurance. *Health Medical Care Services Review* 1: 3–15.

Williams, S.J. 1995. *Essentials of health services*. Albany, NY: Delmar Publishers.

Williams, S.J., and P.R. Torrens. 1993. Influencing, regulating, and monitoring the health care system. In: *Introduction to health services*. 4th ed. S.J. Williams and P.R. Torrens, eds. Albany, NY: Delmar Publishers. pp. 377–396.

Wilson, F.A., and D. Neuhauser. 1985. *Health services in the United States*. 2nd ed. Cambridge, MA: Ballinger Publishing Co.

Wong, M.D. et al. 2001. Effects of cost sharing on care seeking and health status: Results from the medical outcomes study. *American Journal of Public Health* 91, no. 11: 1889–1894.

# Chapter 13

## Health Policy

### Learning Objectives

- To understand the definition, scope, and role of health policy in the United States
- To recognize the principal features of US health policy
- To comprehend the process of legislative health policy
- To become familiar with some of the critical health policy issues in the United States
- To discuss the passage of the Patient Protection and Affordable Care Act of 2010 from a political perspective

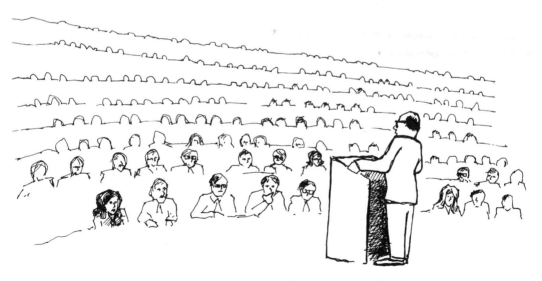

*"Ladies and Gentlemen, to come up with a uniform health policy, we will now break up into 31 different groups."*

## Introduction

Even though the United States does not have a centrally controlled system of health care delivery—at least not yet—it does have a history of federal, state, and local government involvement in health care and health policy. Government involvement in social welfare programs can be traced back to alms-houses and pesthouses, the two well-known government-run institutions of the 19th century (see Chapter 3). Perhaps the most visible policy efforts, however, that continue to have repercussions and will have future implications were the social programs created under the Social Security legislation during Franklin Roosevelt's presidency in the 1940s. Amendments to the Social Security Act later created the massive public health insurance programs, Medicare and Medicaid in 1965 and the more recent Children's Health Insurance Program (CHIP) program in 1997. The government's success in bringing about social change through health policy has given the government a solid footing to engage in further expansion of tax-financed health care. Hence, the government continues to find new opportunities to mold health care delivery through health policy. This chapter defines what health policy is and explores the principal features of health policy in the United States. It describes how legislative policy is developed and provides a policy context for many past developments in health care delivery.

## What Is Health Policy?

Public policies are authoritative decisions made in the legislative, executive, or judicial branch of government intended to direct or influence the actions, behaviors, or decisions of others (Longest 2010). When public policies pertain to or influence the pursuit of health, they become health policies. Therefore, *health policy* can be defined as "the aggregate of principles, stated or unstated, that . . . characterize the distribution of resources, services, and political influences that impact on the health of the population . . ." (Miller 1987).

Public policies are supposed to serve the interests of the public; however, the term "public" has been interpreted differently in the political landscape. At the most general level, the term "public" refers to all Americans. "Public" can also refer to voters or likely voters; that is, the subset of Americans who directly determine the outcomes of political elections. Finally, the term can refer to only those who are politically active. The latter group consists of those Americans who communicate directly with their representatives by either writing or calling, contribute money to politicians or political groups, attend protests or other forums on behalf of a particular interest or candidate, or, in other ways, make their voices and policy preferences heard. People who are older, have more years of education, and have strong party identification are more likely to be politically active.

Legislators and policy makers tend to be responsive to the views or wishes of these active Americans, particularly when they are constituents from within their legislative districts. Conversely, politicians also tend to strongly lean toward supporting policies that agree with their own ideologies or advance their political agendas. Because most policy makers are politicians, policy making and politics are often closely intertwined. The danger is that policy making often

public policy

*policy-for-politics* [handwritten]

becomes highly politicized and becomes hostage to the ideologies of the political party that happens to be in power at a given time. The party in power also exerts considerable peer pressure on its own members to support policies along party lines. Also, the primary concern of most politicians is to get elected or reelected. Hence, certain policies are driven by a strong desire to keep campaign promises or to please some powerful constituent group. The policy-for-politics approach does not ask for or consider the cost-benefit of a proposed policy. Also, party-line politics keep the American public deeply divided on major issues.

## Uses of Policy

### Regulatory Tools

Health policies may be used as *regulatory tools* (Longest 2010). They call on government to prescribe and control the behavior of a particular target group by monitoring the group and imposing sanctions if it fails to comply. Examples of regulatory policies are abundant in the health care system. Federally funded quality improvement organizations (QIOs, formerly peer review organizations), for instance, develop and enforce standards concerning appropriate care under the Medicare program (see Chapter 12). State insurance departments across the country regulate insurance companies and managed care organizations (MCOs) in an effort to protect customers from default on coverage in case of financial failure of the insurer, excessive premiums, and mendacious practices.

Some health policies are "self-regulatory." For example, physicians set standards of medical practice, hospitals accredit one another as meeting the standards that the Joint Commission on Accreditation of Healthcare Organizations has set, and schools of public health decide which courses should be part of their graduate programs in public health (Weissert and Weissert 1996). Similarly, MCOs voluntarily collect and report on quality measures using Health Effectiveness Data and Information Set (HEDIS) data (see Chapter 9) to the National Committee for Quality Assurance, which is a voluntary, nongovernmental agency.

### Allocative Tools

Health policies may also be used as *allocative tools* (Longest 2010). They involve the direct provision of income, services, or goods to certain groups of individuals or institutions. Allocative tools in the health care arena are distributive or redistributive. *Distributive policies* spread benefits throughout society. Typical distributive policies include funding of medical research through the NIH, the development of medical personnel (e.g., medical education through the National Health Service Corps), the construction of facilities (e.g., hospitals under the Hill-Burton program during the 1950s and 1960s), and the initiation of new institutions (e.g., HMOs under the Health Maintenance Organization Act of 1973). *Redistributive policies* are designed to benefit only certain groups of people by taking money from one group and using it for the benefit of another. This system often creates visible beneficiaries and payers. For this reason, health policy is often most visible and politically charged when it performs redistributive functions. Redistributive policies include Medicaid, which takes tax revenue from the more affluent

* Hill-Burton [handwritten]
  - fed. grant to create more hospital beds
  - But, not controlled by fed. gov.

and spends it on the poor in the form of free health insurance. Other redistributive policies include CHIP, welfare, and public housing programs. Redistributive policies, in particular, are believed to be essential for addressing the fundamental causes of health disparities. Expansion of health insurance for the uninsured—proposed under the Patient Protection and Affordable Care Act (ACA) of 2010—is also based on a redistributive approach.

## Different Forms of Health Policies

Health policies often come as a by-product of social policies enacted by the government. For example, the Social Security Act of 1935 was passed mainly as a retirement income security measure for the elderly, but it also contained the Old Age Assistance program that enabled the elderly to pay for services in homes for the aged and boarding homes. After World War II, policies that excluded fringe benefits from income or Social Security taxes and a Supreme Court ruling that employee benefits, including health insurance, could be legitimately included in the collective bargaining process (see Chapter 3) had the effect of promoting employer-sponsored private health insurance. Consequently, employer-based health benefits grew rapidly in the mid-20th century.

The extraordinary growth of medical technology in the United States can also be traced to health policies that directly support biomedical research and encourage private investments in such research. The National Institutes of Health (NIH) had a budget of about $10 million when the agency was established in the early 1930s. Following exponential growth, the proposed fiscal year 2011 NIH budget is $32.2 billion (NIH 2010). Encouraged by policies, such

as patent laws, that permit firms to recoup their investments in research and development, private industry also spends a significant amount on biomedical research and development.

Health policies affect groups or classes of individuals, such as physicians, the poor, the elderly, and children. They can also affect various types of organizations, such as medical schools, health maintenance organizations (HMOs), hospitals, nursing homes, manufacturers of medical technology, and employers. Examples include licensing of physicians and nurses by states; federal certification of health care institutions, enabling them to receive public funds to care for Medicare and Medicaid patients; court decisions that may prevent the merger of two hospitals on the grounds of violating federal antitrust laws; and local ordinances banning smoking in public places.

Statutes or laws, such as the statutory language contained in the 1983 Amendments to the Social Security Act that authorized the prospective payment system (PPS) for reimbursing hospitals for Medicare beneficiaries, are also considered policies. Another example is the certificate-of-need (CON) programs, through which many states seek to regulate capital expansion in their health care systems (see Chapters 5 and 12).

The scope of health policy is limited by the political and economic system of a country. In the United States, where proindividual and promarket sentiments dominate, public policies are likely to be fragmented, incremental, and noncomprehensive. National policies and programs are typically based on the notion that local communities are in the best position to identify strategies that will address their unique needs. However, the type of change that can be enacted at the community level is clearly limited.

## Principal Features of US Health Policy

Several features characterize US health policy, including government as subsidiary to the private sector; fragmented, incremental, and piecemeal reform; pluralistic politics associated with demanders and suppliers of policy; decentralized role of the states; and impact of presidential leadership. These features often act or interact to influence the development and evolution of health policies.

### Government as Subsidiary to the Private Sector

In much of the developed world, national health care programs are built on a consensus that health care is a right of citizenship and that government should play a leading role in the delivery of health care. In the United States, health care has not been seen as a right of citizenship or as a primary responsibility of government. Instead, the private sector has played a dominant role. Traditionally, Americans have been opposed to any major government interventions in health care financing and delivery, except for helping the underprivileged.

A general mistrust of government by Americans goes back to the founding of this nation. The Declaration of Independence defined the new nation in a great protest over government intrusion on personal liberty. It outlined the individual's right to life, liberty, and the pursuit of happiness. The Constitution further limited the powers of government. The fundamental beliefs and values (see Chapter 2) that most Americans still subscribe to evolved from these earlier founding documents.

Generally speaking, the government's role in US health care has grown incrementally, mainly to address perceived problems and negative health consequences for the underprivileged. Also, the most credible argument for policy intervention in the nation's domestic activities begins with the identification of situations in which markets fail or do not function efficiently. Ironically, even though health care in the United States functions under imperfect market conditions (see Chapter 1), problems and issues in health care are often blamed on "the market," which prompts politicians to further regulate health care through policy interventions. For example, cost escalations in the health care delivery system were assumed to reflect on the inability of private parties to control health care costs, which paved the way for various prospective payment methods. Ironically, certain policy interventions have also fueled the growth of health care expenditures, at least indirectly. Widespread legislation across states to reign in managed care's initiatives to contain escalating health care costs is a prime example. Yet, for lack of other cost-control alternatives, several states passed laws to enroll all of their Medicaid beneficiaries in managed care programs. Conversely, voluntary enrollment by Medicare enrollees in the federal Medicare Advantage (Part C) program has not been so successful (see Chapter 9).

Government spending for health care has been largely confined to filling the gaps in areas where the private sector has been either unwilling or unable to address certain issues. For example, court decisions such as *Duggan v. Bowen* and *Olmstead v. L.C.* were largely responsible for promoting large-scale transfers of people with mental illness and disabilities from institutions to community-based settings across the United States. Other policy interventions include various public health measures, such as environmental protection and communicable disease control and preparedness for disasters and bioterrorism. Recent enactment of the ACA of 2010 is another example of gap-filling to expand health insurance coverage for the uninsured.

## Fragmented Policies

Public power in the United States is enormously fragmented. This system follows the design of the founding fathers, who developed a structure of "checks and balances" to limit government's power. Federal, state, and local governments pursue their own policies with little coordination of purpose or programs. The subsidiary role of the government and the attendant mixture of private and public approaches to the provision of health care also resulted in a complex and fragmented pattern of health care financing in which (1) the employed are predominantly covered by voluntary insurance provided through contributions that they and their employers make; (2) the elderly are insured through a combination of private–public financing of Medicare; (3) the poor are covered through Medicaid through a combination of federal and state tax revenues; and (4) special population groups, for example, veterans, American Indians, members of the armed forces, Congress, and employees of the executive branch, have coverage that the federal government provides directly.

## Incremental and Piecemeal Policies

US health policies have been incremental and piecemeal, resulting from compromises involving the resolution of a variety of competing interests. An example is the broadening of the Medicaid program since its start in 1965. In 1984, the first steps were taken to mandate coverage of pregnant women and children in two-parent families who met income requirements and to mandate coverage for all children 5 years old or younger who met financial requirements. In 1986, states were given the option of covering pregnant women and children up to 5 years of age in families with incomes below 100% of the federal poverty level (FPL). In 1988, that option was increased to cover families at 185% of the FPL. In 1997, under CHIP, states were allowed to use Medicaid to extend coverage to uninsured children who otherwise did not qualify for the existing Medicaid program (see Chapter 6). Beginning 2014, when ACA of 2010 is expected to be fully implemented, states must use Medicaid to cover everyone under age 65 with income up to 133% of the FPL. This illustrates how a program is reformed and/or expanded through successive legislative action. When the federal government mandates Medicaid eligibility or benefits, it essentially tells the states to expand their programs to continue receiving federal matching dollars. The Medicare program also expanded incrementally, at first covering only the elderly under Parts A and B in 1965.

## Interest Groups as Demanders of Policy

Health policy outcomes in the United States are heavily influenced by the demands of interest groups and the compromises struck to satisfy those demands. Exhibit 13–1 summarizes the major concerns of dominant interest groups. Powerful interest groups involved in health care politics have historically resisted any major change (Alford 1975). Each group fights hard to protect its own best interests. The system's stability is ensured because most groups are satisfied with the benefits they receive; however,

Exhibit 13–1 Preferences of Selected Interest Groups

**Federal and state governments**
- Cost containment
- Access to care
- Quality of care

**Employers**
- Cost containment
- Workplace health and safety
- Minimum regulation

**Consumers**
- Access to care
- Quality of care
- Lower out-of-pocket costs

**Insurers**
- Administrative simplification
- Elimination of cost shifting

**Practitioners**
- Income maintenance
- Professional autonomy
- Malpractice reform

**Provider organizations**
- Profitability
- Administrative simplification
- Bad debt reduction

**Technology producers**
- Tax treatment
- Regulatory environment
- Research funding

the result for any single group is less than optimal.

Well-organized interest groups are the most effective "demanders" of policies. By combining and concentrating their members'

resources, organized interest groups can dramatically change the ratio between the costs and benefits of participation in the political markets for policy change. These interest groups represent a variety of individuals and entities, such as physicians in the American Medical Association (AMA); senior citizens allied with AARP (formerly called the American Association of Retired Persons); institutional providers, such as hospitals belonging to the American Hospital Association (AHA); nursing homes belonging to the American Health Care Association; and the companies making up the Pharmaceutical Research and Manufacturers of America (PhRMA).

Physicians have often found it hard to lobby for their interests with a single voice because they include so many specialty groups. For example, the American Academy of Pediatrics is involved in advocacy for children's health issues. Other groups include Physicians for a National Health Program, the American Society of Anesthesiologists, and the Society of Thoracic Surgeons. These groups can come together on issues that threaten the interests of the entire group, as in 1992 when Medicare decided to change the reimbursement system from fee for service to a resource-based relative value scale (RBRVS), although the physicians did not prevail.

The policy agendas of interest groups reflect the interests of their members. For example, the AARP advocates programs to expand financing for the elderly. It became a major advocate for prescription drug coverage for Medicare beneficiaries by supporting the Medicare Prescription Drug Improvement and Modernization Act of 2003. Conversely, it may seem surprising that AARP did not oppose the proposed Medicare cuts in the ACA of 2010, perhaps because this organization supports national health care. Still, it was surprising that, for once, it seemed to abandon its main objective to champion the interests of its elderly members. Other examples of interest groups include labor unions, which have become the staunchest supporters of national health insurance. The primary concerns of educational and research institutions and accrediting bodies are embedded in policies that would generate higher funding to support their educational and research activities.

Pharmaceutical and medical technology organizations are concerned with detecting changes in health policy and influencing the formulation of policies concerning approval and monitoring of drugs and devices. Three main factors drive health policy concerns about medical technology: (1) Medical technology is an important contributor to rising health costs, (2) Medical technology often provides health benefits, and (3) The utilization of medical technology also provides economic benefits by creating jobs in health care and other sectors of the economy. These factors are likely to remain important determinants of US policies on medical technology. Another factor driving US technology policy is the policy makers' desire to develop cost-saving technology and to expand access to it. The government is spending more and more money on outcome studies and comparative-effectiveness studies to identify the value of alternative technologies that promise to provide better care at lower cost.

Business also is a major interest group, although it is split, mainly along the lines of large and small employers. American employers' health policy concerns are shaped mostly by the degree to which they provide health insurance benefits to their employees, their employees' dependents, and their retirees. Many small business owners adamantly oppose health policies requiring them to cover employees because they believe they cannot afford it. Employees also pay attention to health policies that affect worker health or the labor–management relations experienced by employers. For example, employers have to comply with federal and state regulations on employee health and well-being and on the prevention of job-related illnesses and injuries. Employers are often inspected by regulatory agencies to ensure that they adhere to workplace health and safety policies.

Other, relatively newer members of the health policy community, represent consumer interests. For example, the tea-party movement representing conservative Americans actively demonstrated in Washington and around the country during the passage of the ACA of 2010, even though their voices went unheard. Consumer representation on the liberal side was noticeably silent, perhaps for two main reasons: (1) It was believed that a liberal majority in Congress and a liberal president were already taking action on their behalf, and (2) the tea-party movement was extensively marginalized in the liberal news media with innuendoes based largely on false reports.

## Pluralistic Suppliers of Policy

In the United States, each branch and level of government can influence health policy. For example, both the executive and legislative branches at the federal, state, and local levels can establish health policies, and the judicial branch can uphold, strike down, or modify existing laws affecting health and health care at federal, state, or local levels.

All three branches of government—legislative, executive, and judicial—are suppliers of policy. Of these, the legislative branch is the most active in policy making, which is particularly evident from policies that take the form of statutes or laws. Legislators play central roles in providing policies demanded by their various constituencies.

Members of the executive branch also act as suppliers of policies. Presidents, governors, and other high-level public officials propose policies in the form of proposed legislation and push legislators to enact their preferred policies. Top executives, as well as executives and managers in charge of departments and agencies of government, make policies in the form of rules and regulations used to implement statutes and programs. In this manner, they interpret congressional interest and, thereby, become intermediary suppliers of policies.

The judicial branch of government also is a policy supplier. Whenever a court interprets an ambiguous statute, establishes judicial precedent, or interprets the Constitution, it makes policy. These activities are not conceptually different from legislators enacting statutes or members of the executive branch establishing rules and regulations for the implementation of the statutes. All three activities concur with the definition of policy, in that they are authoritative decisions made within government to influence or direct the actions, behaviors, and decisions of others.

## Decentralized Role of the States

In the United States, under the theory of federalism, political power is shared between the federal government and the governments in each state. Hence, individual states play a significant role in the development and implementation of health policies. An example is the state governments'

*State power*

dominant role in curtailing the influence of managed care in the delivery of health care. Other examples of states' roles include financial support for the care and treatment of the poor and chronically disabled, oversight of health care practitioners and facilities through state licensure and regulation, training of health personnel (states pay most of the costs to train health care professionals), and authorization of health services available through local governments. Exhibit 13–2 lists the arguments often cited in favor of decentralizing health programs at the state level.

Many of the incremental policy actions have originated in state governments. One action, taken by 24 states, was to create a special program called an "insurance risk pool." This type of program helps people acquire private insurance otherwise unavailable to them because of the medical risks they pose to insurance companies. The program is financed by a combination of individual premiums and taxes on insurance carriers.

Other state-initiated programs were created to address the needs of vulnerable populations. For example, New Jersey developed a program to ensure access to care for all pregnant women. Florida set up a program, called Healthy Kids Corporation, which linked health insurance to schools. Washington developed a special program for the working poor that uses HMOs and preferred provider organizations (PPOs) to provide care within the state's counties. Maine established a program, MaineCare, to offer HMO-based coverage at moderate prices to small businesses with 15 or fewer employees. Minnesota created a program, Children's Health Plan, designed to provide benefits to children up to 9 years of age who lived in families with incomes below

Exhibit 13–2  Arguments for Enhancing States' Role in Health Policy Making

- Americans distrust centralized government in general and lack faith in the federal government as an administrator in particular.
- The federal government has grown too large, intrusive, and paternalistic.
- The federal government is too impersonal, distant, and unresponsive.
- State and local governments are closer to the people and more familiar with local needs; therefore, they are more accessible and accountable to the public and better able to develop responsive programs than federal agencies.
- National standards reduce flexibility and seriously constrain the ability of states to experiment and innovate.
- States are equipped to take on such functions (i.e., more full-time legislators, more professional staffs and bureaucrats).
- States are more likely to implement and enforce programs of their own making.
- States have served as important laboratories for testing different structures, approaches, and programs and for providing insight into the political and technical barriers encountered in enactment and implementation.
- States respond to crises faster.
- It is easier to change a state law than a federal one.
- States are more willing to take risks.

185% of the FPL but who do not qualify for Medicaid. Two states in particular took bold policy initiatives to expand health insurance coverage. In 1989, Oregon embarked on a controversial experiment that expanded Medicaid coverage to more than 100,000 additional people, by reducing the Medicaid benefit package (Bodenheimer 1997). In 2006, Massachusetts passed a universal health insurance program based on employer and employee mandates (see Chapter 14).

There are disadvantages to the dichotomous federal–state approach to policy making. For one, it makes it difficult to coordinate a national strategy in many areas. For example, it is difficult to plan a national disease-control program if some states do not participate or if states do not collect and report data in a uniform manner. States may also interpret federal incentives in ways that jeopardize the policy's original intent. For example, many states took advantage of federal matching grants for Medicaid by including a number of formerly state-funded services under an "expanded" Medicaid program. This allowed states to gain increased federal funding, while providing exactly the same level of services they had provided before. This phenomenon, called Medicaid maximization, although pursued by only a few states, had an impact outside of those states and may have contributed to rising national health care costs in the early 1990s (Coughlin et al. 1999).

## Impact of Presidential Leadership

To pass national policy initiatives, a strong presidential role is almost always necessary. Lyndon Johnson's role in the passage of Medicare and Medicaid, George W. Bush's role in adding prescription drug coverage to Medicare, and the more recent enactment of the ACA of 2010 under Barack Obama are key examples. Presidents have important opportunities to influence congressional outcomes through their efforts to bring about compromises, to engage in political maneuvering, or to take advantage of economic and/or political situations, particularly when policies concern their own preferred agendas.

Ironically, presidents' political agendas often result, years later, in unintended and undesirable consequences. In 1946, Harry Truman took advantage of reports that the nation had severe capacity deficits in the hospital sector and that many Americans across the country were unable to access acute care services. Later, in 1965, Lyndon Johnson dreamed of a "great society" to push his Medicare and Medicaid agenda through Congress. These programs passed through political compromises. However, overbuilding of hospitals and unrestrained use of Medicare and Medicaid sent health care costs through an uncontrolled upward spiral. Paradoxically, just when the nation achieved its goal of 4.5 community hospital beds per 1,000 population in 1980, as envisioned under the Hill-Burton program (see Chapter 8), the government concluded that the Medicare and Medicaid programs were no longer sustainable due to the rapid rise in health care costs. Consequently, Ronald Reagan authorized the PPS method of payment to reduce hospital utilization, which started a downward trend and created a glut of unoccupied hospital beds nationwide. Rising health care costs shortly after Medicare and Medicaid were implemented also presented an economic opportunity for Richard Nixon to pass the Health Maintenance Organization Act in 1973. Nixon also was successful in getting the CON legislation enacted under the National Health Planning and Resources Development Act of 1974. This Act represented an additional effort to restrain rapidly rising health care costs by requiring approvals for new equipment and new hospital construction. In the

1990s, even though Bill Clinton's comprehensive reform efforts failed, his incremental initiatives did succeed in the creation of CHIP and enactment of the Health Insurance Portability and Accountability Act (HIPAA) of 1996.

Moving forward to national health care, Clinton enjoyed a relatively high level of public interest in health care reform (see Chapter 3), but his administration did not act on it quickly enough. Also, ever-changing details of his proposal, which were made public, became overly complex for the people to grasp. Moreover, Americans did not want their taxes increased to pay for health reform.

## Politics of the Patient Protection and Affordable Care Act

The enactment of the ACA of 2010, signed by Barack Obama, became reality following a unique political approach that is perhaps unparalleled in the history of American policy making. Obama used to his benefit the political opportunity of having a solid Democratic majority in both houses of Congress. He had the advantage of strong Democratic leadership of Nancy Pelosi in the House of Representatives and that of Harry Reid in the Senate. Obama had three other factors in his favor: (1) He found a unique economic opportunity, as the nation was in the middle of the worst economic downturn since the Great Depression, with an unemployment rate that exceeded 10%. (2) Obama and his Democratic colleagues ceaselessly bashed former President George W. Bush, laying the blame on him for every malaise that the nation was going through. (3) The insurance industry was portrayed as the villain responsible for rising health care costs. Also, unlike Clinton, Obama and the Democrats kept the details of the plan secret from the public. Pelosi's statement in a televised speech before the Legislative Conference for the National Association of Counties is very revealing when she said, "We have to pass the bill so that you can find out what is in it" (Pye 2010; http://www.youtube.com/watch?v=hV-05TLiiLU). The same Pelosi, only weeks earlier, had bragged "about the transparency of the process that produced the bill" (Roff 2010). During townhall meetings around the country, Obama dodged key issues and gave only vague answers about the "plan." The Obama–Pelosi–Reid trio was strongly determined to pass national health care reform.

Whether there was any genuine attempt on the part of Democrats to make it a bipartisan process is debatable. During the entire process leading to the bill's passage, Republicans were marginalized and kept out of any meaningful debate on health reform. Obama, who arranged a summit with the Republican leadership and proclaimed that he would come to the summit with an open mind, had already released the version of the legislation that had passed the Senate controlled by Democrats. As one commentator put it, "The truth is that Democrats never had any intention of working with Republicans, except to pick off two or three Senators and calling it 'bipartisanship.' This worked for Democrats on the stimulus, and they had hoped to do it again on health care. In the House, three Chairmen—Charlie Rangel, Henry Waxman, and George Miller—holed up last spring to write the most liberal bill they could get through the House. Republicans were told that unless they embraced the 'public option,' there was nothing to discuss" (Wall Street Journal 2010). The president and congressional Democrats criticized Republicans as offering only opposition

and no ideas for health reform, but the Republicans, despite the lack of media attention, introduced three health care bills (see Chapter 14), all of which failed. In the end, the ACA passed without a single Republican vote.

Oberlander (2010) adds other factors that led to the passage of the ACA. Instead of employing different reform strategies, the House introduced a single health reform bill that combined three bills from three House committees, demonstrating greater agreement among Democrats. The final legislation also allowed certain exemptions from individual and employer mandates. Oberlander (2010) also credits weak opposition to the bill from health industry stakeholders. Instead of waging a war against the industry, Obama and congressional Democrats were willing to compromise. By promising millions of newly insured people who would use health care, they received pledges from stakeholders, including PhRMA and the AHA to support health reform. Even the insurance industry and the AMA endorsed the legislation, although the support faded over time. Another key factor for success is the speedy process of pushing the reform through the legislative process. However, a drawback was that the general public was confused about the legislation and was not supportive (Patel and McDonough 2010).

## The Development of Legislative Health Policy

The making of US health policy is a complex process that involves private and public sectors, including multiple levels of government, and reflects (1) the relationship of the government to the private sector, (2) the distribution of authority and responsibility within a federal system of government, (3) the relationship between policy formulation and implementation, (4) a pluralistic ideology as the basis of politics, and (5) incrementalism as the strategy for reform.

## The Policy Cycle

The formation and implementation of health policy occurs in a policy cycle comprising five components: (1) issue raising, (2) policy design, (3) public support building, (4) legislative decision making and policy support building, and (5) legislative decision making and policy implementation. These activities are likely to be shared with Congress and interest groups in varying degrees.

Issue raising is clearly essential in the policy formation cycle. The enactment of a new policy is preceded by a variety of actions that first create a widespread sense that a problem exists and needs to be addressed. The president may form policy concepts from a variety of sources, including campaign information; recommendations from advisers, cabinet members, and agency chiefs; personal interests; expert opinions; and public opinion polls.

The second component of policy making is the design of specific policy proposals. Presidents have substantial resources to develop new policy proposals. They may call on segments of the executive branch of government, such as the Centers for Medicare & Medicaid Services and policy staffs within the Department of Health and Human Services (DHHS). The alternative, preferred by both Kennedy and Johnson, was the use of outside task forces.

In building public support, presidents can choose from a variety of strategies, including major addresses to the nation and

efforts to mobilize their administration to make public appeals and organized attempts to increase support among interest groups. To facilitate legislative decision making and policy support building, presidents, key staff, and department officials interact closely with Congress. Presidents, generally, meet with legislative leaders several mornings each month to shape the coming legislative agenda and identify possible problems as bills move through various committees.

## Legislative Committees and Subcommittees

The legislative branch creates health policies and allocates the resources necessary to implement them. Congress has three important powers that make it extremely influential in the health policy process. First, the Constitution grants Congress the power to "make all laws which shall be necessary and proper for carrying into execution." The doctrine of implied powers states that Congress may use any reasonable means not directly prohibited by the Constitution to carry out the will of the people. This mandate gives it great power to enact laws influencing all manner of health policy. Second, Congress possesses the power to tax, which allows it to influence and regulate the health behavior of individuals, organizations, and states. Taxes on cigarettes, for example, are intended to reduce individual cigarette consumption, whereas tax relief for employer benefits is designed to promote increased insurance coverage for working people. Third, Congress possesses the power to spend. This ability allows for direct expenditures on the public's health through federal programs, such as Medicare and the NIH, but the power to allocate resources also gives Congress the ability to induce state conformance with federal policy objectives. Congress may prescribe the terms with which it dispenses funds to the states, such as mandating the basic required elements of the federal/state-funded Medicaid program.

At least 14 committees and subcommittees in the House of Representatives, 24 in the Senate, and more than 60 other such legislative panels directly influence legislation (Falcone and Hartwig 1991; Morone et al. 2008). The conglomeration of reform proposals that emerge from these committees face a daunting political challenge—separate consideration and passage in each chamber, negotiations in a joint conference committee to reconcile the bills passed by the two houses, and then return to each chamber for approval. In the Senate, 41 of the 100 members can thwart the whole process at any point.

Five committees—three in the House and two in the Senate—control most of the legislative activity in Congress (Longest 2010) and are subsequently discussed.

## House Committees

The Constitution provides that all bills involving taxation must originate in the House of Representatives. The organization of the House gives this authority to the Ways and Means Committee. Hence, the Ways and Means Committee is the most influential by distinction of its power to tax. This committee was the launching pad for much of the health financing legislation passed in the 1960s and early 1970s under the chairmanship of Representative Wilbur Mills (D-AR). Ways and Means has sole jurisdiction over Medicare Part A, Social Security, unemployment compensation, public welfare, and health care reform. It also shares jurisdiction over Medicare Part B with the House Commerce Committee. This committee, formerly Energy and Commerce, has jurisdiction over Medicaid, Medicare Part B, matters of public health, mental health, health personnel, HMOs, foods and drugs, air pollution, consumer products safety, health planning, biomedical research, and health protection.

The Committee on Appropriations is responsible for funding substantive legislative provisions. Its subcommittee on Labor, Health and Human Services, Education, and Related Agencies is responsible for health appropriations. Essentially, this committee holds the power of the purse. The committee and the subcommittee are responsible for allocating and distributing federal funds for individual health programs, except for Medicare and Social Security, which are funded through their respective trust funds.

## Senate Committees

The Committee on Labor and Human Resources has jurisdiction over most health bills, including the Public Health Service Act; the Food, Drug and Cosmetic Act; HMOs; health personnel; and mental health legislation (e.g., Community Mental Health Centers Act). This committee formerly included a subcommittee on Health and Scientific Research, which was used by its then chairman, Senator Edward Kennedy (D-MA) as a forum for debate on whether the United States should have a national health care program. When the full committee came under Republican control in the 1980s, the subcommittee was abolished.

The Committee on Finance and its Subcommittee on Health, similar to the Ways and Means Committee in the House, have jurisdiction over taxes and revenues, including matters related to Social Security, Medicare, Medicaid, and Maternal and Child Health (Title V of the Social Security Act). It is responsible for many of the Medicare and Medicaid amendments, such as QIOs, PPS, and amendments controlling hospital and nursing home costs.

## The Legislative Process

When a bill is introduced in the House of Representatives, the Speaker assigns it to an appropriate committee. The committee chair forwards the bill to the appropriate subcommittee. The subcommittee forwards proposed legislation to agencies that will be affected by the legislation, holds hearings ("markup") and testimonies, and may add amendments. The subcommittee and committee may recommend, not recommend, or recommend tabling the bill. Diverse interest groups; individuals; experts in the field; and business, labor, and professional associations often exert influence on the bill through campaign contributions and intense lobbying. The full House then hears the bill and may add amendments. The bill can be approved with or without amendments. The approved bill is then sent to the Senate.

In the Senate, the bill is sent to an appropriate committee and next forwarded to an appropriate subcommittee. The subcommittee may send the bill to agencies that will be affected. It also holds hearings and testimonies from all interested parties (e.g., private citizens, business, labor, agencies, and experts). The subcommittee votes on and forwards the proposed legislation with appropriate recommendations. Amendments may or may not be added. The full Senate

hears the bill and may add amendments. If the bill and House amendments are accepted, the bill goes to the president. If the Senate adds amendments that have not been voted on by the House, the bill must go back to the House floor for a vote.

If the amendments are minor and noncontroversial, the House may vote to pass the bill. If the amendments are significant and controversial, the House may call for a conference committee to review the amendments. The conference committee consists of members from equivalent committees of the House and Senate. If the recommendations of the conference committee are not accepted, another conference committee is called.

After the bill has passed both the House and Senate in identical form, it is forwarded to the president for signature. If the president signs the legislation, it becomes law. If the president does not sign the legislation, at the end of 21 days, it becomes law unless the president vetoes the legislation. If less than 21 days are left in the congressional session, presidential inaction results in a veto. This is called a "pocket veto." The veto can be overturned by a two-thirds majority of the Congress; otherwise, the bill is dead.

## Policy Implementation

Once legislation has been signed into law, it is not a fait accompli. The new law is forwarded to the appropriate agency of the executive branch, where multiple levels of federal bureaucracy must interpret and implement the legislation. Rules and regulations must be written, detailing what the entities affected by the legislation must do to comply with it. During this process, politicians, interest groups, or program beneficiaries may influence the legislation's ultimate design. Sometimes, the result can differ significantly from its sponsors' intent. The process of policy making is complex enough; its implementation can be quite daunting as well.

The agency publishes proposed regulations in the *Federal Register* and holds hearings on how the law is to be implemented. A bureaucracy, only loosely controlled by either the president or Congress, writes (publishes, gathers comments about, and rewrites) regulations. Then the program goes on to the 50 states for enabling legislation if appropriate. There, organized interests hire local lawyers and lobbyists, and a completely new political cycle begins. Finally, all parties may adjourn to the courts, where long rounds of litigation may shape the final outcome.

## Critical Policy Issues

Most past health policy initiatives have focused on access to care, cost of care, and quality of care. Some Americans contend that they have the right (access) to the best care (quality) at the least expense (cost) despite their level of income or social class. Legislative efforts, on the other hand, have been specific to issues in access (expanding insurance coverage, outreach programs in rural areas), cost containment (PPS, RBRVS), and quality (creating the Agency for Healthcare Research and Quality [AHRQ] and calling for clinical practice guidelines; see Chapter 12).

With the publication of *Healthy People 2010* and *2020*, elimination of health disparities across sociodemographic subpopulations has emerged as a bold policy objective. Since health disparities are caused primarily

by nonmedical factors (see Chapter 2), the advancement of this goal signals a new policy direction that integrates health policy with broader social policies. Although it is highly unlikely that this goal will be fulfilled within the next decade, the promotion of this policy objective reflects a significant government commitment. In the remainder of this section, the three areas of greatest health policy concerns are highlighted.

### Access to Care

Underlying support for government policies that enhance access to care is the social justice principle that access to health care is a right that should be guaranteed to all American citizens. There are two variations on this argument: (1) All citizens have a right to the same level of care, and (2) all citizens have a right to some minimum level of care. Which position the United States should espouse has never been openly debated in the policy circles. In the past, however, access to comprehensive services was aimed primarily at the most needy and underserved populations, as was the case with Medicaid. Medicare, on the other hand, did not incorporate the same level of access, which was limited by high deductibles and copayments and exclusion of certain services (see Chapter 6).

### Providers

Policy issues include ensuring a sufficient number and desirable geographic distribution of various types of providers. The debate over the supply of physicians is an important public policy issue because policy decisions influence the number of persons entering the medical profession, and that number, in turn, has implications for policies related to access and cost. The

Healthy People 2010 2020

number of new entrants into the profession is influenced by programs of government assistance for individual students and by government grants made directly to educational institutions. An increased supply of physicians, particularly specialists, may result in increased health care expenditures because of increased demand for care induced by the physicians. An increased supply of physicians, particularly primary care physicians, is necessary to provide basic health care to the newly insured under any expansion of health insurance coverage. For example, the ACA of 2010 will likely remain ineffective in achieving access goals without increasing the supply of physicians.

One goal on which both Republicans and Democrats seem to agree is preserving community health centers as a safety net for the underprivileged. Consequently, federal support has been boosted. This included doubling of funding over a 5-year period under the Bush Administration and $2 billion in the American Recovery and Reinvestment Act of 2009. Additional funding is slated under the ACA of 2010 (Iglehart 2010a).

## Public Financing

Although a national health care program is seen by many people as the best way to ensure access, the United States has focused, instead, on the needs of particular groups. Hence, we see numerous categorical programs, some of which were discussed in previous chapters, particularly Chapters 6 and 11.

Access continues to be a problem in many communities, partly because health policies enacted since 1983 have focused on narrowly defined elements of the delivery system. The United States has not had a unified strategy of reforming the system based on a policy of integrated services. Whether

the ACA of 2010 will make significant headway in this direction is yet unknown.

## Access and the Elderly

Three main concerns dominate the debate about Medicare policy: (1) Spending should be restrained to keep the program viable, (2) the program is not adequately focused on the management of chronic conditions, and (3) the program does not cover long-term nursing home care. These concerns originate from the assumption that the elderly need public assistance to finance their health care. Under the ACA of 2010, the nation is expected to have its first major government-sponsored long-term care insurance program through the Community Living Assistance Services and Supports (CLASS) provision (Iglehart 2010b).

## Access and Minorities

Minorities are more likely than Whites to face access problems. Hispanics, African Americans, Asian Americans, Native Americans, and Native Hawaiians and Pacific Islanders—to name the most prevalent minorities—all face barriers accessing health care. In some instances, the combination of low-income and minority status creates difficulties; in others, the interaction of special cultural habits and minority status causes problems. With the exception of Native Americans, no other minority population has programs specifically designed to serve its needs. Resolving the problems confronting minority groups would require policies designed to target the special needs of minorities, to encourage professional education programs sensitive to their special needs, and to develop programs to expand the delivery of services to areas populated by minorities.

## Access in Rural Areas

Delivery of health care services in rural communities has always raised the question of how to bring advanced medical care to residents of sparsely settled areas. Financing high-tech equipment for a few people is not cost efficient, and finding physicians who want to live in rural areas is difficult.

In the Omnibus Budget Reconciliation Act (OBRA) of 1986, Congress began to address the particular problems of rural hospitals, with three important provisions. The Act separated the urban and rural pools of funds used to pay for outliers, those cases in which excessive expenditures above the PPS allotment are incurred. It also provided early payments to hospitals with fewer than 100 beds. The designation of critical access hospitals in 1997 under Medicare rules also provided increased reimbursement to small rural hospitals under cost-plus rather than PPS reimbursement.

Chapter 11 discussed various policy attempts that intend to alleviate shortages of health care professionals in rural areas. They include federal designation of health professions shortage areas (HPSA) and funding for the National Health Service Corps. However, the funding covers a limited period of time per physician and does not help alleviate the issue over a longer term. The ACA of 2010 contains provisions to boost the supply of health care workforce and funding for the National Health Service Corps.

## Access and Low Income

Low-income mothers and their children are likely to be uninsured. Many of them also live in medically underserved areas, such as inner cities. Pregnant women in low-income families are far less likely to receive prenatal care than women in higher-income categories. The CHIP program requires periodic reauthorization, which can hamper continuity of services to those enrolled. The ACA of 2010 extends the authorization of CHIP through September 30, 2015.

## Access and Persons with AIDS

People with AIDS can face significant barriers in obtaining insurance coverage, and their illness leads to catastrophic health care expenditures. In 2014, the ACA of 2010 will make it illegal to deny insurance coverage to people with HIV/AIDS. However, because of the many legal requirements that place increased burdens on health insurers, premiums are expected to skyrocket. If this happens, people with HIV/AIDS and others with serious preexisting conditions will be transferred to Medicaid or government-sponsored health insurance exchanges.

In 2003, George W. Bush pledged $15 billion over 5 years to combat HIV/AIDS in developing countries, with a particular focus on Africa. According to the Foundation for AIDS Research (amfAR), Congress has provided significant increases for HIV/AIDS research, care, treatment, and prevention in the United States; however, domestic agencies still lack adequate resources to effectively combat the HIV/AIDS epidemic (amfAR 2007).

## Cost of Care

No other aspect of health care policy has received more attention during the past 20-plus years than efforts to contain health care costs. Cost containment has become a major policy priority because government has

PPS → prospective payment system —→ MAIN WEAPON OF COST CONTROL
• criteria for how much will be paid for a particular service is predetermined

*Critical Policy Issues* 537

a significant role in the financing of health care services. As Chapter 6 points out, the government's main weapon of cost control has been the development of PPS methodologies for all major types of health care services. PPS has achieved success in curtailing inpatient costs, but outpatient costs have continued to escalate. Only limited successes have been achieved in cost containment because direct control over utilization has, so far, proven to be unpopular in the United States, as the experience with managed care pointed out (see Chapter 9). Whether or not public policy can be used to impose explicit rationing in the United States is yet to be seen. The fragmented multipayer system does not lend itself to a centralized policy of cost containment.

## Quality of Care → 6 Areas

Along with access and cost, quality of care is the third main concern of health care policy. In March 2001, the Institute of Medicine (IOM) issued a comprehensive report, *Crossing the Quality Chasm*. Building on the extensive evidence collected by the IOM committee, the report identified six areas for quality improvement: (1) Safety—Patients should be as safe in health care facilities as they are in their homes. (2) Effectiveness—The health care system should avoid overuse of ineffective care and underuse of effective care. (3) Patient centeredness—Respect for the patient's choices, culture, social context, and special needs must be incorporated into the delivery of services. (4) Timeliness—Waiting times and delays should be continually reduced for both patients and caregivers. (5) Efficiency—Health care should engage in a never-ending pursuit to reduce total

costs by curtailing waste, such as waste of supplies, equipment, space, capital, and the innovative human spirit. (6) Equity—The system should seek to close racial and ethnic gaps in health status (Berwick 2002).

## Research on Quality  AHRQ

Funding to evaluate new treatment methods and diagnostic tools has increased dramatically; so has funding for research to measure the outcome of medical interventions and appropriateness of medical procedures. The AHRQ is 1 of 12 agencies within DHHS. Its mission is to improve the quality, safety, efficiency, and effectiveness of health care for all Americans. AHRQ fulfills this mission by developing and working with the health care system to implement information that

- Reduces the risk of harm from health care services by using evidence-based research and technology to promote the delivery of the best possible care.
- Transforms the practice of health care to achieve wider access to effective services and reduce unnecessary health care costs.
- Improves health care outcomes by encouraging providers, consumers, and patients to use evidence-based information to make informed treatment decisions.

Ultimately, AHRQ achieves its goals by translating research into improved health care practice and policy. Health care providers, patients, policy makers, payers, administrators, and others use AHRQ research findings to improve health care quality, accessibility, and outcomes of care (AHRQ 2010). Comparative effectiveness research

(CER) is a more recent undertaking by the AHRQ (see details in Chapter 14).

## Malpractice Reform

The federal government began its actions to relieve the malpractice crisis and devote greater attention to policing the quality of medical care with the Health Care Quality Act of 1986. This legislation mandated the creation of a national database within the DHHS to provide data on legal actions against health care providers. This information helps people recruiting physicians in one state know of actions against those physicians in other states. On the other hand, comprehensive tort reform, so far, has failed to materialize despite a lot of lip service the politicians have given to the need to overhaul the malpractice system. Some states have limited damage awards in malpractice cases, but no uniform national policy has emerged. One main reason is opposition from trial lawyers and consumer groups, who contend that limiting lawsuit awards hurts victims of egregious medical mistakes and reduces incentives to protect patient safety.

## Role of Research in Policy Development

The research community can influence health policy making through documentation, analysis, and prescription (Longest 2010). The first role of research in policy making is documentation; that is, the gathering, cataloging, and correlating of facts that depict the state of the world that policy makers face. This process may help define a given public policy problem or raise its political profile. A second way in which research informs and, thus, influences policy making is through analysis of what does and does not work. Examples include program evaluation and outcomes research. Often taking the form of demonstration projects intended to provide a basis for determining the feasibility, efficacy, or practicality of a possible policy intervention, analysis can help define solutions to health policy problems. The third way in which research influences policy making is through prescription. Research that demonstrates that a course of action being contemplated by policy makers may (or may not) lead to undesirable or unexpected consequences can contribute significantly to policy making.

## Summary

The US health care delivery system is the product of many health policies, which over the years, have brought about incremental changes. Health policies are developed to serve the public's interests; however, public interests are diverse. Interest group politics often have a remarkable influence on policy making. On the other hand, a complex process and divided opinions may leave the public out of even major policy decisions. Although the public wants the government to control health care costs, it also believes that the federal government already controls too much of Americans' daily lives. Presidential leadership and party politics played a major role in the passage of the Patient Protection and Affordable Care Act. Yet, several critical policy issues pertaining to access, cost, and quality remain. Among future challenges, cost containment will be the most daunting. The political feasibility of adopting a public policy to impose explicit rationing in the United States is yet unknown.

---

## Test Your Understanding

### Terminology

*allocative tools*
*distributive policies*
*health policy*

*public policies*
*redistributive policies*
*regulatory tools*

---

## Review Questions

1. What is health policy? How can health policies be used as regulatory or allocative tools?
2. What are the principal features of US health policy? Why do these features characterize US health policy?
3. Identify health care interest groups and their concerns.
4. Why do you think the Clinton health reform failed but the Obama health reform succeeded?
5. What is the process of legislative health policy in the United States? How is this process related to the principal features of US health policy?
6. Describe the critical policy issues related to access to care, cost of care, and quality of care.

---

## REFERENCES

Agency for Healthcare Research and Quality (AHRQ). 2010. *AHRQ annual highlights, 2009.* Available at: http://www.ahrq.gov/about/highlt09.htm. Accessed March 2011.

Alford, R.R. 1975. *Health care politics: Ideology and interest group barriers to reform.* Chicago, IL: University of Chicago Press.

Berwick, D.M. 2002. A user's manual for the IOM's "Quality Chasm" report. *Health Affairs* 21, no. 3: 80–90.

Bodenheimer, T. 1997. The Oregon health plan—Lessons for the nation. *New England Journal of Medicine* 337, no. 9: 651–655.

Coughlin, T. et al. 1999. A conflict of strategies: Medicaid managed care and Medicaid maximization. *Health Services Research* 34, no. 1: 281–293.

Falcone, D., and L.C. Hartwig. 1991. Congressional process and health policy: Reform and retrenchment. In: *Health policies and policy.* 2nd ed. T. Litman and L. Robins, eds. New York: John Wiley & Sons. pp. 126–144.

Foundation for AIDS Research (amfAR). 2007. *Public Policy.* Available at: http://www.amfar.org/cgi-bin/iowa/programs/publicp/record.html?record=9. Accessed December 2008.

Iglehart, J.K. 2010a. Health centers fill critical gap, enjoy support. *Health Affairs*. 29, no. 3: 343–345.

Iglehart, J.K. 2010b. The end of the beginning: Enactment of health reform. *Health Affairs* 29, no. 5: 758–759.

Longest, B.B. 2010. *Health policymaking in the United States*. 5th ed. Ann Arbor, MI: Health Administration Press.

Miller, C.A. 1987. Child health. In: *Epidemiology and health policy*. S. Levine and A. Lillienfeld, eds. New York: Tavistock Publications.

Morone J.A. et al. 2008. *Health policies and policy*. 4th ed. New York: Delmar.

National Institutes of Health (NIH). 2010. *Summary of the FY 2011 President's Budget*. Available at: http://officeofbudget.od.nih.gov/pdfs/FY11/Summary%20of%20the%20FY%202011%20 Presidents%20Budget.pdf. Accessed March 2011.

Oberlander, J. 2010. Long time coming: Why health reform finally passed. *Health Affairs* 29, no. 6: 1112–1116.

Patel, K., and J. McDonough. 2010. From Massachusetts to 1600 Pennsylvania Avenue: Aboard the health reform express. *Health Affairs* 29, no. 6: 1106–1111.

Pye, J. 2010. Pelosi: "We have to pass the bill so that you can find out what is in it." Available at: http://www.unitedliberty.org/articles/5233-pelosi-we-have-to-pass-the-bill-so-that-you-can-find-out-what-is-in-it. Accessed March 2011.

Roff, P. 2010. Pelosi: Pass health reform so you can find out what's in it. *US News and World Report: Politics*. Available at: http://www.usnews.com/opinion/blogs/peter-roff/2010/03/09 /pelosi-pass-health-reform-so-you-can-find-out-whats-in-it. Accessed March 2011.

Wall Street Journal. 2010. Republicans and ObamaCare. *Wall Street Journal-Eastern Edition* March 23: A20.

Weissert, C., and W. Weissert. 1996. *Governing health: The politics of health policy*. Baltimore: Johns Hopkins University Press.

# PART V

---

# System Outlook

# Chapter 14

## The Future of Health Services Delivery

### Learning Objectives

- To identify the major forces of change and how they may affect health care delivery
- To understand the precedents of the Patient Protection and Affordable Care Act of 2010
- To assess the future of health reform and alternatives
- To explore the dilemmas of universal access, preexisting conditions, and costs
- To discuss the components necessary to build a delivery infrastructure for the future
- To understand the special skills needed by future nurses, physicians, and other health care workers
- To evaluate the future of long-term care
- To appreciate the role of international cooperation in dealing with global threats
- To obtain an overview of new frontiers in clinical technology
- To survey the unfolding of evidence-based health care and comparative effectiveness research

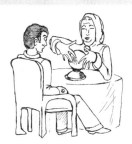

*"Will the U.S. have universal health insurance?"*

## Introduction

The future outlook of health care delivery in the United States is predicated on major current developments and the course these developments might take in the foreseeable future. On the other hand, any attempts to project the future of health care provoke more questions than answers. For instance, the major provisions contained in the Patient Protection and Affordable Care Act (ACA) of 2010 do not go into effect until 2014, and the law itself is being challenged legally. The future often turns out differently than people anticipate (Kenen 2011), and this could happen to the ACA of 2010.

When we look at health care delivery as an institution in and of itself, several external factors can be identified that would exert powerful influences for this institution to change and conform. Certain forces, such as demographic trends, project a foreseeable course, based on which some predictions can be made. For other external factors, even short-term predictions are difficult. For instance, it is impossible to predict the future course of the US economy and the rate of unemployment, both of which directly affect employer-based health insurance.

Future change also relies on historical precedents. Certain fundamental features of US health care delivery, such as a largely private infrastructure and the society's fundamental values (discussed in Chapters 2 and 3), have, in the past, resisted any proposals for a sweeping transformation of health care. Yet, certain historical precedents have also been used as a springboard for current change, and they will no doubt influence future change as well.

## Forces of Change

Six main types of forces can be identified to help inform a need for change and the direction of change that might occur. The same forces can also help us understand why certain changes have occurred. The six forces, however, often interact in complex ways, and these interactions can create opportunities for change. How those opportunities are either garnered or forgone determines the nature of change. American beliefs and values can be regarded as an overarching factor that runs across all six forces and lends a certain degree of stability to the health care system through a moderating effect on the other forces. Of the following six forces, economic and political factors are perhaps the most dominant.

### Social and Demographic Forces

Factors such as shifts in the demographic composition of the population, cultural factors, and lifestyles affect not only the need for health care services but also how those needs will be met. The elderly, vulnerable populations, and people with certain health conditions all present varied needs. An equally challenging factor, however, is how population shifts affect the composition of the health care workforce because health care delivery is labor intensive. People needing health care services have to depend on others who have the qualifications and the motivation to render needed services. Future immigration will affect both the demand and supply factors affecting health care delivery. Cultural factors, also based on the rate and quality of immigration, will continue to slowly transform health care delivery. For example, language and other cultural barriers affect both the patient and caregiver. Language training and posting of signs in different languages are only one small piece of the more complex cultural puzzle. Personal lifestyles significantly impact the future of wellness, prevention, health promotion, and the burden placed on financing and delivery of health care because of the prevalence of unhealthy lifestyles and behaviors. Similarly, dealing with chronic conditions among the elderly will require a shift in focus away from acute care toward prevention, disease management, and expansion of community-based long-term care.

## Economic Forces

Economic forces include factors such as the economy, unemployment, and globalization. Periods of economic growth and recession come and go in waves, some stronger than others and some more lasting than others. Depending on which way the tide is turning, the ebb and flow of the economy either empowers or disempowers almost everyone: the consumers, the employers, and certainly the politicians. There is a tendency to spend more than usual when good economic times roll on. Entitlements become more generous, as was the case with the addition of Part D to Medicare. The gross domestic product (GDP) was on the rise between 2002 and 2003 and 2003 and 2004, when Part D was added to Medicare. Paradoxically, when the economy "turns south," politicians' appetites for spending do not seem to abate. Then President George W. Bush, for example, obtained Congressional approval to create an economic stimulus package, amounting to $168 billion in 2008, when it became

clear that the economic downturn could be severe. President Barack Obama beat all-time records by spending $787 billion in the American Recovery and Reinvestment Act of 2009, shortly after he got into office. In addition, an ambitious health care legislation was passed in 2010 under the pretext of giving health insurance coverage to all Americans and saving money at the same time. On November 17, 2009, the CBS News proudly announced, "It's another record-high for the U.S. National Debt, which today topped the $12-trillion mark (yes, that is trillion with a 't'). Divided evenly among the U.S. population, the debt amounted to $38,974.34 for every man, woman, and child" in the United States (Knoller 2009). It is anyone's guess if, when, and how an ever-mounting debt will be repaid to foreign nations by American taxpayers. Health care will not be left unaffected by a debt crisis. High unemployment in the United States translates into a greater number of uninsured Americans. During the 2007–2009 recession, the unemployment rate in the United States topped 10%, the highest it had been in 26 years. It is estimated that, during this period, 5 million Americans lost employment-based health insurance (Holahan 2011). Globalization also seems to have negatively impacted employment in America, as US manufacturers in certain, mainly nonspecialized, industries have outsourced production to foreign subcontractors (Drayse 2008). Other effects of globalization are subsequently discussed in this chapter.

## Political Forces

Chapter 13 discusses the role of politics and its influence on health policy. Policies that affect education at home, as well as immigration policies, can determine not only the number but also the qualifications needed for the future health care workforce. The history of health care in the United States and in other countries is replete with examples of major changes brought about through political will. Politics serves a nation best when it is subservient to the people's will. However, Americans remain divided on major policy issues, and health care is one such issue. It is anyone's guess whether the ACA of 2010 would have passed or failed had there been adequate transparency and public debate.

## Technological Forces

It is widely believed that technological innovation in medical sciences will continue to revolutionize health care. Americans strongly favor ongoing innovation, availability, and use of new technology. The high cost of research and development and subsequent costs of unrestrained use of technology, however, do raise questions about how long this can continue, given that each year the United States spends an increasing share of its national economic production on health care. Yet, certain technologies will promote a greater degree of self-reliance and also achieve cost efficiencies in certain areas of health care. However, the overall effect of technology is to increase costs unless it is accompanied by utilization control measures.

## Informational Forces

Information technology (IT) has numerous applications in health care delivery, as Chapter 5 points out. IT has also become an indispensable tool for managing today's

health care organizations. The application of IT in health care is still evolving. Garnering IT's full potential will continue well into the future.

## Ecological Forces

New diseases, natural disasters, and bioterrorism have major implications for health care delivery. These factors have global consequences. Major catastrophes will increasingly require global cooperation and sharing of resources.

# Precedents of Health Reform

Many people have viewed a lack of health insurance for Americans as the most pressing issue in health care delivery. Hence, more recently, the term "health reform" has been associated with the expansion of health insurance. In current debates, the ACA of 2010 and any alternative proposals are being referred to as health reform. Expansion of health insurance under the ACA of 2010 is based on two major historical state-based initiatives, both of which have been perceived as highly successful: The Oregon Health Plan and the Massachusetts Health Plan.

## The Oregon Health Plan

The state of Oregon embarked on a bold initiative in the late 1980s to extend health insurance coverage to uninsured Oregonians. At that time, the uninsurance rate in Oregon was 18%. The Oregon Health Plan was formed over several years through successive pieces of legislation. In the end, reform incorporated three main components:

(1) Expansion of Medicaid to cover people who previously did not qualify. Delivery of services was mainly through managed care, which now covers roughly 75% of Medicaid clients in Oregon. The cost for Medicaid expansion was to be paid by rationing services. Oregon's model of rationing revolved around the creation of a list of medical services. A state-appointed Health Services Commission reduced over 10,000 medical procedures to a list of 709 medical conditions and their related treatments. The list was prioritized, according to the "net benefit" of each condition/treatment pair (Oberlander et al. 2001). (2) The Oregon Medical Insurance Pool was established as a state agency with state funding to offer health insurance to people who could not buy coverage because of preexisting conditions. (3) An *employer mandate* in which employers are legally required to help pay for their employees' coverage was installed. The Oregon Plan required employers to provide medical insurance to all employees working 17.5 hours or more per week and to cover their dependents as well. The law had a *play-or-pay* provision in which employers must either provide their employees health insurance (play) or pay into a public health insurance program. In Oregon's case, the latter was envisioned as a special state insurance fund that would offer coverage to workers not covered by their employers. This play-or-pay provision, however, never materialized because the federal Employee Retirement Income Security Act (ERISA) of 1974 exempts self-insured businesses from state insurance regulations and taxes. ERISA prevents states from requiring employers to provide health coverage or to spend any particular amount on health coverage (Steuerle and Van de Water 2009).

Obtaining exemption from ERISA has proven very difficult. Oregon, for one, was unable to obtain federal exemption.

Hawaii is the only state to have this exemption for its employer mandate. The state passed its employer mandate (not a true play-or-pay) law in 1974 and was able to get a limited exemption from ERISA. In Hawaii, employers must provide most employees with health insurance and must make a prescribed contribution to that insurance rather than pay a tax (Steuerle and Van de Water 2009).

## The Massachusetts Health Plan

In April 2006, Massachusetts became the first state to break the gridlock between Democrats and Republicans and passed a bipartisan plan that intended to achieve nearly universal coverage in the state. The reform has four main features: (1) An individual mandate (implemented at the end of 2007) requires all state residents to have health insurance or face legal penalties. The penalty amounted to the loss of a taxpayer's state income tax exemption, or roughly $900 in 2008 (Chandra et al. 2011). (2) The employer mandate requires all employers with more than 10 workers to offer, at a minimum, a Section 125 cafeteria plan that permits workers to purchase health insurance with pretax dollars (The Henry J. Kaiser Family Foundation 2006). Massachusetts law requires that employers make a "fair and reasonable" contribution to their employees' insurance or pay a fee called a "fair share provision" (RAND 2011). By playing (pun intended) on play or pay, but without calling it as such, it appears that Massachusetts has been able to skirt around ERISA. (3) Large government subsidies enable low-income individuals to buy insurance under a feature called Commonwealth Care. People whose incomes are less than the federal poverty level (FPL) have their premiums paid by the state. Those earning up to 300% of the FPL pay a subsidized premium. (4) At the core of the plan is the reorganization of a large part of the state's private insurance system into a "single market" structure with uniform rules and a central clearinghouse, or connector, to facilitate the purchase and administration of private health insurance coverage. Only plans approved by the state's insurance department may be sold through the connector (Haislmaier and Owcharenko 2006). The connector creates a common risk pool for small-group and individual consumers. Mandates, along with spreading risk over a larger population, counteract adverse selection and favorable risk selection, which lessens cost shifting that occurs when uncompensated care is delivered (Gostin and Connors 2010).

The plan has achieved some successes. The Massachusetts public has favorable views of the plan (Blendon et al. 2008). Even a large number of physicians (70%) in Massachusetts support the plan (SteelFisher et al. 2009). The prevalence of uninsurance fell to 12-year lows in Massachusetts, from 11.5% in 1996 to 3.5% in 2008. The overall prevalence of unmet needs because of inability to afford health care fell from 9.2% in 1996 to 7.2% in 2008. However, this was not the case for middle-income earners, Hispanics, Blacks, and those in fair to poor health (Clark et al. 2011). Hence, some of the most vulnerable population groups did not benefit. It also appears that socioeconomic barriers still persist. Clark and colleagues (2011) noted that people with the lowest incomes were much less likely than those with higher incomes to

obtain age-appropriate mammography, Pap smears, colorectal cancer screening, and cholesterol screening. Health care expenditures remain, by far, the biggest challenge in Massachusetts.

## The Patient Protection and Affordable Care Act

The ACA of 2010 is a massive and complex piece of legislation. Without a doubt, the law represents the most ambitious transformation of the US health care delivery system since the creation of Medicare and Medicaid in 1965. For the future, it remains to be seen whether the ACA of 2010 contains the seeds for pushing the system toward a *single-payer plan* in which the financing of health care is in the government's hands. Features of the ACA of 2010 are pointed out throughout this book as they have applied to the various topics of discussion.

The main features of insurance expansion in the health reform law are based on the health plans implemented in Oregon and Massachusetts. During his public appearances to promote the plan, President did not mention Oregon presumably because that would have immediately associated it with rationing of health care and Medicaid, which is viewed as a welfare program by most Americans. Instead, Obama mainly referred to the plan in Massachusetts, perhaps to make his health reform appealing to conservative voters because the Massachusetts Health Plan was hatched and implemented when Mitt Romney, a Republican, was the governor.

The political maneuvering used in the passage of the ACA of 2010 is discussed in Chapter 13. Insurance expansion in the law mainly covers six features: (1) Individual mandates and penalties for not having health insurance, starting in 2013.

(2) Employer mandate to offer coverage or pay a "free rider" tax. This applies to employers with 50 or more employees. (3) Expansion of Medicaid to cover all people at or below 133% of the FPL\* and to continue the Children's Health Insurance Program (CHIP) through 2019, as well as premium subsidies for people with incomes up to 400% of the FPL. (4) States must establish health insurance exchanges (equivalent to the connector in Massachusetts) through which small groups and individuals can purchase health insurance. (5) A sliding scale tax credit for small businesses with fewer than 25 workers. (6) Outlaw denial of health insurance to people with preexisting medical conditions in 2014. In the meantime, people with preexisting conditions can enroll in a temporary federal program.

How much the plan will end up costing will not be known for several years. By that time, the current administration would have been gone from the White House, and many members of Congress would also have left office. In other words, dealing with problems and issues will be shifted onto the shoulders of someone else, who most likely had nothing to do with the creation of this massive program.

There are other implications pertaining to access. As pointed out in previous chapters, the dream of universal access to health care is untenable unless accompanied by supply-side rationing. The extent of rationing will depend on the cost of producing health care services. Because of a high focus on specialty care and use of technology, health care production is much

costlier in the United States, compared to other nations. Hence, *universal access*— the ability of every, or nearly all, citizens to obtain health care when needed—cannot be achieved without massive rationing. Rationing is easier to achieve in a government-run program than in a private system. Yet, to some extent, a constrained capacity to deliver health care will act as its own rationing mechanism.

Medicaid expansion is a main feature of ACA of 2010. Medicaid enrollment is expected to grow by 16 million people by 2019, an increase of more than 25% (Cunningham 2011). The shortage of primary care physicians (PCPs) will be a major barrier to access. The access dilemma is compounded by the fact that states with the smallest number of PCPs per capita overall, generally in the South and Mountain West, will also see the largest percentage increases in Medicaid enrollment (Cunningham 2011).

The effect of expanding Medicaid has also been studied recently. The researchers, Allen and colleagues (2010), found a high degree of adverse selection—people with worse health status than others were the most likely to enroll. On the one hand, Medicaid does help people who need health care the most and who may also be least able to afford it. From a financing perspective, Medicaid expansion will shift the increased financial burden from the federal government to the states.

## The Future of Health Reform

The legal challenges to the ACA of 2010 were referred to in Chapter 3. Hence, the future of this law remains uncertain, even though certain provisions of the law have already been implemented.

---

\*Medicaid currently covers only children under the age of 6 and pregnant women whose family income is at or below 133% of the FPL. Eligibility for others is decided by each state, based on people's assets and income.

## What If?

What if the law gets repealed? Or significantly altered? Or funding to implement it gets slashed? These are big questions that will be decided from 2012 onward. Much will depend on whether, in 2012, the Democratic Party maintains control of the Senate and whether Obama, the champion of health reform, retains the presidency.

Regardless, the seeds for health reform have been sown. Health reform can no longer remain a dead issue because a relatively significant number of Americans will be upset at the prospect of losing their "free" health care under the ACA of 2010. Not tackling health care reform would be tantamount to political suicide for the Republicans, leaving the Republicans no choice but to replace ACA of 2010 with an alternative plan.

## Possible Reform Alternatives

Possible alternatives for the future can come from the three bills or proposals that were introduced or proposed by the Republicans in 2009, namely, the Patients Choice Act of 2009, the Health Care Freedom Plan (a proposal), and the Empowering Patients First Act. The combined main features of these plans are:

1. Establish state-based health care exchanges to facilitate the individual purchase of private health insurance and create a market where private health plans compete for enrollees based on price and quality. A second option is to create a national market for health insurance to allow individuals to purchase health insurance plans across state lines. The exchanges provide greater information rather than act as purchasing mechanisms.

2. Allow automatic enrollment in employer's health plans, and create tax incentives for small businesses for auto-enrollment.

3. Give tax credits or vouchers to individuals to purchase health insurance.

4. Provide block grants to states to develop innovative models that ensure affordable health insurance coverage for Americans with preexisting medical conditions.

5. Replace Medicaid with a program to provide grants to states for (a) acute medical care assistance to otherwise qualified blind or disabled individuals, foster care children, low-income women with breast or cervical cancer, certain tuberculosis-infected individuals, and certain individuals covered under the existing Medicaid program and (b) long-term care services and support for qualified disabled and elderly populations. A second option is to give Medicaid beneficiaries the choice to either remain in Medicaid or purchase private health insurance through vouchers.

6. Establish and implement a competitive bidding mechanism to promote competition among Medicare Advantage plans and strengthen programs that help prevent Medicare fraud and abuse.

7. Amend the Public Health Service Act to require supplementing the cost of private health insurance for eligible low-income families through the distribution of supplemental debit cards, which may be used for costs associated with health care and provide direct support in accessing health care.

8. Repeal the CHIP program.

9. Develop a national, strategic plan for preventive health and for health promotion and disease prevention activities consistent with such a plan.

10. Tort reform that will develop mechanisms for the resolution of disputes concerning injuries allegedly caused by health care providers and reduce predatory and frivolous malpractice lawsuits.

11. Assure that consumers have access to price information prior to treatment so they can make informed decisions about their care.

The Internet is likely to play a major role in the purchase of health insurance regardless of whether it is through exchanges or directly from insurers. Internet-based *e-health plans* will enable consumers to tailor plans according to individual needs, obtain instant quotes, and make online purchases. "Consumer choice," "affordability," "cost effectiveness," and "better value" will continue to be used as buzzwords to entice consumers into private or public options.

## The Dilemma of Universal Coverage

Neither the ACA of 2010 nor the alternative proposals previously discussed achieve universal coverage. However, the ACA of 2010 seems to come much closer to achieving that goal, even though it would also leave approximately 23 million Americans uninsured. Hawaii and Oregon have the longest-running programs that attempted to eliminate the uninsured in these two states. In Oregon, despite the expansion of Medicaid and rationing of care, 15.6% of the state's population was uninsured in 2006 (Office for Oregon Health Policy and Research 2007). In Hawaii, 8% of the total

population was estimated to be uninsured in 2009, according to the Henry J. Kaiser Family Foundation (Kaiser undated).

Achieving universal coverage would require a single-payer system, according to the Physicians for a National Health Program, an organization supported by a small percentage of physicians. A single-payer plan would place the responsibility for financing health care with one entity, most likely the federal government. One major advantage of this system is that all Americans and lawful residents would be entitled to benefits regardless of individual or family income. Private insurance plans and government entitlement programs (i.e., Medicaid, Medicare, TriCare, and the Federal Employee Health Benefits Program) would no longer be necessary under a single-payer system, although the market for some private insurance will remain for those desiring coverage beyond what a basic government plan might offer. Given that the United States has largely a private infrastructure for health care delivery, an American single-payer system would resemble the system in Canada (see Chapter 1). Costs would be contained through supply-side rationing, but higher taxes and open rationing of health services would be highly resisted by the American public.

## The Dilemma of Preexisting Medical Conditions

Offering health insurance to people with poor health status but without charging them more through higher premiums has been criticized on equity grounds. Actually, disregarding risk in underwriting is contrary to the general principles of insurance. When underwriting disregards risk rating, it makes premiums go up for everyone. Conversely, as pointed out in Chapter 6, it creates a problem for high-risk individuals because they may be unable to obtain coverage at affordable prices. To address this problem, a number of states (approximately 35) created *high-risk pools* that target people with preexisting conditions who are unable to get employer-sponsored or individual coverage and who do not qualify for public insurance programs. Premiums have been kept at affordable levels through federal subsidies to the states. High-risk pools have been successful in extending insurance to over 200,000 Americans in 2009, according to the National Association of State Comprehensive Health Insurance Plans. The ongoing issue, of course, has been that not all states have created these pools, so many Americans have been left without the ability to obtain health insurance.

The ACA of 2010 temporarily relies on a federal program, which is likely to use existing state pools as well until 2014, when insurers will be required to offer health insurance to everyone regardless of preexisting conditions. It will be interesting to see how this will be achieved without a significant rise in insurance premiums for everyone.

## The Cost Dilemma

Since it is too late to turn back the clock on health reform, the nation will have to deal with the abject realities of how it will be paid for. "The Obama administration's budget displays an unsustainable debt spiral over the next decade" (Holtz-Eakin and Ramlet 2010). Regardless of which direction health reform eventually goes, cost control will be the key to any program's long-term sustainability. To save the Medicare program from bankruptcy, several changes to reduce costs

are proposed in the ACA of 2010. This is a step in the right direction. The law also proposes various other savings. Cutler (2010), for instance, thinks that various efficiencies featured in the law will save $450 billion over one decade. The Congressional Budget Office (CBO) has also projected that the law will have a modest effect on reducing the nation's burgeoning deficit. There is, however, no dearth of speculation and controversy about cost savings.

Holtz-Eakin and Ramlet (2010) have done their own math and concluded that cost-saving projections are "built on a shaky foundation of omitted costs, premiums shifted from other entitlements, and politically dubious spending cuts and revenue increases." At this point no one can be sure of the fiscal outcomes; however, Tennessee and Massachusetts can, perhaps, give a glimpse into the future.

Tennessee has recently dropped 200,000 people from TennCare, as the Medicaid program in Tennessee is called. Although Tennessee residents have complained about losing the safety net and the residents' inability to obtain needed health care, the state must deal with a $400 million budget gap (Wadhwani 2010).

In Massachusetts, health care expenditures continue to rise at a rate much faster than the national average. Since 2006, total state health care spending has increased 28%; insurance premiums have increased by 8–10% per year, nearly double the national average (Tanner 2009). As for the Medicaid program, in 2006, the state spent approximately $1 billion on Medicaid, subsidies for medium-to-lower earners, and other health care programs. By 2010, the spending rose to $1.75 billion (Tully 2010). That is an average annual rate of increase of 15%. Even the *New York Times* commented, "The day of reckoning has arrived.... Thanks to new taxes and fees imposed..., the health plan's jittery finances have stabilized for the moment. But government and industry officials agree that the plan will not be sustainable over the next 5 to 10 years if they do not take significant steps to arrest the growth of health spending" (Sack 2009).

Lamm and Blank (2005) cogently stated that universal coverage is feasible, but, to financially sustain such a system, Americans will have to "give up a cherished dream: the dream of total, universal care for any ailment freely available on demand." Hence, a change in mind-set is necessary. As Paulus and colleagues (2008) have proposed, the underpinnings for a change in philosophy should be to seek value in health care. It necessitates asking the questions What do we propose to get in return for what we pay? and How much should we pay for what we should reasonably expect to get? The pillars of a value-driven system will be individual responsibility for one's own health, self-management support, patient activation, preventive services, health education, and an infrastructure based on primary care. An infrastructure built on these pillars has the potential to return the biggest dividends in improving health at a reasonable cost.

# Delivery Infrastructure of the Future

Any reform efforts remain grossly deficient without reforming the health care infrastructure. An inadequate infrastructure will lead to access bottlenecks for millions, which is likely to invite further policy intervention and government control. Currently, about 50% of physicians accept Medicaid patients

into their practices (Cunningham and May 2006). The main reason is low reimbursement and delays in receiving payment from Medicaid after services have been delivered. Because Medicaid expansion will cover an additional 16 million Americans under the ACA of 2010 (Cunningham 2011), physicians are likely to receive mandates to deliver services to Medicaid patients without favoring privately insured patients. Physicians who refuse will be charged with discrimination. Even with such mandates, access will be restricted regardless of the source of insurance because the delivery system will get overloaded. With an overloaded primary care system, whether the currently overloaded emergency care system will see any relief is another lingering unanswered question.

To translate the expansion of health insurance into access for all and, yet, achieve the goal of affordability will require (1) a vastly expanded network of primary care and gatekeeping and (2) a greater degree of engagement by consumers in their own health. Achievement of these objectives necessitates a major change in the current health care infrastructure. The concepts of patient-centered medical home and community-oriented primary care (presented in Chapter 7) are steps in the right direction, but the use of these models is still in its infancy. A major hurdle has been the shortage of PCPs and primary care nurses in the United States. Also, physicians and nurses will have to be trained to practice in a wellness-oriented model of primary care delivery. In the future, the delivery system will evolve to replace periodic encounters between patients and providers by an ongoing relationship that includes remote monitoring of health status and virtual consultations (Adler et al. 2009).

## Implementing the Medical Home Model

Four critical issues have been identified in the implementation of the medical home model:

1. Qualifying a physician practice as a medical home—A valid tool should capture the capabilities a medical practice should have to qualify as a medical home. This can help medical practices focus on the most important activities that would improve care. Research shows that four key primary care elements—accessibility, continuity, coordination, and comprehensiveness—positively affect health outcomes, satisfaction, and costs. An ideal qualification tool would ensure that medical homes are built on a firm foundation of these four pillars (O'Malley et al. 2008).

2. Matching patients to medical homes— For medical homes to achieve their potential to improve care, payers must link each eligible patient to a medical home practice in a way that ensures transparency, fairness, and matching of clinical needs. Equally important are adequate choice and awareness of the medical home model for patients. Also, physicians must be able to predict the additional revenue they can expect for acting as a medical home (Peikes et al. 2008).

3. Information exchange—There must be effective mechanisms for exchanging clinical information with patients and providers outside of the medical home. Adequate information exchange is necessary for care coordination across providers, care settings, and clinical conditions (Maxfield et al. 2008). This is because healing relationships grow in number and complexity when patients face serious or chronic illnesses. These patients have connections with multiple clinicians (Epstein et al. 2010). Accordingly, health care organizations should support more loosely affiliated "communities of care" besides individual clinician–patient relationships (Ubel et al. 2005).

4. Paying for medical homes—Existing payment systems do not compensate physicians for important activities such as care coordination and patient education. One major challenge is to determine an ideal array of services that result in high quality and efficient patient care. Another challenge is that care coordination activities are difficult to itemize, may occur outside face-to-face encounters, and can vary in type and intensity across different patients. Hence, an effective payment system would require some sort of capitation fees (Pham et al. 2008).

## Implementing Community-Oriented Primary Care

Community-oriented primary care (COPC) incorporates a population-based approach to identifying and addressing community health problems. Health must be incorporated into every aspect of society and daily life. That means nurturing children early in their lives, eating healthy food, getting sufficient exercise, and living in healthy homes and communities (Williams 2010). A system of health care delivery based on COPC would require developments on at least four fronts:

1. Primary care must take a central place in the delivery of health services. However, it will also require a refocus on how physicians are trained. Competencies needed for future practice include an understanding of the patients' community, delivery of care within rural settings, and chronic disease management (Dent et al. 2010).

2. The biomedical model that has dominated both research and health professionals' education must be broadened to include a stronger element of the social and behavioral sciences (Engle 1977).

3. Primary and secondary prevention (see Chapter 2) must be appropriately linked in a clinical setting with population-based health programs. Primary and secondary prevention, as well as certain aspects of tertiary prevention, are essential elements of primary care.

4. Public health functions must be strengthened as an adjunct to clinical interventions because clinicians alone cannot deal with most population-based health problems. Community organizations, such as schools, social service agencies, churches, and employers, must become partners in strengthening public health programs (Lee 1994).

## Lessons from the Vermont Blueprint

In 2006, Vermont launched a program called Vermont Blueprint for Health. The pilot program has been shifting to a statewide program since the passage of the ACA of 2010. In essence, the Vermont Blueprint integrates the medical home model and COPC. It is based on a foundation of medical homes supported by community health teams and an integrated information technology infrastructure. Each community health team is staffed by five full-time equivalent employees and led by a registered nurse to serve a population of approximately 20,000. The teams offer individual care coordination, health and wellness coaching, and behavioral health counseling. For the program to be financially successful, there must be a measurable reduction in avoidable emergency department visits and hospitalizations (Bielaszka-DuVernay 2011).

## The Role of Patient Activation

Informed by earlier research, Kravitz (2008) concluded that Americans are of two minds when it comes to health care. One mind embraces the continuity, comprehensiveness, and coordination afforded by an ongoing primary care relationship; the other doubts and questions whether the PCP's judgment can be fully relied on. Hence, the patient's own mind-set greatly influences utilization decisions about medical care. Besides the choices patients make regarding utilization, daily management of a person's own health care profoundly affects utilization, costs, and outcomes.

Many experts acknowledge that improvements in quality, cost containment, and reductions in low-value care will not occur without more informed and engaged consumers. *Patient activation* refers to a person's ability to manage his or her own health and utilization of health care. The challenge is that activation levels differ considerably across socioeconomic and health status characteristics. For example, among all insurance groups, people enrolled in Medicaid are the least activated (Hibbard and Cunningham 2008). Information and support may help close some of the gaps among various population groups, such as racial and ethnic minorities. Achieving this goal will require a close relationship, partnership, and mutual respect between providers and patients.

# Future Workforce Challenges

An adequate and well-trained workforce is a critical component of the health care delivery infrastructure. Chapter 4 discusses some of the workforce-related issues and challenges. This section highlights future needs and recommendations for change.

## The Nursing Profession

In 2008, The Robert Wood Johnson Foundation (RWJF) and the Institute of Medicine (IOM) launched a 2-year initiative to respond to the need to assess and transform the nursing profession. A committee was assigned the task of producing a report that would make recommendations for an action-oriented blueprint for the future of nursing. Four recommendations have been put forth (National Academy of Sciences 2010):

1. Nurses should practice to the full extent of their education and training. Uniformity on the scope of practice for advance practice nurses, who have master's or doctoral degrees, currently does not exist across states because of varying licensing and practice rules. Also, current residency programs for nurses focus primarily on acute care. To address future

needs, residency programs must be developed and evaluated in community settings.

2. Nurses should achieve higher levels of education and training through an improved education system that promotes seamless academic progression. Increased clinical demands call for higher levels of education and training. Patient needs have become more complicated, and nurses need to attain requisite competencies to deliver high-quality care. These competencies include leadership, health policy, system improvement, research in evidence-based practices, teamwork and collaboration, and competency in specific content areas, including community health, public health, and geriatrics. Nurses are also being called on to fill expanding roles and to master technological tools and information management systems, while collaborating and coordinating care across teams of health professionals.

3. Nurses should be full partners with physicians and other professionals in redesigning health care. Being a full partner involves taking responsibility for identifying problems and areas of system waste, devising and implementing improvement plans, tracking improvement over time, and making necessary adjustments to realize established goals.

4. Effective workforce planning and policy making require better data and improved information systems. Data collection and analysis should drive a systematic assessment and projection of workforce requirements by role,

skill mix, region, and demographics to inform changes in nursing practice and education.

## Training of Primary Care Physicians

The shortage of PCPs and its exacerbation in the future is only one aspect of the challenge that must be addressed. Caudill and colleagues (2011) argue that the PCPs trained today will not have the requisite skills to fulfill their contemplated responsibilities because of a variety of factors. Future health care demands—mainly because of a growing number of people with complex chronic conditions—will require PCPs to function as "comprehensivists." These comprehensivists will need to be experts in (1) anticipating, preventing, and managing the progression and/or complications of common complex conditions; (2) managing complex pharmacology; (3) understanding end-of-life issues and medical ethics; (4) coordinating care; and (5) leading health care teams. Their practice environments will need to contain the elements and systems to support comprehensive care, such as advanced information systems. Comprehensivists will also need to be able to direct and coordinate a health care team that includes expertise in patient education, mental health and behavioral modification, physical and occupational therapy, pharmacy, and home health. Care delivery will have to be consistent with evidence-based medicine, while incorporating the patient's values (Caudill et al. 2011).

To train future PCPs, education must be more efficient, integrated, and longitudinal. Time must be created for medical students to learn essential elements of patient safety and quality, teamwork in the health care environment, health maintenance, and continuity of care, without sacrificing fundamental knowledge. Education must become learner centered, with shared responsibility and decision making as a primary model for patient-centered care. A pay-for-educational-performance and outcomes model, with organizational bundling of educational costs, may need to be piloted in a similar way to the piloting of new care delivery models (Caudill et al. 2011).

## Training in Patient-Centered Care

The IOM identified *patient-centered care* as one of the main elements of high-quality care. It defined patient-centered care as "respecting and responding to patients' wants, needs and preferences, so that they can make choices in their care that best fit their individual circumstances" (IOM 2001). Communication skills are a fundamental component of this approach to care. Patient-centered communication seeks to increase the health professionals' understanding of patients' individual needs, perspectives, and values; gives patients the information they need to participate in their care; and builds trust and understanding. Decisions about care should be made collaboratively and in the patient's best interest. The patient-centered approach has a positive impact on outcomes, such as patient satisfaction, adherence to treatment regimen, and self-management of chronic conditions. Communication skills should be taught in a systematic way, including practice and constructive feedback (Levinson et al. 2010). One of the most frequently used systems to analyze physician–patient communication is the Roter Interaction Analysis System (RIAS), which also has been used for developing training programs in patient-centered communication for practitioners in primary care settings (Helitzer et al. 2011).

## Training in Geriatrics

Based on current trends, a shortage of health care professionals schooled in geriatrics is a critical challenge. Although coverage of geriatric issues at medical schools has been increasing, only about 9,000 practicing physicians in the United States (2.5 geriatricians per 10,000 elderly) have formal training in geriatrics. Without sustained efforts to improve training, this number is expected to drop to 6,000 in the future. Among nurses, fewer than 0.05% have advanced certification in geriatrics (CDC/Merck 2004).

The elderly use the majority of home health care services and nursing home care, about one-half of hospital inpatient days, and approximately one-quarter of all ambulatory care visits. Growth of the elderly population will impose increased demands on the health care delivery system, which has, thus far, ignored the need for specialized geriatrics training. Evidence shows that care of older adults by health care professionals prepared in geriatrics yields better physical and mental outcomes without increasing costs (Cohen et al. 2002).

Current trends in the education and training of health care professionals shows that future demand will far outstrip the supply of physicians, nurses, therapists, social workers, and pharmacists with geriatrics training. This problem is compounded due to a shortage of faculty in colleges and universities who are trained in geriatrics. Only 600 medical school faculty out of 100,000 list geriatrics as their primary specialty. Due to this and, perhaps, other reasons, only 3% of medical students take any elective geriatric courses. In other disciplines as well, such as nursing, pharmacy, and dentistry, the majority of educational curricula do not require geriatric training. For example,

60% of nursing schools have no geriatric faculty (CDC/Merck 2004). A shortage of workforce members prepared in geriatrics affects all settings, but it especially affects long-term care providers who serve large numbers of frail elderly. Geriatrics training is also important in other types of health services, such as oncology, neurology, rehabilitation, and critical care (Kovner et al. 2002). Even though there are encouraging signs that initiatives are being taken by educational institutions in recognition of a critical deficit in geriatric training, to date, few concrete efforts have been made.

## The Future of Long-Term Care

Financing and delivery of long-term care will remain a major challenge. The good news is that long-term care is typically needed later in life. Even though the first wave of baby boomers started retiring in 2011, they are not likely to need professional long-term care services until 2025 or later. However, the system must be reformed before that time comes. In their report to the National Commission for Quality Long-Term Care, Miller and Mor (2006) identified six main areas of concern that must be addressed: financing, resources, infrastructure, workforce, regulation, and information technology.

### Financing

Most middle-class families are unprepared to meet long-term care expenses. Most people think that Medicare would pay for their long-term care needs. But, as Chapters 6 and 10 point out, Medicare covers only short-term, postacute care. It is estimated that less than 10% of the elderly have private long-term care insurance (Burke et al. 2005).

Unless policy initiatives are established to promote long-term care health insurance plans, the public sector will see its expenditures grow rapidly. Purchasing long-term care insurance is both expensive and confusing. The CBO (2004) recommended improving the way private markets for LTC insurance currently function. For instance, private insurance could be made more attractive to consumers by standardizing insurance policies to allow competing policies to be more easily compared. Currently, state insurance regulations do not require insurance carriers to offer policies that conform to particular design standards. Standardized policies could also stimulate price competition among insurers and help keep premiums lower than they would otherwise be. However, reform is also needed in a public financing system, particularly within Medicaid, that pays for the bulk of long-term care costs. The Deficit Reduction Act (DRA) of 2005 tightened Medicaid eligibility rules. The law also extended the time period for asset transfers, called the look-back period, to qualify for Medicaid (Crowley 2006). In 2004, Medicaid and Medicare financed roughly 60% of all long-term care costs (CBO 2004). Without reform, these programs will put enormous financial pressure on the future working population.

## Resources

Financing for long-term care in the United States used to be heavily tilted in favor of institutional rather than community-based services. The Home and Community Based Waiver (HCBW) program (see Chapter 10) has achieved some successes in moving patients out of nursing homes to receive community-based care. However, research shows that Medicaid spending, which covers a substantial share of long-term care expenses, has actually increased, not decreased. It appears that the waivers may actually induce more people to enter the Medicaid program (Amaral 2010).

## Infrastructure

The institutional long-term care sector has been going through a cultural change that has led to the creation of enriched living environments in nursing homes. New architectural designs, living arrangements, and worker and patient empowerment are improving the quality of life in nursing facilities that have adopted the innovative models, such as Eden Alternative, Green House Project, and Wellspring. Over time, traditional living and care arrangements will be replaced by these and other innovative models (for an overview of these models, refer to Singh 2010 and Chapter 8).

## Workforce

The aging of America will shrink the overall pool of workers. Experts think that this will have a particularly drastic effect on the health care sector and long-term care in particular because of low pay and hard work. Between 2000 and 2010 alone, a deficit of 1.9 million direct care workers was estimated (DHHS 2003).

## Regulation

Many experts see fundamental contradictions between the existing regulatory mechanisms that address quality issues in nursing facilities through periodic inspections and sanctioning and regulations that require the same nursing facilities to implement quality improvement programs. Also, one of the most disconcerting aspects of government regulation of long-term care is its inconsistent application, both within and across regions over time (Miller and Mor 2006). These issues need to be resolved.

## Information Technology

Interoperable IT systems (discussed in Chapter 5) will enable providers to track patients' care across hospitals, nursing homes, home health agencies, and physicians' offices. Such systems are particularly critical in long-term care because the elderly frequently make transitions between long-term care and nonlong-term care settings. Currently, such transitions rarely occur smoothly because of high rates of missing or inaccurate information (Miller and Mor 2006).

## Global Threats and International Cooperation

The prevention and control of infectious diseases will continue to pose major challenges. These and other threats can affect people globally. Examples include natural disasters, such as the earthquake and tsunami that killed thousands in Japan in March 2011; industrial accidents, such as the oil rig explosion in the Gulf of Mexico in April 2010; and large-scale bioterrorism, which has not yet occurred, but global unrest amid the rise of extremism makes it a real possibility in the future. Often, such events occur without warning. Large-scale devastation, such as that caused by the Haiti earthquake in January 2010, can severely strain a nation's capacity to deal with mass casualties and rebuilding efforts. Increasingly,

disasters will require international assistance, cooperation, and joint efforts.

Increase in air travel resulted in the spread of Severe Acute Respiratory Syndrome (SARS) from China to Canada in 2003 and of polio virus from India to northern Minnesota in 2005 (Milstein et al. 2006). These examples highlight the importance of early identification of infectious threats and subsequent rapid response to prevent further spread, which is often difficult without international cooperation (Johns et al. 2011). Many medical advances that physicians and patients take for granted, including cancer treatment, surgery, transplantation, and neonatal care, are endangered by increasing antibiotic resistance of infectious agents and a distressing decline in the antibiotic research and development pipeline (Infectious Disease Society of America 2004). Antibiotic resistance is both a public health and security threat. Virtually all of the antibiotic resistant pathogens that exist naturally can be bioengineered through forced mutation or cloning. Also, existing pathogens could be genetically manipulated to make them resistant to available antibiotics. Currently, international efforts, including the establishment of a Transatlantic Task Force for Antimicrobial Resistance, are under way (Hughes 2011). Efforts to strengthen global health security include disease surveillance for outbreaks of international importance and urgency, exchange of technical information on new pathogens, and early warning and control of serious animal disease outbreaks. The latter is important because of the 2003–2005 outbreak of the H5N1, avian influenza, in Asia.

International cooperative efforts include the Biological Weapons Convention (BWC) and the International Health Regulations

(IHR). As a treaty among participating nations, the BWC bans development, production, stockpiling, or otherwise acquiring/retaining microbial or other biological agents or toxins. It also covers weapons, equipment, or means of delivery designed to use biological agents for hostile purposes or in armed conflict. It also promotes common understanding and effective action on biosecurity, national implementation measures, suspicious outbreaks of disease, disease surveillance, and codes of conduct for scientists. The IHR constitute an international legal instrument that is binding on 194 countries. IHR's aim is to help the international community prevent and respond to acute public health risks that have the potential to cross borders and threaten people worldwide. Such crises can result from emerging infections like SARS or a new human influenza pandemic. The IHR can also apply to other public health emergencies, such as chemical spills, leaks and dumping, or nuclear meltdowns (WHO 2008).

Adequate delivery of health care to millions around the world depends on an adequate and well-trained workforce. Worldwide, there is a shortage of nearly 4.3 million health workers. Moreover, 57 countries, 39 of which are in Africa, have fewer than 23 health workers for every 10,000 population. Even some of Asia's burgeoning economies, such as India and Indonesia, can face a health care crisis in the event of a major disaster. The problem in many countries is compounded by an unequal distribution of workers, lack of training, and international migration of health professionals from poor countries to rich countries. Also, in spite of the pivotal role that community health workers play in scaling up essential services, this workforce

category does not receive adequate support in most nations (Chatterjee 2011).

# New Frontiers in Clinical Technology

Despite its association with cost escalation, technological progress will continue. Increased efforts in technology assessment (see Chapter 5) will go hand in hand with new innovations. To what extent clinical decisions will be influenced mainly by cost effectiveness of technology, however, remains an open question.

The Institute for the Future (2000) predicted that eight types of medical technologies would especially affect future delivery of patient care: rational drug design, advances in imaging, minimally invasive surgery, genetic mapping and testing, gene therapy, vaccines, artificial blood, and xenotransplantation. Ongoing progress has occurred in several of these areas, and, more recently, advances in regenerative medicine have come to the forefront.

1. Rational drug design is a step beyond the painstaking and costly random search for new pharmaceuticals that is characterized by trial and error. Now, scientists can study the structure and composition of a receptor or enzyme and actually design new chemicals or molecular entities that bind to the receptor or enzyme. Rational drug design will shorten the drug discovery process. The chief candidates for this process are drugs to treat neurological and mental disorders and antiretroviral therapies for HIV/AIDS, encephalitis, measles, and influenza.

2. Imaging technologies have made one of the most dramatic advances in health care mainly because of the exponential growth in the performance of silicon devices (Busse 2006). Current research focuses on four areas: (a) Finding new energy sources and focusing an energy beam to avoid damage to adjacent tissue and to minimize residual damage. (b) Use of microelectronics in digital detectors and advances in the contrast media for a finer detection of abnormalities. (c) Faster and more accurate analysis of images using 3-D technology. (d) Improvements in display technology to produce higher resolution displays. The rise of modern neuroscience and the rapid development of new technologies for imaging, treating, and modulating neural function are leading to an increased emphasis on the brain as the central site for health intervention. The use of neuroimaging in understanding pain is only one area of intervention. Discovery and treatment of minor strokes and early detection of Alzheimer's are two of the other areas where neuroimaging will improve treatment options (Adler et al. 2009).

3. The latest advances in minimally invasive surgery include image-guided brain surgery, minimal access cardiac procedures, and the endovascular placement of grafts for abdominal aneurysms. The overall impact of minimally invasive procedures on cost efficiency and the patients' quality of life from early recovery assures the growth of this technology and the growth of ambulatory surgicenters.

Robotic surgery will also continue to play an increasing role to ensure precision.

4. Genetic mapping has enabled the identification of a wide range of genes that can cause complex diseases, such as diabetes, cancer, heart disease, Huntington's disease, and Alzheimer's disease. The discovery of genetic susceptibility to certain diseases will improve preventive techniques. The term *genometrics* is used for the association of genes with specific disease traits. Human genome has also opened the way for the new field of *molecular medicine*, a branch of medicine that deals with the understanding of the role that genes play in disease processes and treatment of diseases through gene therapy.

5. Gene therapy is a therapeutic technique in which a functioning gene is inserted into targeted cells to correct an inborn defect or provide the cell with a new function. The future challenge in this area is to develop methods that discriminately deliver enough genetic material to the right cells. Cancer treatment is receiving much attention as a prime candidate for gene therapy since current techniques (surgery, radiation, and chemotherapy) are effective in only one-half the cases.

6. Vaccines have traditionally been used prophylactically to prevent specific infectious diseases, such as diphtheria, smallpox, and whooping cough. However, the therapeutic use of vaccines in the treatment of noninfectious diseases, such as cancer, has

opened new fronts in medicine. At the same time, development of new vaccines for emerging infectious diseases remains on the research agenda. Making vaccines safer for wide-scale preventive use against bioterrorism in which such agents as smallpox and anthrax may be used will also be an ongoing pursuit.

7. Research will continue on the development of fluids that, in many instances, could be used as substitutes for real blood in transfusions, particularly in war and in natural disasters, when supplies may fall short.

8. Transplantation of organs is one of the 20th century's greatest medical advances. It treats a life-threatening chronic disease by replacing the diseased organ. However, a critical shortage of transplantable tissues remains a major concern. *Xenotransplantation* in which animal tissues are used for transplants in humans is a growing research area.

9. Regenerative medicine is the first truly interdisciplinary field that utilizes and brings together nearly every field in science. This new field holds the realistic promise of regenerating damaged tissues and organs in vivo (in the living body) through reparative techniques that stimulate previously irreparable organs into healing themselves. Regenerative medicine also enables scientists to grow tissues and organs in vitro (in the laboratory) and safely implant them when the body is unable to be prompted into healing itself. This revolutionary technology has the potential to develop therapies for previously untreatable diseases and conditions. Examples of diseases regenerative medicine can cure include diabetes, heart disease, renal failure, osteoporosis, and spinal cord injuries. Virtually any disease that results from malfunctioning, damaged, or failing tissues may be potentially cured through regenerative medicine therapies (DHHS 2005).

## Care Delivery in the Future

Gossink and Souquet (2006) paint a picture of what medical care in the future may look like. This will be achieved mainly through advancements in medical imaging, molecular medicine, and distant monitoring. Medical care will shift its focus from the acute phase of illness to prevention and aftercare. Lifestyle, family history, and genetic factors will be used to develop a patient's risk profile. Patients with an elevated risk profile will be regularly screened for possible onset of acute disease and to follow the course of chronic disease. Some screening will be possible at home with the patient in wireless contact with the physician. If molecular diagnosis detects disease, the extent and location of the disease will be assessed through molecular imaging. Image-guided, minimally invasive procedures will be used if surgery is recommended. Pharmaceutical treatment will be individualized. A feedback system will determine needed drug dosage by a continuous measurement of drug concentration at the targeted site in the body. Miniature implanted devices will take over damaged body functions. Regenerative medicine and cell therapy will revive organs, such as a damaged heart. If needed, complete artificial organs, such as the pancreas, liver, and even heart, could be implanted. Physicians will be able to continuously monitor the condition of elderly patients with chronic conditions and could be dispatched in case of an emergency.

# Evidence-Based Health Care and Beyond

Over several years, mounting evidence showed that high-spending providers did not necessarily deliver better outcomes. The goal of evidence-based medicine (EBM) has been to increase the value of medicine. Quality of care can actually be improved while reducing costs—thus, increasing the value of medical care—by reducing misuse and overuse (Slawson and Shaughnessy 2001). The tools for the practice of EBM have been developed for several years, mainly in the form of clinical practice guidelines (see Chapter 12). Evidence-based practice guidelines are intended to represent "best practices" and "proven therapies." Halm and colleagues (2007) reported a remarkable reduction in the proportion of patients undergoing carotid endarterectomy (a surgical procedure that removes the inner lining of the carotid artery if it has become thickened or damaged by plaque) for inappropriate reasons. However, EBM's full potential has not yet been realized, and work in this area will be ongoing.

*Comparative effectiveness research* (CER) is a more novel concept in which a chosen intervention is guided by scientific evidence of how well it would work, compared to other available treatments. The American Recovery and Reinvestment Act of 2009 allocated $1.1 billion for this type of research. Further, the ACA of 2010 called for the creation of a Patient-Centered Outcomes Research Institute.

# Strategies for Evidence-Based Care

Future strategies to improve guidelines and protocols and their adherence include:

- Health care leaders must continue to emphasize the adoption of evidence-based guidelines.

- Ongoing development of computer-based models incorporating EBM will facilitate multidisciplinary caregiving based on best practices by various practitioners, including physicians and nurses.

- Ongoing clinical trials will be the backbone of EBM. Adherence to clinical guidelines is higher when the recommendations are supported by evidence from randomized controlled trials (Leape et al. 2003).

- Guidelines and protocols must be revised and kept current to incorporate new scientific evidence when warranted.

- Future practice guidelines must incorporate economic analysis to promote the delivery of cost-effective health care.

- Financial incentives, including provider payments and patient cost sharing, must be restructured. Reimbursement methods should focus on paying for best achievable outcomes and the most effective care over the course of treatment instead of paying for units of service (Gauthier et al. 2006).

# Strategies for Comparative Effectiveness Research

The key steps involved in CER are (1) identify new and emerging clinical interventions, (2) review and synthesize current medical research, (3) identify gaps between existing medical research and the needs of clinical practice, (4) promote and generate new scientific evidence and analytic tools, (5) train and develop clinical researchers, (6) translate and disseminate research findings to diverse stakeholders, and (7) reach out to stakeholders via a citizens forum (AHRQ 2011).

Etheredge (2010) has suggested that our collective knowledge about comparative effectiveness will grow more quickly if we can draw on the voluminous information contained in clinical trial databases and on other clinical research data sets, rather than on new CER studies alone. Problems of noncomparability notwithstanding, if existing information can be extracted in a meaningful way, CER could then be used to fill research gaps.

Future priorities for CER include the capacity to conduct experimental and quasi-experimental comparative studies; evaluation of broad, system-level strategies, such as benefit designs and payment reforms; focus on population subgroups, including vulnerable groups, most likely to benefit from a given intervention; dissemination of research results; and the actual use of evidence in the delivery of care (Benner et al. 2010). At present, much remains unknown about how CER will be conducted for example, whether or not it will invite participation from important stakeholders, such as physicians.

Americans support research that would provide information on treatment options. Conversely, public support for research is contingent upon how medical evidence will be used in practice. The public remains opposed to the use of research for allocation of resources or for mandating certain treatment decisions (Gerber et al. 2010). The public's attitudes may well become the biggest obstacle to cost-efficient delivery of health care in the future and to any attempts by the government to mandate certain types of care or to ration services.

## Summary

Health care delivery in the United States continues to change. Political factors played a major role in the passage of the ACA of 2010, but its survival is not certain. Future directions in health care will be determined mainly by political, economic, social, technologic, informational, and ecological changes. American beliefs and values and the will of the people will also steer health care in a direction that is currently difficult to foresee. However, the plight of the uninsured and the nation's ability to deliver what Americans have come to expect from the health care system will continue to pose major challenges. This is particularly true in the wake of a mounting national debt that many economists think is likely to reach a point of crisis.

Some attempts have been made to strengthen the delivery infrastructure, to make it more responsive to the growing population of people with chronic conditions and to improve community health. Shortage of primary care physicians and nurses, as well as the critical need to train the workforce to effectively function in an environment that focuses more on chronic than acute care, remains an obstacle that must be overcome for the system to address future health needs in a changing demographic landscape. The financing and delivery of long-term care will put further strains on the system.

International threats have emerged as a result of globalization. Rapid response to deal with infectious diseases that can quickly spread around the world, natural disasters, and man-made threats of terrorism will increasingly require global assistance, cooperation, and joint efforts. Resistance of infectious agents to antibiotics also poses global concerns. Many developing and underdeveloped countries face critical shortages of trained health care workers.

Despite its association with cost escalation, technologic progress will continue, but technology assessment will also play an increasing role. Imaging technology, minimally invasive surgery, genetic mapping, regenerative medicine, information systems, and home monitoring of patients will help shape the delivery of medical care in a way never before imagined. Standardized protocols for practitioners will continue to be informed by scientific evidence that will include comparative effectiveness research.

## Test Your Understanding

### Terminology

comparative effectiveness
    research
e-health plans
employer mandate
genometrics

high-risk pools
molecular medicine
patient activation
patient-centered care
play or pay

single-payer plan
universal access
xenotransplantation

## Review Questions

1. Explain the six main forces that will determine future change in health care.
2. Briefly discuss the historical precedents on which the Patient Protection and Affordable Care Plan of 2010 was based.
3. In what way should the delivery infrastructure change to meet the needs of a larger number of insured Americans?
4. What is patient activation? What are the main challenges in activation?
5. What recommendations have been made to transform the nursing profession?
6. What training is needed for primary care physicians to become "comprehensivists"?
7. What are some of the main reasons behind the deficits in geriatric training?
8. What are the main challenges faced by long-term care in the future?
9. Give an overview of what new technology might achieve in the delivery of health care.
10. What role does international cooperation play in globalization?
11. What can be done to achieve greater adoption of evidence-based medicine in the delivery of health care?
12. What attitudes do Americans have toward medical research and its use?

# REFERENCES

Adler, R. et al. 2009. *Healthcare 2020*. Palo Alto, CA: Institute for the Future.

Agency for Healthcare Research and Quality (AHRQ). 2011. *What is comparative effectiveness research?* Available at: http://www.effectivehealthcare.ahrq.gov/index.cfm/what-is-comparative-effectiveness-research1/. Accessed January 2011.

Allen, H. et al. 2010. What the Oregon health study can tell us about expanding Medicaid. *Health Affairs* 29, no. 8: 1498–1506.

Amaral, M.M. 2010. Does substituting home care for institutional care lead to a reduction in Medicaid expenditures? *Health Care Management Science* 13, no. 4: 319–333.

Benner, J.S. et al. 2010. An evaluation of recent federal spending on comparative effectiveness research: Priorities, gaps, and next steps. *Health Affairs* 29, no. 10: 1768–1776.

Bielaszka-DuVernay, C. 2011. Vermont's blueprint for medical homes, community health teams, and better health at lower cost. *Health Affairs* 30, no. 3: 383–386.

Blendon, R.J. et al. 2008. Massachusetts health reform: A public perspective from debate through implementation. *Health Affairs* 27: W556–W565.

Burke, S.P. et al. 2005. *Developing a better long-term care policy: A vision and strategy for America's future*. Washington, DC: National Academy of Social Insurance.

Busse, F. 2006. Diagnostic imaging. In: *Advances in healthcare technology: Shaping the future of medical care*. G. Spekowius and T. Wendler, eds. Dordrecht, The Netherlands: Springer. pp. 15–34.

Caudill, T. et al. 2011. Health care reform and primary care: Training physicians for tomorrow's challenges. *Academic Medicine* 86, no. 2: 158–160.

Centers for Disease Control and Prevention/Merck Institute of Aging and Health (CDC/Merck). 2004. *The state of aging and health in America, 2004*. Available at: http://www.cdc.gov/aging/. Accessed March 2007.

Chandra, A. et al. 2011. The importance of the individual mandate—Evidence from Massachusetts. *New England Journal of Medicine* 364, no. 4: 293–295.

Chatterjee, P. 2011. Progress patchy on health-worker crisis. *Lancet* 377, no. 9764: 456.

Clark, C.R. et al. 2011. Lack of access due to costs remains a problem for some in Massachusetts despite the state's health reforms. *Health Affairs* 30, no. 2: 247–255.

Cohen, H.J. et al. 2002. A controlled trial of inpatient and outpatient geriatric evaluation and management. *New England Journal of Medicine* 346, no. 12: 906–912.

Congressional Budget Office (CBO). 2004. *Financing long term care for the elderly*. Washington, DC: CBO.

Crowley, J.S. 2006. *Medicaid long-term care services reforms in the Deficit Reduction Act*. Washington, DC: The Henry J. Kaiser Family Foundation.

Cunningham, P.J. 2011. *State variation in primary care physician supply: Implications for health reform Medicaid expansions*. Research Brief No. 19. Washington, DC: Center for Studying Health System Change.

Cunningham, P.J., and J.H. May. 2006. *Medicaid patients increasingly concentrated among physicians*. Tracking Report No. 16. Washington, DC: Center for Studying Health System Change.

Cutler, D. 2010. Analysis and commentary: How health care reform must bend the cost curve. *Health Affairs* 29, no. 6: 1131–1135.

Dent, M.M. et al. 2010. Chronic disease management: Teaching medical students to incorporate community. *Family Medicine* 42, no. 10: 736–740.

Department of Health and Human Services (DHHS). 2003. *The future supply of long-term care workers in relation to the aging baby boom generation, Report to Congress.* Washington, DC: Department of Health and Human Services.

Department of Health and Human Services (DHHS). 2005. *2020: A new vision—A future for regenerative medicine.* Washington, DC: Department of Health and Human Services.

Drayse, M.H. 2008. Globalization and regional change in the U.S. furniture industry. *Growth and Change* 39, no. 2: 252–282.

Engle, G.L. 1977. The need for a new medical model: A challenge for biomedicine. *Science* 196, no. 1: 127–136.

Epstein, R.M. et al. 2010. Why the nation needs a policy push on patient-centered health care. *Health Affairs* 29, no. 8: 1489–1495.

Etheredge, L.M. 2010. Creating a high-performance system for comparative effectiveness research. *Health Affairs* 29, no. 10: 1761–1767.

Gauthier, A. et al. 2006. *Toward a high performance health system for the United States.* New York: The Commonwealth Fund.

Gerber, A.S. et al. 2010. The public wants information, not board mandates, from comparative effectiveness research. *Health Affairs* 29, no. 10: 1872–1881.

Gossink, R., and J. Souquet. 2006. Advances and trends in healthcare technology. In: *Advances in healthcare technology: Shaping the future of medical care.* G. Spekowius and T. Wendler, eds. Dordrecht, The Netherlands: Springer. pp. 1–14.

Gostin, L.O., and E.E. Connors. 2010. Health care reform in transition. *Journal of the American Medical Association* 303, no. 12: 1188–1189.

Haislmaier, E.F., and N. Owcharenko. 2006. The Massachusetts approach: A new way to restructure state health insurance markets and public programs. *Health Affairs* 25, no. 6: 1580–1590.

Halm, E.A. et al. 2007. Has evidence changed practice? Appropriateness of carotid endarterectomy after the clinical trials. *Neurology* 68, no. 3: 187–194.

Helitzer, D.L. et al. 2011. A randomized controlled trial of communication training with primary care providers to improve patient-centeredness and health risk communication. *Patient Education & Counseling* 82, no. 1: 21–29.

The Henry J. Kaiser Family Foundation (Kaiser). Undated. *Hawaii: Facts at-a-glance.* Available at: http://www.statehealthfacts.org/profileglance.jsp?rgn=13#. Accessed May 2011.

The Henry J. Kaiser Family Foundation. 2006. *Massachusetts health care reform plan.* Available at: http://www.kff.org. Accessed April 2006.

Hibbard, J.H., and P.J. Cunningham. 2008. *How engaged are consumers in their health and health care, and why does it matter?* Research Brief No. 8. Washington, DC: Center for Studying Health System Change.

Holahan, J. 2011. The 2007–09 recession and health insurance coverage. *Health Affairs* 30, no. 1: 145–152.

Holtz-Eakin, D., and M.J. Ramlet. 2010. Analysis and commentary: Health care reform is likely to widen federal budget deficits, not reduce them. *Health Affairs* 29, no. 6: 1136–1141.

Hughes, J.M. 2011. Preserving the lifesaving power of antimicrobial agents. *Journal of the American Medical Association* 305, no. 10: 1027–1028.

Infectious Disease Society of America. 2004. *Bad bugs, no drugs.* Alexandria, VA: Infectious Disease Society of America.

Institute for the Future. 2000. *Health and health care 2010: The forecast, the challenge.* San Francisco, CA: Jossey-Bass Publishers.

Institute of Medicine (IOM). 2001. *Crossing the quality chasm: A new health system for the 21st century.* Washington, DC: National Academies Press.

Johns, M.C. et al. 2011. A growing global network's role in outbreak response: AFHSC-GEIS 2008–2009. *BMC Public Health* 11 (Suppl. 2): S3.

Kenen, J. 2011. Dx on the preexisting condition insurance plan. *Health Affairs* 30, no. 3: 379–381.

Knoller, M. 2009. *National debt now tops $12 trillion.* CBS News: Political Hotsheet, November 17, 2009. Available at: http://www.cbsnews.com/8301-503544_162-5686644-503544.html. Accessed March 2011.

Kovner, C.T. et al. 2002. Who cares for older adults? Workforce implications of an aging society. *Health Affairs* 21, no. 5: 78–89.

Kravitz, R.L. 2008. Beyond gatekeeping: Enlisting patients as agents for quality and cost-containment. *Journal of General Internal Medicine* 23, no. 10: 1722–1723.

Lamm, R.D., and R.H. Blank. 2005. The challenge of an aging society. *The Futurist* July–August: 23–27.

Leape, L.L. et al. 2003. Adherence to practice guidelines: The role of specialty society guidelines. *American Heart Journal* 145, no. 1: 19–26.

Lee, P.R. 1994. Models of excellence. *Lancet* 344, no. 8935: 1484–1486.

Levinson, W. et al. 2010. Developing physician communication skills for patient-centered care. *Health Affairs* 29, no. 7: 1310–1318.

Maxfield, M. et al. 2008. Medical homes: The information exchange challenge. In: *Making medical homes work: Moving from concept to practice.* P.B. Ginsburg, ed. Washington, DC: Center for Studying Health System Change.

Miller, E.A., and V. Mor. 2006. *Out of the shadows: Envisioning a brighter future for long-term care in America.* Providence, RI: Brown University.

Milstein, J.B. et al. 2006. The impact of globalization on vaccine development and availability. *Health Affairs* 25, no. 4: 1061–1069.

National Academy of Sciences. 2010. *The future of nursing: Leading change, advancing health.* Washington, DC: The Institute of Medicine.

Oberlander, J. et al. 2001. Rationing medical care: Rhetoric and reality in the Oregon health plan. *Canadian Medical Association Journal* 164, no. 11: 1583–1587.

Office for Oregon Health Policy and Research. 2007. *Profile of Oregon's uninsured, 2006.* Available at: http://www.oregon.gov/OHPPR/RSCH/docs/uninsuredprofile.pdf?ga=t. Accessed March 2011.

O'Malley, A.S. et al. 2008. Qualifying a physician practice as a medical home. In: *Making medical homes work: Moving from concept to practice*. P.B. Ginsburg, ed. Washington, DC: Center for Studying Health System Change.

Paulus, R.A. et al. 2008. Continuous innovation in health care: Implications of the Geisinger experience. *Health Affairs* 27, no. 5: 1235–1245.

Peikes, D. et al. 2008. Matching patients to medical homes: Ensuring patient and physician choice. In: *Making medical homes work: Moving from concept to practice*. P.B. Ginsburg, ed. Washington, DC: Center for Studying Health System Change.

Pham, H.H. et al. 2008. Paying for medical homes: A calculated risk. In: *Making medical homes work: Moving from concept to practice*. P.B. Ginsburg, ed. Washington, DC: Center for Studying Health System Change.

RAND. 2011. Overview of employer mandate. The RAND Corporation. Available at: http://www.randcompare.org/policy-options/employer-mandate. Accessed March 2011.

Sack, K. 2009. Massachusetts faces costs of big health care plan. Available at: http://www.nytimes.com/2009/03/16/health/policy/16mass.html. Accessed March 2009.

Singh, D.A. 2010. *Effective management of long-term care facilities*. 2nd ed. Sudbury, MA: Jones & Bartlett Publishers.

Slawson, D.C., and A.F. Shaughnessy. 2001. Using "medical poetry" to remove the inequities in health care delivery. *Journal of Family Medicine* 50, no. 1: 51–65.

SteelFisher, G.K. et al. 2009. Physicians' views of the Massachusetts health care reform law—A poll. *New England Journal of Medicine* 361, no. 19: 39.

Steuerle, C.E., and P.N. Van de Water. 2009. *Administering health insurance mandates*. Available at: http://www.nasi.org/usr_doc/Administering_Health_Insurance_Mandates.pdf. Accessed March 2011.

Tanner, M. 2009. *Massachusetts miracle or Massachusetts miserable: What the failure of the "Massachusetts Model" tells us about health care reform*. Briefing Paper no. 112. Washington, DC: CATO Institute.

Tully, S. 2010. *5 painful health-care lessons from Massachusetts*. Available at: http://money.cnn.com/2010/06/15/news/economy/massachusetts_healthcare_reform.fortune/index.htm. Accessed March 2011.

Ubel, P.A. et al. 2005. Misimagining the unimaginable: The disability paradox and health care decision making. *Health Psychology* 24 (4 Suppl.): S57–S62.

Wadhwani, A. 2010. *Tennessee removes about 100,000 people from Medicaid rolls*. Available at: http://www.kaiserhealthnews.org/Stories/2010/April/08/TennCare.aspx. Accessed March 2011.

Williams, D.R. 2010. Beyond the Affordable Care Act: Achieving real improvements in Americans' health. *Health Affairs* 29, no. 8: 1481–1488.

World Health Organization (WHO). 2008. *What are the International Health Regulations?* Available at: http://www.who.int/features/qa/39/en/index.html. Accessed March 2011.

# Glossary

**Academic medical center:** A term commonly used when one or more hospitals organize around a medical school. Apart from the training of physicians, research activities and clinical investigations become an important undertaking in these institutions.

**Access:** The ability of persons needing health services to obtain appropriate care in a timely manner. Can you get medical care when you need it? If yes, you have access to medical care. Access is not the same as health insurance coverage, although insurance coverage is a strong predictor of access for **primary care** services.

**Accountable care organization (ACO):** An integrated group of providers who are willing and able to take responsibility for improving the overall health status, care efficiency, and satisfaction with care for a defined population.

**Acquired immune deficiency syndrome (AIDS):** The occurrence of immune deficiency caused by the **HIV** virus.

**Activities of daily living (ADLs):** The most commonly used measure of disability. ADLs determine whether an individual needs assistance to perform basic activities, such as eating, bathing, dressing, toileting, and getting into or out of a bed or chair. See **functional status** and **IADLs**.

**Actuary:** A person professionally trained in the technical aspects of insurance and related fields, particularly in the mathematics of insurance, such as the calculation of premiums, reserves, and other values.

**Acupuncture:** Use of long, thin needles passed through the skin to specific reflex points to treat chronic pain or to produce regional anesthesia.

**Acute care:** Short-term, intense medical care for an illness or injury usually requiring hospitalization. See **subacute care**.

**Administrative costs:** Costs that are incidental to the delivery of health services. These costs are not only associated with the billing and collection of claims for services delivered but also include numerous other costs, such as time and effort incurred by employers for the selection of insurance carriers, costs incurred by insurance and managed care organizations to market their products, and time and effort involved in the negotiation of rates.

**Adult day care:** A community-based, long-term care service that provides a wide range of health, social, and recreational services to elderly adults who require supervision and care while members of the family or other informal caregivers are away at work.

**Advanced practice nurse (APN):** A general name for nurses who have education and clinical experience beyond that required of an RN. APNs include four areas of specialization in nursing: clinical nurse specialists (CNSs), certified registered nurse anesthetists (CRNAs), nurse practitioners (NPs), and certified nurse midwives (CNMs).

**Adverse selection:** A phenomenon in which individuals who are likely to use more health care services than others due to poor health enroll in health insurance plans in greater numbers, compared to people who are healthy. See **favorable risk selection**.

**Affective disorders:** A group of disorders characterized by severe mood changes, often accompanied by a manic or depressive syndrome.

**Agency for Healthcare Research and Quality (AHRQ):** A federal agency within the Department of Health and Human Services whose mission is to improve the quality, safety, efficiency, and effectiveness of health care through research activities.

**AIDS:** Acquired immune deficiency syndrome. The occurrence of immune deficiency caused by the **HIV** virus.

**Allied health:** A broad category that includes services and professionals in many health-related technical areas. Allied health professionals include technicians, assistants, therapists, and technologists.

**Allopathy:** A philosophy of medicine that views medical treatment as active intervention to counteract the effects of disease through medical and surgical procedures that produce effects opposite those of the disease. See **homeopathy** and **osteopathy**.

**Alternative medicine:** Also called "alternative and complementary medicine." Nontraditional remedies, for example, **acupuncture, homeopathy, naturopathy, biofeedback, yoga exercises, chiropractic**, and herbal therapy.

**Alzheimer's disease:** A progressive degenerative disease of the brain producing loss of memory, confusion, irritability, severe loss of functioning, and ultimately death. The disease is named after German neurologist, Alois Alzheimer (1864–1915).

**Ambulatory:** Refers to the ability to move about at will.

**Ambulatory care:** Also referred to as **outpatient services**. Ambulatory care includes (1) care rendered to patients who come to physicians' offices, outpatient departments of hospitals, and health centers to receive care; (2) outpatient services intended to serve the surrounding community (community medicine); and (3) certain services that are transported to the patient.

**Ancillary services:** Hospital or other **inpatient services** other than room and board and professional medical services, such as physician and nursing care. Examples include radiology, pharmacy, laboratory, bandages and other supplies, and physical therapy.

**Anesthesiology:** Administration of drugs for the prevention or relief of pain during surgery.

**Angioplasty:** The reconstruction or restructuring of a blood vessel by operative means or nonsurgical techniques, such as balloon dilation or laser.

**Anorexia nervosa:** A mental disturbance characterized by self-imposed starvation because the patient may claim to feel fat even when emaciated.

**Antiretroviral:** A drug that stops or suppresses the activity of a retrovirus, such as HIV.

**Antitrust:** Federal and state laws that make certain anticompetitive practices illegal. These practices include price fixing, price discrimination, exclusive contracting arrangements, and mergers among competitors.

**Arthroscope:** An **endoscope** for examining the interior of a joint.

**Assignment:** The practice under which a physician agrees to accept whatever the insurer (generally **Medicaid** and **Medicare**) will pay. A physician not on assignment will **balance bill** the patient for the amount remaining after the insurer has paid.

**Atherosclerosis:** A form of hardening of the arteries caused by accumulation of substances such as fatty deposits.

**Audiology:** Identification and evaluation of hearing disorders and correction of hearing loss through **rehabilitation** and **prostheses**.

**Baby boom:** A sudden, large increase in the birth rate, especially that of the United States after World War II from 1946 through 1964. Baby boomers, as this generation is often referred to, comprise about 77 million adults.

**Balance bill:** Billing of the leftover sum by the **provider** to the patient after insurance has only partially paid the charge initially billed.

**Beneficiary:** Anyone covered under a particular health insurance plan.

**Benefit period:** Under **Medicare** rules, benefits for an inpatient stay are based on a benefit period. A benefit period is determined by a spell of illness beginning with hospitalization and ending when the beneficiary has not been an inpatient in a hospital or a skilled nursing facility for 60 consecutive days.

**Biofeedback:** A training program that uses relaxation and visualization to develop the ability to control one's involuntary nervous system as an aid to reducing stress, lowering blood pressure, and alleviating headaches.

**Blue Cross:** An independent, nonprofit membership corporation providing protection against the cost of hospital care on a service basis in a limited geographic area.

**Blue Shield:** An independent, nonprofit membership corporation providing protection against the cost of outpatient and surgical care on a service basis in a limited geographic area.

**Bulimia:** A mental disturbance that leads to bouts of overeating followed by induced vomiting.

**Capitation:** A reimbursement mechanism under which the provider is paid a set monthly fee per **enrollee** (sometimes referred to as per member per month or **PMPM** rate) regardless of whether or not an enrollee sees the provider and regardless of how often an enrollee sees the provider.

**Cardiology:** Medical science pertaining to study of the heart and its diseases.

**Cardiopulmonary resuscitation (CPR):** Medical procedure used to restart a patient's heart and breathing when the patient has suffered a heart failure.

**Carve out:** The assignment through contractual arrangements of specialized services to an outside organization because these services are not included in the contracts MCOs have with their providers or the **MCO** does not provide the services.

**Case management:** An organized approach to evaluating and coordinating care, particularly for patients who have complex, potentially costly problems that require a variety of services from multiple **providers** over an extended period.

**Case mix:** An aggregate of the severity of conditions requiring medical intervention. Case-mix categories are mutually exclusive and differentiate patients according to the extent of resource use.

**Catastrophic care:** Medical care needed when a patient suffers a major injury or life-threatening illness that requires expensive long-term treatment.

**Categorical programs:** Public health care programs designed to benefit only a certain category of people.

**Centers for Disease Control and Prevention (CDC):** The federal public health agency in the United States.

**Centers for Medicare & Medicaid Services (CMS):** Federal agency that administers the Medicare and Medicaid programs.

**Certificate of need (CON):** Control exercised by a government planning agency over expansion of medical facilities, for example, determination of whether a new facility should be opened in a certain location, whether an existing facility should be expanded, or whether a hospital should be allowed to purchase major equipment.

**Certified nurse midwives:** RNs with additional training from a nurse-midwifery program in areas such as maternal and fetal procedures, maternity and child nursing, and patient assessment. CNMs deliver babies, provide family planning education, and manage gynecological and obstetric care. They can substitute for obstetricians/gynecologists in prenatal and postnatal care. See **Nonphysician practitioners** (NPPs).

**Charge:** The amount a **provider** bills for rendering a service. See **cost**.

**Children's Health Insurance Program (CHIP):** A joint federal–state program established as Title XXI of the Social Security Act under the 1997 Balanced Budget Act. CHIP provides health insurance for children from low-income families who do not qualify for **Medicaid**.

**Chiropractic:** A system of medicine, based on manipulation of the spine, physiotherapy, and dietary counseling to treat neurological, muscular, and vascular problems. Chiropractic care is based on the belief that the body is a self-healing organism.

**Chiropractor:** A licensed practitioner who has completed the Doctor of Chiropractic (DC) degree. Chiropractors must be licensed to practice. Requirements for licensure include completion of an accredited program that awards a Doctor of Chiropractic (DC) and an examination by the state chiropractic board.

**Chronic condition (chronic disease):** A medical condition that persists over time. Chronic diseases may lead to a permanent medical condition that is nonreversible and/or leaves residual disability.

**Churning:** A phenomenon in which people gain and lose health insurance coverage multiple times.

**Claim:** A demand for payment of covered medical expenses sent to an insurance company.

**Clinical practice guidelines (medical practice guidelines):** Standardized guidelines in the form of scientifically established protocols, representing preferred processes in medical practice.

**Clinical trial:** A research study, generally based on random assignments, designed to study the effectiveness of a new drug, device, or treatment.

**Closed panel:** Also called "closed network," "in network," or "closed access." A health plan that pays for services only when provided by physicians and hospitals on the plan's **panel**.

**Community health center (CHC):** Local, nonprofit, community-owned health care providers serving low-income and medically underserved communities.

**Community hospital:** Nonfederal (i.e., VA and military hospitals are excluded), short-term, general or special hospital whose services are available to the public.

**Community rating:** Same insurance rate for everyone, as opposed to **experience rating**.

**Comorbidity:** Presence of more than one health problem in an individual.

**Comparative effectiveness research (CER):** A concept in which a chosen medical intervention is guided by scientific evidence on how well it would work compared to other available treatments.

**Competition:** Rivalry among sellers for the purpose of attracting customers.

**Concurrent utilization review:** A process that determines, on a daily basis, the length of stay necessary in a hospital. It also monitors the use of ancillary services and ensures that the medical treatment provided is appropriate and necessary.

**Continuous quality improvement (CQI):** See **total quality management**.

**Continuum:** A range or spectrum of health care services from basic to complex.

**Copayment (coinsurance):** A portion of health care charges that the insured has to pay under the terms of his or her health insurance policy. See **deductible**.

**Cost:** What it costs the provider to produce a service. See **charge**.

**Cost efficiency (cost effectiveness):** A service is cost efficient when the benefit received is greater than the cost incurred to provide the service. See **efficiency**.

**Cost-plus:** Reimbursement to a **provider** based on **cost** plus a factor to cover the value of capital.

**Cost sharing:** Sharing in the cost of health insurance premiums by those enrolled and/or payment of certain medical costs out of pocket, such as **copayments** and **deductibles**.

**Cost shifting (cross-subsidizing):** In general, shifting of costs from one entity to another as a way of making up losses in one area by charging more in other areas. For example, when care is provided to the uninsured, the **provider** makes up the cost for those services by charging more to the insured.

**Cost-utility analysis:** Analysis that includes the use of **quality-adjusted life years**.

**Covered lives:** People enrolled in a managed care plan. See **enrollees**.

**Critical access hospital (CAH):** Medicare designation for small rural hospitals with 25 beds or fewer that provide emergency medical services besides short-term hospitalization for patients with noncomplex health care needs. CAHs receive **cost-plus** reimbursement.

**Critical pathways:** Outcome-based, patient-centered case management tools that are interdisciplinary, facilitating coordination of care among multiple clinical departments and caregivers. A critical pathway identifies planned medical interventions in a given case, along with expected outcomes.

**Custodial care:** Nonmedical care provided to support and maintain the patient's condition and the essentials of daily living, generally requiring no active medical or nursing treatments.

**Deductible:** The portion of health care costs that the insured must first pay (generally up to an annual limit) before insurance payments kick in. Insurance payments may be further subject to **copayment**.

**Deemed status:** A designation used when a hospital, by virtue of its accreditation by the Joint Commission or the American Osteopathic Association, does not require separate certification from the DHHS to participate in the Medicare and Medicaid programs.

**Defensive medicine:** Excessive medical tests and procedures performed as a protection against malpractice lawsuits, otherwise regarded as unnecessary.

**Delirium:** A state of mental confusion and excitement often accompanied by disorientation, illusions, or hallucinations.

**Dementia:** A brain disorder characterized by progressive mental deterioration with loss of memory. **Alzheimer's disease** is one disorder that leads to severe dementia.

**Denial of claim:** Refusal by a **payer** to reimburse a **provider** for services rendered.

**Dental assistants:** Usually work for dentists in the preparation, examination, and treatment of patients.

**Dental hygienists:** Work under the supervision of dentists and provide preventive dental care, including cleaning teeth and educating patients on proper dental care.

**Dentist:** A professional who diagnoses and treats dental problems related to the teeth, gums, and tissues of the mouth.

**Department of Health and Human Services (DHHS):** The principal US federal agency responsible for protecting the health of all Americans and providing essential human services.

**Dependency:** (1) A person's reliance on another for assistance with common daily functions, such as bathing and grooming. See **activities of daily living**. (2) Children's reliance on adults, such as parents or school officials, to recognize and respond to their health needs.

**Dermatology:** Medical science pertaining to the study of the skin and its diseases.

**Developmental disability:** A physical incapacity that generally accompanies **mental retardation** and often arises at birth or in early childhood.

**Developmental vulnerability:** Rapid and cumulative physical and emotional changes that characterize childhood and the potential impact that illness, injury, or untoward family and social circumstances can have on a child's life-course trajectory.

**Diagnosis-related group (DRG):** A diagnostic category associated with a fixed payment to an acute care hospital under the **prospective payment system**.

**Diminishing marginal returns:** A term used in economics that, in the health care context, means that, at a certain point, additional deployment of health care resources in a given situation will become less effective in achieving the desired outcome.

**Disability:** Physical or mental handicap—partial or total—resulting from sickness or injury.

**Discharge planning:** Part of the overall treatment plan designed to facilitate discharge from an inpatient setting. It includes, for example, an estimate of how long the patient will be in the hospital, what the expected outcome is likely to be, whether any special requirements will be needed at discharge, and what needs to be facilitated for postacute continuity of care.

**Disease management:** Used primarily by health **plans**, this is a population-oriented strategy involving patient education, training in self-management, ongoing monitoring of the disease process, and follow-up aimed at people with chronic conditions, such as diabetes, asthma, depression, and coronary artery disease.

**Disparities:** Differences in the quality of health care or the health outcomes of different groups of people (e.g., racial/ethnic, socioeconomic, gender) that are not due to access-related factors or clinical needs, preferences, and appropriateness of interventions.

**Do-not-resuscitate (DNR) orders:** Advance directives telling medical professionals not to perform **CPR**. Through DNR orders, patients can have their

wishes known regarding aggressive efforts at resuscitation.

**Durable medical equipment (DME):** Supplies and equipment not immediately consumed, such as **ostomy** supplies, wheelchairs, and oxygen tanks.

**Durable power of attorney:** A written document that provides a legal means for a patient to delegate authority to another to act on the patient's behalf, even after the patient has been incapacitated.

**Dyspnea:** Difficult or labored respiration; shortness of breath.

**Effectiveness (efficacy):** Health benefits of a medical intervention.

**Efficiency:** Provision of higher-quality and more appropriate services at a lower cost, generally measured in terms of benefits relative to costs. See **cost efficiency**.

**E-health:** Health care information and services offered over the Internet by professionals and nonprofessionals alike.

**E-therapy:** Any type of professional therapeutic interaction that makes use of the Internet to connect qualified mental health professionals and their clients.

**Electronic health records: Information technology** applications that enable the processing of any electronically stored information pertaining to individual patients for the purpose of delivering health care services.

**Eligibility:** The process of determining whether a patient qualifies for benefits, based on such factors as age, income, and veteran status.

**Emergency department:** Hospital facilities for the delivery of unscheduled **outpatient** services to patients whose conditions require immediate care. Emergency departments must be staffed 24 hours a day.

**Emergent condition:** An acute condition that requires immediate medical attention.

**Employer mandate:** A legal requirement for employers to help pay for their employees' health insurance.

**Enabling services:** Services that enable people to receive medical care that otherwise would not be received despite insurance coverage, for example, transportation and translation services.

**Encephalitis:** Inflammation of the brain.

**Encephalography:** X-ray examination of the brain.

**Endemic:** A disease restricted to a local region. See **epidemic** and **pandemic**.

**Endoscope:** An instrument consisting of a tube and an optical system used for observing the inside of a hollow organ or cavity.

**Enrollee:** A person enrolled in a health plan, especially in a managed care plan.

**Enteral:** Within or by way of the intestine.

**Entitlement:** A health care program to which certain people are entitled. For example, almost everyone at 65 years of age is entitled to Medicare because of contributions made through taxes. **Medicaid**, conversely, is a **welfare program**.

**Epidemic:** An outbreak of an infectious disease that spreads rapidly and affects many individuals within a population. See **endemic** and **pandemic**.

**Epidemiology:** The study of the distribution and determinants of health, health-related behavior, disease, disorder, and death in a population group.

**Etiology:** Study of the causes of disease or dysfunction.

**Evidence-based medicine:** Use of current best evidence from published research in medical decision making.

**Exclusive provider plan:** A health plan that is very similar to those offered by preferred provider organizations, except that use is restricted to in-network providers.

**Experience rating:** Setting of insurance rates based on a group's actual health care expenses in a prior period. This allows healthier groups to pay less. See **community rating**.

**Family medicine:** A branch of medical practice based on a core of knowledge to function as the primary provider of health care and to perform the roles of patient management, problem solving, counseling, and coordination of care.

**Favorable risk selection:** Also called "risk selection." A phenomenon in which healthy people are disproportionately enrolled into a health plan. See **adverse selection**.

**Fee for service:** Payment of separate fees to physicians for each service performed, such as examination, administering a test, and hospital visit. The physician sets the fees.

**Fee schedule:** A schedule of fees for various health care services.

**First-dollar insurance:** Health care coverage with no **cost sharing**.

**Flat-of-the-curve medicine:** Medical care that produces relatively little or no benefit for the patient because of **diminishing marginal returns**.

**Formulary:** A list of acceptable prescription drugs approved by a health plan.

**Fraud:** Intentional filing of false billing claims or cost reports and provision of services that are not medically necessary.

**Fringe benefits:** A term loosely denoting life insurance, health insurance, or pension benefits provided in whole or in part by an employer to its employees.

**Functional status:** A person's ability or inability to cope with the **activities of daily living**.

**Gatekeeper:** A primary care physician who functions as the provider of first contact to deliver primary care services and to make referrals for specialty care.

**Gatekeeping:** The use of primary care physicians to coordinate health care services needed by an enrollee in a managed care plan.

**Gene therapy:** A therapeutic technique in which a functioning gene is inserted into targeted cells to correct an inborn defect or provide the cell with a new function.

**Generalist:** A physician in family practice, general internal medicine, or general pediatrics. See **specialist**.

**Genometrics:** The association of genes with specific disease traits.

**Geriatrics:** A branch of medicine that deals with the problems and diseases that accompany aging.

**Gerontology:** Study of the aging process and the special problems associated with aging.

**Global budget:** A plan of total expenditures in a health care system established in advance.

**Globalization:** Various forms of cross-border economic activities driven by global exchange of information, production of goods and services more economically in developing countries, and increased interdependence of mature and emerging world economies.

**Gross domestic product (GDP):** A measure of all the goods and services produced by a nation in a given year.

**Group policy:** An insurance policy purchased by an organization or association as a benefit to its employees or members. Typical groups are employers, union or trade organizations, and professional associations.

**Head Start:** A federal government-funded program that provides child development services to children in low-income families, including services in education, health care, nutrition, and mental health.

**Health informatics:** The application of information science to improve the efficiency, accuracy, and reliability of health care services. Health informatics requires the use of **information technology** (IT) but goes beyond IT by emphasizing the improvement of health care delivery.

**Health maintenance organization (HMO):** A type of managed care organization that provides comprehensive medical care for a predetermined annual fee per enrollee.

**Health professional shortage area (HPSA):** A federal designation indicating an area has shortages of primary medical care, dental, or mental health providers. HPSAs may be urban or rural areas, population groups, or medical or other public facilities.

**Health reimbursement arrangement (HRA):** An account set up and funded by an employer that can be used by an employee or a retiree to pay for health care expenses.

**Health-related quality of life (HRQL):** In a composite sense, HRQL includes a person's own perception of health, ability to function, role limitations stemming from physical or emotional problems, and personal happiness during or subsequent to disease experience.

**Health Resources and Services Administration (HRSA):** A federal agency of the Department of Health and Human Services whose mission is to improve access to health care services for people who are uninsured, isolated, or medically vulnerable.

**Health technology assessment:** Any process of examining and reporting properties of a medical technology used in health care, such as safety, effectiveness, feasibility, and indications for use, cost, and cost effectiveness, as well as social, economic, and ethical consequences, whether intended or unintended.

**Healthcare Effectiveness Data and Information Set (HEDIS):** The standard for reporting quality information on managed care plans.

**Hemiplegia:** Paralysis of one-half of the body.

**Hemodialysis:** A mechanical procedure used to cleanse the blood by removing toxic chemicals in patients who have lost the function of one or both kidneys.

**Holistic medicine:** A philosophy of health care that emphasizes the well-being of every aspect of a person, including the physical, mental, social, and spiritual aspects of health.

**Home health services:** Services such as nursing, therapy, and health-related **homemaker** or social services brought to patients in their own homes because such patients are generally unable to leave their homes safely to get the care they need.

**Homemaker services:** Nonmedical support services given to a homebound individual, for example, bathing, food preparation, house repairs, and shopping.

**Homeopathy:** A system of medicine based on the theory that "like cures like," meaning large doses of substances that produce symptoms of a disease in healthy people can be administered in small and diluted doses to cure the same illness. The system was founded in the late 18th century by a German physician, Samuel Hahnemann (1755–1843). See **allopathy**.

**Horizontal integration:** A growth strategy in which an organization extends its core product or service. See **vertical integration**.

**Hospice:** A cluster of special services for the dying, which blends medical, spiritual, legal, financial, and family-support services. The venue can vary from a specialized facility to a nursing home to the patient's own home.

**Hospitalist:** A physician who specializes in the care of hospitalized patients.

**Human immunodeficiency virus (HIV):** Human immunodeficiency virus. A virus that can destroy the immune system and lead to **AIDS**.

**Huntington's disease:** A disease of the central nervous system that slowly diminishes an individual's ability to walk, think, talk, and reason. Eventually, the person becomes completely dependent on others for care.

**Hypertension:** High blood pressure.

**Iatrogenic illness (injury):** Illness or injury caused by the process of medical care.

**Incidence:** The number of new cases of a disease in a defined population within a specified period.

**Indemnity plan:** An insurance plan that provides reimbursement to the insured regardless of the expenses actually incurred. For example, a predetermined cash amount is paid to the beneficiary per procedure or per day in the hospital. The insured is responsible for paying the provider.

**Independent practice association (IPA):** A legal entity that physicians in private practice can join so that the organization can represent them in the negotiation of managed care contracts.

**Information technology (IT):** Technology used for the transformation of data into useful information. IT involves determining data needs, gathering appropriate data, storing and analyzing the data, and reporting the information generated in a user-friendly format.

**Informed consent:** A fundamental patient right to make an informed choice regarding medical treatment based on full disclosure of medical information by the providers.

**Inpatient services:** Services delivered on the basis of an overnight stay in a health care institution.

**Instrumental activities of daily living (IADLs):** A person's ability to perform household and social tasks, such as home maintenance, cooking, shopping, and managing money. See **activities of daily living (ADLs)**.

**Insured:** The individual who is covered for risk by insurance.

**Insurer:** An insurance agency or managed care organization that offers insurance.

**Integrated delivery system (IDS):** A network of organizations that provides or arranges to provide a coordinated continuum of services to a defined population and is willing to be held clinically and fiscally accountable for the outcomes and health status of the population serviced.

**Interest group:** An organized sector of society, such as a business association, citizen group, labor union, or professional association, whose main purpose is to protect members' interests through active participation in the policy-making process.

**Internal medicine:** General diagnosis and treatment for problems involving one or more internal organs in adults.

**International Classification of Diseases, 9th Version, Clinical Modification (ICD-9-CM):** The official system of assigning codes to diagnoses and procedures.

**Joint Commission on Accreditation of Healthcare Organizations (JCAHO):** Also called "joint commission." A private, nonprofit organization that sets standards and accredits most of the nation's general hospitals and many of the long-term care facilities, psychiatric hospitals, substance abuse programs, outpatient surgery centers, urgent care clinics, group practices, community health centers, hospices, and home health agencies.

**Laparoscopy:** A minimally invasive surgical procedure in which one or more tiny incisions are made instead of one large incision. Surgery is performed by inserting long, slender instruments through the openings, along with tiny cameras attached to special tubes, called endoscopes, to view the surgery. Examples of its use are gallbladder removal, appendectomies, and hernia repairs.

**Licensed practical nurses (LPNs):** Called licensed vocational nurses (LVNs) in some states. Nurses who have completed a state-approved program in practical nursing and a national written examination. They often work under the supervision of RNs to provide patient care. See **Registered nurses**.

**Life expectancy:** Actuarial determination of how long, on average, a person of a given age is likely to live.

**Lifetime cap:** The maximum amount of money a health insurance policy will pay over the lifetime of the insured.

**Lithotripsy:** A technique in which kidney and gallbladder stones are pulverized by shockwaves. This procedure eliminates the need for invasive surgery.

**Living will:** A legal document in which a patient puts into writing what his or her preferences are regarding treatment during terminal illness and the use of life-sustaining technology. It is a directive instructing a physician to withhold or discontinue medical treatment when the patient is terminally ill and unable to make decisions.

**Long-term care:** A variety of individualized, well-coordinated services that are designed to promote the maximum possible independence for people with functional limitations. These services are provided over an extended period to meet the patients' physical, mental, social, and spiritual needs, while maximizing quality of life.

**Long-term care hospital (LTCH):** A special type of long-stay hospital described in section 1886(d)(1)(B)(iv) of the Social Security Act. LTCHs must meet Medicare's conditions of participation for acute (short-stay) hospitals and must have an average length of stay greater than 25 days. LTCHs serve patients who have complex medical needs and may suffer from multiple chronic problems requiring long-term hospitalization.

**Low birth weight:** A weight of less than 2,500 grams at birth.

**Magnet hospital:** A special designation by the American Nurses Credentialing Center, an affiliate of the American Nurses Association, to recognize quality patient care, nursing excellence, and innovations in professional nursing practice in hospitals.

**Magnetic resonance imaging (MRI):** The use of a uniform magnetic field and radio frequencies to study body tissue and structure.

**Maldistribution:** An imbalance (i.e., surplus in some but shortage in others) of the distribution of health professionals, such as physicians, needed to maintain the health status of a given population at an optimum level. Geographic maldistribution refers to the surplus in some regions (such as metropolitan areas) but shortage in other regions (such as rural and inner city areas) of needed health professionals. Specialty maldistribution refers to the surplus in some specialties (such as physician specialists) but shortage in others (such as primary care).

**Mammography:** The use of breast X-ray to detect unsuspected breast cancer in asymptomatic women.

**Managed care:** A system that integrates the functions of financing, insurance, delivery, and payment and uses mechanisms to control costs and utilization of services.

**Margin:** (Total revenues – Total costs)/ Total revenues. Generally shown as a percentage.

**Market justice:** A distributional principle according to which health care is most equitably distributed through the market forces of supply and demand rather than government interventions. See **social justice**.

**Means-tested program:** A program in which **eligibility** depends on income.

**Medicaid:** A joint federal–state program of health insurance for the poor.

**Medical loss ratio:** The percentage of premium revenue spent on medical expenses.

**Medical model:** Delivery of health care that places its primary emphasis on the treatment of disease and relief of symptoms instead of prevention of disease and promotion of optimum health.

**Medical practice guidelines:** See **clinical practice guidelines**.

**Medically underserved area (MUA):** A federal designation for a geographic area that has a shortage of personal health services for its residents.

**Medically underserved population (MUP).** A federal designation for a group of persons who face economic, cultural, or linguistic barriers to health care.

**Medicare:** A federal program of health insurance for the elderly, certain disabled individuals, and people with end-stage renal disease.

**Medigap:** Commercial health insurance policies purchased by individuals covered by Medicare to insure the expenses not covered by Medicare.

**Mental retardation:** Significantly subaverage, general intellectual functioning, existing concurrently with deficits in adaptive behavior and manifested during the developmental period.

**Metropolitan statistical area (MSA):** The US Bureau of Census has defined an MSA as a geographic area that includes at least (1) one city with a population of 50,000 or more or (2) an urbanized area of at least 50,000 inhabitants and a total MSA population of at least 100,000 (75,000 in the New England Census Region).

**Minimum data set (MDS):** An assessment instrument used for determining the **case mix** in a **skilled nursing facility**.

**Monopoly:** A market dominated by a single supplier for a unique product or service.

**Monopsony:** A market dominated by a single buyer.

**Moral hazard:** Consumer behavior that leads to a higher utilization of health care services because people are covered by insurance.

**Morbidity:** Sickness.

**Mortality:** Death.

**Multihospital system:** Operation of two or more hospitals owned, leased, sponsored, or contractually managed by a central organization.

**Myocardial infarction:** Heart attack.

**National Committee on Quality Assurance (NCQA):** A private organization that accredits managed care organizations and establishes standards for reporting quality.

**National Health Service Corps (NHSC):** Administered by HRSA, the NHSC recruits health professionals to work in medically underserved rural and urban communities. Education loan repayment is a major incentive for providers to join the NHSC.

**Naturopathy:** A system of medicine based on such natural remedies as nutrition, use of herbs, massage, and **yoga exercises**.

**Neonatal:** Refers to the first 28 days after birth.

**Neurology:** Branch of medicine that specializes in the nervous system and its diseases.

**New morbidities:** Dysfunctions, such as drug and alcohol abuse, family and neighborhood violence, emotional disorders, and learning problems, from which older generations do not suffer.

**Nonphysician practitioners (NPPs):** Clinical professionals who practice in many areas similar to those in which physicians practice but who do not have an MD or a DO degree. NPPs are sometimes called midlevel practitioners because they receive less advanced training than physicians but more training than RNs.

**Nonprofit (organization):** Also called "not for profit." A private organization, such as a hospital, that operates under Internal Revenue Code, Section 501(c)(3). These organizations are tax exempt. In exchange for tax exemption, they must provide some defined public good, such as service, education, or community welfare, and not distribute profits to any individuals.

**Nosocomial infections:** Infections acquired while receiving health care.

**Nurse practitioners (NPs):** Individuals who have completed a program of study leading to competence as RNs in an expanded role. NP specialties include pediatric, family, adult, psychiatric, and geriatric programs. The primary function of NPs is to promote wellness and good health through patient education. Their traditional nursing role has expanded to include taking patients' comprehensive health histories, assessing health status, performing physical examinations, and formulating and managing a care regimen for acutely and chronically ill patients. See **nonphysician practitioners (NPPs)**.

**Nursing facility (NF):** A nursing home (or part of a nursing home) certified to provide services to Medicaid beneficiaries. See **skilled nursing facility**.

**Obesity:** For adults, it is defined as a body mass index (BMI) of 30 or greater. BMI is calculated by dividing a person's body weight in kilograms by the square of his or her height in meters. See **overweight**.

**Obstetrics/gynecology:** Diagnosis and treatment relating to the sexual and reproductive system of women using surgical and nonsurgical techniques.

**Occupational therapy:** Therapy to help people improve their ability to perform tasks in their daily living and working environment.

**Oncology:** Medical specialty dealing with cancers and tumors.

**Ophthalmology:** The branch of medicine specializing in the eye and its diseases.

**Opportunistic infection:** An infection that occurs when the body's natural immune system breaks down.

**Optometrist:** A professional who possesses a Doctor of Optometry degree and has passed a written and clinical state board examination. An optometrist provides vision care—examination, diagnosis, and correction of vision disorders.

**Organized medicine:** Concerted activities of physicians, mainly to protect their own interests, through such associations as the American Medical Association (AMA).

**Organization for Economic Cooperation and Development (OECD):** A forum of approximately 30 countries, including all Western European nations, the United States, Canada, New Zealand, Australia, Japan, and others, committed to a market economy. Representatives of member nations meet and discuss global economic and social policies.

**Orphan drugs:** Certain new drug therapies for conditions that affect fewer than 200,000 people in the United States.

**Orthopedics:** Branch of medicine dealing with the skeletal system (i.e., bones, joints, muscles, ligaments, and cartilage).

**Osteopathy:** A medical philosophy based on the holistic approach to treatment. It uses the traditional methods of medical practice, which include pharmaceuticals, laboratory tests, X-ray diagnostics, and surgery, and supplements them by advocating treatment that involves correction of the position of the joints or tissues and emphasizes diet and environment as factors that might destroy natural resistance. See **allopathy**.

**Osteoporosis:** Loss of bone density.

**Ostomy:** Surgically formed artificial opening for bowel discharge.

**Otitis media:** Inflammation of the middle ear.

**Outcome:** The end result of health care delivery; often viewed as the bottom-line measure of the effectiveness of the health care delivery system.

**Out-of-pocket costs:** Costs of health care paid by the recipient of care. For an individual covered by health insurance, these costs generally include the **deductible**, **copayments**, cost of excluded services, and costs in excess of what the insurer has determined to be "customary, prevailing, and reasonable."

**Outpatient services:** As opposed to **inpatient services**, outpatient services include any health care services that are not provided based on an overnight stay in which room and board costs are incurred. See **ambulatory care**.

**Overutilization (overuse):** Utilization of medical services, the cost of which exceeds the benefit to consumers or the risks of which outweigh potential benefits.

**Overweight:** For adults, it is defined as a body mass index (BMI) of 25 or greater. BMI is calculated by dividing a person's body weight in kilograms by the square of his or her height in meters. See **obesity**.

**Package pricing:** Bundling of fees for an entire package of related services.

**Palliative:** Serving to relieve or alleviate, such as pharmacologic pain management and nausea relief.

**Pandemic:** Relating to the spread of disease in a large segment of the population. See **endemic** and **epidemic**.

**Panel:** Providers selected to render services to the members of a managed care plan constitute its panel. The plan generally refers to them as "preferred providers."

**Paramedic:** Health care workers other than physicians who work as emergency medical technicians.

**Parenteral nutrition:** The full name is "total parenteral nutrition" (TPN). It infuses nutrients and water into the veins through a catheter, bypassing the gastrointestinal tract.

**Parkinson's disease:** A chronic disease of the nervous system characterized by tremor and muscular debility. Named after the British physician, James Parkinson (1755–1824).

**Pathology:** Study of the nature and cause of disease that involves changes in structure and function.

**Patient-centered care:** Delivery of health care that respects and responds to patients' wants, needs and preferences so that they can make choices in their care that best fit their individual circumstances.

**Pay for performance:** A reimbursement plan that links payment to quality and efficiency as an incentive to improve the quality of health care and to reduce costs.

**Payer:** The party who actually makes payment for services under the insurance coverage policy. In most cases, the payer is the same as the insurer.

**Pediatrics:** General diagnosis and treatment for children.

**Per diem:** A type of reimbursement mechanism for inpatient care in a health care institution. The reimbursement comprises a flat rate for each day of inpatient stay.

**Per member per month (PMPM):** Refers to a capitated rate. See **Capitation**.

**Perinatal:** Referring to the time period from the 28th week of pregnancy through 28 days after birth.

**Pharmaceutical care:** A mode of pharmacy practice in which the pharmacist takes an active role on behalf of patients, which includes giving information on drugs and advice on their potential misuse and assisting prescribers in appropriate drug choices. In so doing, the pharmacist assumes direct responsibility collaboratively with other health care professionals and with patients to achieve the desired therapeutic outcomes.

**Pharmacist:** A professional who has graduated from an accredited pharmacy program that awards a Bachelor of Pharmacy or Doctor of Pharmacy degree and has successfully completed a state board examination and a supervised internship.

**Pharmacology:** Body of science dealing with drugs, their nature, properties, and effects.

**Phlebotomy:** Drawing of blood by using a syringe and needle.

**Physical therapy:** The evaluation and treatment of physical problems resulting from injury or disease, including problems with joint motion, muscle strength, endurance, and heart and lung function.

**Physician assistants (PAs):** Professionals who work in a dependent relationship with a supervising physician to provide comprehensive medical care to patients. The major services provided by PAs include evaluation, monitoring, diagnostics, therapeutics, counseling, and referral. See **nonphysician practitioners (NPPs)**.

**Physician extenders:** Also called **nonphysician practitioners (NPPs)**.

**Physician–hospital organization (PHO):** A legal entity formed between a hospital and a physician group to achieve shared market objectives and other mutual interests.

**Plan:** A health insurance plan.

**Plastic surgery:** Surgery for the restoration, repair, or reconstruction of body structures.

**Play or pay:** A type of **employer mandate** in which employers must choose to provide health insurance to employees ("play") or contribute, generally a certain percentage of payroll costs, to a government-administered fund ("pay") to provide health insurance for all who are not covered by their employers.

**Podiatrists:** Professionals who treat patients with foot diseases or deformities.

**Point of service (POS):** A managed care plan that allows its members to decide at the time they need medical care (at the point of service) whether to go to a **provider** on the panel or to pay more to receive services out of network.

**Policy:** The document that sets out the insurance contract.

**Postneonatal:** The period between 28 days and 1 year after birth. See **neonatal**.

**Postpartum:** Occurring after childbirth.

**Practice profiling:** Use of provider-specific practice patterns and comparing individual practice patterns to some norm.

**Preadmission screening:** The assessment of an individual's functional status by a trained health professional prior to institutional placement to determine whether alternative community services would be more appropriate.

**Preexisting condition:** A physical and/or mental condition that existed before the effective date of an insurance policy.

**Preferred provider organization (PPO):** A type of managed care organization that has a **panel** of preferred providers who are paid according to a discounted **fee schedule**. The enrollees do have the option to go to out-of-network providers at a higher level of **cost sharing**.

**Premium:** The insurer's charge for insurance coverage; the price for an insurance plan.

**Prepaid plan:** A contractual arrangement under which a provider must provide all needed services to a group of members (or **enrollees**) in exchange for a fixed monthly fee paid in advance to the provider on a per-member basis (called **capitation**).

**Prevalence:** The number of cases of a given disease in a given population at a certain point in time.

**Primary care:** Basic and routine health care provided in an office or clinic by a **provider** (physician, nurse, or other health care professional) who takes responsibility for coordinating all aspects of a patient's health care needs. An approach to health care delivery that is the patient's first contact with the health care delivery system and the first element of a continuing health care process.

**Primary care case management (PCCM):** A managed care arrangement in which a state contracts directly with primary care providers, who agree to be responsible for the provision and/or coordination of medical services for Medicare recipients under their care.

**Primary prevention:** In a strict epidemiological sense, it refers to prevention of disease, for example, health education, immunization, and environmental control measures.

**Prior approval:** A form of **utilization review** in which an insurance company requires a **provider** to get permission from the insurance company before providing care (usually surgery).

**Program of All-Inclusive Care for the Elderly (PACE):** An example of the integrated care model of long-term care case management for clients who have been certified as eligible for nursing home placement. It has had a high success rate of keeping clients in the community.

**Prospective payment system (PPS):** Criteria for how much will be paid for a particular service is predetermined, as opposed to "retrospective payment" in which the amount of **reimbursement** is determined on the basis of costs actually incurred.

**Prospective utilization review:** A process that determines the appropriateness of utilization before the care is actually delivered.

**Prosthesis:** An artificial device used to enhance lost functioning. Examples include artificial limbs and hearing aids.

**Provider:** Any entity that delivers health care services and can either independently bill for those services or is tax supported. Common examples of providers include physicians, dentists, optometrists, and therapists in private practices; hospitals, diagnostic and imaging clinics; and suppliers of medical equipment (e.g., wheelchairs, walkers, ostomy supplies, oxygen).

**Provider-induced demand:** Artificial creation of demand by providers that enables them to deliver unneeded services to boost their incomes.

**Psychiatry:** Branch of medicine that specializes in mental disorders.

**Psychologists:** Mental health professionals who must be licensed or certified to practice. Psychologists may specialize in such areas as clinical, counseling, developmental, educational, engineering, personnel, experimental, industrial, psychometric, rehabilitation, school, and social psychology.

**Psychosomatic ailments:** Disorders in which emotional distress is converted into physical symptoms.

**Psychotropic medication:** A category of medications that affect psychic function, behavior, or experience.

**Public health:** A wide variety of activities undertaken by state and local governments to ensure conditions that promote optimum health for society as a whole.

**Quad-function model:** The four key functions necessary for health care delivery: financing, insurance, delivery, and payment.

**Quality-adjusted life year (QALY):** The value of one year of high-quality life, used as a measure of health benefit.

**Quality assessment:** Process of defining quality and deciding how quality is to be measured according to established standards.

**Quality assurance:** The process of ongoing quality measurement and using the results of assessment for ongoing quality improvement. See **total quality management**.

**Quality improvement organization (QIO):** A private organization composed of practicing physicians and other health care professionals in each state that is paid by the **Centers for Medicare & Medicaid Services** under contract to review the care provided to Medicare beneficiaries.

**Quality of life:** (1) Quality of life refers to factors considered important by patients, such as environmental comfort, security, interpersonal relations, personal preferences, and autonomy in making decisions when institutionalized. (2) It also includes overall satisfaction with life during and following a person's encounter with the health care delivery system.

**R&D:** Research and development.

**Radiology:** The branch of medicine that involves the use of radioactive substances, such as X-rays, to diagnose, prevent, and treat disease.

**Rationing:** Any process of limiting the utilization of health care services. Rationing can be achieved by price, waiting lists, or deliberately limiting access to certain services.

**Registered nurses:** Nurses who have completed an associate's degree (ADN), a diploma program, or a bachelor's degree (BSN) and are licensed to practice.

**Rehabilitation:** Therapies that restore lost functioning or maintain the current levels of functioning and prevent further decline.

**Reimbursement:** The amount insurers pay to a **provider**. The payment may only be a portion of the actual **charge**.

**Reinsurance:** Acceptance by an insurer, called the reinsurer, of all or part of the risk underwritten by another insurer.

**Reliability:** Reflects the extent to which repeated applications of a measure produce the same results.

**Residency:** Graduate medical education in a specialty that takes the form of paid on-the-job training, usually in a hospital.

**Resident:** (1) Patient in a nursing home or some other long-term care facility. (2) Physician in **residency**.

**Resource-based relative value scale (RBRVS):** A system instituted by Medicare for determining physicians' fees. Each treatment or encounter by the physician is assigned a "relative value" based on the time, skill, and training required to treat the condition.

**Resource utilization groups (RUGs):** A classification system designed to differentiate nursing home patients by their levels of resource use.

**Respiratory therapy:** Treatment for various acute and chronic lung conditions, using oxygen, inhaled drugs, and various types of mechanical ventilation.

**Respite care:** A service that provides temporary relief to informal caregivers, such as family members.

**Retrospective reimbursement:** Setting of reimbursement rates based on costs actually incurred.

**Retrospective utilization review:** A review of **utilization** after services have been delivered.

**Risk adjustment:** Any adjustment made for people who are likely high users of health care services, for example, adjustment of payments based on the proportion of high-risk patients.

**Risk contracting:** In managed care, the concept of **capitation**, when applied to high-risk groups, such as the elderly, is sometimes referred to as risk contracting. All covered services are provided for a fixed monthly premium per enrollee.

**Risk factor:** An environmental element, personal habit, or living condition that increases the likelihood of developing a particular disease or negative health condition in the future.

**Risk management:** Limiting risks against lawsuits or unexpected events.

**Risk pool:** A pool of high-risk individuals offered health insurance in some states at a subsidized **premium**.

**Risk selection:** See **favorable risk selection.**

**Safety net:** Programs, generally government financed, that enable people to receive health care services when they lack private resources to pay for them. Without these programs, many people would have to forgo the services. For example, **Medicaid** becomes a safety net for **long-term care** services once a patient has exhausted private funds (see **spend-down**). **Community health centers** are safety net providers for many uninsured and vulnerable populations.

**Secondary care:** Routine hospitalization, routine surgery, and specialized outpatient care, such as consultation with specialists and **rehabilitation**. Compared to **primary care**, these services are usually brief and more complex, involving advanced diagnostic and therapeutic procedures.

**Secondary prevention:** Efforts to detect disease in early stages to provide a more effective treatment, for example, screening.

**Self-insure:** A large company may act as its own insurer by collecting premiums and paying claims. Such businesses most often purchase **reinsurance** against unusually large claims.

**Self-referral:** Physicians order services from laboratories or other medical facilities in which they have a direct financial interest, usually without disclosing this conflict of interest to the patient.

**Service plan:** A **plan** that provides the **insured** with specified health care services. It pays the hospital or physicians directly, except for the **deductible** and **copayments,** which the insured pays.

**Single-payer plan:** A health care reform proposal in which the financing of health care is in the government's hands.

**Skilled nursing care:** Medically oriented care provided mainly by a licensed nurse under the overall direction of a physician.

**Skilled nursing facility (SNF):** A nursing home (or part of a nursing home) certified to provide services under **Medicare.** See **nursing facility (NF)**.

**Small area variations:** Unexplained variations in the treatment patterns for similar patients and medical conditions.

**Smart card:** A credit card-like device with an embedded computer chip and memory to hold personal medical information that can be accessed and updated at a hospital or physician's office.

**Social health maintenance organization (S/HMO):** An example of the integrated care model of long-term care case management that coordinates long-term care and acute care services for Medicare beneficiaries who voluntarily enroll in the program.

**Social justice:** A distribution principle, according to which health care is most equitably distributed by a government-run national health care program. See **market justice**.

**Socialized medicine:** Any large-scale government-sponsored expansion of health insurance or intrusion in the private practice of medicine.

**Specialist:** A physician who specializes in specific health care problems, for ex-ample, **anesthesiologists, cardiologists,** and **oncologists**. See **generalist**.

**Speech therapy:** Therapy focusing on individuals with communication problems, including using the voice correctly, speaking fluently, and feeding or swallowing.

**Spend-down:** A requirement under most Medicaid programs that individuals spend their assets down to a predetermined level to be eligible for benefits.

**Spina bifida:** A deformity of the spine.

**Subacute care:** Technically complex services that are beyond traditional **skilled nursing care**.

**Supplemental Food Program for Women, Infants, and Children (WIC):** The program was created on September 26, 1972, as an amendment to the Child Health Nutrition Act of 1966, with the objective of providing sufficient nutrition for pregnant women, mothers, infants, and children.

**Supplemental Security Income (SSI):** A federal program of income support for the disabled, including mental illness and some infectious diseases.

**Supply-side rationing:** Also called "planned rationing" that is generally carried out by a government to limit the availability of health care services, particularly expensive technology.

**Surgicenter:** A freestanding, ambulatory surgery center that performs various types of surgical procedures on an outpatient basis.

**Swing bed:** A hospital bed used for acute care or skilled nursing care, depending on fluctuations in demand.

**Teaching hospital:** A hospital with an approved residency program for physicians.

**Technology assessment:** See **health technology assessment**.

**Telehealth:** Although, in general the terms, **telemedicine** and telehealth can be used interchangeably, in a stricter sense, telehealth encompasses educational, research, and administrative uses, as well as clinical applications that involve nurses, psychologists, administrators, and other nonphysicians.

**Telematics:** A term used to describe the combination of information and communications technology to meet user needs.

**Telemedicine:** Use of telecommunications technology that enables physicians to conduct two-way, interactive video consultations or transmit digital images, such as X-rays and MRIs, to other sites.

**Telemetry:** Remote monitoring, such as monitoring cardiac function, from a central station.

**Tertiary care:** The most complex level of care. Typically, tertiary care is institution-based, highly specialized, and highly technological. Examples include burn treatment, transplantation, and coronary artery bypass surgery.

**Tertiary prevention:** Interventions that would prevent complications from **chronic conditions** and prevent further illness, injury, or disability.

**Third-party administrator (TPA):** An administrative organization, other than the employee benefit **plan** or health care **provider**, that collects premiums, pays **claims**, and/or provides administrative services.

**Third-party payers:** In a multipayer system, the payers for covered services, for example, insurance companies, managed care organizations, and the government. They are called third parties because they are neither the providers nor the recipients of medical services.

**Total care:** In the context of long-term care delivery, total care focuses on recognizing any health care need that may arise and ensuring that the need is evaluated and addressed by appropriate clinical professionals.

**Total parenteral nutrition (TPN):** A liquid mixture pumped directly into the bloodstream, providing a balance of essential nutrients.

**Total quality management (TQM):** TQM creates an environment in which all aspects of health services within an organization are oriented to patient-related objectives and the production of desirable health outcomes. It holds the promise of not only improving quality but also increasing efficiency and productivity by identifying and implementing less costly ways to provide services. This system is viewed as an ongoing effort to improve quality. Hence, it is also referred to as **continuous quality improvement (CQI)**.

**Trauma center:** An emergency unit specializing in the treatment of severe injuries.

**Triage:** A system of prioritizing treatment when demand for medical care exceeds supply.

**Uncompensated care:** Charity care provided to the uninsured who cannot pay.

**Underinsurance:** Medical insurance coverage considered inadequate to cover the costs of a major illness.

**Underutilization:** Occurs when medically needed health care services are withheld. This is especially true when potential benefits are likely to exceed the cost or risks.

**Underwriting:** A systematic technique used by an **insurer** for evaluating, selecting (or rejecting), classifying, and rating risks.

**Universal access:** The ability of all citizens to obtain health care when needed. It is a misnomer because timely access to certain services may still be a problem because of **supply-side rationing**.

**Universal coverage:** Health insurance coverage for all citizens.

**Upcoding:** A fraudulent practice in which a higher-priced service is billed when a lower-priced service is actually delivered.

**Urgent care center:** A **walk-in clinic** generally open to see patients after normal business hours in the evenings and weekends without having to make an appointment.

**Urology:** The branch of medicine concerned with the urinary tract in both sexes and the sexual/reproductive system in males.

**Utilization:** Extent to which health care services are actually used.

**Utilization review (UR):** A process by which an insurer reviews decisions by physicians and other **providers** on how much care to provide.

**Validity:** The validity of a measure denotes the extent to which it actually assesses what it purports to measure. If a measure reflects the quality of care, improvements in quality should yield a higher score for improved quality and vice versa.

**Venous stasis:** Stagnation of normal blood flow causing swelling and pain, generally in the legs.

**Ventilator:** A mechanical device for artificial breathing. The ventilator (or mechanical respirator) forces air into the lungs.

**Vertical integration:** Linking of services that are at different stages in the production process of health care. Examples include a hospital system that acquires a firm that produces medical supplies or a physician group practice or a hospital that launches hospice, long-term care, or ambulatory care services. See **horizontal integration**.

**Voluntary hospital:** A **nonprofit** hospital.

**Voucher:** The voucher approach to health insurance reform relies on individual decisions to purchase health insurance. Tax credits are issued in advance to individuals in the form of vouchers with which to offset the costs of purchasing health insurance.

**Walk-in clinic:** A freestanding, **ambulatory** clinic in which patients are seen without appointments on a first come, first served basis.

**Welfare program:** A **means-tested program** for which only people below certain income levels qualify. **Medicaid** is a welfare program. See **entitlement**.

**Workers' compensation:** Employer-paid benefit that compensates workers for medical expenses and wages lost due to work-related injuries or illnesses.

**Xenotransplantation:** Also called "xenografting." Transplanting of animal tissue into humans.

**Yoga exercises:** Using physical postures and regulation of breathing to treat certain chronic conditions and to achieve overall health benefits.

# Index

Page numbers followed by *t* or *f* indicate tables or figures, respectively. Page numbers in *italics* indicate exhibits.